ACUTE MEDICINE

2nd EDITION

DECLAN O'KANE, MD, FRCP

Consultant Physician

Scion

© **Scion Publishing Limited, 2018**

Second edition first published 2018

First edition published 2015

A CIP catalogue record for this book is available from the British Library.

ISBN 978 1 907904 91 2

Scion Publishing Limited

The Old Hayloft, Vantage Business Park, Bloxham Road, Banbury OX16 9UX, UK

www.scionpublishing.com

Important Note from the Publisher

The information contained within this book was obtained by Scion Publishing Ltd from
sources believed by us to be reliable. However, while every effort has been made to ensure
its accuracy, no responsibility for loss or injury whatsoever occasioned to any person acting
or refraining from action as a result of information contained herein can be accepted by
the authors or publishers.

Readers are reminded that medicine is a constantly evolving science and while the authors
and publishers have ensured that all dosages, applications and practices are based on
current indications, there may be specific practices which differ between communities.
You should always follow the guidelines laid down by the manufacturers of specific
products and the relevant authorities in the country in which you are practising.

Typeset by Medlar Publishing Solutions Pvt Ltd, India

Printed in the UK

Contents

Preface xv
Abbreviations xvii

01	**Resuscitation**	**1**
1.1	Introduction	1
1.2	Initiating resuscitation	1
1.3	Basic life support: UK Guidelines 2015	2
1.4	Advanced life support: UK Guidelines 2015	4
1.5	Treatment of shockable rhythms (VF/pulseless VT)	5
1.6	Treatment of non-shockable rhythms (asystole/PEA)	6
1.7	Reversible causes of cardiac arrest	6
1.8	Resuscitation issues	7
1.9	Drugs for cardiac arrest	9
1.10	Special cases in resuscitation	9
1.11	Return of spontaneous circulation (ROSC)	10
1.12	Bradycardia management: be prepared to pace	11
1.13	Tachycardia management: be prepared to DC shock	12
1.14	Emergency DC cardioversion	14
1.15	Emergency pericardiocentesis	14
1.16	Automated implantable cardioverter defibrillator (AICD)	15
1.17	Adult choking algorithm	16

02	**The acutely ill patient**	**17**
2.1	Levels of care	17
2.2	National early warning scores	17
2.3	Clinical risk and response	18
2.4	ABCDE assessment	18
2.5	Getting senior help: advice before you call for advice	19
2.6	Phone protocols	19
2.7	Advanced airways management	20
2.8	Tracheostomy/laryngectomy emergencies	21
2.9	Assessing and managing fluid balance	21
2.10	Fluid replacement regimens	24
2.11	Venous access: choosing a venous cannula	25
2.12	Acid–base balance and blood gas interpretation	25
2.13	Assessment of shocked patient	27
2.14	Immediate actions in a shocked patient	28
2.15	Quick review of different forms of shock	28
2.16	Acute heart failure/cardiogenic shock	29
2.17	Vasopressors and inotropes	33
2.18	Anaphylactic/anaphylactoid shock	34
2.19	Toxic shock syndrome	35
2.20	Hypovolaemic shock	36
2.21	Systemic inflammatory response syndrome/sepsis/severe sepsis	37

| 2.22 | Haemorrhagic shock | 41 |
| 2.23 | Massive transfusion protocol | 42 |

03   Cardiology emergencies   45

3.1	Anatomy and physiology	45
3.2	Chest pain assessment	46
3.3	Chest pain differentials	47
3.4	Palpitations	48
3.5	Syncope and transient loss of consciousness (TLOC)	49
3.6	Differentials of syncope/transient loss of consciousness (TLOC)	50
3.7	Sudden cardiac death	53
3.8	Acute coronary syndrome	54
3.9	Stable angina	63
3.10	Arrhythmias	64
3.11	Tachyarrhythmias	65
3.12	Monomorphic ventricular tachycardia	66
3.13	Polymorphic ventricular tachycardia (torsades de pointes)	67
3.14	Supraventricular tachycardia	68
3.15	Symptomatic bradycardia	69
3.16	Atrial fibrillation	72
3.17	Aortic dissection	74
3.18	Acute myocarditis	76
3.19	Acute pericarditis	78
3.20	Pericardial effusion/tamponade	79
3.21	Severe (malignant) hypertension	81
3.22	Infective endocarditis	83
3.23	Cardiomyopathy	85

04   Respiratory emergencies   87

4.1	Pathophysiology	87
4.2	Oxygen therapy	88
4.3	Acute breathlessness	90
4.4	Acute stridor	93
4.5	Acute respiratory failure	94
4.6	NIV protocol and settings	97
4.7	Invasive ventilation	98
4.8	Massive haemoptysis	99
4.9	Acute respiratory distress syndrome (ARDS)	100
4.10	Acute exacerbation of COPD	101
4.11	Acute severe asthma	104
4.12	Pneumothorax	106
4.13	Pleural effusion	109
4.14	Pneumonia	110
4.15	*Pneumocystis* pneumonia	113
4.16	Empyema	114
4.17	Pulmonary embolism and deep vein thrombosis	114

4.18	Lung 'white out'	119
4.19	Lung abscess	120

05 Endocrine and diabetic emergencies 121

5.1	Primary hypoadrenalism (Addisonian crisis)	121
5.2	Hypoglycaemia	123
5.3	Hyperkalaemia	124
5.4	Hypokalaemia	125
5.5	Hypercalcaemia	126
5.6	Hypocalcaemia	127
5.7	Myxoedema coma	128
5.8	Thyroid storm/thyrotoxic crisis	129
5.9	Pituitary apoplexy	131
5.10	Hyponatraemia	132
5.11	Hypernatraemia	134
5.12	Hypophosphataemia	135
5.13	Hyperphosphataemia	135
5.14	Hypomagnesaemia	135
5.15	Hypermagnesaemia	135
5.16	Lactic acidosis	136
5.17	Acute porphyria	136
5.18	Diabetic ketoacidosis	137
5.19	Hyperosmolar hyperglycaemic state (HHS)	141
5.20	Diabetic foot infections	142
5.21	Diabetes and surgery	142
5.22	Variable rate intravenous insulin infusion	143
5.23	Diabetes care in emergencies	145

06 Gastroenterology emergencies 147

6.1	Acute diarrhoea	147
6.2	Constipation	148
6.3	Dyspepsia	150
6.4	Upper gastrointestinal bleeding	151
6.5	Lower gastrointestinal bleeding	156
6.6	Acute abdomen	158
6.7	Acute abdomen – surgical causes	159
6.8	Acute abdomen – medical causes	159
6.9	Gastric outlet obstruction/pyloric stenosis	161
6.10	Acute severe colitis	162
6.11	*Clostridium difficile* colitis	164
6.12	Intestinal obstruction	165
6.13	Acute colonic pseudo-obstruction	166
6.14	Acute bowel ischaemia	166
6.15	Acute diverticulitis	167
6.16	Re-feeding syndrome	167
6.17	Ingested foreign bodies and food impactions	168

07	**Hepatobiliary emergencies**	**171**
7.1	Jaundice	171
7.2	Acute liver failure	171
7.3	Viral hepatitis	174
7.4	Alcoholic hepatitis	175
7.5	Alcoholic ketoacidosis	176
7.6	Alcohol abuse	176
7.7	Zieve's syndrome	177
7.8	Delirium tremens/alcohol withdrawal	178
7.9	Decompensated cirrhosis, ascites and spontaneous bacterial peritonitis	179
7.10	Hepatorenal syndrome	180
7.11	Hepatic encephalopathy	181
7.12	Chronic liver disease	183
7.13	Liver abscess	183
7.14	Gallstone disease and local complications	184
7.15	Acute cholangitis	185
7.16	Acute pancreatitis	186

08	**Haematological emergencies**	**191**
8.1	Anaemia	191
8.2	Severe thrombocytopenia	192
8.3	Heparin-induced thrombocytopenia	194
8.4	Disseminated intravascular coagulation	195
8.5	Sickle cell crisis	195
8.6	Haemolytic uraemic syndrome	197
8.7	Thrombotic thrombocytopenic purpura	199
8.8	Bleeding disorders and reversal of anticoagulation	200
8.9	Bleeding on warfarin	201
8.10	Bleeding on heparin	201
8.11	Bleeding on direct oral anticoagulants	202
8.12	Bleeding on/after thrombolysis	202
8.13	Blood transfusion and blood products	202
8.14	Which blood/plasma product?	203
8.15	Cross-matching	204
8.16	Acute transfusion reactions	205
8.17	Indications for irradiated blood	206
8.18	Immunocompromised patients	206
8.19	Plasmapheresis/plasma exchange (PLEX)	207

09	**Infectious disease emergencies**	**209**
9.1	Pyrexia of unknown origin	209
9.2	Assessment of the febrile traveller	210
9.3	Falciparum malaria	212
9.4	Traveller's diarrhoea	214
9.5	Tick typhus	214
9.6	Rocky Mountain Spotted fever	214
9.7	Schistosomiasis (Katayama fever)	215

9.8	Dengue	215
9.9	Viral haemorrhagic fever	215
9.10	Chikungunya	216
9.11	Plague/tularaemia	216
9.12	Brucellosis	216
9.13	*Pseudomonas* infection	217
9.14	Q fever	217
9.15	Anthrax	217
9.16	Leptospirosis	217
9.17	Listeriosis	218
9.18	Botulism	218
9.19	Clostridial infection	219
9.20	Acute bacterial sepsis	219
9.21	Measles	219
9.22	Chickenpox/varicella zoster virus (Shingles)	219
9.23	Mumps infection	220
9.24	Herpes simplex 1 and 2	220
9.25	Infectious mononucleosis	220
9.26	Cytomegalovirus	221
9.27	Influenza	221
9.28	Severe acute respiratory syndrome	221
9.29	Middle Eastern respiratory syndrome	222
9.30	Zika virus infection	222
9.31	Needlestick injury	222
9.32	Tuberculosis (*Mycobacterium tuberculosis*)	223
9.33	HIV/acquired immunodeficiency syndrome	224
9.34	Syphilis	227
9.35	Oropharyngeal bacterial infections	227
9.36	Diphtheria	228
9.37	Lemierre's syndrome (*Fusobacterium necrophorum*)	228
9.38	Meticillin sensitive/resistant *Staph. aureus*	229
9.39	Bacterial resistance: VRE, ESBL, CRE/CRO	229
9.40	Gastroenteritis and similar infections	230
9.41	*E. coli* infections	230
9.42	*Staphylococcal* food poisoning	230
9.43	*Shigella dysenteriae*	231
9.44	Enteric fever (typhoid/paratyphoid)	231
9.45	*Bacillus cereus*	231
9.46	Cholera	231
9.47	Giardiasis	231
9.48	Amoebiasis	232
9.49	Neurocysticercosis	232
9.50	Tetanus	232
9.51	Lyme disease	233

10	**Renal and urological emergencies**	**235**
10.1	Pathophysiology	235
10.2	Haematuria	235
10.3	Reduced urinary output (anuria/oliguria)	237
10.4	Acute kidney injury	237

10.5	Chronic kidney disease	242
10.6	Urinary tract infection	243
10.7	Renal obstruction (obstructive uropathy)	244
10.8	Nephrolithiasis	245
10.9	Ischaemic priapism	247

11	**Neurological emergencies**	**249**
11.1	Neuroscience and neuroanatomy	249
11.2	Clinical assessment	252
11.3	Patterns of weakness	253
11.4	Coma	256
11.5	Acute headache	262
11.6	Primary headaches	263
11.7	Secondary headaches	264
11.8	Acute delirium/confusion	265
11.9	Viral encephalitis	268
11.10	Rabies	269
11.11	Acute bacterial meningitis	269
11.12	Acute viral (aseptic) meningitis	272
11.13	Cerebral abscess	272
11.14	Septic cavernous sinus thrombosis	273
11.15	Idiopathic intracranial hypertension	273
11.16	Seizures: status epilepticus	274
11.17	Non-convulsive status epilepticus	278
11.18	Neuroleptic malignant syndrome	279
11.19	Cerebrovascular disease	279
11.20	Transient ischaemic attacks	279
11.21	Ischaemic stroke	282
11.22	Haemorrhagic stroke	288
11.23	Subarachnoid haemorrhage	290
11.24	Cerebral hyperperfusion syndrome	295
11.25	Subdural haematoma	295
11.26	Epidural haematoma/head trauma	296
11.27	Guillain–Barré syndrome	297
11.28	Myasthenia gravis	299
11.29	Acute cord injury	300
11.30	Acute transverse myelitis	302
11.31	Acute dystonic reactions	302
11.32	Acute vertigo	303
11.33	Bell's palsy/Ramsay Hunt syndrome	305
11.34	Acute demyelination	306
11.35	Acute peripheral mononeuropathy	307
11.36	Motor neurone disease (amyotrophic lateral sclerosis)	307
11.37	Dementias	308
11.38	Acute hydrocephalus and shunts	308
11.39	Managing raised intracranial pressure	309
11.40	Cerebral oedema	311
11.41	Neurosurgical options	311

12	**Rheumatological emergencies**	**313**
12.1	Septic arthritis	313
12.2	Osteomyelitis	313
12.3	Reactive arthritis	314
12.4	Acute gout and pseudogout	314
12.5	Rheumatoid arthritis	315
12.6	Trauma and fractures in elderly	316
12.7	Proximal femoral fracture	316
12.8	Fractured pubic ramus	316

13	**Ophthalmological emergencies**	**319**
13.1	Acute visual loss	319
13.2	Red eye	320
13.3	Neuro-ophthalmology	321
13.4	Giant cell (temporal) arteritis	322

14	**Toxicology emergencies**	**325**
14.1	Reduce absorption or increase excretion/elimination of toxins	325
14.2	Supportive management of specific issues	326
14.3	Intralipid therapy	330
14.4	(High dose) Insulin–glucose euglycaemic therapy	330
14.5	Amphetamine ('speed') and 3,4 MDMA ('ecstasy') toxicity	331
14.6	Beta-blocker toxicity	331
14.7	Benzodiazepine toxicity	331
14.8	Calcium channel blocker toxicity	332
14.9	Sodium valproate toxicity	332
14.10	Carbon monoxide toxicity	333
14.11	Cocaine toxicity	333
14.12	Local anaesthetic toxicity	334
14.13	Cyanide toxicity	334
14.14	Digoxin toxicity	334
14.15	Ethanol (C_2H_5OH) toxicity	335
14.16	Ethylene glycol toxicity	335
14.17	Methanol toxicity	336
14.18	Gamma hydroxybutyrate (GHB) toxicity	336
14.19	Insulin toxicity	337
14.20	Iron (ferrous sulphate) toxicity	337
14.21	Lithium toxicity	337
14.22	Monoamine oxidase inhibitors toxicity	338
14.23	Neuroleptics toxicity	338
14.24	Direct (novel) oral anticoagulants toxicity	338
14.25	Non-steroidal anti-inflammatory drugs (NSAIDs) toxicity	338
14.26	Opioid/opiate toxicity	339
14.27	Organophosphate/carbamates toxicity	339
14.28	Paracetamol (acetaminophen) toxicity	340
14.29	Paraquat toxicity	342

14.30	Chloroquine/quinine toxicity	342
14.31	Salicylate toxicity	343
14.32	SSRI/SNRI toxicity	343
14.33	Tricyclic antidepressant toxicity	344
14.34	Theophylline toxicity	344
14.35	Body packers ('mules')	344
14.36	Cannabis toxicity	345
14.37	Sulphonylurea toxicity	345
14.38	Methaemoglobinaemia	345
14.39	Phenobarbital toxicity	346
14.40	Carbamazepine toxicity	346
14.41	Lead, arsenic, mercury, thallium (heavy metal) toxicity	346

15	**Medical emergencies in pregnancy**	**347**
15.1	Medical problems in pregnancy	347
15.2	Pharmacology in pregnancy	347
15.3	Amniotic fluid embolism	348
15.4	Hypertension in pregnancy	348
15.5	Eclampsia and pre-eclampsia	349
15.6	Diabetes in pregnancy	350
15.7	Acute hepatobiliary disease in pregnancy	350
15.8	Diagnoses and management of liver disease in pregnancy	351
15.9	Pulmonary embolism and pregnancy	352
15.10	Acute severe asthma in pregnancy	353
15.11	Status epilepticus in pregnancy	353
15.12	Cardiac disease in pregnancy	354
15.13	Inflammatory bowel disease and pregnancy	354

16	**Oncological emergencies**	**355**
16.1	Malignancy-related hypercalcaemia	355
16.2	Tumour lysis syndrome	355
16.3	Hyperviscosity syndrome	355
16.4	Brain tumour	356
16.5	Neutropenic sepsis	357
16.6	Malignant superior vena caval obstruction	358
16.7	Severe nausea and vomiting	359
16.8	Malignant spinal cord compression	359

17	**Miscellaneous emergencies**	**361**
17.1	Abnormal gaits	361
17.2	Falls with no altered consciousness	361
17.3	Fat embolism	362
17.4	Air embolism	363
17.5	Refeeding syndrome	363
17.6	Accidental hypothermia	363
17.7	Malignant hyperpyrexia	365
17.8	Acute rhabdomyolysis	365

17.9	Painful leg	366
17.10	Acute limb ischaemia	367
17.11	Abdominal aortic aneurysm	368

18	**Dermatological emergencies**	**369**
18.1	Introduction	369
18.2	Toxic epidermal necrolysis/Stevens–Johnson syndrome	369
18.3	Cellulitis/erysipelas, bites, surgery	370
18.4	Erythroderma (exfoliative dermatitis)	370
18.5	Severe (erythrodermic/pustular) psoriasis	371
18.6	Necrotising fasciitis	371
18.7	Other important rashes for acute physicians	372

19	**General management**	**373**
19.1	Enteral feeding	373
19.2	Parenteral feeding	374
19.3	Pain management	374
19.4	WHO pain ladder	375
19.5	Using opiates and other analgesics	376
19.6	Venous thromboembolism prevention	377
19.7	Duties of a doctor	378
19.8	Medical errors, harm and duty of candour	379
19.9	Never events – events that should 'never' occur	379
19.10	Risk management and risk register	379
19.11	Duty of candour	380
19.12	Discharging patients safely	380
19.13	Self-discharge	382
19.14	Suicidal patients	382
19.15	Common law and Mental Health Act	383
19.16	Mental capacity	384
19.17	Managing opiate addicts	384
19.18	Driving and disease	385
19.19	Do not attempt cardiopulmonary resuscitation (DNACPR)	387
19.20	End of life care	387
19.21	Palliative care drugs	389
19.22	Roles and responsibilities after death	391
19.23	Death certification	392
19.24	Managing inpatients with pressure sores and ulcers	395
19.25	Rehabilitation, function and discharge	395
19.26	Drains and tubes	396
19.27	Surgical problems and referrals	396

20	**Procedures**	**399**
20.1	Checks before any procedure	399
20.2	Venepuncture	399
20.3	Chest drain insertion	400
20.4	Central venous line insertion	404

20.5	Lumbar puncture	407
20.6	Abdominal paracentesis	409
20.7	Arterial blood gas	410
20.8	Nasogastric tube insertion	411

21	**Normal laboratory values**	**413**
21.1	Clinical chemistry values	413
21.2	Haematology values	415
21.3	CSF values	416

22	**Emergency drugs (use with *BNF*)**	**417**
22.1	Prescribing and side effects abbreviations	417
22.2	Antibiotic prescribing advice	417
22.3	Commonly used and emergency drugs	418
22.4	Important drug interactions and metabolism	439
22.5	Potentially fatal drug errors	440
22.6	Prescribing warfarin	440
22.7	Steroids	441

| Index | | 443 |

Preface

I wrote this book for my own needs, to have a reference for the questions that come up when dealing with acutely unwell medical patients. I was conscious that the answers could often not be found quickly and readily. I hope it will be useful for others at all levels, especially the on-call Medical SPR. Emergency department doctors and others may also find it useful. It is a quick reference of 'what and why' that covers common and not so common emergencies. It is compact and facts can be found quickly. I am very aware of the frailties of human memory and decision-making. A simple checklist at hand can hopefully enhance safety and clinical care. Included at the back is a quick emergency drug reference where drug information is consolidated to avoid repetition. This does not replace the *British National Formulary* (*BNF*) which has now been released as a free app and is the best source of prescribing information. Despite great care, we may have errors of omission or fact. This is not a cookbook to slavishly follow, but a guide to help the reader to analyse a difficult situation with a framework and some salient facts. Lastly, this is a book by a generalist. It is not meant to replace experts. All difficult cases benefit from early expert help – this book should aid the dialogue. To some the information will be new, and to others it is simply a reminder. It needs to be compact and concise so let us not waste further words or space.

 ## Acknowledgments

I'd like to thank my wife and my two girls for their love, patience and support. This book is dedicated to the memory of my good friend, Jeremy Sherman FRCS. In my training I was fortunate to work for many wonderful hard-working clinicians. I am particularly indebted to Professor Jennifer Adgey CBE and the late Dr James I. Coyle. I'd like to thank those who have read the manuscript and made helpful suggestions and additions including Dr Jacob F. de Wolff, Dr Andrew Solomon, Dr Pad Boovalingam, Dr Omar Kirresh, Dr Peter Rhead and Dr Christopher Miller, and Dr V Srinivasan and Dr Abdul Elmarimi for their kind help. Any remaining errors are mine. If you have any comments, questions or suggestions, please write to me at drokane@gmail.com. Errata will be available at www.scionpublishing.com/acutemed.

 ## Updates to the 2nd edition

Almost all subjects have been edited and updated. Interesting topics such as the use of intralipid therapy in toxicology and management of inhaled cyanide have been added, along with new articles on transverse myelitis and demyelination. There have been multiple other updates and references to national and international guidelines, including stroke and resuscitation. The challenge has been to add quality without adding quantity.

Declan O'Kane, September 2017

Disclaimer

Every effort has been made in preparing this publication to provide accurate and up to date information in accord with accepted standards and practice at the time of publication. The author can make no warranties that the information contained herein is totally free from error, not least because clinical standards are constantly changing. The author therefore disclaims all liability for direct or consequential damages resulting from the use of material within this publication. Readers are recommended to check all drugs doses, indications and C/I and interactions used with the *BNF* or drug data-sheet prior to use. If a reader is unsure what to do then they should seek support from their senior medical adviser. Patients should seek help from their own doctor/healthcare provider.

Decision making for the medical registrar

The first medical registrar year is tough and stressful, but with the years it gets easier and more enjoyable: you recognise the same patterns and problems like a chess puzzle and the solutions become easier to resolve in seconds, and you can solve other people's puzzles for them. Sometimes, however, a problem is completely new so you need to sit down and work it out from first principles and/or ask for help from someone who may have encountered the situation before. Referrals will come thick and fast – regard these as compliments to your skills in problem-solving. Get help once you have thought (time allowing) it through yourself and presented your plan. If you are unhappy or concerned call for advice. Share diagnostic dilemmas and don't sit on them. Don't go home without resolving your concerns. As consultants we constantly discuss interesting and difficult cases. Good medical practice is about reflection and seeking feedback. Good luck.

Abbreviations

AAA	abdominal aortic aneurysm	APKD	adult polycystic kidney disease
ABC	airway, breathing and circulation	APL	antiphospholipid
		APLS	antiphospholipid syndrome
ABCDE	ABC + disability, exposure	APML	acute promyelocytic leukaemia
ABG	arterial blood gas		
ABU	asymptomatic bacteriuria	APS	antiphospholipid syndrome
ACA	anterior cerebral artery	APTT	activated thromboplastin time
ACE	angiotensin converting enzyme	AR	aortic regurgitation
		ARB	angiotensin-II receptor blocker
Ach	acetyl choline	ARDS	acute/adult respiratory distress syndrome
ACOMM	anterior communicating artery		
ACS	acute coronary syndrome	ARF	acute respiratory failure
ACTH	adrenocorticotrophic hormone	ART	antiretroviral therapy
		ARVC	arrhythmogenic right ventricular cardiomyopathy
ADA	adenosine deaminase		
ADEM	acute disseminated encephalomyelitis	AS	aortic stenosis
		ASD	atrial septal defect
ADLs	activities of daily living	ASO(T)	antistreptolysin O (titre)
AED	automated external defibrillators/anti-epilepsy drug	AST	aspartate aminotransferase
		ATN	acute tubular necrosis
		AV	arteriovenous / atrioventricular
AF	atrial fibrillation		
AFB	acid fast bacilli (TB)	AVM	arteriovenous malformation
AFLP	acute fatty liver of pregnancy	AVNRT	atrioventricular nodal re-entrant tachycardia
aHUS	atypical haemolytic uraemic syndrome		
		AVPU	awake, voice, pain, unresponsive
AICD	automated implantable cardioverter–defibrillator	AVRT	atrioventricular re-entrant tachycardia
AIDP	acute inflammatory demyelinating polyneuropathy	AXR	abdominal X-ray
		BAL	bronchoalveolar lavage
		BBB	bundle branch block
AIDS	acquired immunodeficiency syndrome	BD/bd	twice daily or 12 h
		BE	base excess
AKI	acute kidney injury	BiPAP	bilevel positive airway pressure
ALA	alanine aminotransferase		
ALF	acute liver failure	BJP	Bence–Jones protein
ALI	acute lung injury	BMS	bare metal stents
ALP	alkaline phosphatase	BNP	B-type natriuretic peptide
ALS	advanced life support	BP	blood pressure
ALT	alanine aminotransferase	BUN	blood urea nitrogen
AMAN	acute motor axonal neuropathy	BVM	bag–valve mask
		CABG	coronary artery bypass grafting
AMTS	abbreviated mental test score		
ANA	antinuclear antibody	CAD	coronary artery disease
ANCA	antineutrophil cytoplasmic antibody	CBG	capillary blood glucose
		CC	chest compression
ANP	atrial naturietic peptide		

CCB	calcium channel blocker	DNACPR	do not attempt cardiopulmonary resuscitation
CCF	congestive cardiac failure		
CEA	carcinoembryonic antigen/ carotid endarterectomy	DOAC	direct oral anticoagulant (previously NOAC)
CFU	colony-forming units	DOB	date of birth
CHB	complete heart block	DPG	2,3-diphosphoglycerate
CI-AKI	contrast-induced acute kidney injury	DRESS	drug rash with eosinophilia and systemic symptoms
CIDP	chronic inflammatory demyelinating polyneuropathy	DSA	digital subtraction angiography
		DVT	deep vein thrombosis
CIS	clinically isolated syndrome	DWI	diffusion weighted imaging
CK	creatine kinase	EBV	Epstein–Barr virus
CKD	chronic kidney disease	ECG	electrocardiogram
CLO test	Campylobacter-like organism test (rapid urease test)	ECMO	extracorporeal membrane oxygenation
CMP	cardiomyopathy	EEG	electroencephalogram
CMV	cytomegalovirus	EF	ejection fraction
CO	cardiac output	ELISA	enzyme-linked immunosorbent assay
COPD	chronic obstructive pulmonary disease		
		EMA	endomysial antibodies
CPAP	continuous positive airway pressure	EMG	electromyography
		EPAP	expiratory positive airway pressure
CPR	cardiopulmonary resuscitation		
CRH	corticotropin-releasing hormone	EPO	erythropoietin
		EPS	electrophysiological study
CRP	C-reactive protein	ERCP	endoscopic retrograde cholangiopancreatography
CRT	cardiac resynchronization therapy		
		ESBL	extended-spectrum beta-lactamases
CSF	cerebrospinal fluid		
CSM	carotid sinus massage	ESR	erythrocyte sedimentation rate
CSU	catheter sample urine		
CTG	cardiotocogram	EST	exercise stress test
CTPA	computed tomography pulmonary angiogram	ESWL	extracorporeal shock wave lithotripsy
		EVD	external ventricular drainage
CVP	central venous pressure	EWS	early warning score
CVST	cerebral venous sinus thrombosis	FBC	full blood count
		FEV	forced expiratory volume
CXR	chest X-ray	FFP	fresh frozen plasma
DAPT	dual antiplatelet therapy	FMF	familial Mediterranean fever
DBP	diastolic blood pressure	FSH	follicle stimulating hormone
DCM	dilated cardiomyopathy	FVC	forced vital capacity
DCR	damage control resuscitation	G5	5% glucose (dextrose)
DES	drug-eluting stents	GBS	Guillain–Barré syndrome
DHEA	dehydroepiandrosterone	GBM	glomerular basement membrane
DI	diabetes insipidus		
DIC	disseminated intravascular coagulation	GCA	giant cell arteritis
		GCS	Glasgow Coma Score
DKA	diabetic ketoacidosis	GFR	glomerular filtration rate
DM	diabetes mellitus		

GGT	gamma-glutamyl transpeptidase	HUS	haemolytic uraemic syndrome
GH	growth hormone	IABP	intra-aortic balloon pump
GHB	gamma-hydroxybutyric acid	IAH	impaired awareness of hypoglycaemia
GI	gastrointestinal		
GN	glomerulonephritis	IBD	inflammatory bowel disease
GORD	gastro-oesophageal reflux disease	IBS	irritable bowel syndrome
		ICA	internal carotid artery
GRACE	Global Registry of Acute Coronary Events	ICH	intracerebral haemorrhage
		ICP	intracranial pressure
GTT	glucose tolerance test	ICS	intercostal space
GvHD	graft-versus-host disease	IGF-1	insulin-like growth factor 1
H	headache	IHD	ischaemic heart disease
HAART	highly active antiretroviral therapy	IJV	internal jugular vein
		IM	intramuscular route
HAP	hospital-acquired pneumonia	IMA	inferior mesenteric artery
HAS	human albumin solution	INR	international normalized ratio
HBV	hepatitis B virus	IP	incubation period
HCM	hypertrophic cardiomyopathy	IPAP	inspiratory positive airway pressure
HCV	hepatitis C virus		
HDU	high dependency unit	ITP	immune (idiopathic) thrombocytopenic purpura
HELLP	syndrome of haemolysis, elevated LFTs, low platelets		
		IVC	inferior vena cava
HF	heart failure	IVDU	IV drug user
HHS	hyperosmolar hyperglycaemic state	IVIG	intravenous immunoglobulin
		IVII	intravenous insulin infusion
HHT	hereditary haemorrhagic telangiectasia	IVT	intravenous thrombolysis
		IVU	intravenous urogram
5-HIAA	5-hydroxyindoleacetic acid	Ix	investigations
HIT(T)	heparin-induced thrombocytopenia +/− thrombosis	JVP	jugular venous pressure
		KUB	kidneys, ureter, bladder
		LA	left atrium
HIV	human immunodeficiency virus	LAD	left axis deviation/left anterior descending
HOCM	hypertrophic cardiomyopathy	LAFB	left anterior fascicular block
HONK	hyperosmolar non-ketotic state	LBBB	left bundle branch block
		LCA	left coronary artery
HPTHM	hyperparathyroidism	LCHAD	long-chain 3-hydroxyacyl-coA dehydrogenase
HR	heart rate (ventricular rate)		
HRCT	high resolution CT	LDH	lactate dehydrogenase
HRS	hepatorenal syndrome	LFT	liver function test
HRT	hormone replacement therapy	LIMA	left internal mammary artery
HSC	haemopoietic stem cell	LMN	lower motor neuron
HSE	herpes simplex encephalitis	LMWH	low molecular weight heparin
hsTn	high sensitivity troponin	LOC	loss of consciousness
HSV	Herpes simplex virus	LP	lumbar puncture
HTIG	human tetanus immunoglobulin	LPFB	left posterior fascicular block
		LTOT	long term oxygen therapy
		LV	left ventricle
HTLV	human T cell lymphotropic virus	LVAD	LV assist device
		LVEDP	LV end diastolic pressure

LVEF	LV ejection fraction	NC	nasal cannula
LVF	left ventricular failure	NCS	nerve conduction studies
LVH	left ventricular hypertrophy	NCSE	non-convulsive status epilepticus
LVOT	LV outflow tract		
MAHA	microangiopathic haemolytic anaemia	NDI	nephrogenic diabetes insipidus
MAOI	monoamine oxidase inhibitor	NEAD	non-epileptic attack disorder
MAP	mean systemic arterial pressure	NEWS	National Early Warning Score
		NG	nasogastric
MAT	microscopic agglutination test/multifocal atrial tachycardia	NIH	National Institute for Health
		NIPPV	non-invasive positive pressure ventilation
MCA	middle cerebral artery	NIV	non-invasive ventilation
MCH	mean cell haemoglobin	NMO	neuromyelitis optica
MCV	mean cell volume	NMS	neuroleptic malignant syndrome
MDAC	multidose activated charcoal		
MEN	multiple endocrine neoplasia	NOAC	new/novel oral anticoagulant (see DOAC)
MERS	Middle Eastern respiratory syndrome		
		NOS	nitric oxide synthase
MG	myasthenia gravis	NRTI	nucleoside reverse transcriptase inhibitors
MGUS	monoclonal gammopathy of undetermined significance		
		NS	0.9% normal saline
MI	myocardial infarction	NSAID	non-steroidal anti-inflammatory drug
MIC	minimum inhibitory concentration		
		NSTEMI	non-ST elevation MI
MLF	medial longitudinal fasciculus	N&V	nausea and vomiting
MND	motor neurone disease	NVE	native valve endocarditis
MODS	multiple organ dysfunction syndrome	OCP	oral contraceptive pill
		OGD	oesophagogastroduodenos-copy
MPO	myeloperoxidase		
MR	mitral regurgitation	OGTT	oral glucose tolerance test
MRCP	magnetic resonance cholangiopancreatography	OPs	organophosphates
		PA	pernicious anaemia/posterior–anterior
MRSA	meticillin-resistant *Staphylococcus aureus*		
		PAF	paroxysmal atrial fibrillation
MS	multiple sclerosis/mitral stenosis	PAN	polyarteritis nodosa
		PAWP	pulmonary artery wedge pressure
MSH	melanocyte-stimulating hormone		
		PBC	primary biliary cirrhosis
MSU	mid-stream urine/monosodium urate	PBG	porphobilinogen
		PCA	posterior cerebral artery
MT	mechanical thrombectomy	PCC	prothrombin complex concentrates
MTP	massive transfusion protocol		
MTS	mental test score	PCI	percutaneous coronary intervention
MUMS	migraine with unilateral motor symptoms		
		PCOMM	posterior communicating artery
MVP	mitral valve prolapse		
Mx	management	PCP	*Pneumocystis carinii* pneumonia
NAAT	nucleic acid amplification test		
NAC	*N*-acetyl cysteine	PCWP	pulmonary capillary wedge pressure
NBM	nil by mouth		

PE	pulmonary embolism	RA	rheumatoid arthritis/right atrium
PEEP	positive end-expiratory pressure	RAA	renin–angiotensin–aldosterone
PEFR	peak expiratory flow rate	RAD	right axis deviation
PEG	percutaneous endoscopic gastrostomy / polyethylene glycol	RAS	renal artery stenosis/reticular activating system
		RAST	radioallergosorbent test
PEJ	percutaneous endoscopic jejunostomy	RBBB	right bundle branch block
		RBC	red blood cell
PEP	post-exposure prophylaxis	RCA	right coronary artery
PET	pre-eclamptic toxaemia/ positron emission tomography	RCVS	reversible cerebral vasoconstriction syndrome
PFO	patent foramen ovale	RF	respiratory failure/rheumatoid factor
PFTs	pulmonary function tests		
PICA	posterior inferior cerebellar artery	RIF	right iliac fossa
		ROSC	return of spontaneous circulation
PICC	peripheral inserted central catheter		
		RPGN	rapidly progressive glomerulonephritis
PICH	primary intracerebral haemorrhage		
		RR	respiratory rate
PMC	primary motor cortex	RRT	renal replacement therapy
PML	progressive multifocal leucoencephalopathy	RSV	respiratory syncytial virus
		RTA	renal tubular acidosis/road traffic accident
PMR	polymyalgia rheumatica		
PNH	paroxysmal nocturnal haemoglobinuria	RV	right ventricle
		RVH	right ventricular hypertrophy
POTS	postural orthostatic tachycardia syndrome	Rx	treatment
		SACD	sub-acute combined cord degeneration
PPCI	primary percutaneous coronary intervention		
		SAH	subarachnoid haemorrhage
PPD	purified protein derivative	SAN	sinoatrial node
PPE	plasma protein electrophoresis/ personal protective equipment	SARS	severe acute respiratory syndrome
PPI	proton pump inhibitor	SBP	systolic blood pressure/ spontaneous bacterial peritonitis
PPM	permanent pacemaker		
PRES	posterior reversible encephalopathy syndrome		
		SC	subcutaneous route/sickle cell
PRL	prolactin level	SCD	sudden cardiac death
PSA	prostate specific antigen	SDH	subdural haematoma
PSC	primary sclerosing cholangitis	SE	status epilepticus/side effect
PSM	pansystolic murmur	SIADH	syndrome of inappropriate ADH secretion
PT	prothrombin time		
PTH	parathyroid hormone	SIRS	systemic inflammatory response syndrome
PTX	pneumothorax		
PUD	peptic ulcer disease	SJS	Stevens–Johnson syndrome
PUO	pyrexia of unknown origin	SLE	systemic lupus erythematosus
PVD	peripheral vascular disease	SMA	superior mesenteric artery
PVE	prosthetic valve endocarditis	SMX	sulfamethoxazole
PVL	plasma viral load	SOB	shortness of breath
Px	prevention or prophylaxis	SOFA	sepsis-related organ failure assessment
QDS	four times a day or 6-hourly		

SOL	space-occupying lesion	TSH	thyroid stimulating hormone
SPECT	single photon emission	TSS	toxic shock syndrome
	computed tomography	TTE	transthoracic echocardiogram
SR	sinus rhythm	TTG	tissue transglutaminase
SSP	secondary spontaneous	TTP	thrombotic thrombocytopenic
	pneumothorax		purpura
STEMI	ST elevation MI	TVR	target vessel revascularisation
STI	sexually transmitted infection	U&E	urea/creatinine and
SUDEP	sudden unexpected death		electrolytes
	in epilepsy	UFH	unfractioned heparin
SUND	sudden unexpected nocturnal	ULN	upper limit of normal
	death	UMN	upper motor neuron
SVC	superior vena cava	URTI	upper respiratory tract
SVR	systemic vascular resistance		infection
SVT	supraventricular tachycardia	USS	ultrasound scan
T1DM	type 1 diabetes mellitus	UTI	urinary tract infection
T2DM	type 2 diabetes mellitus	V/Q	ventilation/perfusion
TAB	temporal artery biopsy	VATS	video-assisted thoracoscopic
TACI	total anterior circulation infarct		surgery
TACO	transfusion-associated	VB	variceal bleed
	circulatory overload	VBG	venous blood gas
TB	tuberculosis	VDRL	venereal disease research
TCA	tricyclic antidepressant		laboratory
TdP	torsades de pointes	VEGF	vascular endothelial growth
TDS	three times a day		factor
TEN	toxic epidermal necrolysis	VF	ventricular fibrillation
TF	typhoid fever	VIHE	valproate-induced
TFTs	thyroid function tests		hyperammonaemic
TIA	transient ischaemic attack		encephalopathy
TIBC	total iron binding capacity	VKA	vitamin K antagonist
TIMI	thrombolysis in MI	VRE	vancomycin resistant
TIPS	transjugular intrahepatic		enterococcus
	portosystemic shunt	VRIII	variable rate IV insulin infusion
TLOC	transient loss of consciousness	VSD	ventricular septal defect
TMP	trimethoprim	VT	ventricular tachycardia
TNF	tumour necrosis factor	VTE	venous thromboembolism
TOE	transoesophageal	vWF	von Willebrand factor
	echocardiogram	VZV	varicella zoster virus
TPHA	*Treponema pallidum* serology	WBI	whole bowel irrigation
TPN	total parenteral nutrition	WCC	white cell count
TPO	thyroid peroxidase	WG	Wegener's granulomatosis
TRAb	TSH receptor antibodies	WPW	Wolff–Parkinson–White
TRALI	transfusion associated lung		syndrome
	injury	ZIG	zoster immune globulin

01 Resuscitation

1.1 Introduction

- Ensure you are up to date with BLS and ALS courses. See your national guidelines, e.g. UK/US/European guidelines online. There is much in common in guidelines. The things that differ are due to a lack of evidence and so either way is defensible. Watch the videos on resuscitation at the UK Resuscitation Council site.
- It is difficult to perform trials on resuscitation and much is extrapolated from basic theory and laboratory and animal experiments. Guidelines are just that and experienced clinicians who know and understand the evidence or lack of evidence can deviate to a degree.
- Resuscitating an unresponsive pulseless apnoeic patient can be stressful and it is never as simple as a basic algorithm suggests. It is not uncommon to find yourself trying to cope with a collapsed patient wedged in a toilet cubicle. All you can do is your best. Such a patient is certifiable as dead and you cannot make that situation any worse. In a small number of cases you can make a significant difference.
- Are you unsure of the rhythm – could it be VF? If so, do not hesitate to defibrillate. If there is **any** delay in defibrillation then get good quality CPR going, at least using chest compressions. *Survival depends on the immediate initiation of chest compressions and early defibrillation if rhythm is shockable.*
- As soon as you arrive use the ABCs to quickly determine the basics – check the **Airway** is not obstructed, look for **Breathing** whilst palpating a major pulse to assess the **Circulation**. Commence chest compressions as quickly as possible; hopefully someone else will already have done so. Your concern is whether unresponsiveness is due to circulatory collapse or not. If unsure start CPR. It is less harmful to CPR a patient who turns out to have a pulse to delay CPR in a pulseless patient. If possible let someone else do CPR as you take stock and look at the bigger picture. This is a very useful reason for the ABCs – to buy you some thinking and information-gathering time.
- Once you have the defibrillator leads on, look at the rhythm and assess if it is shockable. If shockable then shock and treat for VT/VF. Go through the standard list of treatable causes, ensuring effective CPR continues.

1.2 Initiating resuscitation

- Is there a 'do not resuscitate' form in the notes? Check for advanced directive or community DNACPR order. Are patient's wishes expressed? If you can't be sure then start and continue resuscitation as long as is reasonable. See DNACPR ▶Section 19.19. Reassess and take senior advice especially in a young or hypothermic or overdosed patient. Stop when continuing is considered futile.
- Those without a DNACPR should be for resuscitation. However, new guidance states that "if the healthcare team is as certain as it can be that a person is dying as an inevitable result of underlying disease or a catastrophic health event, and CPR would not re-start the heart and breathing for a sustained period, CPR should not be attempted" (*Decisions Relating to CPR* 3e (BMA, Resus Council (UK), RCN) 2016). I would still expect there to be an emphasis to make reasonable attempts to discuss with family and attempt to discuss DNACPR if death was predictable.
- Emphasis should be on cardiac arrest prevention and so care should be instigated pre-arrest when reversible factors can be dealt with. If a patient is *in extremis* and

pre-arrest, then call the arrest team early before the patient is pulseless. The ABC assessment gives you time to think of your plan. Delegate roles.

- If you are leading the arrest, then ask others to get venous/intraosseous access and obtain notes. Determine the ceiling of care. Contact your senior if unsure or unclear. Send away extra staff if there are demands elsewhere. Extra hands might be more productive seeing other sick patients and preventing cardiac arrests elsewhere.
- Stop once you all feel that continuing is futile. Thank the team. Complete audit sheets and record all in the patient notes. Arrange to talk with family. Do a self-debrief: anything you would do differently or better? Seek feedback and add to your PDP.
- **Favourable outcome:** witnessed arrest; in-hospital; early effective CPR; shockable rhythm; early defibrillation; hypothermia (e.g. submerged in icy water).

1.3 Basic life support: UK Guidelines 2015

- **Safety:** make sure you, the victim and any bystanders are safe.
- **Response:** check victim for a response. Gently shake shoulders and ask loudly: "Are you all right?". If responds leave in the position in which you find him, provided no further danger; get help if needed; reassess regularly.
- **Airway:** open the airway. Turn victim onto back. Place your hand on forehead and gently tilt head back; with your fingertips under the point of the victim's chin, lift the chin to open the airway.
- **Breathing:** look, listen and feel for normal breathing for no more than 10 seconds. In the first few minutes after cardiac arrest, a victim may be barely breathing, or taking infrequent, slow and noisy gasps. Do not confuse this with normal breathing. If you have any doubt whether breathing is normal, act as if it is they are not breathing normally and prepare to start CPR. Call for help and Arrest Team.
- **Send for AED:** send someone to get an AED if available. If you are on your own, do not leave the victim, start CPR.
- **Chest compressions (CCs):** kneel by the patient. Place the heel of one hand on the lower sternum. Place heel of your other hand on top of the first hand. Interlock the fingers of your hands and ensure that pressure is not applied over the patient's ribs. Keep your arms straight. Do not apply any pressure over the upper abdomen or the bottom end of the bony sternum. Position your shoulders vertically above the patient's chest and press down on the sternum to a depth of 5–6 cm. After each CC, release all the pressure on the chest without losing contact between your hands and the sternum; repeat at a rate of 100–120 per min.
- **Give rescue breaths:** after 30 compressions open the airway again using head tilt and chin lift and give 2 rescue breaths. Pinch the soft part of the nose closed, using the index finger and thumb of your hand on the forehead. Allow the mouth to open, but maintain chin lift. Take a normal breath and place your lips around his mouth, making sure that you have a good seal. Blow steadily into the mouth while watching for the chest to rise, taking about 1 second as in normal breathing; this is an effective rescue breath. Maintaining head tilt and chin lift, take your mouth away from the victim and watch for the chest to fall as air comes out. Take another normal breath and blow into the victim's mouth once more to achieve a total of two effective rescue breaths. Do not interrupt CCs by more than 10 seconds to deliver two breaths. Then return your hands without delay to the correct position on the sternum and give a further 30 chest compressions. Continue with CCs and rescue breaths in a ratio of 30:2. If you are untrained or unable to do rescue breaths, give CC-only CPR at a rate of at least 100–120 per min.

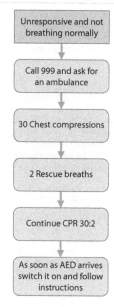

Basic life support algorithm.

Reproduced with permission from the Resuscitation Council (UK) 2015.

- **If an AED arrives:** switch it on. Attach the electrode pads on the patient's bare chest. If more than one rescuer is present, CPR should be continued while electrode pads are being attached to the chest. Follow the spoken/visual directions. Ensure that nobody is touching the patient while the AED is analysing the rhythm. If a shock is indicated, deliver shock but ensure that nobody is touching the patient, push shock button as directed (fully automatic AEDs will deliver the shock automatically), immediately restart CPR at a ratio of 30:2. Continue as directed by the voice/visual prompts. If no shock is indicated, immediately resume CPR. Continue as directed by the voice/visual prompts.
- **Continue CPR:** do not interrupt resuscitation until you become exhausted or the patient is definitely waking up, moving, opening eyes and breathing normally. It is rare for CPR alone to restart the heart. Only if you are certain the person has recovered continue CPR.
- **Recovery position:** if certain the patient is breathing normally but still unresponsive, place in the recovery position. Remove the patient's glasses, if worn, kneel beside the patient and make sure that both legs are straight. Place the arm nearest to you out at right angles to his body, elbow bent with the hand palm-up. Bring the far arm across the chest, and hold the back of the hand against the patient's cheek nearest to you. With your other hand, grasp the far leg just above the knee and pull it up, keeping the foot on the ground. Keeping his hand pressed against cheek, pull on the far leg to roll the patient towards you on to side. Adjust the upper leg so that both the hip and knee are bent at right angles. Tilt the head back to make sure that the airway remains open. If necessary, adjust the hand under the cheek to keep the head tilted and facing downwards to allow liquid material to drain from the mouth. Check breathing regularly. Be prepared to restart CPR immediately if the patient deteriorates or stops breathing normally.

- **American guidance 2015** for the single rescuer is to initiate chest compressions before giving rescue breaths (C–A–B for chest compression (100–120 per min)–airway–breathing rather than A–B–C) to reduce delay to first compression. The single rescuer should begin CPR with 30 compressions then 2 breaths. All lay rescuers should, at a minimum, provide chest compressions for victims of cardiac arrest.

1.4 Advanced life support: UK Guidelines 2015

New points: minimise all interruptions to chest compression (CCs) to less than 5 seconds when attempting defibrillation or tracheal intubation by preplanning and coordination. Waveform capnography can identify return of spontaneous circulation. Peri-arrest ultrasound can help identify reversible causes. Extracorporeal life support techniques may be used as a rescue therapy in selected patients where standard ALS measures are not successful.

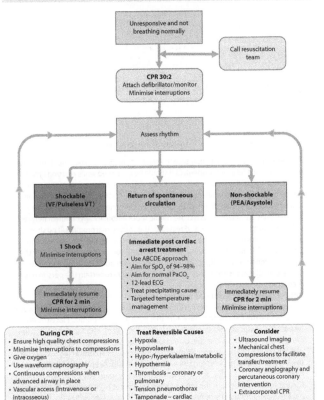

Advanced life support algorithm.
Reproduced with permission from the Resuscitation Council (UK) 2015.

1.5 Treatment of shockable rhythms (VF/pulseless VT)

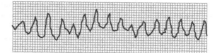

Ventricular fibrillation.

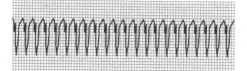

Pulseless VT (pVT).

- **Confirm cardiac arrest:** signs of life and normal breathing. If trained to do so, check for breathing and pulse simultaneously. Call resuscitation team. Perform uninterrupted CCs while applying defibrillation/monitoring pads – one below the right clavicle and the other in the V6 position in the midaxillary line. Plan and communicate pausing CCs for rhythm analysis. Stop CCs; confirm VF/pVT from the ECG. This pause in CCs should be brief and no longer than 5 seconds. Resume CCs immediately; warn all rescuers other than the individual performing the CCs to "stand clear" and remove any oxygen delivery device as appropriate. The designated person selects energy on the defibrillator and presses the charge button. Use at least 150 J for the first shock, the same or a higher energy for subsequent shocks. If unsure of the correct energy level for a defibrillator choose the highest available energy. Ensure person giving the CCs is the only person touching the patient. Once the defibrillator is charged and the safety check is complete, tell rescuer doing the CCs to "stand clear"; when clear, give the shock. After shock delivery immediately restart CPR using a ratio of 30:2, starting with CCs. Do not pause to reassess the rhythm or feel for a pulse. The total pause in CCs should be brief and no longer than 5 seconds. Continue CPR for 2 min; the team leader prepares the team for the next pause in CPR. Pause briefly to check the monitor. If VF/pVT, repeat steps above and deliver a second shock. If VF/pVT persists, repeat steps above and deliver a third shock. Resume CCs immediately. Give ADRENALINE 1 mg IV and AMIODARONE 300 mg IV while performing a further 2 min CPR. Withhold adrenaline if there are signs of return of spontaneous circulation (ROSC) during CPR. Repeat this 2 min CPR – rhythm/pulse check – defibrillation sequence if VF/pVT persists. Give further ADRENALINE 1 mg IV after alternate shocks (i.e. approximately every 3–5 min). If organised electrical activity compatible with a cardiac output is seen during a rhythm check, seek evidence of ROSC (check for signs of life, a central pulse and end-tidal CO_2 if available). If there is ROSC, start post-resuscitation care. If there are no signs of ROSC, continue CPR and switch to the non-shockable algorithm. If asystole is seen, continue CPR and switch to the nonshockable algorithm. Consider a further dose of AMIODARONE 150 mg IV after 5 defibrillation attempts. LIDOCAINE 1 mg/kg may be used as an alternative if amiodarone is not available but do not give lidocaine if amiodarone has been given already.
- **Waveform capnography:** can enable ROSC to be detected without pausing CCs. It may help avoid bolus injection of adrenaline after ROSC has been achieved. Several human studies have shown that there is a significant increase in end-tidal CO_2 when

ROSC occurs. If ROSC is suspected during CPR withhold adrenaline. Give adrenaline if cardiac arrest is confirmed at the next rhythm check.

- **Adrenaline** (epinephrine): regardless of the arrest rhythm, after the initial adrenaline dose has been given, give further 1 mg doses of adrenaline every 3–5 min until ROSC is achieved; in practice, this will be about once every two cycles of the algorithm. If signs of life return during CPR (e.g. purposeful movement, normal breathing or coughing), or there is an increase in end-tidal CO_2, check the monitor; if an organised rhythm is present, check for a pulse. If a pulse is palpable, start post-resuscitation care. If no pulse is present, continue CPR.
- **Witnessed, monitored VF/pVT:** if a patient has a monitored and witnessed cardiac arrest in the catheter laboratory, coronary care unit, a critical care area or whilst monitored after cardiac surgery, and a manual defibrillator is rapidly available: confirm cardiac arrest and shout for help. If the initial rhythm is VF/pVT, give up to three quick successive (stacked) shocks. Rapidly check for a rhythm change and, if appropriate, ROSC after each defibrillation attempt. Start CC and continue CPR for 2 min if the third shock is unsuccessful.
- **Precordial thump:** unlikely to cardiovert. Consider only when it can be used without delay whilst awaiting the arrival of a defibrillator in a monitored VF/pVT arrest. Using the ulnar edge of a tightly clenched fist, deliver a sharp impact to the lower half of the sternum from a height of about 20 cm.

1.6 Treatment of non-shockable rhythms (asystole/PEA)

- **Pulseless electrical activity** (PEA): cardiac arrest in the presence of electrical activity (other than VT) that would normally be associated with a palpable pulse. Often have some mechanical myocardial contractions, but not enough to produce a detectable pulse or BP. PEA can be caused by reversible conditions that can be treated if they are identified and corrected. Survival with asystole or PEA is unlikely unless a reversible cause can be found and treated effectively.
- **Asystole:** check the ECG for P waves as patient may respond to cardiac pacing when there is ventricular standstill with continuing P waves. There is no value in attempting to pace true asystole.
- **Treatment of PEA and asystole:** start CPR 30:2. Give ADRENALINE 1 mg IV as soon as intravascular access is achieved. Continue CPR 30:2 until the airway is secured – then continue CCs without pausing during ventilation. Recheck the rhythm after 2 min: if electrical activity compatible with a pulse is seen, check for a pulse and/or signs of life and if a pulse and/or signs of life are present, start post-resuscitation care. If no pulse and/or no signs of life are present (PEA or asystole): continue CPR, recheck the rhythm after 2 min and proceed accordingly. Give further ADRENALINE 1 mg IV every 3–5 min (during alternate 2 min loops of CPR). If VF/pVT at rhythm check, change to shockable side of algorithm.

1.7 Reversible causes of cardiac arrest

- **Hypoxia:** ensuring airway patent, adequate ventilation, maximal FiO_2 during CPR with BVM or intubation. Check adequate chest rise and bilateral breath sounds. Check ET tube is not misplaced in a bronchus or the oesophagus. ▶ Section 4.5.
- **Hypovolaemia:** PEA caused by hypovolaemia is usually due to severe haemorrhage. Clues may be trauma, GI bleeding or signs of ruptured AAA. Stop the haemorrhage and restore intravascular volume with fluid and blood products. Other causes include anaphylaxis and other causes of shock. Needs IV access x2, IV fluids (normal saline (NS)). Blood if severe haemorrhage (O-neg). See Haemorrhagic shock ▶ Section 2.22.

- **Hyperkalaemia:** if suspect K$^+$ >6.5 mmol/L give 10 ml 10% CALCIUM GLUCONATE IV and 10 U INSULIN with 50 ml 50% GLUCOSE over 15 mins. ▶Section 5.3.
- **Hypocalcaemia/calcium channel blocker toxicity:** 10 ml 10% CALCIUM GLUCONATE IV. ▶Section 5.6.
- **Hypoglycaemia:** GLUCAGON 1 mg IM/SC and if IV access 50 ml 50% GLUCOSE or equivalent must be given. ▶Section 5.2.
- **Hypothermia:** drowning, exposure. Rectal temperature. Rewarm. Hypothermia is neuroprotective. Do not stop until patient rewarmed and resuscitation fails. ▶Section 17.6.
- **Coronary thrombosis** is the most common cause of sudden cardiac arrest. Even if ROSC has not been achieved, consider primary PCI when feasible continuing CPR. For ACS ▶Section 3.8.
- **Pulmonary embolism:** mechanical circulatory obstruction, consider immediate thrombolysis and CPR even in cases requiring in excess of 60 min of CPR. Consider performing CPR for 60–90 min before stopping. In some, surgical or mechanical thrombectomy can be considered. For PE ▶Section 4.17.
- **Tension pneumothorax:** trauma associated or ventilated patient. Clinical/ultrasound diagnosis. Do not wait for CXR. Insert needle in 2nd interspace on affected resonant side (trachea deviated away). Diagnostic 'hiss' hopefully as decompresses. BP should improve. Insert chest drain. ▶Section 4.12.
- **Tamponade:** signs (raised JVP, low BP) obscured by the arrest itself. Suspected if penetrating chest trauma, anticoagulants, recent MI or cardiac intervention. May need resuscitative thoracotomy or needle pericardiocentesis. Ultrasound is diagnostic. ▶Section 3.20.
- **Toxins:** look for evidence of drugs taken and treat accordingly. Local anaesthetic or lipophilic drug cardiotoxicity consider 100 ml IV bolus of 20% intralipid emulsion in a 70 kg adult followed by an infusion and continue good quality CPR. See intralipid in toxicology chapter (▶Sections 14.6 & 14.8).

1.8   Resuscitation issues

- **Mechanical chest compression** devices not recommended unless having to transport patient or to relieve other members of the team during prolonged arrests.
- **Use of ultrasound imaging:** focused echo/USS can help diagnose and treat potentially reversible causes of cardiac arrest. Challenging to perform during CPR. A sub-xiphoid probe position is recommended. Placement of the probe just before compressions are paused for a planned rhythm assessment enables a well-trained operator to obtain views within 10 seconds. Can diagnose tamponade, PE, hypovolaemia, PTX. Absence of any cardiac motion is highly predictive of death.
- **Blood gas values:** during cardiac arrest are misleading and bear little relationship to the tissue acid–base state. Analysis of central venous blood may provide a better estimation of tissue pH.
- **Oxygen during defibrillation:** remove oxygen mask or nasal cannulae to at least 1 m away from the patient's chest during defibrillation. Leave the ventilation bag connected to the tracheal tube or other airway adjunct or disconnect the ventilation bag from the tracheal tube and move it at least 1 m from the patient's chest during defibrillation.
- **Airway management and ventilation:** options are no airway and no ventilation (compression-only CPR), compression-only CPR with the airway held open (with or without supplementary oxygen), mouth-to-mouth breaths, mouth-to-mask, bag-mask ventilation with simple airway adjuncts, supraglottic airways (SGAs), and tracheal intubation (inserted with the aid of direct laryngoscopy or

videolaryngoscopy, or via a SGA). Patients who remain comatose post resuscitation will usually require intubation. Personnel skilled in advanced airway management should attempt laryngoscopy and intubation without stopping chest compressions; a brief pause in chest compressions may be required as the tube is passed through the vocal cords, but this pause should be less than 5 seconds. In the absence of these, use bag-mask ventilation and/or an SGA until appropriately experienced and equipped personnel are present.

- **Basic airway manoeuvres and airway adjuncts:** assess the airway. Use head tilt and chin lift, or jaw thrust to open the airway. Simple airway adjuncts (oropharyngeal or nasopharyngeal airways) can help to maintain an open airway. If risk of cervical spine injury, use jaw thrust or chin lift with manual in-line stabilisation of the head and neck by an assistant. If life-threatening airway obstruction persists despite effective application of jaw thrust or chin lift, add head tilt in small increments until the airway is open; establishing a patent airway takes priority over concerns about a potential cervical spine injury.

- **Ventilation:** artificially ventilate as soon as possible if spontaneous ventilation is inadequate or absent. Expired air ventilation (rescue breathing) FiO_2 is only 0.17 so aim to ventilate with oxygen-enriched air. Consider pocket resuscitation mask with mouth-to-mask ventilation and supplemental oxygen. A two-person technique for bag-mask ventilation is preferable. Deliver each breath over 1 second and give a volume that corresponds to normal chest movement; this represents a compromise between giving an adequate volume, minimising the risk of gastric inflation, and allowing adequate time for CC. During CPR with an unprotected airway, give two ventilations after each sequence of 30 CCs. Once intubated, ventilate the lungs at a rate of about 10 breaths/min.

- **Alternative airway devices:** an **endotracheal** tube is the optimal method of managing the airway during cardiac arrest. However, it is not without its difficulties in insertion. Several alternative airway devices have been used for airway management during CPR. These include the classic laryngeal mask airway (cLMA), the laryngeal tube (LT) and the i-gel, and the LMA supreme (LMAS). **Laryngeal mask airway (LMA):** easy to insert and ventilation is more efficient and easier than BVM. If gas leakage is excessive, chest compression will have to be interrupted to enable ventilation. Can give some airway protection. **Tracheal intubation:** should be attempted only by trained personnel able to carry out the procedure with a high level of skill and confidence. No intubation attempt should interrupt CCs for more than 5 seconds. Use an alternative airway technique if tracheal intubation is not possible. After intubation, tube placement must be confirmed and the tube secured adequately. **Videolaryngoscopy:** used increasingly as it enables a better view of the larynx and increases success rate of intubation. May be useful during CPR. **Confirmation of correct placement of ET tube:** end-tidal CO_2 detectors that include a waveform graphical display (capnographs) are the most reliable for verification of tracheal tube position during cardiac arrest. If not available observe chest expansion bilaterally, listen over lung fields bilaterally in the axillae (breath sounds should be equal and adequate) and over the epigastrium (breath sounds should not be heard). **Cricothyroidotomy:** if it is impossible to ventilate an apnoeic patient with a bag-mask, or to pass a tracheal tube or alternative airway device, delivery of oxygen through a cannula or surgical cricothyroidotomy may be life saving. A tracheostomy is contraindicated in an emergency, as it is time consuming, hazardous and requires considerable surgical skill and equipment.

1.9 Drugs for cardiac arrest

There is a paucity of good evidence. Drugs are of secondary importance to high quality uninterrupted CC and early defibrillation.

- **Adrenaline** (epinephrine): no evidence for survival to hospital discharge, only improved short-term survival. Trials are ongoing.
- **Antiarrhythmics:** no drug shown to increase survival to discharge. Amiodarone increases survival to admission. Ongoing trial comparing amiodarone to lidocaine.
- **Vascular access during CPR:** Get vascular access if possible. Peripheral venous cannulation is quicker, easier to perform and safer. If drugs given then give a 20 ml flush and elevate the limb for 10–20 sec to facilitate drug delivery to the central circulation.
- **Intraosseous route:** if no IV access then consider intraosseous (IO) route. Effective route in adults. Plasma concentrations comparable with IV injection. Sternal IO route comparable with IV adrenaline. Several IO devices are available using humerus, proximal or distal tibia, and sternum. Use as per local experience and skills and kit.
- **Extracorporeal cardiopulmonary resuscitation** (ECPR): should be considered as a rescue therapy for those patients in whom initial ALS measures are unsuccessful and/or to facilitate specific interventions (e.g. coronary angiography and percutaneous coronary intervention (PCI) or pulmonary thrombectomy for massive pulmonary embolism). Requires vascular access and a circuit with a pump and oxygenator and can provide a circulation of oxygenated blood to restore tissue perfusion. Can be a bridge to allow treatment of reversible underlying conditions. This is extracorporeal life support (ECLS), and more specifically extracorporeal CPR (ECPR). Can improve survival when there is a reversible cause for cardiac arrest (e.g. ACS/PE, severe hypothermia, poisoning). Useful if cardiac arrest is witnessed, the individual receives immediate high quality CPR, and ECPR is implemented early (e.g. within 1 h of collapse) including when instituted by emergency physicians and intensivists.
- **Duration of resuscitation attempt:** if resuscitation is unsuccessful the team leader should discuss stopping CPR with the team. Requires a careful assessment of the likelihood of success. It is reasonable to continue if the patient remains in VF/pVT, or there is a potentially reversible cause that can be treated. The use of mechanical compression devices and ECPR techniques make prolonged attempts at resuscitation feasible in selected patients. It is generally accepted that asystole for more than 20 min in the absence of a reversible cause and with ongoing ALS constitutes a reasonable ground for stopping further resuscitation attempts. Guidance is that resuscitation may be discontinued if all of the following apply: (1) 15 min or more has passed since the onset of collapse, (2) no bystander CPR was given before arrival of the ambulance, (3) there is no suspicion of drowning, hypothermia, poisoning/overdose, or pregnancy, (4) asystole is present for more than 30 sec on the ECG monitor screen.

Do not interrupt CPR unless definite signs of recovery. Keep pauses as short as possible. Plan and coordinate interruptions so they are as short as possible. Compression-only CPR where unable/unwilling to give rescue breaths.

1.10 Special cases in resuscitation

- **Post-cardiac surgery cardiac catheterisation:** cardiac arrest where CCs difficult. Give 3 quick consecutive 'stacked' (repeated) shocks before starting CCs. Consider re-sternotomy (reopening the sternal wound) to exclude tamponade. Internal defibrillation with paddles. Direct cardiac compression can be given to the heart. Use 20 J in cardiac arrest but only 5 J if supported on cardiopulmonary bypass.

- **Post drowning:** immediately start CPR and 15 L/min O_2; ROSC prior to hospital suggests better prognosis. Look for and treat high K^+ with fresh water drowning. Look for and manage compounding issues, e.g. associated hypothermia/exposure, drug overdose or suicide attempt. Duration of hypoxia is the most critical survival factor.

- **Post electrocution:** extensive burns can affect face, neck and airway. CPR because patient may be in VF or asystole with early intubation if possible. Asystole is seen after DC shock and VF after AC shock (mains supply). Check for secondary spinal injury or other trauma. Muscle paralysis can cause respiratory failure (reduced FVC <1.5 L). Fluid resuscitation as tissue/muscle damage. Ensure good diuresis, watch for AKI and check CK and K^+.

- **Cardiac arrest in pregnancy:** Caesarean section within 5 min of the cardiac arrest can save mother and baby. Call maternal cardiac arrest team and obstetrician immediately and note time. After 20 weeks aortocaval compression left lateral tilt (right side high and left side low). Use a fixed wedge or a large gravid uterus can be manually displaced to the left. Optimal CCs in higher position on sternum. Ventilate: BVM 100% O_2 and monitor capnography. Optimal airway control. Follow ALS algorithm using same drugs. Place IV access above diaphragm (not femoral) and give IV fluids as needed. *Defibrillation is regarded as safe throughout pregnancy.* Remove fetal monitors during defibrillation. If you suspect *magnesium toxicity* stop it and give 10 ml IV 10% CALCIUM GLUCONATE. If no ROSC within 4 min then emergency Caesarean section and aim to deliver within 5 min of resuscitation commencing. Delivery can be life saving for mother and fetus and may improve a desperate situation. **Possible causes:** bleeding coagulopathy, DIC, sepsis, acute MI, concealed haemorrhage – placental abruption, ectopic pregnancy, rupture or dissection of aneurysms, pulmonary embolus (thrombolysis if life-threatening PE), amniotic fluid embolism (immediate Caesarean), anaesthetic complication, known or new cardiac disease, HTN, pre-eclampsia/eclampsia, placenta abruptio/placenta praevia. Discuss an urgent management plan for these if ROSC – most are obstetric.

1.11 Return of spontaneous circulation (ROSC)

- **ROSC:** diagnose if palpable central pulse or sudden increase in end-tidal CO_2 trace. (Continuous quantitative waveform capnography for monitoring of ET tube placement is a useful marker that identifies ROSC.) If signs of ROSC then complete assessment: ABC. O_2/ventilation. You bring the patient back from death so the immediate questions are why the cardiac arrest and anticipate possible complications. Get an ECG, ABG, U&E, troponin. Again ask why. Get a 12-lead ECG. Is it STEMI needing primary PCI/thrombolysis, acute PE needing thrombolysis, hyperkalaemia needing calcium and insulin/glucose?

- **Stabilise: ABC: high FiO_2** can now be reduced to give O_2 as per BTS guidance. Check FBC, U&E, ABG, CXR, 12-lead ECG, Mg^{2+}, Ca^{2+}, troponin, lactate. Of these the ECG is the most useful as a large MI should be evident. If STEMI then PPCI is the next approach if stable.

- **Induced hypothermia** may be neuroprotective. Indicated in those comatose following ROSC due to VF arrest. Involves cooling to 32–34°C for 12–24 h or longer post-ROSC. Evidence in non-VF arrest lacking but is used in comatose patients after either form of arrest. Methods include cooling blankets and ice bags as well as ice-cold isotonic infusion. Up to 3 L has been given in some trials.

- **Glycaemic control:** aim for glucose control of 6–11 mmol/L. Avoid hypoglycaemia which can cause or exacerbate brain injury.
- **Coagulopathy:** watch for signs and check APTT, FBC, PT, platelets, fibrinogen if any doubt.
- **Hypotension:** treat (SBP <90 mmHg) by addressing cause with a choice of inotrope and/or vasopressor, e.g. (▶Section 2.17 on inotropes). Fluids: 1–2 L of NS or Ringer's lactate. Chilled to 4°C for induced hypothermia. Other vasopressors are listed later.
- **Post-arrest myocardial dysfunction:** may be related to an underlying STEMI but a period of hypoperfusion can result in temporarily impaired pump function for up to 72 h which can be bridged with DOBUTAMINE and intra-aortic balloon pump if required.
- **Low BP** and shock may be partly driven by a SIRS type mechanism with a drop in systemic vascular resistance and in these cases NORADRENALINE infusion may be useful – take expert advice (and ▶Section 2.17 on inotropes). This is best delivered within an ITU setting with access to invasive monitoring.
- **Arrhythmias:** see below for management of tachy-/bradyarrhythmias.
- **Seizures and myoclonic jerks:** can be seen post-ROSC in up to 10% of patients. These can be managed conservatively but if significant and frequent then may consider anticonvulsants. Clonazepam can be used for myoclonus as well as valproate.
- **Oxygen: 15 L/min** with a non-rebreather mask gives an FiO_2 of about 90% and is recommended in cardiac arrest and shock, but should be reduced post-arrest to avoid O_2 toxicity. Follow BTS guidance. Watch O_2 saturation. Watch for CO_2 retention, which can only be diagnosed by ABG.
- **SBP goal is >100 mmHg.** Use fluids, an arterial line, and pressors/inotropes (noradrenaline and dobutamine) as needed. Coronary angiography is strongly recommended for patients with ST elevation or new LBBB. Though the guidelines recognise that evidence is limited, they also recommend consideration of PCI for other patients without a known non-cardiac source.
- **Electrolytes:** keep potassium between 4.0 and 4.5 mmol/L. Monitor BM and avoid tight glucose control, particularly hypoglycaemia.

1.12 Bradycardia management: be prepared to pace

Do not give atropine to patients with cardiac transplants. Denervated hearts do not respond to vagal blockade by atropine, which may cause paradoxical sinus arrest or high-grade AV block in these patients.

Causes: physiological (e.g. during sleep, in athletes), cardiac causes (e.g. AV block or sinus node disease), non-cardiac causes (e.g. vasovagal, hypothermia, hypothyroidism, hyperkalaemia), drugs (e.g. beta-blockade, diltiazem, digoxin, amiodarone).

Management: see algorithm below. Give up to 6 × 0.5 mg (3 mg) of ATROPINE, ISOPRENALINE 5 mcg/min IV, ADRENALINE 2–10 mcg/min. Give IV GLUCAGON if a beta-blocker or calcium channel blocker is a likely cause of the bradycardia. DIGIBIND if due to digoxin toxicity. IV THEOPHYLLINE (100–200 mg by slow IV injection) for bradycardia complicating acute inferior wall myocardial infarction, spinal cord injury or cardiac transplantation. **US (AHA) guidance:** ADRENALINE/EPINEPHRINE 2–10 mcg/min or DOPAMINE 2–10 mcg/kg per minute. Also see bradycardia ▶Section 3.15.

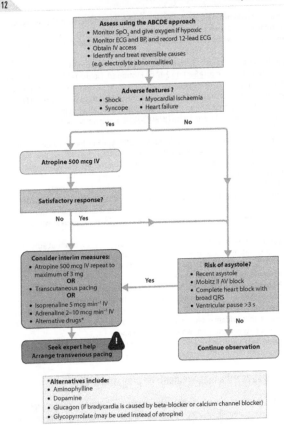

Adult bradycardia algorithm.
Reproduced with permission from the Resuscitation Council (UK) 2015.

1.13 Tachycardia management: be prepared to DC shock

Assess: ABCDE. Give O_2 if appropriate and obtain IV access. Monitor ECG, BP, SpO_2, record 12-lead ECG. Troponin. Check U&E.

Management: if unstable (i.e. has adverse features likely to be caused or made worse by the tachycardia, e.g. shock, syncope, chest pain/ischaemia, heart failure) synchronised cardioversion is the treatment of choice. Uncommon for tachycardia to cause compromise significantly with rate 100–150 per min unless existing cardiorespiratory disease. If cardioversion fails to restore sinus rhythm, and the patient remains unstable, give AMIODARONE 300 mg IV over 10–20 min and re-attempt electrical cardioversion. The loading dose of AMIODARONE may be followed by an infusion of 900 mg over 24 h. Management of SVT and VT also detailed in cardiology chapter (tachyarrhythmias, ▶ Sections 3.11–16).

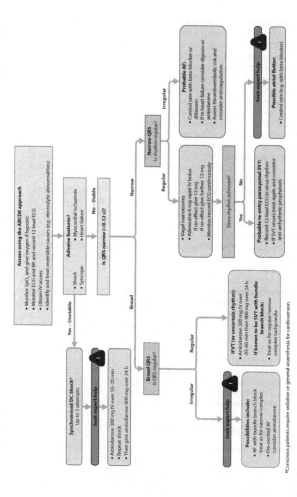

Tachycardia algorithm.

Reproduced with permission from the Resuscitation Council (UK) 2015.

1.14 Emergency DC cardioversion

- **Indication:** DC cardioversion (if we treat VF it is called defibrillation) should be considered in all fast and unstable tachyarrhythmias. Usually the ventricular rate is >150/min. If there is chest pain, pulmonary oedema, syncope or shock due to the arrhythmia.
- **Contraindications: these are relative.** For elective DCC digitalis toxicity is a concern as it can cause ventricular arrhythmias – usually 1 or 2 doses omitted if elective. DCC does not reverse sinus tachycardia or multifocal atrial tachycardia. Concerns about non-anticoagulated AF of duration >48 h and embolic/stroke risk needs to be weighed against the need for improving haemodynamics. Ideally a TOE to identify left atrial appendage thrombus should be done. This may not be practical or feasible or available in the emergency situation. Take expert advice. In these cases some form of rate control rather than rhythm control may be tried, but DC cardioversion is quick and often effective.
- **Sedation:** enlist help of anaesthetist to protect airway. If conscious needs sedation, e.g. MIDAZOLAM 2.5 mg slow IV (max 7.5 mg) is the sedation of choice and provides amnesia and sedation. ANNEXATE and airway control and bag-valve mask should be available for oversedation. Written consent if possible. Use pulse oximetry and ECG monitoring via the pads. Remove nitrate patches. Ensure good IV access. Remove oxygen at shock.
- **DC cardioversion:** place pads on the chest (anterior posterior may be preferred for AF). Broad complex or AF use a biphasic shock of 120–150 J or monophasic 200 J; for atrial flutter or SVT, use 70–120 J. Ensure that the defibrillator is 'synced' with the R wave of the QRS complexes. There is a sync button which does this and a bright dot appears on the R wave – this avoids shocking on a T wave and inducing VF. Give 3 successive shocks if there is no immediate cardioversion, giving up to full energy available. Ensure you warn all before giving the shock. If no success, consider repeating after AMIODARONE 150–300 mg slow IV over 20 min. Post procedure recovery position as tolerated until wakes up.
- **Elective cardioversion for AF:** those on warfarin should have evidence of levels of INR within the therapeutic window for the past 4 weeks prior to the procedure. Evidently in the emergency situation this is waived, but therapeutic LMWH should be given if not anticoagulated and continued for 4 weeks post procedure, irrespective of outcome. In some cases a TOE showing absence of thrombus in the left atrial appendage can suggest that elective cardioversion can proceed without pre-existing anticoagulation. Take advice if unsure.
- **Complications:** skin soreness like a sunburn over the pads, arrhythmias, stroke (DC cardioversion may precipitate systemic emboli from intracardiac thrombus) especially in AF which is not anticoagulated, failure is seen in many with AF but more successful in VT and atrial flutter and SVT, mild troponin rises.

1.15 Emergency pericardiocentesis

- **Relative contraindications** need to be balanced with urgency and risks of inaction. These are uncorrected bleeding disorders, e.g. low platelets, ↑INR. A long needle is passed using a sub-xiphoid approach under strict asepsis and local anaesthesia, with echo/ultrasound control, aspirating with needle at 30° to skin with the patient sitting up at 45° angle, aiming for tip of the left shoulder.
- **Connect a 20 or 50 ml syringe to the spinal needle,** and aspirate 5 ml of IV NS into the syringe. While advancing the needle, the occasional injection of up to 1 ml of NS helps to keep the needle lumen patent. Seldinger technique is used and a wire is passed; once the pericardial space is entered then a floppy soft-tipped guide-wire is passed into the space and around the heart. A pig tailed or soft straight

multiperforated sterile drainage catheter is inserted over the wire and the wire removed. This allows rapid drainage and improved BP.
- **Take senior advice** if available and transfer patient to cardiology centre as soon as possible. Drainage of large effusions, especially if chronic ones, must be evacuated very slowly; otherwise, there may be acute ventricular dilation or pulmonary oedema.
- **Complications:** PTX, damage to myocardium, coronary vessels, arrhythmias, pulmonary oedema.

 ## Automated implantable cardioverter defibrillator (AICD)

AICDs often function as a pacemaker, but can also deliver low-energy synchronised cardioversion and high-energy defibrillation shocks that successfully terminate 99% of ventricular fibrillation attacks. Indications are as follows (patient on chronic, best medical therapy and have a reasonable expectation of survival with good functional status for >1 y).

Level A evidence
- LVEF ≤35% due to prior MI who are at least 40 days post-MI and NYHA Functional Class II or III.
- LV dysfunction due to prior MI who are at least 40 days post-MI, LVEF ≤30%, and NYHA Functional Class I.
- Survivors of cardiac arrest due to VF or haemodynamically unstable sustained VT after evaluation with reversible causes excluded.

Level B evidence
- Non-ischaemic DCM who have an LVEF ≤35% and NYHA Functional Class II or III.
- Non-sustained VT due to prior MI, LVEF <40%, and inducible VF or sustained VT at EPS (electrophysiological study).
- Structural heart disease and spontaneous sustained VT, whether haemodynamically stable or unstable.
- Syncope of undetermined origin with clinically relevant, haemodynamically significant sustained VT or VF induced at EPS.

- **Cardiac arrest with AICD:** these patients are at high risk of cardiac arrest. If AICD senses a shockable rhythm it will fire a 40 J shock internally which may cause pectoral muscle contraction. Shocks to rescuers doing CPR are minimal, especially if wearing gloves. Generally produces a maximum of 8 possible discharges. Place shock pads away from AICD, e.g. antero-posterior: left precordium to below left scapula. A magnet placed over the AICD will disable any of its activity. Ask cardiology to deactivate in end of life care.
- **Patients with AICDs receiving shocks:** those who have received shocks need a full assessment of their clinical status and device function. Shocks are a red flag for clinical events. Even if inappropriate there is a related increased mortality. Shocks are unpleasant, causing psychological distress, anxiety, and decreased quality of life. Catheter ablation of arrhythmias may be needed. Specialist assessment is needed.
- **Ongoing SVT/AF/VT with haemodynamic compromise:** ignore presence of the AICD and treat. Consider external DC shock, IV amiodarone and/or beta-blockers (if haemodynamically tolerated). To shock avoid placement of paddles in the skin area over the AICD pocket. If possible, attempt an anterior–posterior electrode position.
- **Repetitive AICD shocks without a tachyarrhythmia or due to tachyarrhythmia** (atrial or ventricular) that is haemodynamically well tolerated by the patient: place a magnet over the device to inhibit further shock delivery.
- **Contact with the patient during AICD discharge:** is harmless but gloves (1–2) decrease conductivity and attenuate potential discomfort.

1.17 Adult choking algorithm

- **Choking** usually when eating. Patient clutches neck/chest and unable to speak. Can be wheezing and stridor. May become unconscious. If conscious with airway obstruction give 5 back blows then 5 abdominal thrusts: if signs suggest mild airway obstruction then encourage coughing, but do nothing else. But if signs of severe airway obstruction and conscious give up to five back blows. Stand to the side and slightly behind the patient. Support the chest with one hand and lean the victim well forwards so that when the obstructing object is dislodged it comes out of the mouth rather than goes further down the airway. Give up to five sharp blows between the shoulder blades with the heel of your other hand.
- **Check to see if each back blow has relieved the airway obstruction.** If this fails, then give up to five abdominal thrusts. Stand behind the patient and put both arms round the upper part of his abdomen. Lean the victim forwards. Clench your fist and place it between the umbilicus and the bottom end of the sternum. Grasp this hand with your other hand and pull sharply inwards and upwards. Repeat up to five times. If the obstruction is still not relieved, continue alternating five back blows with five abdominal thrusts. If unconscious start CPR. Help the patient carefully to the ground. Call an ambulance immediately. Begin CPR. Those trained and experienced in feeling for a carotid pulse should initiate CPR even if a pulse is present in the unconscious choking victim.
- **Following successful treatment** for choking, foreign material may nevertheless remain in the upper or lower respiratory tract and cause complications later. Patients with a persistent cough, difficulty swallowing, or with the sensation of an object being still stuck in the throat should therefore be referred for an immediate ENT opinion.

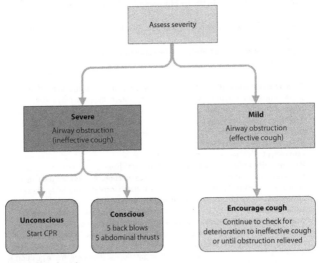

Adult choking algorithm.
Reproduced with permission from the Resuscitation Council (UK) 2015.

02 The acutely ill patient

2.1 Levels of care

- **Introduction:** Clinicians need to classify patients according to their needs to enable best possible care in the most appropriate part of the hospital. These have been designated as differing levels and you should know the terminology.

- **Level 0:** Normal ward care in acute hospital, e.g. IV therapy. Observations less frequently than every 4 h.
- **Level 1:** Patients at risk of deteriorating, or those recently relocated from higher levels of care, whose needs can be met on an acute ward with additional advice and support from the critical care team, e.g. observations more than every 4 h, tracheostomy, CVP line, chest drain, continuous infusion of insulin, PCA, post-op.
- **Level 2 (HDU):** Patients requiring detailed observation or intervention including support for a single failing organ system or post-op care and those 'stepping down' from higher levels of care. Hourly monitoring, needing FiO_2 >0.5 by face mask.
- **Level 3 (ITU):** Patients requiring advanced respiratory support alone or basic respiratory support together with support of at least two organ systems. This level includes all complex patients requiring support for multi-organ failure.

The care delivered depends on several factors. These include the skills of the nurses predominantly and the skill mix, i.e. appropriately trained nurses, their seniority and the number of healthcare assistants available. The ratio of skilled staff to patients is fundamental in allowing time for the correct level of care and observation. When a patient is sick (i.e. there is need for one or more organ support – cardiac, renal, pulmonary, etc.) there is a need to move the patient to a level of care that is appropriate, which may mean moving them to the medical assessment unit (MAU) or to an HDU or ITU bed. For the latter two groups of patients it is good to involve critical care outreach as early as possible.

2.2 National early warning scores

- Studies have shown that those needing ITU have had major derangements in SaO_2, HR, respiratory rate and BP many hours before escalation. The aim is to identify these patients and react in a more timely fashion to improve outcome. Sick patients are sliding metaphorically along an icy slope to the edge of the cliff over many hours and are potentially salvageable. Cardiac arrest patients have progressed and fallen off the cliff and hit the ground where resuscitation outcomes are so much worse.
- Early warning scores provide a 'track-and-trigger' system to efficiently identify and respond to patients who present with or develop acute illness and to assess and manage using an ABCDE approach. The RCP has developed National Early Warning Scores (NEWS). There is also a recommendation that escalation communication uses the SBAR protocol. NEWS should be an aid and not a substitute for competent experienced clinical judgment.

Parameter	0	+1	+2	+3
Resp rate/min	12–20	9–11	21–44	≥25 or ≤8
SpO₂* (%)	≥96	94–95	92–93	≤91
Temp (°C)	36.1–38.0	35.1–36.0 or 38.1–39.0	≥39.1	≤35
Systolic BP (mmHg)	111–219	101–110	91–100	≤90 or >220
Pulse rate (bpm)	51–90	41–50 or 91–110	111–130	≥131 or ≤40
Conscious	A	A	A	VPU
Supplemental O₂	No		Yes	

*For patients with known Type 2 respiratory failure due to COPD, recommended BTS target saturations of 88–92% should be used. These patients will still 'score' if their O₂ sats are below 92% unless the score is 'reset' by a competent clinical decision-maker and patient-specific target O₂ saturations are prescribed and documented on the chart and in the clinical notes. Note that a high systolic BP does not score until it is 220 mmHg.

2.3 Clinical risk and response

- **Low risk** (0–4): should prompt assessment by a trained nurse who decides if a change to frequency of clinical monitoring or an escalation of clinical care is required.
- **Medium risk** (5–6 or a RED score): needs an urgent review by a clinician competent to assess acute illness – ward-based doctor or acute team nurse, who can escalate to a team with critical care skills as required.
- **High risk** (≥7): prompts emergency assessment by a clinical team/critical care outreach team with critical care competencies and there is usually transfer of the patient to a higher dependency care area.
- **Exceptions:** extreme values in one physiological parameter (e.g. HR <40 bpm, or a RR <8 per min or temp <35°C) should not be ignored and on its own requires urgent clinical evaluation.

Reference: Royal College of Physicians (2012) National Early Warning Score (NEWS): Report of a working party. London: RCP.

2.4 ABCDE assessment

While assessing ABCDE get help from nursing or other medical staff, work quickly to get IV access send bloods done, ABG and ECG and arrange a portable CXR, depending on the assessment. It is helpful if one can be the doing the tasks and the other can be thinking about what is going on and what needs to be done. In all emergencies, one person needs to be leading and thinking of the underlying diagnosis and management.

Important signs of impending demise: increased HR, low HR, increased RR, low or falling BP, cold peripheries, oliguria or anuria, fall in GCS (coma) or new confusion, cyanosis, distress, silent chest.

Focus	Assessment, warning signs and actions
Airway	**Ideal:** normal speech and no added airways noises. **Warning:** reduced GCS <9, paradoxical chest movements, wheeze, snoring, drooling, grunting, stridor **Actions:** chin lift, jaw thrust, removal of foreign bodies, oropharyngeal airway, suction visible debris, recovery position, intubation, treat any suspected anaphylaxis
Breathing	**Ideal:** talks in full sentences, comfortable, RR 12–20. SaO_2 >94–98%. **Warning:** RR <8 or >20 and tired. Wheeze, reduced chest expansion one side – dull or resonant, silent chest, accessory muscles, cyanosis, tracheal deviation. **Possible actions:** O_2 15 L/min unless COPD. Urgent portable CXR and ABG, SALBUTAMOL 2.5 mg Neb for wheeze, FUROSEMIDE 50 mg IV/GTN for pulmonary oedema, chest drain for PTX, CPAP, NIV, cough assist device, ventilation, IV antibiotics
Circulation	**Ideal:** cap refill <2 sec. HR 50–90 bpm. SBP 120–140 mmHg. Urine output 40 ml/h. Normal heart sounds, no murmurs. **Warning:** cold shut down, peripheral cyanosis, SBP <90 mmHg or >220 mmHg. ↑JVP. Urine output <40 ml/h. **Possible actions:** repeated 250 ml NS fluid bolus. IV antibiotics. ECG, ECHO, PCI/thrombolysis (ACS/PE), LMWH (PE), inotropes, balloon pump. Transfusion if bleeding and/or correct coagulopathy
Disability	**Ideal:** normal GCS orientated. **Warning:** low GCS, confused, comatose, pupil signs, Cheyne–Stokes. Check plantars. Use **A**lert, **V**oice, **P**ain, **and U**nresponsive. **Possible actions:** check and give glucose if needed. Naloxone for opiates. IV ANTIBIOTIC/ACICLOVIR for CNS infection
Exposure	**Ideal:** full examination. **Warning:** top to toe exam. Meningism, peritonitis, hypothermia, fractures, spinal injury, palpate all over. Bruising, pain, PR exam if spinal injury. **Actions:** cautious rewarming, watch observations, bloods
End of life	Some are dying and the appropriate action should be a communication with patient and/or family and DNR discussions and a personalised care plan for the dying. HDU and ITU are inappropriate and patients need good holistic compassionate care with families and loved ones.
DEFGH	**D**on't **E**ver **F**orget **G**lucose or **H**eroin (opiates) if comatose

2.5   Getting senior help: advice before you call for advice

- Seeking help from seniors, peers or other disciplines is a key skill at all levels. Pre-call organisation is crucial. It depends on what time is available. If *in extremis* get the notes, observations and call quickly whilst others continue to manage the patient. If more time, get the notes and make a quick summary list of clinical details. Get lab results, imaging and pathology and make a summary note. Check notes, drug chart, fluid balance and observations charts and bring all of this to the phone with you. Know SaO_2, BP, HR, FiO_2, IV drugs and infusions.
- What was premorbid state and the patient's wishes? If the patient had stated they did not want intubation and ventilation for a chronic worsening lung condition then best to confirm this before calling ITU (ring the family if needed for baseline and other such information if you think it will alter the escalation decision). Personalising the case aids recall and makes the patient memorable, e.g. a "73 year old retired teacher". Use SBAR – see below.

2.6   Phone protocols

Often A calls B and for some reason the line breaks down. B then tries to ring A whilst A tries to ring B with much confusion, frustration and time wasted. Have an agreed telephone policy, e.g. the initial caller alone must always try to re-establish the line.

You will also at times be the recipient of phone calls. Those calling you will have different skills and experiences. If things just do not sound right, then you must go and see for yourself. If you can try to prioritise the call then do so. Tell the staff how long it will take you to attend, if possible. If you need an ECG then they can have this done for you by the time you arrive or have given PRN analgesia or other interventions that may help the situation.

SBAR communication tool

- **Situation:** identify yourself and your role. Identify the name, age and sex of patient. What is the immediate concern to resolve or request? e.g. *"I need a CT head"*.
- **Background:** explain clinical context. What has happened? Reason admitted. Main past medical history. Relevant medications, procedures, resus status, other input already taken. Relevant lab results. e.g. *"A 73 year retired schoolteacher on warfarin for AF fell and struck his head and is now drowsy with a GCS of 9. If the CT shows an SDH or ICH I will reverse anticoagulation immediately and refer to neurosurgeons"*.
- **Assessment:** latest observations and NEWS. Bring the notes and observations charts and lab results to the phone with you. *"He now has a GCS of 9 which was 12 when seen in A&E. His INR was 4 on admission. Vitamin K and PCC have been given"*.
- **Recommendation:** for nursing staff explain what you need – if you feel that patient needs to be seen now, or it can be dealt with in 20 min, or an hour. If it is an SHO/Registrar/ST calling a consultant, follow the above advice.

2.7 Advanced airways management

Methods for airway support

- **Endotracheal intubation:** a bridging measure to allow treatment/recovery. Elective intubation is much safer than emergency intubation. Ensure adequate preparation. Ensure pre-oxygenated with 100% O_2 before commencing. Intubation must only be by appropriately trained personnel. Rapid sequence induction (RSI) will require sedation with an induction agent e.g. propofol, which is commonly used but can drop BP. Used with neuromuscular blocker such as suxamethonium. Analgesia may also be given.
- **Tracheostomy:** preferred in those needing ongoing airways protection. Better tolerated and more comfortable than endotracheal tube. Less sedation is required. Less dead space to ventilate and airways resistance is reduced. It avoids many of the upper airways complications of an ET tube. Those with tracheostomies are sometimes managed in step-down units outside an HDU/ITU facility. Ensure nursing and medical staff are trained in their use.
- **Oropharyngeal airway:** the Guedel is J-shaped and is passed between teeth into oropharynx. Usually rotated 180° from pointing up to pointing down during insertion over tongue. Often used when BVM ventilation being used. In a semi-comatose patient a nasopharyngeal airway is better tolerated.
- **Nasopharyngeal airway:** used in semi-comatose patient who is making satisfactory attempts at breathing. Can place patient in the recovery position with O_2 and a nasopharyngeal airway and monitor closely. The main contraindication is basal skull fracture (major trauma, CSF, coma, should be seen on CT). General advice is to choose the size of nasopharyngeal airway to match the width of the patient's little finger or nares. Average height females require a size 6 Portex and males a size 7. Lubricate the end with KY jelly. They go straight back into the nasal cavity and turn downward towards the posterior pharynx. Insert into largest nares. Attach a safety pin at the nose end to prevent further tube movement into airway.

2.8 Tracheostomy/laryngectomy emergencies

- **Discussion:** a tracheostomy is a tube inserted directly into the trachea through which the patient can breathe or be mechanically ventilated. Insertion is beyond this text; only ongoing management and emergencies are covered here. Tracheostomies relieve upper airway obstruction and provide airway protection. They enable weaning from mechanical ventilation, to allow long-term ventilation and to provide assistance in removing respiratory tract secretions. Early post-insertion complications include *haemorrhage, loss of the airway, blockage or complete or partial tracheostomy tube displacement*.
- **Long-term complications** include tracheomalacia, tracheal stenosis. The tube should be kept clean and secure. Key information is whether the patient has a patent upper airway, meaning that it is anatomically possible for the upper airway to connect to the trachea and thus allow ventilation by this route. *Those with a laryngectomy and stoma do not have a patent upper airway.* The following equipment should be immediately available for all patients with a tracheostomy *in situ*, regardless of which ward they are managed on. Self-inflating BVM, O_2 with face-masks (non-rebreathing type) and tracheostomy masks, working suction and suction catheters, intubation equipment (including bougie) and a range of endotracheal tubes, laryngeal mask airway (LMA) device, dilating tracheostomy forceps, spare tracheostomy inner-tube appropriate for tracheostomy in place (i.e. dedicated to the patient and their tracheostomy). Staff should be competent in management of tracheostomy and complications.
- **If unwell and hypoxic** then apply oxygen to face and mouth if patent upper airway. Laryngectomy patients have an end stoma and cannot be oxygenated via mouth or nose. All other patients should have oxygen applied to the face. Management of a blocked laryngectomy involves tracheal suction and intubation of the laryngeal stoma. Call arrest team and for anaesthetic support urgently if airway compromised. Assess patency, ABCDE approach as ever, consider passing suction catheter to see where blockage is and remove any debris.

References: National Tracheostomy Safety Project website, www.tracheostomy.org.uk/

2.9 Assessing and managing fluid balance

Being able to quickly assess hydration is fundamental to managing disease. Clinical context is important as well as clinical signs. Patients on a general ward can have very poorly recorded I/O charts. Weight is very useful especially if you have been recording them on the admission or previous admissions. A litre of water is 1 kg. Rapid changes in weight are usually losses or gains of water.

- **Dehydration:** sunken eyes, dry mouth and reduced skin turgor, complains of thirst. With time becomes obtunded. ↓BP, postural ↓BP, weak low volume pulse, ↑HR. Reduced body weight. ↓Urine output ↓urinary Na. ↑Hb, ↑urea more so than creatinine, hypernatraemia if free water loss. May be a cause e.g. vomiting, diarrhoea, obstructed fluid-filled bowel, polyuria, sweating, fistulae. CVP low. Fluid balance chart shows net loss (if accurate and all I/O recorded). Management is appropriate fluid replacement. Is it just water depletion or salt too and other electrolytes? Stop diuretics. Manage stomas or other losses.
- **Overhydration:** ↑JVP, gravitational dependent oedema, ascites, anasarca, breathless if CCF. Normal BP or hypertension, ↑HR if in CCF. Increased body weight. Normal/↑urine output and urine Na. Bloods normal unless pre-existing disease. Low Na possible. Evident cause e.g. ↑intake, liver/cardiac/renal failure/nephrotic syndrome. CVP raised. Fluid balance chart shows net gain (if accurate and all I/O recorded). Manage fluid restriction, diuretics. Match losses + 500 ml orally if possible.
- **Euvolaemic:** warm, well filled. BP and HR normal. Body weight unchanged. Normal urine output. Normal I/O. Bloods normal.

Assessment

- Examine for hypovolaemia. Seek help if still unsure (it can be difficult) about volume status especially when complex, e.g. where there is ongoing organ failure (e.g. cardiac/renal/liver) or sepsis, pyrexia and drains losing fluids.
- Examine the notes – cause of admission, past history, procedures? Examine the chart – drugs, observations, pyrexia, BP, HR, urine output, output of drains, all of which should be stored within the fluid balance chart. What has preceded the assessment? Surgery, new drugs given?
- Do not hang your diagnosis on one sign – the fluid balance chart may be badly completed, a ↑JVP might suggest RV infarction or a PE and a need for filling rather than overload, a CVP line may be blocked or erroneously measured, a BP might be recorded in an arm with atherosclerotic arteries and be misleadingly low so check other side. Healthy scepticism is always wise, especially when appearance of patient and signs don't match.
- Fluid losses may be hidden unless looked for, e.g. ascites and intestinal luminal or generalised oedema can contain significant fluid losses. During sepsis and inflammation increased fluid can be found in the interstitium and this depletes the circulating volume.
- Other ways to assess fluid balance is measuring urine output, which is a crude measure of renal perfusion. Oliguria/anuria where there is no evidence of post renal obstruction suggests renal water and sodium retention and even incipient AKI. Many resort to using the JVP but this is not without its limitations and potential complications and should be reserved for the patient on HDU/ITU.
- The physiological response to volume loss is the release of ADH and free water retention. There is sodium retention through the RAA mechanism. Stress/surgery and pain also cause cortisol and ADH release. The hypovolaemic patient is typically vasoconstricted with cold peripheries, mild ↑HR and dry mucous membranes, typically oliguric with a low urinary sodium.
- **Other losses:** the values here are very rough with wide variation and generally all prescriptions of IV fluids must take into account renal/cardiac function, latest blood results, fluid balance status, drugs prescribed.

Gastrointestinal losses

Fluid	Vol. (L/day)	Na (mmol/L)	K (mmol/L)	Cl (mmol/L)	HCO_3 (mmol/L)
Saliva	1–1.5	50	15	30	90
Gastric aspirate	1–2.5	60	10	140	0
Bile	0.5–1.0	200	10	50	40
Pancreatic juice	1–2	120	10	40	100
Small bowel secretions	2–3	140	10**	Variable	Variable

** ↑in inflammatory conditions.

Replacing losses

Situation	Choice of replacement (NS = 0.9% normal saline)
General GI losses	Replace with equivalent volumes of oral rehydration (if mild and able to drink) and/or IV NS, and treat cause
Significant diarrhoeal losses	These tend to contain significant amounts of K (e.g. 40 mmol/L) and so low K can occur which may well worsen any ileus and other problems. Potassium should be monitored and replaced with oral rehydration (if mild and able to drink) and/or IV NS with potassium, and treat cause
Fistulae and overactive ileostomies	Loss of chloride and bicarbonate – replace with oral rehydration (if mild and able to drink) and/or IV NS, and treat cause
Systemic sepsis with 3rd space losses	Replace with oral rehydration (if mild and able to drink) and/or IV NS, and treat cause
Pyrexia, sweating Insensible losses	Replace with oral rehydration (if mild and able to drink) and/or IV NS, and treat cause

Normal oral intake is best. Involve dietician if calorific or other needs identified. Ensure adequate access and able to hold beaker or use straw or other handheld devices. Good nursing/health care assistance if unable to swallow. Short term consider NG tube and longer term consider PEG tube placement. IV fluids only when above routes are unsatisfactory. If enteral replacement is not possible then IV fluids to consider are described below.

Choice of fluids

Fluid	Comments
5% GLUCOSE (G5)	Solution that uses glucose (sugar) as the solute to make it isotonic. Hypotonic once glucose (solute) metabolised by the body's cells. Used to replace free water loss, e.g. severe hypernatraemia secondary to diabetes insipidus. 1 L contains 50 g glucose.
0.9% NaCl (NS)	Crystalloid high in Na content. *First line for hypovolaemic shock.* Can cause a hyperchloraemic metabolic acidosis. Short half-life. Remains in the vascular space for only 15 min. In the UK the favoured choice of most physicians.
GLUCOSE– saline	A hybrid containing 0.18% NaCl (only one-fifth of the concentration of NS) and 4% GLUCOSE. Again it has a short half-life and remains in the vascular space for only minutes.
Hartmann's (lactated Ringer's)	Isotonic crystalloid solution containing NaCl, KCl, $CaCl_2$ and sodium lactate all dissolved in sterile water. *Indicated for shock.* Distributed equally throughout the extracellular space and is rapidly lost from the intravascular space. Favoured choice of anaesthetists. Contains a high level of Na (at 131 mmol/L) and little K (at 5 mmol/L), and there is a small amount of calcium (2 mmol/L). The 29 mmol/L of lactate may be helpful for buffering acidosis. It does have a lower Cl concentration than normal saline (111 mmol/L rather than 154 mmol/L).
Plasmalyte (PL148)	Similar to Hartmann's and is a 'balanced' crystalloid solution. It mimics human plasma in its content of electrolytes, osmolality and pH. Has buffer capacity with anions such as acetate, gluconate, and even lactate that are converted to bicarbonate, CO_2, and water. It can manage volume and electrolyte deficit and acidosis. Excess leads to fluid overload. Contains magnesium. Few studies on its use in trauma or hypovolaemic shock. No evidence that it is superior to other crystalloids for the prehospital management of traumatic hypovolaemia.
Gelofusine	Colloid formed from gelatin. Remains for longer within intravascular compartment. May cause histamine release and rash and bronchospasm. No evidence superior to crystalloids.

There has been much discussion about the relative merits of crystalloids versus colloids in critically ill patients. The use of 4% albumin appears to increase mortality, especially in trauma. There is no evidence that crystalloids are better or worse than colloids but crystalloids should be used first line. Crystalloids include 0.9% NaCl (abbreviated here as NS) or Hartmann's. First line in volume replacement and in fluid challenge. Normal saline solution can cause hyperchloraemic acidosis and there is possibly increased use of renal replacement therapy and AKI. There is evidence more for the use of balanced fluids such as Ringer's lactate particularly in septicaemic shock. There may be less metabolic acidosis with balanced crystalloids rather than normal saline solution. In some trials balanced crystalloids were associated with lower in-hospital mortality compared with normal saline solution. Other fluids used in volume replacement are: **colloid**, which contains starch-like substances (e.g. dextran or Gelofusine), **blood and blood products** which remain in the vascular space for longer – red cells have O_2-carrying capacity, platelets and white cells have additional important functions.

Fluid	Na mmol/L	K mmol/L	Cl mmol/L	Mg mmol/L	Ca mmol/L	Lactate mmol/L	Osmolality mOsm/L
0.9% saline (NS)	154	0	154	0	0	0	308
0.18% saline 4% glucose	30	0	30	0	0	0	284
0.45% saline 5% glucose	77	0	77	0	0	0	405
Gelofusine	154	0	154	0	0	0	274
Hartmann's	131	5	111	0	2	29	278
Plasmalyte 148	140	5	98	1.5	0	acetate 27	297
5% glucose (G5)	0	0	0	0	0	190 kcal/L	278

Osmosis: Water moves to dilute any solvent. If the interstitium and blood is hypertonic then water moves out of cells into the vascular space. If the blood is hypotonic it moves into cells and can cause cellular oedema and more worrying, cerebral oedema (Hyponatraemia ▶ Section 5.10).

2.10 Fluid replacement regimens

These are usually for people having no oral or enteral intake, such as those who are post-operative or comatose, e.g. stroke patients. They should only be used transiently and feeding issues should be contemplated, because there is no significant calorific intake here. When patients are perioperative and on IV fluids then electrolytes should be checked at least every 24–48 h, or more often if there is any abnormality or any additional factors or deterioration. Avoid excessive fluid replacement in those with cardiac failure or renal failure and take expert advice if unsure. In an uncomplicated average patient requiring fluid replacement, titrate Na, H_2O, and K added by weight, U&E result, recorded fluid balance input and output, clinical examination and co-morbidities.

Normal daily fluid and electrolyte requirements: 25–30 ml/kg/d water = 1 mmol/kg/day sodium, potassium, chloride, 50–100 g/day glucose (1 L 5% glucose = 50 g glucose). Reassess and monitor the patient. Stop IV fluids when no longer needed. Nasogastric fluids or enteral feeding are preferable when maintenance needs are more than 3 days.

NOTE: NS (0.9% Saline)and G5 (5% Glucose) are used as simple shorthand here but must be written out in full in clinical practice. Normal daily fluid and electrolyte requirements: 25–30 ml/kg/d water = 1 mmol/kg/day sodium, potassium, chloride, 50–100 g/day glucose (1 L 5% Glucose = 50 g glucose). Reassess and monitor the patient. Stop IV fluids when no longer needed. Nasogastric fluids or enteral feeding are preferable when maintenance needs are more than 3 days. Can be given as 1 N-Saline and 2 L 5% Glucose at rate of 1 L/10 hrs. Traditional 3 L/day may be excessive.

Potassium replacement

Normal needs 60–100 mmol/day. May be omitted or reduced in the first 1–2 days post-surgery or where there is significant trauma/burns/blood transfusions as tissue damage will release potassium. In those on potassium infusions check levels at least daily. Maintain between 3.5–5 mmol/L, (4–5 mmol/L on the CCU). Take advice if unsure. See hypokalaemia ▶ Section 5.4 or hyperkalaemia ▶ Section 5.3 if situation requires. Most potassium-containing fluids come prepared, e.g. with NS or G5. **Potassium must never be given quickly IV due to risks of cardiac arrest. Ward areas may give infusions of up to 10 mmol/h e.g. 40 mmol/L in 500–1000 ml over 4 h for severe hypokalaemia. Critical care areas can give 20 mmol/h with close ECG/K monitoring. All must be given by infusion pump and closely monitored.**

Venous access: choosing a venous cannula

Poiseuille showed that small increases in cannula diameter = large increases in flow. A pink Venflon is unsuitable to resuscitate a patient needing volume replacement. Ideally one or more grey 16G would be used. Flow rates can double if pressure on the bag of up to 300 mmHg is used. Flow is proportional to radius^4 (Poiseuille's law) so a small increase in radius can greatly improve flow and vice versa. Flow is inversely proportional to length and so central lines with long catheters impair flow and are inappropriate for rapid volume replacement. They also carry a higher risk of infection and complications than peripheral lines.

Colour and size	Flow (ml/min)	Time to infuse 1000 ml NS (min)	Uses
Yellow 24G			Paediatric
Blue 22G		22	Thin fragile veins
Pink 20G	50	15	IV drugs and IV fluids routine use
Green 18G	100	10	Blood transfusions and IV fluids. Rapid infusion needed insert 2 if possible or 16G/14G
Grey 16G	200	6	Rapid IV infusion, hypovolaemic shock, ruptured AAA, haemorrhagic shock
Brown or orange 14G	360	3.5	Rapid blood transfusion, PPH, ectopic pregnancy, AAA, haemorrhagic shock

Acid–base balance and blood gas interpretation

- **Introduction:** we are all net producers of acid, which is excreted both by the kidneys and by removing CO_2 from the lungs. To assess acid–base balance we can measure an ABG. Once primary respiratory cause excluded then VBG will give us pH and $[HCO_3^-]$ which may be enough. The pH is the product of renal and respiratory function and metabolic activity and buffering systems.

Normal ABG values (note 1 kPa = 7.6 mmHg)

- **pH 7.35–7.45** if >7.45 alkalosis, <7.35 acidosis, H^+ >45 nmol/L acidosis, H^+ <35 nmol/L alkalosis
- PCO_2 **35–45 mmHg (4.6–6 kPa)** PCO_2 >6.5 kPa and hypoxia = type 2 RF (▶Section 4.5)
- PO_2 **80–100 mmHg (11–13 kPa)** Hypoxia PO_2 <8 kPa respiratory failure (▶Section 4.5)
- SaO_2 **95–100% (BTS 94–98% acceptable, 88–92% if COAD)**
- HCO_3 **22–26 mmol:** changes here are slow and renally driven over hours or days. High [HCO_3] may suggest chronic Type 2 RF
- **Base deficit:** −2 to + 2 normal; <−5 metabolic acidosis; <−10 severely ill
- **Anion gap (AG):** (Na+K) − (Cl + HCO_2); normal <12 mmol/L

- **Interpretations of acid–base disturbances:** determine the primary derangement, e.g. CO_2 retention with respiratory failure or a low HCO_3 with high anion gap and methanol ingestion. The body will try to respond with secondary corrections. Secondary corrections: an abnormality in pH leads to compensatory changes. Acidosis is detected in brainstem (medulla) and peripheral chemoreceptors and leads to increased ventilation and the excretion of CO_2 from the lungs; this takes minutes. There is also bicarbonate retention in the kidneys; this takes hours to days.
- **Measure anion gap** (AG) which is [cations] − [anions] and is normally 12 +/− 2 mmol/L. An anion is a negatively charged ion such as phosphate, sulphate, organic acids or negatively charged proteins. Cations = [Na + K]; anions = [Cl + HCO]; some equations omit the small K contribution. Normally, measured [cations (+ve ions)] > [anions (−ve ions)], so there is a normally an 'anion gap'.
- **Osmolar:** rarely, you will need to measure the calculated and laboratory calculated osmolar gap when indicated – usually with a ↑anion gap metabolic acidosis.
- **Alveolar–arterial PO_2 gradient:** PAO_2–PaO_2. PAO_2 = (FiO_2 × (76−47) − (PaO_2/0.8). An increase suggests shunting. Normal = 4–10.
- **Base excess:** a calculated number (normal −2 to +2) the primary data is used to predict the pH in normal blood in the presence of the PCO_2 measured so if the PCO_2 ↑, then the predicted ↓pH, and vice versa. BE then calculates the amount of acid or base needed to change the predicted pH to the pH measured. This is the base deficit/excess. It is an estimate of 'metabolic' as opposed to 'respiratory' disturbance. A base excess <−2 indicates metabolic acidosis; a BE >+2 indicates metabolic alkalosis.
- **Pathophysiology:** the pH = −log [hydrogen ions]. pH varies from 1 (acidic) to 14 (highly alkaline), with neutrality being 7. Blood is alkaline with a pH of 7.35–7.45. Gastric acid pH = 1. Ketone bodies are water-soluble, fat-derived fuels that are used by many tissues for energy generation when there is limited glucose availability. The brain becomes especially dependent upon ketones for fuel when plasma glucose levels are inadequate. Henderson–Hasselbalch equation. Note PCO_2 dependent on lung function getting rid of CO_2. Hyperventilating lowers $PaCO_2$, hypoventilation leads to a rise in $PaCO_2$.
- **Interpretation:** (1) Look at pH; normal pH may be compensated. pH <7.35: acidosis; pH >7.45: alkalosis; (2) Look at PCO_2. PCO_2 >6.0 kPa: hypercarbia suggests type 2 RF PCO_2 <4.6 kPa: hyperventilation may be triggered by metabolic acidosis; (3) Look at HCO_3 22–26 mmol/L: normal. <22: met. acidosis. >26: met. alkalosis or renal compensation of a resp. acidosis (4) Look at anion gap if metabolic acidosis. If AG >12 mmol/L suggests increased acid production or failure to excrete it. AG 3–12 mmol/L – usually due to a loss of HCO_3 ions (balanced by increased Cl).

Typical blood gas abnormalities

Term	ABG	Causes and management
Met. acidosis with ↑anion gap	*Primary issue is* HCO_3 <22 mmol/L, pH <7.35, AG >12 mmol/L	**Clinical:** hyperventilation or Kussmaul breathing. **Causes:** AKI, lactic acidosis, diabetic or alcoholic ketoacidosis, methanol, CO, cyanide, metformin, paraldehyde, iron, ethylene glycol, salicylates. Measure osmolar gap to identify ethylene glycol, methanol, alcohol excess.
Met. acidosis with normal anion gap	*Primary issue is* HCO_3 <22 mmol/L, pH <7.35, AG <12 mmol/L	**Clinical:** hyperventilation/Kussmaul breathing. **Causes:** RTA, diarrhoea, small intestinal fistula, pancreatic alkali losses, carbonic anhydrase inhibitors, ureterenterostomy, rapid hydration with NaCl, Addison's disease.
Met. alkalosis	Primary issue is HCO_3 >28 mmol/L, pH >7.45, $PaCO_2$ normal	**Clinical:** paraesthesia, tetany. **Causes:** antacids, dialysis, milk-alkali syndrome, pyloric stenosis/gastric outlet obstruction with vomiting, Bartter's syndrome, adrenogenital syndromes, Cushing's syndrome, Conn's syndrome.
Resp. acidosis	*Primary issue is* PCO_2 >6 kPa, pH <7.35, normal or compensated rise HCO_3	**Clinical:** hypoventilating, drowsy, hypoxic. **Causes:** chest disease, e.g. asthma, COPD, airway obstruction, hypoventilation, respiratory nerve or muscle weakness.
Resp. alkalosis	*Primary issue is* $PaCO_2$ <4.7 kPa, pH >7.45, normal HCO_3	**Clinical:** paraesthesia, tetany. **Causes:** hyperventilation (anxiety), asthma, CCF, hypoxia, PE, ventilation/perfusion mismatch, aspirin/salicylate overdose.

2.13 Assessment of shocked patient

- **Definition:** shock is a clinical syndrome with generalised tissue hypoxia due to reduced O_2 delivery or increased extraction. It may be worsened by anaemia, reduced cardiac output, pyrexia, hypoxaemia. ↓BP can be the first sign of a serious acute illness, e.g. MI, sepsis, haemorrhage, Addison's, anaphylaxis.
- **Clinical syndrome:** pale, sweating, cold, clammy, confused, obtunded, ↑HR, ↓SBP <90 mmHg. Tachypnoea, oliguric, ↑JVP – cardiogenic shock, PE, RV failure, tamponade. Warm peripheries, bounding pulse, hypo- or hyperthermia, sepsis, rash, erythema.

Clinical severity assessment score

- **Class 1:** 10–15% blood volume loss. Physiological compensation and no clinical changes appear.
- **Class 2:** 15–30% blood volume loss. Partial compensation. Postural ↓SBP, generalised vasoconstriction, urine output <30 ml/h. Identify and treat to prevent progression.
- **Class 3:** 30–40% blood volume loss. Decompensating shock with ↓BP. HR >120, tachypnoea, urine output <20 ml/h, confused.
- **Class 4:** 40% blood volume loss. Marked ↓BP, ↑HR and tachypnoea. Anuria, comatose. Irreversible shock heading to multi-organ failure. Rapid intervention for any recovery.
- **Pathophysiology: in shock** O_2 extraction increases, but anaerobic lactic acidosis can occur. Sepsis causes release of bacteria and other molecules with vasodilatation. Increased cardiac output, capillary permeability and hypovolaemia. Reduced oxidative phosphorylation, ATP and cell pump dysfunction. Progressive downward spiral of multi-organ failure and death.

- **Findings:** mean arterial pressure: <60 mmHg and systolic BP <90 mmHg. Lactate: >4 mmol/L (elevated value correlates with high 28-day mortality). Cardiac output: <2.2 L/min/m^2 (except sepsis). Urinary catheter: oliguric unless polyuria state, e.g. HHS/ DKA.
- **Initial investigations:** FBC: Hb normal or ↓Hb if bleeding, ↑Hb if fluid loss alone, ↑WCC. U&E: AKI, dehydration, consider prerenal, renal, post-renal. Troponin: MI/sepsis. ↑D-dimer with DIC/DVT/PE non-specific, ↑lactate can guide severity. **Echocardiogram:** assess LV, valves, exclude pericardial fluid/blood collection or vegetations. **CXR:** widened mediastinum in dissection; cardiomegaly can suggest heart failure or pericardial effusion, look for consolidation, tension PTX, collapse, malignancy, oedema. 12-lead ECG: arrhythmias, ischaemia, infarction, electrolyte changes, cardiomyopathy. Sepsis screen: blood cultures, urinalysis, sputum, USS for fluid collection/liver abscess. **Arterial blood gases:** metabolic or respiratory acidosis, or both. AXR for acute abdomen, bowel obstruction or perforation suspected.
- **Supporting investigations: CTPA or V/Q scan:** exclude PE. CT may show lung and aortic pathology. **CT abdomen:** if suspected AAA, pancreatitis or suspected retroperitoneal bleeding or fluid collection or bowel obstruction or ischaemia. **Abdominal–pelvic USS:** renal obstruction, cholecystitis, jaundice, liver abscess or pelvic collection. **Coagulation screen:** DIC: ↓fibrinogen, platelets and ↑APTT ↑PT. **Invasive monitoring** such as CVP and pulmonary artery (capillary) wedge pressure (PAWP) can be useful when the type of shock is not clear, e.g. PE where PAWP is normal and ↑CVP, LVF where ↑PAWP and CVP normal or elevated and cardiac tamponade where PCWP and ↑CVP. **Urgent endoscopy:** for diagnosis and therapy of suspected upper GI bleed.

2.14 ▶ Immediate actions in a shocked patient

- **Immediately** (1) Get good IV access, e.g. ×2 antecubital fossa green/brown/grey Venflons, good access to monitoring, e.g. intra-arterial lines on HDU, O$_2$ to give sats 94–98%. Get ECG, CXR, send FBC/U&E/LFT/lactate and cultures and consider troponin and D-dimer. Cross-match if haemorrhage. If ↓BP and unsure if volume depleted give 250 ml NS IV over 5–10 min and see if HR and BP improves. (2) Get help if patient expiring, even summoning arrest team if periarrest. If no bleeding, inpatient, no MI on ECG then think PE or sepsis. But keep reviewing. You may rationally treat multiple aetiologies, e.g. sepsis and PE until the diagnosis is confirmed. (NS = 0.9% Saline and G5 = 5% Glucose).
- **Good venous access is key.** A grey Venflon (16) can give 1 L NS over 6 min and a brown or orange can give 1 L NS over 3.5 min – the lines of choice in volume loss. However, 2 green Venflons is far better than nothing and may be easier than a larger bore cannula in a shocked constricted patient. Central access takes time and flow is not great and is difficult in underfilled patients. The femoral vein is always worth trying and, short-term, can give good access. Once you get access ensure it is protected and not pulled out in the melee of sorting out a sick patient. If you are able to get a patient to an HDU/ITU setting and there is time then an arterial line should be considered, especially if there is a plan to use inotropes.

2.15 ▶ Quick review of different forms of shock

- **Cardiogenic shock** ▶ Section 2.16: impaired heart function. Get Echo/CXR: consider risk factors for ACS. 'Pump or valve failure', ACS, myocarditis, CMP, drug toxicity (calcium channel or beta-blocker overdose), VT, CHB, tachy/bradyarrhythmias, valve failure: acute MR, AR, MS, AS. **Clinical:** obtunded, cold peripheries, oliguria, postural ↓BP, dizziness, presyncope, drowsiness, confusion, ↑HR, rapid breathing (acidotic). CRT (press over nailbed for 5 s) abnormal if >2 s for pink colour to return.

Management: cautious fluid challenge, CXR to confirm pulmonary oedema, ECG useful ST/T wave changes, ↑troponin, ↑CK. STEMI needs urgent PCI/thrombolysis, consider inotropes, e.g. DOBUTAMINE, consider IABP, can BP tolerate nitrates/loop diuretics? Can I get an echo? Inferior MI and RV dysfunction may need volume loading. Get senior help quickly.

- **Obstructive shock:** obstructed atrial heart filling. Get Echo/CXR. **Causes:** pulmonary embolism, cardiac tamponade, tension PTX (▶Section 4.12), constrictive pericarditis. **Clinical:** as above ↑JVP. Muffled heart sounds with tamponade, hyper-resonant hemithorax, deviated trachea with tension PTX. Obvious DVT with PE. **Management:** get ABG. Dimer. Bedside Echo, CXR. 14 gauge IV cannula 2nd/3rd ICS for tension PTX and chest drain, LMWH and thrombolysis for PE. Pericardiocentesis for tamponade can be lifesaving. Give fluids.

- **Non-haemorrhagic hypovolaemic shock:** ▶Section 2.20: **causes:** water/fluid loss. non-haemorrhagic – cholera, DKA, HHS, pancreatitis, Addison's disease, diabetes insipidus, dehydration, over diuresis, severe vomiting and diarrhoea. **Clinical:** thirst, oliguria, fluid loss – severe urine or GI fluid loss (diarrhoea, vomiting), polyuria, loss into interstitium – anaphylaxis. **Management:** treat DKA/HHS/↑Ca. Treat diabetes insipidus. Oral/IV rehydration therapy for cholera or GI loss. Adrenal: IV HYDROCORTISONE 50–100 mg + start 1 L NS.

- **Haemorrhagic hypovolaemic shock:** ▶Section 2.22: **causes:** think AAA, GI bleed, retroperitoneal, obvious traumatic lesion, fractured pelvis, femur. **Clinical:** as above + sign of bleeding (internal/external), e.g. pulsatile bleeding, AAA, melena, Grey Turner, Cullen signs, thigh haematoma, psoas haematoma, ectopic pregnancy. **Management:** elevate legs, IV access, transfuse 2–4 U blood. O-negative if critical. Reverse coagulopathy – PCC (Beriplex/Octaplex) for warfarin. Fresh frozen plasma is often necessary with coagulopathy. Vitamin K. Praxbind for Dabigatran. Fluid resus. with NS. Leaking AAA: vascular urgent surgical consult for repair GI bleed: upper/lower endoscopic therapy or laparotomy. Bedside USS and beta-hCG if ectopic suspected and laparotomy.

- **Distributive sepsis, anaphylaxis:** ▶Sections 2.18 & 2.21. Fluid moves into extravascular space. **Clinical:** warm vasodilated peripheries, ↓BP, oliguria, ↑HR, confusion, rapid breathing (acidotic). DBP drops more quickly than SBP. Anaphylaxis (drug, transfusion, sting, nut allergy): flushed, wheeze, urticarial. Sepsis: meningococcal sepsis with purpura, retained tampon. **Management:** raised legs, IV fluids: NS. Sepsis: IV antibiotics + start 1 L NS and NORADRENALINE. Anaphylaxis: IM ADRENALINE + HYDROCORTISONE + IV fluids + nebs.

- **Neurogenic shock:** exclude sepsis and other causes first. **Causes:** vasodilation due to loss of sympathetic tone, rare. Usually in trauma setting. Spinal anaesthesia. **Clinical:** acute cord injury usually cervical. Paraparesis, ↓HR, warm dry skin, priapism, sensory level, vasodilation, hypoventilation. **Management:** consider volume and noradrenaline, isoprenaline or pacing for severe ↓HR, stabilise spine. Trauma team assessment.

2.16 Acute heart failure/cardiogenic shock

- **About:** perilous peri-arrest state needing rapid action and senior help. Mortality is 70%. A bedside echocardiogram confirms the diagnosis and possible aetiology. Acute heart failure and cardiogenic shock differ by degrees of cardiac dysfunction.
- **Aetiology:** failure of the LV leads to forward failure and failure to perfuse organs. Backward failure due to rise in LA pressure, PA pressure, and then CVP. Increased pressure moves fluid into the interstitium and alveoli. There is perfusion without oxygenation (V/Q mismatch) and so hypoxia. Mitral stenosis causes pulmonary oedema but LV function is normal. Chronic mitral regurgitation better tolerated as left atrium has dilated so lower LVEDP.

- **Diagnosis:** systolic and diastolic heart failure can coexist: severely impaired tissue perfusion and PCWP >18 mmHg. Cardiogenic shock when MAP <60 mmHg or SBP <90 mmHg. Systolic: reduced ejection fraction <0.4 or <40%. Diastolic: failure to fill non-compliant ventricle. Like trying to inflate a stiff balloon.

Causes of cardiogenic pulmonary oedema and shock

- **Acute coronary syndromes:** Chest pain and NSTEMI/STEMI with LV impairment due to Left Main stem or LAD disease or Acute MR. Check 12-lead ECG. If acute escalate for reperfusion with PPCI/thrombolysis which can cause instant improvement. Check troponin.
- **Pre-existing cardiac disease:** with new or fast AF, ischaemia or infarction, fluid overload, new medications (negative inotropes, NSAIDs).
- **Precipitants:** missed medications, e.g. diuretics, co-morbidities, pneumonia, excess alcohol, fluid overload, arrhythmias, ischaemia.
- **Cardiomyopathy or myocarditis:** possible potential recovery with supportive management.
- **Valve failure:** aortic stenosis (murmur fades when shocked), mitral stenosis (loud S1 and MDM and AF), severe aortic regurgitation (widening pulse pressure and loud EDM, endocarditis), severe mitral regurgitation (loud PSM, papillary muscle infarction or endocarditis).
- **Arrhythmias:** fast AF, VT, CHB reducing cardiac output.
- **Cardiac tamponade:** impaired diastolic filling reduces output. Needs echo and pericardiocentesis.
- **Hypertensive crisis:** rare but consider renal artery stenosis or phaeochromocytoma.
- **Neurogenic:** SAH, ICH, traumatic cord lesion.

Clinical

- BP usually normal or low <90/60 mmHg. Occasionally high – hypertensive crisis.
- Severe dyspnoea, cyanosed, agitated, low volume pulse with cold peripheries. Pink frothy sputum and haemoptysis, and dyspnoea, oliguria. Triple rhythm, S3, pulsus alternans, ↑HR, AF.
- Right heart failure: ↑JVP, dependent oedema, ascites, hepatomegaly.
- High output cardiac failure – AV fistula, Paget's disease is very rare nowadays.
- NYHA grading of breathlessness: I. No symptoms, II. Symptoms with moderate exercise. III. Symptoms with minimal exercise. IV. Symptoms at rest.

Investigations

- **FBC/U&E:** ↓Hb AKI/CKD. ↑LFTs ↑PT with severe liver congestion.
- **ABG:** type 1 RF, lactate >2.0 mmol/L.
- **Biomarker:** ↑Troponin, ↑CKMB: with NSTEMI/STEMI or myocarditis.
- **ECG:** arrhythmia, ↓voltage, ST↑ (STEMI consider PCI) ↓ST – NSTEMI/USA. New LBBB, true posterior MI. RBBB may suggest PE or ASD. Low voltage QRS tamponade.
- **CXR:** pulmonary oedema, cardiomegaly and increased upper lobe venous markings, bat wing oedema, Kerley B lines, bilateral pleural effusion.
- **BNP/NT-proBNP:** BNP >500 pg/ml or NT-proBNP >2000 pg/ml suggests heart failure. BNP <100 pg/ml makes heart failure unlikely. Levels correlate with impairment of left ventricular function.
- **Echocardiogram:** LV or RV dysfunction, assess valve integrity and exclude tamponade or VSD. Aortic stenosis severe if mean gradient >40 mmHg or area <1 cm^2.
- **Swan–Ganz:** may be attempted if diagnosis or management uncertain.
- **Cardiac catheterisation:** image coronary vessels looking for occluded vessel, culprit lesion, poor LV, severe AR, dilated root. Can perform angioplasty, stenting.

General management

- **Sit patient up. ABC O₂** if needed as per BTS guidance. Analgesia: DIAMORPHINE 2.5–5 mg or MORPHINE 5–10 mg IV + METOCLOPRAMIDE 10 mg IV antiemetic can relieve chest pain/dyspnoea. Treat any cause, e.g. cardiovert patient in sustained VT or Fast AF or PCI/lysis the STEMI, or balloon pump and cardiac surgery for the valve disease.
- **LOOP DIURETIC:** FUROSEMIDE 50–100 mg IV when SBP >110 mmHg. More modest doses of IV FUROSEMIDE venodilate and cause diuresis without further reducing the BP. BUMETANIDE 1–2 mg IV is an alternative.
- **NITRATES:** (do not use if low BP) give SL GTN 800 mcg (2 sprays) and then consider IV GTN if SBP >100 mmHg. Titrate to pain, breathlessness and BP.
- **HDU/CCU/ITU** bed with cardiac monitoring, physiological monitoring, urinary catheter. Venous/arterial line. Give O₂ as per BTS guidelines and reassess after ABG. May be a role for CVP line.
- **ACUTE CORONARY SYNDROME:** ▶ Section 3.8. If STEMI then reperfusion by PCI or thrombolysis can dramatically improve LV function.
- **SALBUTAMOL 2.5–5.0 mg** neb stat. and PRN if any bronchospasm. Can worsen ↑HR.
- **AMINOPHYLLINE 250 mg IV over 30 min loading dose** has been used but much less nowadays as concerns over arrhythmias. Consider only if significant element of bronchospasm.
- **Arrhythmias:** if in AF then consider loading with DIGOXIN or AMIODARONE via a large or central cannula. AMIODARONE for VT with SBP >90 mmHg, otherwise DC shock for any tachyarrhythmia and ↓BP or LVF.
- **Anticoagulate** with LMWH if patient in AF or LV thrombus.
- **Inotropes:** BP <90 mmHg. Consider low dose DOPAMINE 5–10 mcg/kg/min is usually first line. No evidence of benefit. Dopamine and dobutamine are the drugs of choice to improve cardiac contractility, with dopamine the preferred agent in patients with hypotension.

Specific additional issues

- **Severe hypertension:** manage with IV nitrates/IV diuretics.
- **Avoid drugs** which can worsen heart failure, e.g. calcium channel blockers such as verapamil, antiarrhythmics, NSAIDs, COX-2 inhibitors, steroids.
- **Ultrafiltration:** veno-venous isolated ultrafiltration can remove fluid but usually reserved for those unresponsive or resistant to diuretics or in severe renal failure.
- **Cardiac tamponade:** globular heart on CXR. Urgent bedside echo if available. Consider needle pericardiocentesis.
- **Hypovolaemia or RV failure or PE:** a fluid challenge may help with CVP monitoring if possible. Patients often feel better lying flat. Give 0.9% SALINE/Colloid 200 ml aliquots IV over 10–15 min and reassess HR and BP.
- **CPAP:** where available it can improve oxygenation. Start at 5 and increase as needed to 10–12 cmH₂O. Check ABG 30 min and 1 h post-CPAP. When changing pressure turn flow up in 2 cmH₂O steps at 2–3 min intervals over the first 10–15 min. CPAP can improve oxygenation but may compromise venous return.
- **Intubation and ventilation:** will reduce work of breathing and O₂ demand so mechanical ventilation should be considered.
- **Intra-aortic balloon pump (IABP):** 25–50 ml elongated helium-filled balloon inserted via the femoral artery and placed distal to the left subclavian artery, but proximal to the renal arteries. Balloon inflates with diastole and deflates with early systole. Improves cerebral and coronary perfusion and myocardial oxygenation in cardiogenic shock and acute LVF, refractory unstable angina and ischaemic

ventricular arrhythmias via the augmentation of the intrinsic 'Windkessel effect', whereby potential energy stored in the aortic root during systole is converted to kinetic energy with the elastic recoil of the aortic root. Most coronary perfusion is in diastole. **C/I:** significant aortic regurgitation, aortic arch aneurysm or suspected aortic dissection or severe peripheral vascular disease. It is thrombogenic and patients should be anticoagulated with heparin. Problems are suboptimal timing of inflation and deflation of the balloon produces haemodynamic instability. Timing should ensure balloon inflates as systolic pressures fall with a second pressure rise in diastole which then falls off presystole. The balloon can be set to assist every beat (1:1) or less often (1:2, 1:4, or 1:8). Adjust inflation and deflation timing both of which can be late or early. Oliguria may occur if the balloon lies too distal and occludes renal vessels. The balloon causes haemolysis. Never switch the balloon off while *in situ*.

- **Ventricular assist devices:** provide bridging cardiac support. Requires cardiopulmonary bypass. Various different types. Bridge to transplant or recovery or revascularisation.
- **VTE prophylaxis:** advocated because high risk of DVT/PE.

Stabilised heart failure

Maximise vasodilator therapy (ACE inhibitor/ARB) before increasing diuretic therapy.

- **ACE inhibitors,** e.g. RAMIPRIL 1.25 mg start lowest dose and titrate gradually up to full dose over several weeks + beta-blockers (once stable), e.g. carvedilol. In those with EF <40%, reduces the risk of hospitalisation and the risk of premature death. If ACE inhibitors not tolerated, usually due to cough, consider angiotensin II receptor blockers, e.g. candesartan. Monitor U&E for renal dysfunction and hyperkalaemia. Contraindicated in pregnancy and renal artery stenosis.
- **Diuretics:** FUROSEMIDE 40–80 mg OD or BUMETANIDE 1–2 mg OD ($\downarrow$K), often combined with aldosterone antagonists, should be considered in those who are breathless with minimal exertion and worse. Monitor U&E.
- **Thiazide:** METOLAZONE 5–10 mg OD is a particularly potent thiazide diuretic given orally, reserved for short periods for those with intractable volume overload. Given under close supervision.
- **Consider stopping:** Verapamil, Diltiazem, alpha-blockers, Class I antiarrhythmics, NSAIDs.
- **Angiotensin receptor antagonists:** usually for those who cannot tolerate ACE inhibitor. Consider titrating up the dose. Can cause $\uparrow$K. Monitor U&E.
- **Aldosterone antagonists: Spironolactone/Eplerenone:** in NYHA III/IV failure (symptoms at rest or minimal exercise). Can be added to conventional treatment including an ACE inhibitor/ARB (87%) and a beta-blocker (75%). Spironolactone can cause $\uparrow$K and worsening renal function. Eplerenone is a similar drug with proven benefits post-MI and in heart failure but with less gynaecomastia.
- **Beta-blockers:** e.g. **Carvedilol, Bisoprolol,** or **Metoprolol** have shown benefit in clinical trials. Start low and slowly titrate dose up. These should not be started until patient stable otherwise they can lead to worsening of condition. Nebivolol is recommended for stable mild–moderate heart failure in patients over 70 years old.
- **Ivabradine:** inhibits I_f channels in SAN. Consider to reduce the risk of hospitalization in patients in sinus rhythm with an EF <35%, a heart rate remaining >70/min, and persisting symptoms despite maximal standard treatment.
- **Hydralazine and oral nitrates** for those who do not tolerate ACE inhibitor/ARB.
- **Digoxin:** for those with heart failure and AF. Evidence that it reduces hospitalisations.
- **Non-pharmacological:** exercise rehabilitation programmes have been shown to improve functional capacity. Combine with salt restriction and weight loss and smoking cessation.

- **Revascularisation:** consider angiogram and revascularisation by PCI or CABG.
- **Automated implantable cardioverter–defibrillator** if at high risk for lethal arrhythmias.
- **Anticoagulation: Warfarin/direct oral anticoagulant** if in AF or thromboembolic event or cardioembolic source. Start LMWH and warfarinise. Role in dilated cardiomyopathy is debatable. Consider direct oral anticoagulants for non-valvular AF. Heart failure increases risk of stroke with AF.
- **Cardiac resynchronization therapy** indicated if LVEF <35%, sinus rhythm, LBBB with a QRS >150 ms, and NYHA functional Class II–IV on guideline-directed medical therapy.
- **Surgery:** CABG where appropriate, valve surgery (aortic or mitral valve repair or replacement) where appropriate, repair of LV aneurysms, ventricular assist devices mentioned above, transplantation is considered in end-stage cardiac failure in those suitable.
- **Hospitalised patients with anaemia and coronary heart disease** should have a trigger Hb of 70–80 g/L. No evidence for EPO-like agents or use of IV iron in this population (*Ann Intern Med* 2013;159:746).

Reference: European Society of Cardiology (2012) *ESC guidelines for the diagnosis and treatment of acute and chronic heart failure.*

2.17 Vasopressors and inotropes

- **Discussion:** patients presenting with cardiogenic and distributive and septic shock are managed with vasoactive drugs and inotropes. Inotropes are usually sympathomimetic agents that can affect heart rate (chronotropic), and heart contractile function (inotropic). Some may also have vasopressor effects to increase systemic vascular resistance (Noradrenaline, Adrenaline) and others may lower SVR, e.g. Dobutamine. Vasoactive agents and inotropes can improve physiological measurements, but there is no evidence that they improve outcome. They may cause harm. Vasopressors can change the systemic and pulmonary vascular resistance. This can alter flow to skin, muscles and other organ groups. In shock the emphasis is to maintain cerebral, coronary and renal perfusion, often at the cost of flow to skin and other less vital areas. Effects depend on the production of intracellular secondary messengers. Adrenergic receptors act through G proteins. It is suggested that multiple agents at low dose are preferable in cardiac disease. Vasopressin in low or moderate doses can spare catecholamines and inotropes are not generally indicated in end-stage heart failure. Usage of these IV inotropic and chronotropic agents is usually restricted to the ITU, CCU or HDU because these drugs need close and careful monitoring and adjusting, usually on the basis of invasive monitoring. Other physical methods to improve flow include **intra-aortic balloon pump**. These may be used in cardiogenic shock. Anti-shock suits are sometimes used pre-hospital in hypovolaemia.
- **Cardiogenic shock:** DOBUTAMINE low dose is an inotrope and is first line. DOPAMINE medium dose increases HR and is a positive inotrope but may increase O_2 demand. ADRENALINE and NORADRENALINE may help. MILRINONE/LEVOSIMENDAN WITH NORADRENALINE in those with RV dysfunction or elevated pulmonary resistance has been suggested and VASOPRESSIN if MAP remains < 65 mmHg. (*Rev Port Cardiol* 2016;35(12):681–695).
- **Septicaemic shock:** ensure adequate fluid replacement before using inotropes. NORADRENALINE to maintain MAP ≥65 mmHg following adequate volume replacement. DOPAMINE is second line. VASOPRESSIN may be considered for salvage therapy. HYDROCORTISONE for those who fail to respond.

2.18 Anaphylactic/anaphylactoid shock

- **About:** severe and potentially life threatening systemic reaction. Can occur in an acute and unexpected manner and can recur, so on-going monitoring for 6–12 h needed. Over 50% of the intravascular volume can shift to extravascular space.
- **Aetiology:** pre-current episode antigen exposure causes IgE antibody generation. Later re-exposure produces mast cell degranulation due to antigen cross-linking IgE-releasing histamine. Histamine activates receptors with massive release of cytokines and chemokines. Increases postcapillary venule permeability and fluid loss into interstitium. Oedema and low BP exacerbated by vascular smooth muscle relaxation. Release of vasoactive mediators causes laryngeal/pharyngeal/bronchial oedema or bronchospasm and/or ↓BP. Anaphylactoid reactions are identical but not IgE-mediated e.g. opiates, radiocontrast, NSAIDs.
- **Causative agents:** drugs (e.g. penicillin), radiological contrast media, insect bites/stings, eggs, fish, peanuts. Latex allergy (e.g. gloves, tourniquets, and sphygmomanometer cuffs). Consider if allergic reaction occurs during a medical or dental procedure. Blood products. IV immunoglobulin to those with selective IgA deficiency. NSAIDs, ACE inhibitor and Alteplase can cause angioedema/angioneurotic oedema. Aspiration of a hydatid cyst.
- **Clinical:** comes on over minutes with ↓BP, flushing, itching, and urticaria. Chest pain, ↑HR or ↓ HR, incontinence. Laryngeal oedema causing stridor and hoarseness, staccato cough. Wheeze and bronchoconstriction. Periorbital itching. Skin flushing, erythema. Urticaria (not seen with C1 esterase deficiency) or oedema. Abdominal pain, colic, diarrhoea and vomiting, angioedema. Facial swelling, lips, nasal itching, sneezing. Metallic taste in mouth, confusion.
- **Investigations:** FBC: increased WCC. Increased CRP if sepsis/malignancy/inflammatory cause considered. Mast cell tryptase: initial, after 1–2 h and 24h/follow up. Normally <1 ng/ml. Post-anaphylaxis >100 ng/ml. Normal levels do not exclude anaphylaxis and can be seen with food-induced allergy. ECG: SR, ↑HR, ST/T wave changes, new AF. Infection screen: blood/urine cultures. C1 esterase inhibitor deficiency is a rare cause of angioedema without urticaria. Check C4 and C1 inhibitor levels because treatment for this condition is different. Allergy testing: allergen skin testing; RAST identifies specific IgE.
- **Differential:** vasovagal syncope, sepsis, scombroidosis (high histamine in ingested fish), systemic mastocytosis (elevated tryptase), carcinoid syndrome (urine high HIAA). Panic attack, causes of syncope/presyncope, causes of breathlessness. Red man syndrome after IV vancomycin. Monosodium gluconate ingestion: skin warm and feels burning, headache, nausea, bronchospasm. No urticarial/angioedema or ↓BP.
- **Management:** remove cause: stop drug infusion, blood or blood product, remove bee sting. Lie patient flat with legs elevated: if symptoms + low BP. Get good IV access ×2 and start 1 L NS over 20–60 min and fluid replacement as needed to fill vascular space. **ABCs:** 15 L/min Oxygen reservoir mask if shocked as per BTS guidelines. Check ABG. Monitor BP, HR, SaO₂ and ECG. Crash Call Senior Anaesthetists and ENT (if stridor) for help if any concerns of airway obstruction and oedema or any stridor, severe bronchospasm or respiratory compromise. Give ADRENALINE 0.5 ml of 1/1000 (0.5 mg) IM into anterolateral thigh using a blue/green needle in adults if there are systemic signs – wheeze, stridor, respiratory distress, or shock. Also give HYDROCORTISONE 100–200 mg IV. SALBUTAMOL 2.5–5.0 mg Neb for wheeze and dyspnoea which may be repeated. CHLORPHENAMINE 10 mg slow IV/IM (H₁ blocker) and (H₂ blockade) RANITIDINE 50 mg IV over 5 min. Persisting bronchospasm AMINOPHYLLINE 250 mg IV over 20 min loading dose (if not on

theophyllines). Adrenaline reduces histamine release and causes cutaneous vasoconstriction (which can reduce absorption of the bee sting or other allergen). Repeat dose after 5–10 min if poor response. Do not give adrenaline subcutaneously. IM route post-thrombolysis is safer than IV and a muscle haematoma is unlikely to be significant with such a small volume but apply pressure over the injection site to help haemostasis. Benefits may be lifesaving. If still no improvement with airway oedema or bronchospasm and symptoms worsening consider anaesthetic review for intubation and mechanical ventilation, invasive monitoring and inotropes.

- **Second line:** GLUCAGON 2–10 mg slow IV in G5 (protect airway in case of vomiting), followed by IV infusion 50 mcg/kg/h for persisting ↓BP if patient is bradycardic on high dose of beta-blockers (bypasses β-adrenergic receptor and directly activates adenylyl cyclase). VASOPRESSIN when ↓BP not responsive to ADRENALINE.
- **Discharge and follow-up:** Monitor for 6–12 h post full recovery to ensure no late biphasic reactions. Continue PREDNISOLONE 40 mg PO OD for 3 days along with an antihistamine. Discharge with 2 EPIPENS each containing ADRENALINE 0.3 mg for IM usage with instructions on how to self-administer a dose. The second EPIPEN is in case one injector fails or patient needs a second dose. Teach to only use Epipen if anaphylaxis occurs with difficulty breathing or becoming faint. Give self-injection in the lateral thigh. It may be given through clothing, avoiding seams and pockets. Hold needle in place for 10 s to ensure the adrenaline dose has been delivered completely. Check the patient's injection technique regularly to ensure doing it correctly (there are self-teach videos on youtube.com). Long term patient should wear a medic-alert bracelet. All need referral to specialist for allergy clinic/immunology opinion and identification of cause and antigen avoidance. Skin testing is more rapidly obtained, cheaper and sensitive for allergy testing. Immunotherapy is useful in those with IgE-mediated disease.

2.19 Toxic shock syndrome

Otherwise healthy patients with rapid onset fever, rash, ↓BP, erythema, diarrhoea due to toxins from *Staphylococcus aureus* or *Streptococcus pyogenes*. Can cause organ failure, limb loss and death.

- **About:** toxic shock syndrome (TSS) is very rare but potentially fatal. Early signs may be subtle. Septic focus may be a minor skin trauma, post-surgical wound, or tampon or menses. Beware low BP, rash, erythema, fever and diarrhoea. Spot it and act quickly. Superantigens overstimulate B/T cells with cytokine storm.
- **Aetiology:** Staphylococcal toxic shock syndrome toxin 1 (TSST-1) acts as a super antigen and causes release of cytokines (TNF, interleukin-1, M protein and gamma interferon). Induces huge immune response and overstimulation of Th cells. Streptococcal: usually group A beta-haemolytic with high mortality. Due to Toxins A and B acting as super antigens. There may be evidence of soft tissue infection and necrosis, e.g. necrotising fasciitis or pneumonia or bacteraemia.
- **Clinical:** signs are initially subtle and then inexorable decline in healthy adult. Headache, high fever, nausea, vomiting, abdominal pain, severe muscle pain, tenderness. Profuse watery diarrhoea and erythroderma – more likely Staphylococcal. SBP <90 mmHg and increased HR and warm peripheries possibly. Vaginal examination for retained tampon or a simple infected wound. Later after 1–2 weeks: desquamation of the palms and soles. Seen in menstruation or postpartum, females using barrier contraceptives. Postoperative patients, varicella or herpes zoster infection. Patients with chemical or thermal burns.

- **Investigations:** FBC: ↑neutrophil, ↑WCC, thrombocytopenia. U&E: ↑urea/creatinine, ↑lactate, ↑CRP, ↑CK, ↑AST. LFT: low albumin, low calcium. Clotting: coagulopathy – ↑APTT but PT and fibrinogen normal unless DIC. Blood/urine/sputum dipstick and cultures. CXR: look for infection.
- **Complications:** AKI, rhabdomyolysis, acute liver failure, limb loss, circulatory collapse. DIC mortality is 5%.
- **Differentials:** severe Group A Strep. infections (scarlet fever, necrotising fasciitis, toxic shock-like syndrome), Kawasaki syndrome, Staphylococcal scalded skin syndrome, Rocky Mountain spotted fever, leptospirosis, meningococcaemia, Gram-negative sepsis, viral syndromes (e.g. measles, adenoviral infection, certain enterovirus infections, dengue), severe allergic drug reactions.
- **Management:** move to ITU bed (non-contagious). ABC: O₂ as per BTS guidelines. Invasive monitoring. Aggressive fluid resuscitation (5–10 L per day) with IV crystalloids and colloids due to the extreme ↓BP and diffuse capillary leak. Wound decontamination: drain or debride the lesion, remove foreign material, irrigate copiously. Recent surgical wounds should be explored and irrigated even when signs of inflammation are absent. Inotropes, e.g. DOPAMINE and/or NORADRENALINE may be needed when euvolaemic. Antibiotics: FLUCLOXACILLIN 2 g 6 h IV +/– CLINDAMYCIN 1.2 g 12 h IV. VANCOMYCIN 1–1.5 g 12 h IV may be needed. High dose IV Ig 400 mg/kg has been used for streptococcal TSS to neutralise super antigens and opsonise streptococci. Steroids: consider HYDROCORTISONE 50 mg IV 6 h in those with refractory shock despite adequate antimicrobial therapy and resuscitation.

Reference: see www.toxicshock.com.

2.20 Hypovolaemic shock

- **About:** primary water/salt loss. For blood loss see Haemorrhagic shock ▶Section 2.22.
- **Causes:** severe gastroenteritis, HHS, DKA, cholera, burns, over diuresis, diabetes insipidus: cranial or nephrogenic, high Ca, heat stroke, surgical drains and stomas losing excessive fluids which are unreplaced, Addison's disease, major burns, erythroderma.
- **Clinical:** assess state of hydration. Reduced skin turgor, cold, clammy, cold peripheries. ↑HR, postural ↓BP, obtunded, reduced capillary return. Oliguria, progressive confusion and coma.
- **Investigations:** FBC: Hb initially normal and may fall. APTT/PT: look for coagulopathy. U&E: ↑urea (GI bleed or AKI/CKD), ↑creatinine (AKI/CKD), ↑K if AKI or haemolysis. ABG: hypoxia ↓PO₂ <8 kPa, ↓HCO₃, ↑lactate >4.0 mmol/L. Others: calcium, cortisol and SynACTHen test.
- **Management:** (G5 = 5% Glucose, NS = 0.9% Saline) IV access (2 green/grey Venflons antecubital fossa), baseline bloods, urinary catheter, physiological monitoring. Look for and manage cause. Watch for AKI. Consider central venous line and HDU with monitoring. Give antibiotics immediately if sepsis is possible. Volume replacement rate depends on the clinical state, age, cardiac status, renal function and suspected deficit: 1 L (20 ml/kg) Crystalloid e.g. NS IV over 15–30 min depending on BP, then 1 L over 1 h and replace in response to clinical change. If there is concern over volume overload then consider 200 ml NS fluid challenges and reassessment. Replace electrolytes as needed. Ensure Hb >10 g/dl. Manage Na and K levels. Body weight can help manage fluid status. Determine if there is any steroid deficiency, e.g. Addison's disease, and give HYDROCORTISONE 100 mg IV and then IM 6 hourly if suspected as longer effect for steroid replacement. If there is diabetes insipidus investigate if either cranial or nephrogenic. Consider ADH (Vasopressin) if cranial diabetes insipidus.

2.21 Systemic inflammatory response syndrome/sepsis/ severe sepsis

Systemic inflammatory response syndrome (SIRS) ▸ sepsis ▸ severe sepsis ▸ death. This can happen over anything from hours to days.

- **Introduction:** care was changed with the RIVERS trial in 2001 [3] about early goal-directed therapy which was refuted by the recent ProCESS study in 2014 [2] showing no benefit with EGDT. However, all agree that early diagnosis of septic shock is essential. In ProCESS all had 2 L of fluid before being entered into trial. 75% had antibiotics prior to randomization. Prognosis much better than RIVERS. Further trials are ongoing.
- **Systemic inflammatory response syndrome (SIRS):** may be due to generic systemic response to infection, trauma, malignancy, inflammation. Severe infections can manifest as a systemic inflammatory response. Non-infective causes too such as inflammation, acute pancreatitis, severe trauma, ischaemia etc. Causes may be multiple, e.g. cholangitis + acute pancreatitis.
- **Clinical:** classically warm or cool peripheries, delirium, and be obtunded and agitated, deterioration can be rapid with rigors, fever or hypothermia, vomiting, diarrhoea. ↓BP <90/60 mmHg, ↓volume central pulse, purpura (meningococci), macular rash (toxic shock syndrome).

Diagnosis of sepsis-related syndromes

- **Systemic inflammatory response syndrome:** ≥2 of (1) WCC <4 × 10⁹/L or WCC >12 × 10⁹/L or WCC >10% immature neutrophils, (2) Core temp <36°C or >38°C (3) RR >20/min (4) PaCO₂ <4.3 kPa, (5) HR >90 bpm. These are not specific for infection. Clinical acumen should be used.
- **Sepsis** = SIRS + a presumed or confirmed infectious process.
- **Severe sepsis** = SIRS + evidence of organ dysfunction as shown by one or more of these: (1) unexplained/lactic acidosis, (2) CNS: obtunded, coma, (3) renal failure: creatinine >177 μmol/L, (4) urine output <0.5 ml/kg/h, (5) liver failure: bilirubin >34 μmol/L, (6) Plt <100 × 10⁹/L, INR >1.5, (7) respiratory: hypoxia, SpO₂ <90%, (8) CVS: cardiac failure, arrhythmias.
- **Septic shock** = severe sepsis + refractory SBP <90 mmHg despite fluid resuscitation and/or inotropes.

New sepsis 3 definitions (JAMA, 2016;315(8))

- **Sepsis is now defined as a 'life-threatening organ dysfunction due to a dysregulated host response to infection'.** Previous definition above was not infection specific. While recognition and treatment of the infectious trigger is important, attention is now focused on the host response and the related organ dysfunction. The key element of sepsis-induced organ dysfunction is defined by an acute change in total SOFA (Sepsis-related Organ Failure Assessment) score ≥2 points consequent to infection. A simple bedside score ('qSOFA', for quick SOFA) has been proposed, which incorporates ↓BP (SBP ≤100 mmHg), altered mental status and respiratory rate >22/min: the presence of at least 2 of these criteria strongly predicts the likelihood of poor outcome in out-of-ICU patients with clinical suspicion of sepsis. **Septic shock** is now defined as a subset of sepsis includes factors such as the need for vasopressors to obtain a MAP ≥65 mmHg and an increase in lactate concentration >2 mmol/L, despite adequate fluid resuscitation.
- **Pathophysiology:** infected causes induced by endo/exotoxins. Release of cytokines (TNF, IL-1, IL-6) and inducible NOS relaxes vascular smooth muscle and bradykinin. This is opposed by IL-4 and IL-10 which reduce TNF-alpha, IL-1, IL-6, and IL-8. Result is hypoxaemia, hypovolaemia, vasodilation and capillary leak. There is a fall in SVR with increased CO and SBP <90 mmHg and a fall in DBP and warm extremities

with a good capillary refill. Non-vital organs are hypoperfused at the expense of heart, kidneys, liver, and brain. With a severe insult the actual SIRS may lead to severe ↓BP and end-organ damage, a pro-coagulant state and eventually **multiple organ dysfunction syndrome** (MODS). Therapeutic regimens try to reverse this. Compounded by subcellular mitochondrial level dysfunction with reduced O_2 extraction, despite adequate supply, exacerbating tissue acidosis and production of lactate. Critically low perfusion of the gut is also key in the further downward spiral leading to multi-organ failure. Loss of integrity of the gut leads to the release of further cytokines and the entry of more organisms.

Clinical presentation may be masked in those who are on steroids or immunosuppressives. They may be more ill than they appear and this must be borne in mind in terms of escalating therapy for sepsis.

Infective screening in sepsis

- Have a logical system and work top to toe in symptoms and signs.
- **General:** malaise, fever, night sweats, weight loss give idea of onset.
- **Neurology:** meningitis, encephalitis, abscess, vasculitis. Get CT/MRI/LP.
- **Respiratory:** chest signs for cough, fever, pneumonia, empyema, TB.
- **Urinary:** renal angle tenderness, urinary symptoms. Urinalysis.
- **Hepatobiliary:** RUQ pain, jaundice, pale stools, positive Murphy's sign.
- **Peritonism:** appendicitis, paralytic ileus, abdominal.
- **Endocarditis:** new murmurs, stigmata, recent cardiac operations/interventions.
- **Dermatology:** abscesses, boils – check perineum, cellulitis, and burns.
- **Gynaecology:** pelvic pain, STI, retained tampons.
- **Foreign bodies:** new heart valves, catheter, central line, hip replacement.
- **Immunosuppression:** neutropenia, myelodysplasia, haematological malignancy, HIV.
- **Sore throat:** tonsillitis, peri-tonsillar abscess, Lemierre's syndrome, glandular fever.
- **Foreign travel:** viral illness (dengue, VHF), malaria, HIV conversion.
- **CNS infection:** headache, seizure, encephalopathy, focal signs, cold sores.
- **Joint pain/back/bone pain:** septic joint, prosthesis, osteomyelitis, brucellosis.

Clinical assessment for symptoms and signs of septic sources

- **Non-infectious causes of SIRS:** pancreatitis, liver failure and cirrhosis, bowel ischaemia, infarction or perforation, any major surgery (general or obstetric), trauma and tissue damage, malignancy, transfusion reaction, GI bleed/haemorrhagic shock, drug reaction, systemic vasculitis, myocardial infarction, skin reactions (TEN, SJS), seizures.
- **Potential complications of SIRS:** DIC (↓fibrinogen, ↑clotting times, ↓platelets), respiratory failure/ARDS (hypoxia), acute kidney injury, multi-organ failure, GI bleeding/stress ulcer, anaemia, coagulopathy, DVT and VTE, hyperglycaemia, electrolyte disturbances.
- **Final thoughts:** always ask about foreign travel. Malaria, dengue or viral haemorrhagic fever.

The top sepsis killers are *Neisseria meningitides* (meningitis/septicaemia), *Staph. aureus* (boils, endocarditis, bone, joint), *Strep. pneumoniae* (pneumonia, sepsis, meningitis) and *Strep. pyogenes* (cellulitis, pharyngitis). If these turn up on culture take urgent advice on treatment.

Investigations

- **FBC:** ↓Hb, WCC and platelets up or down with sepsis. ↑CRP/ESR. **↑Lactate** >4 mmol/L with sepsis. **↑Procalcitonin:** levels with bacterial infection. May be used to help diagnose bacterial infection and decide about starting or stopping antibiotic treatment. Variable availability. **ABG:** metabolic acidosis +/− respiratory failure.
- **Infection screen: blood cultures:** aerobic/anaerobic before antibiotics. 2 blood cultures from 2 sites 20 min apart. Where common skin contaminants may easily be interpreted as pathogens (such as patients with prosthetic heart valves) patients should have 3× blood cultures from different sites 20 min apart to help the interpretation of cultures that are positive for skin contaminants such as coagulase negative Staph. Ensure good skin decontamination and asepsis. **Urine:** urinalysis and culture. **Thick/thin blood films** if malaria suspected. **Faeces:** send for culture if diarrhoea. **Effusions:** diagnostic tap any pleural or ascitic fluid.
- **CT/MRI head + CSF:** LP if meningitis/encephalitis considered and safe.
- **Skin: take scrapings if any haemorrhagic lesions.** Swab any infected sites or infected lines or pressure sores or wounds.
- **Abdominal/pelvic USS/MRI/CT:** show infected fluid collections, liver, pelvic abscesses.
- **CXR:** pneumonia may show consolidation/effusion/empyema.

Sepsis six actions at a glance

- **Give 15 L/min O_2:** as per BTS (reduce if CO_2 retaining).
- **Take blood cultures:** 2 good quality blood cultures (not from the Venflon insertion) using strict asepsis within 45 min (aerobic and anaerobic bottles) before antimicrobial therapy. Consider respiratory tract, urinary tract, intra-abdominal, joint infection, CNS, endocarditis, line infection.
- **Start IV antibiotics:** e.g. TAZOCIN appropriate to likely cause.
- **Start IV fluid resuscitation:** administer 30 ml/kg crystalloid for ↓BP or lactate ≥4 mmol/L.

If still ↓BP apply vasopressors to get MAP ≥65 mmHg.

- **Check lactate level:** (also request FBC, U&E, LFT, clotting (INR and APTT) and glucose if not yet done) repeat later to see if improving. Other bloods: creat. >177, bili. >34, Plt <100, INR >1.5, urine output <0.5 ml/kg/h, SpO₂ less than 90% suggest poor outcome and get expert help. Transfuse red cells if haematocrit <30%.
- **Monitor urine output/h:** consider catheter. Dip urine and send MSU/CSU.

Reference: www.survivingsepsis.org.

Management

- **ABC:** give 15 L/min high FiO_2 if shocked as per BTS guidelines. Consider ITU/HDU admission if severe sepsis, i.e. before patient is shocked. Involve clinical outreach. Severity: lactate >4 mmol/L and base deficit of −5 to −10 being moderately severe and −10 or worse suggests severely ill. **Intubation and ventilation:** reduces work of breathing and helps oxygenation and is appropriate in selected patients.
- **Circulation:** establish IV access. CVP line if really needed (concerns regarding overfilling/cardiac failure). HDU intra-arterial BP monitoring if possible. Watch FBC, U&E, lactate and ABG. Transfusion to get Hct >30%. Closely monitor urine output (catheterization also excludes post-renal obstruction if AKI).
- **Those with signs of hypoperfusion (low BP, lactate >4 mmol/L) should receive** 30 ml/kg of IV Crystalloid (NS or Hartmann's solution or Ringer's lactate) in first 3 h (approximately 2 L in a 70 kg adult). Repeated 250 ml saline boluses titrated to response. The typical patient may need 4–6 L of fluid in total within 24 h. Repeated assessment is key. Among critically ill adults with sepsis, resuscitation with balanced fluids, e.g. Ringer's lactate, has been associated with a lower risk of in-hospital mortality and is probably the fluid of choice. A trial comparing crystalloids is needed.

- **Treat infection:** take blood cultures before antibiotics with strict asepsis. Avoid taking as part of cannula insertion which is notoriously unreliable with false positives. Then **antibiotics must be given within 1 h of arrival** when an infected aetiology is suspected. These can be stopped if a non-infective aetiology becomes apparent. The markers above are sensitive but non-specific. If no allergy and renal function normal then consider TAZOCIN 4.5 g 4–6 h IV +/− GENTAMICIN 5 mg/kg IV if hospital-acquired. If penicillin-allergic then give MEROPENEM 8 h IV. Consider VANCOMYCIN 1–1.5 g 12 h IV for MRSA. Consider CEFTRIAXONE 1–2 g 12 h IV for suspected meningococcal infection. If MRSA considered then IV VANCOMYCIN. Delayed administration increases mortality. Haematological malignancies: consider IV antifungal agents. Combination therapy (at least two classes of antibiotics to cover a known or suspected pathogen) for patients with septic shock. Combination therapy should not routinely be used for patients without shock.
- **Blood transfusion:** consider blood transfusion if Hb less than 7 g/dL or actively bleeding or myocardial ischaemia. Transfusion at a higher Hb if there are other co-morbidities. Target 7.0–9.0 g/dL. Give platelets if count is <10 000/mm³ or <20 000/mm³ with bleeding.
- **Surgical consult and management:** if abscesses or pus collections or necrotising fasciitis or acute abdomen or suspected perforation or intra-abdominal sepsis. Consider TAZOCIN 4.5 g 8 h IV.
- **Inotropes/vasopressors:** use vasopressors for ↓BP not responding to fluid resuscitation to aim for a mean arterial pressure >65 mmHg. Aim for a CVP >8 mmHg and central venous O_2 saturation (SvO_2) >70%, or mixed venous O_2 saturation (SvO_2) >65%. Consider NORADRENALINE +/− ADRENALINE. Noradrenaline is the first choice for patients who need vasopressors. Vasopressin or Adrenaline can be added. For patients who remain unstable, dobutamine is recommended.
- **Steroids:** HYDROCORTISONE 50 mg IV 6 h in those with refractory shock which has not responded within 1 h of antimicrobial therapy and fluid and inotropic resuscitation.
- **Non-infective SIRS:** cause and management is usually apparent. Fluids, oxygenation, critical care monitoring and focused therapies and interventions are key.
- **Blood glucose:** target blood glucose level 4.0–8.2 mmol/L. Consider a VRIII if hyperglycaemia. Avoid hypoglycaemia.
- **Human activated C protein** was previously advocated in selected severe sepsis cases in ITU. *In vivo* activated protein C (APC) has antithrombotic, antifibrinolytic and anti-inflammatory properties, and its use has been discontinued.
- **Other considerations: in all patients ensure:** analgesia, nutrition (oral or NG preferable), pressure care.
- **Sodium bicarbonate** should not be used for most patients with pH ≥7.15.
- **VTE prophylaxis:** is important.
- **Stress ulcer prophylaxis:** with PPI or RANITIDINE 150 mg BD.

Multiorgan dysfunction due to severe sepsis

- **Pulmonary:** acute lung injury and ARDS.
- **Cardiac:** myocardial dysfunction but vasodilation; drop in peripheral resistance causes increased cardiac output.
- **GI tract:** breakdown in normal mucosal integrity. The large surface area for nutritional uptake becomes a large area for entry of bacteria from the gut lumen. The liver is overwhelmed and is also dysfunctional. Systemic entry of toxins and bacteria to the pulmonary and systemic circulations. Develop ileus, pancreatitis, ischaemic colitis and acalculous pancreatitis and GI haemorrhage.
- **Renal/hepatic:** AKI, and progressive kidney and liver failure.
- **Neurological:** progressive coma.

References: [1] Identifying sepsis early: www.scottishintensivecare.org.uk/education/ise.pdf. Surviving Sepsis Campaign Guidelines 2012: www.survivingsepsis.org. [2] ProCESS trial. *N Engl J Med* 2014;370:1683. [3] Rivers, E. *N Engl J Med* 2001;345:1368.

2.22 Haemorrhagic shock

> With acute traumatic blood loss aim for an SBP >80 mmHg or palpable radial pulse or cerebration. Give small boluses of 250 ml of fluid crystalloid and TRANEXAMIC ACID and reassess.

- **Introduction:** trauma is the commonest cause of young deaths worldwide after HIV/AIDS. Death is usually due to brain injury or exsanguination. The current strategy is that of *damage control resuscitation* (DCR) with concepts such as *permissive hypovolaemia*. Reduced administration of crystalloid has seen a reduction in mortality. Crystalloids and colloids increase BP, dilute clotting factors, destabilise formed clots and lead to further bleeding. They have no significant O_2 carrying capacity. In reducing initial fluid challenge there is a balance in allowing on-going tissue hypoperfusion but maintaining haemostasis and clot control.
- **Major haemorrhage is defined as loss requiring a >2–4 unit transfusion.** Young patients can often cope with loss with physiological reserve and can look better than expected. They can then suddenly decompensate. These patients must be identified early so that appropriate fluid strategies are applied. BP is usually the physiological parameter that defines shock, but cardiac output is also important and determines tissue O_2 delivery. A normal BP may simply be a product of ↑SVR with a ↓CO (remember BP = CO × PR). A bleeding patient with signs of shock already has a significant blood loss.

Sources of bleeding

- **'Bleeders come first':** in a bleeding patient check FBC and clotting profile and treat any coagulopathy/significant thrombocytopenia. The immediate risks of bleeding in a shocked patient override thrombotic risks even in those with prosthetic metal heart valves or previous PE. Take haematological advice if needed.
- **Trauma:** needs trauma management and direct compression and control of bleeding points (further explanation is beyond the scope of this text). Retroperitoneal, long bone and pelvic fractures, haemothorax. Splenic.
- **Ruptured spleen:** abdominal trauma. Increased risk with splenomegaly or glandular fever. Requires urgent laparotomy. Urgent USS or CT abdomen.
- **Abdominal aortic aneurysm:** pulsatile expansile mass + abdominal or back pain. Needs urgent resuscitation and vascular referral and laparotomy. If clinical suspicion high then surgery may proceed on clinical suspicion alone. Otherwise urgent USS or CT abdomen.
- **Upper GI bleed:** ▶ Section 6.4. Is it variceal or non-variceal bleeding? If patient is moribund then it becomes a potential surgical issue and laparotomy is needed to arrest bleeding. May be a delay in melena appearing.
- **Ectopic pregnancy:** fertile female, abdominal pain, missed period, positive β-hCG. Needs urgent surgery.
- **Retroperitoneal bleeding:** palpable mass in abdomen, pelvis, bruising round umbilicus or flanks. Can be seen especially if anticoagulated. Urgent USS or CT abdomen. Reverse anticoagulation.
- **Cryptic shock** is found in those with normal BP and pulse despite significant blood loss. Blood pressure is also directly related to blood loss. Where there is brain injury a higher SBP >90 mmHg is advocated. Avoid a coagulopathy and ensure haemostasis maintained using a ratio of 1 FFP to 1–2 units packed cells from the start. Platelets also given. Consider giving fibrinogen. TRANEXAMIC ACID 1 g IV over 10 min

then TRANEXAMIC ACID 1 g 8 h slow IV reduces clot breakdown, shown to reduce mortality if commenced <3 h of injury.

Reference: Harris T, *et al*. Early fluid resuscitation in severe trauma. *BMJ*, 2012; 345:e5752.

2.23 Massive transfusion protocol

- Massive haemorrhage and resuscitation can result in a refractory coagulopathy. Trauma patients do better if given blood components and transfused early. Give red cells, FFP, cryoprecipitate and platelets as Trauma or Shock Packs in those with massive bleeding, such as those with surgical or medical life-threatening haemorrhage needing over 10–20 units of RBCs in 24 h. Surgical control of haemorrhage with volume resuscitation using fluids and blood components is needed. Once bleeding controlled, a restrictive approach to blood product transfusion is preferred because of the risks and negative outcomes of transfusion such as multiple organ failure, systemic inflammatory response syndrome, TRALI, increased infection, and increased mortality. Increased ratios of plasma and platelets to RBCs and their timely administration are thought to improve outcome in trauma, decrease coagulopathy and transfusion requirements based on retrospective data. Large volumes of plasma are required to correct coagulopathy, so early administration is best and may limit consumptive coagulopathy and thrombocytopenia, and the need for blood and blood products. Limiting the use of isotonic crystalloid will avoid a dilutional coagulopathy. Limiting the use of 0.9% SALINE IV may prevent further acidosis. Evidence is growing for use of point of care coagulation testing to guide haemostatic therapy. Standard coagulation tests such as PT, APTT, INR, platelet count, and fibrinogen usually require 30–60 min for results to be available. For massive transfusion patients requiring acute interventions, results of standard coagulation tests may not be an accurate reflection of coagulation function. Measurement of platelet count and fibrinogen only provides absolute amounts, not functional activity and may overestimate the levels.

- **Resuscitation targets:** hypotensive resuscitation (aim for SBP 80–100 mmHg) until haemorrhage is controlled. If there is concern for traumatic brain injury then higher SBP acceptable. Monitor base deficit and lactate levels to assess adequacy of resuscitation. Correct electrolytes, e.g. high K from large volume of RBCs, low Ca from citrated anticoagulants, and Na and Cl abnormalities from crystalloid resuscitation. Aim for Hb 7–9 g/dL, PT and APTT within normal range (APTT/INR >1.5 give 4 FFP). Aim for platelet count >80×10⁹/L (<30 give 2 units platelets, <80 give 1 unit platelets). Aim for fibrinogen level >1 g/L (<1 g/L then 2 cryoprecipitate). Give 10–20 ml 10% CALCIUM GLUCONATE by slow IV injection if low ionised calcium level.

- **Additional notes:** maintain/achieve normothermia. Avoid/correct acidaemia. Avoid/treat ↓Ca. In obstetric haemorrhage FFP use may be delayed because patients are hypercoagulable. Use forced air warmers and rapid infusion devices where indicated. Warfarin reversal: give VITAMIN K 10 mg slow IV and Prothrombin Complex Concentrates (Octaplex/Beriplex). ↓Platelets or dysfunction or on antiplatelets consider giving additional platelets – take haematology advice. Heparin: heparin has short half-life and protamine causes significant ↓BP. Consider protamine with care and reluctance – it may have some effect with LMWH. Give PROTAMINE IV slowly. Direct oral anticoagulants: Factor Xa inhibitors (e.g. rivaroxaban, apixaban) can be reversed with Prothrombin Complex concentrate. Seek advice from haematologist. Dabigatran (Pradaxa) can be reversed with Idarucizumab (PRAXBIND).

- **Bleeding and prosthetic heart valves:** worst case scenario is a metal mitral ball and cage valve (aortic and newer tilting-disc valves lower risk) which has an annual risk of thromboembolism of 30% if anticoagulation is stopped. Other valves have a much lower incidence, possibly 12% per annum, of thromboembolism. In patients with potentially life threatening acute bleeds, anticoagulation must be stopped temporarily/completely reversed as the risk of death by exsanguination will be significantly higher. In ischaemic stroke the advice from national guidelines for patients with metal valves is to switch to antiplatelets for a week and then restart anticoagulation. For those with haemorrhagic stroke the risks need to be finely balanced but again anticoagulation should be reversed completely acutely for at least 1–2 weeks.

Massive transfusion protocol (MTP) (follow local guidance)

- **Establish good IV access ×2.** Give blood products through warmer. ABC. High flow O_2, 1 L NS initially over 10–20 min unless pulmonary oedema. Send cross-match and bloods. Constantly reassess fluid balance and status. Repeat bloods (FBC, PT, APTT, fibrinogen, U&E, calcium) every 30 min.
- **Consider if immediate surgery indicated to stop bleeding.** Try to focus management on assessment and cause as well as replacement. Liaise with laboratory to ensure packs arrive as needed.
- **Contact blood bank** with patient name, gender, DOB or approximate age and hospital number if known, location. Give brief clinical details, on warfarin, heparin, DOAC, pregnant or not.
- **Bleeding:** TRANEXAMIC ACID 1 g IV over 10 min + 1 g slow IV 8 h. VITAMIN K 5–10 mg IV +/– PCC (Octaplex or Beriplex) if on warfarin. PRAXBIND for Dabigatran. 4 factor PCC for other DOACs until specific drugs become available.
- **Blood bank should send: Shock pack 1:** (4 U uncrossmatched O RhD negative red cells). **Shock pack 2:** (6 U red cells, 4 FFP, 1–2 platelets + 1 cryoprecipitate). Send bloods. **Shock pack 3** (6 U red cells, 2 FFP, 1–2 platelets + 1 cryoprecipitate). Send bloods.
- Discuss with haematology about recombinant Factor VIIa/fibrinogen concentrate.
- **Continue as clinically indicated.** Reassess situation constantly and if MTP ceases at any time then tell switchboard to stand down. Continue with further shock packs until stand down. Identify specific cause of shock and determine any specific remedies.

03 Cardiology emergencies

3.1 Anatomy and physiology

- **Heart:** The heart is a 4 chamber muscular pump forcing blood around parallel pulmonary and systemic circulations. The direction of flow from atria to ventricles to aortic and pulmonary arteries is controlled by valves which allow only one-way flow. Size is that of a clenched fist enveloped in a layer of fibrous pericardium within the pericardial sac. It is suspended by the major vessels. It lies between the lungs and behind the sternum. Inferiorly the surface is formed by the right ventricle and left ventricle and part of the right atrium posteriorly. The inferior surface is in contact with the diaphragm. Posteriorly lies the base of the heart formed by the left atrium in close contact with the descending aorta and oesophagus. The two atria act as storage vessels for blood returning to the heart. The two ventricles act as pumps. On the left side the left atrium receives oxygenated blood from the lungs from the four pulmonary veins. The left atrium and left ventricle are separated by the semilunar mitral valve. The mitral valve has anterior and posterior leaflets. The left ventricle pumps blood into the systemic circulation and has a thick muscular wall. On the right side the right atrium receives deoxygenated blood from the systemic circulation from the inferior and superior vena cava. The right atrium and ventricle are separated by the tricuspid valve, which has three leaflets. Blood is ejected with systole across the pulmonary valve into the pulmonary artery. Right-sided pressures are low and the RV is thin walled compared with the left. The right border of the heart is formed almost entirely by the right atrium. The left border of the heart is formed almost entirely by the left ventricle with the left atrial appendage superiorly. The base or posterior surface is formed almost entirely by the left atrium which is closely opposed to the oesophagus (important for transoesophageal echo). Inferior or diaphragmatic surface of the heart is made up by the right and left atrium.

- **Coronary arteries:** Left coronary artery: arises from the left aortic sinus. It forms the left main stem and branches almost immediately into the left anterior descending (LAD) artery which travels between RV and LV towards the apex and the circumflex. Left anterior descending (LAD) (anterior intraventricular): the LAD gives off the diagonal branches (D1), diagonal branches (D2) and septal branches. Supplies anterior 2/3rd of IV septum and a major portion of left ventricular walls. Circumflex artery (CX), which lies in the left AV groove between the LA and LV, supplies the vessels of the lateral wall of the left ventricle. CX gives off the posterior descending artery (PDA) (10% of patients have a left dominant circulation in which the CX also supplies) and the obtuse marginal branches. Right coronary artery is the first branch of the aorta and arises from the anterior aortic sinus and runs in the AV groove between RA and RV. It gives off the acute marginal branch which runs along the margin of the RV above the diaphragm, Sinus node branch in 60% (otherwise supplied by the CX) and AV node branch and continues as the posterior descending artery (RCA dominant) in over 65% which supplies the inferior wall of the LV and inferior part of the septum. Blood flow in coronary arteries is maximal during diastole when the ventricle relaxes and oxygen extraction is near maximal so increased demand requires increased flow so any significantly partially obstructive lesion (>70%) will cause ischaemia. Slowing the heart lengthens diastole which aids coronary perfusion. Devices such as intra-aortic balloon pumps improve coronary perfusion.

- **Physiology:** Cardiac output (CO) is about 5 L/min. CO = stroke volume × heart rate. In the normal heart ventricular performance measured as CO depends on adequate stretching of the myocytes and appropriate LV filling. In heart failure excess filling cannot be accommodated. Contractility of the heart measured as that fraction ejected from LV per systole and is normally >60%. The ability to move blood also depends on afterload made up of systemic vascular resistance (SVR). Blood pressure (BP) = CO × SVR. SVR is maintained by vasoconstrictors, e.g. angiotensin II and aldosterone. Mean arterial BP = (SBP−DBP)/3 + DBP.

- **Answering bleep:** What are the patient's observations? If inpatient, why in hospital? What is the EWS, are they comfortable, distressed, breathless, ↓BP, tachycardic, hypoxic as all need instant attention. Get IV access, bloods and give O_2. If IHD then give GTN (400–800 mcg) 2 sprays sublingual or equivalent unless SBP <110 mmHg. ECG to be done immediately and attend. Telemetry especially if HR <60 or >100. Look for arrhythmia. If peri-arrest then consider arrest team. On arrival think life-threatening causes – quick examination. Ensure defibrillator is to hand in case of unstable tachyarrhythmias.

3.2 Chest pain assessment

- **Note:** the immediate killers are acute MI, aortic dissection, tension PTX and PE. Acute diagnosis and management of these must be your first concern. Always look at ECG and check troponin if suspicious. Recent warning to consider ACS in younger patients with a history of Kawasaki disease who may have large coronary artery aneurysms.
- **Cardiac:** ACS pain is central and heavy radiating to arms or jaw, but may be atypical even pleuritic or chest wall tenderness. Silent in diabetics and elderly. Elderly may present as a fall or confusion. Patient may be pale, sweaty and terrified looking with a large STEMI.
- **Aorta:** could this be an aortic dissection? History of HTN, tearing pain into back. BP disparity in arms. The lower BP arm has a compromised ipsilateral subclavian. Unfolded aorta on CXR, aortic regurgitation. If so, need urgent CT aorta and avoid any anticoagulants.
- **Lungs:** pain more likely to be pleuritic. Significant risk factors for PE + hypoxia or signs of DVT. Signs of chest infection, pain pleuritic? Get a CXR to exclude PTX and consolidation or rib fracture. May need CTPA.
- **Oesophagus:** has patient had an oesophageal stricture dilated or any procedure? Oesophageal perforation. GORD symptoms, oesophagitis.
- **Chest wall:** sternal fracture, rib fractures, Bornholm's disease.
- **Chest pain killers:** PE, tension PTX, ACS, tamponade, aortic dissection, and ruptured oesophagus.

Who to admit (NICE 2015): chest pain and admission?

- Clinical features suggest a potentially life-threatening cause of chest pain, such as ACS, PE, dissection, oesophageal rupture, PTX, etc.
- RR >30 breaths/min, HR >130 bpm, SBP <90 mmHg, or DBP <60 mmHg (unless this is normal for them), O_2 sats <92%, or central cyanosis (if the person has no history of chronic hypoxia). Altered level of consciousness, Temp >38.5°C.
- Suspected ACS who have current chest pain, have signs of complications (such as pulmonary oedema), pain-free now, but have had chest pain in the last 12 h and have an abnormal electrocardiogram (ECG) or an ECG is not available (see Management while awaiting admission).

Management

- **Support:** O_2 (BTS guidelines). Get IV access. Bed rest, telemetry. Ensure access to defibrillation. Consider causes and exclude ACS.

- **Check 12-lead ECG:** ST elevation and STEMI or new LBBB: cardiology consult for primary PCI/thrombolysis. Non-specific ST/T changes suggest NSTEMI. Saddle-shaped ST elevation throughout all leads except aVr, suggests pericarditis. In PE, ↑HR and S1Q3T3 may be seen but often non-specific.
- **Check FBC, U&E, troponin and D-dimer** (if indicated). Dimer not needed if high probability of PE. Doing dimers without any PE risk assessment is not recommended. Note that Troponin may be elevated in aortic dissection, PE and myocarditis.
- **Check ABG** if breathless or low saturations. Arrange CXR and look for oedema, mediastinal widening, consolidation, PTX, fibrosis, or apical shadowing or mass.
- If pain considered cardiac give sublingual **2 sprays of GTN (800 mcg) or GTN 500 mcg tablet SL** if SBP >110 mmHg and reassess. If pain is severe then give DIAMORPHINE **2.5–5 mg IV or MORPHINE 5–10 mg IV** with an antiemetic, usually METOCLOPRAMIDE 10 mg slow IV.
- If ACS possible, then consider **ASPIRIN 300 mg PO** and follow local guidance, which should be for PPCI if there is a STEMI; for further Management see *Section 11.2*. If aortic dissection then avoid anticoagulation and arrange CT chest ▶ *Section 3.17*. If PE considered and no contraindication then anticoagulate; ▶ *Section 4.17*.

3.3 Chest pain differentials

- **Acute coronary syndrome:** Central heavy chest pain with radiation into arms/jaw. Risk factors: smoker, HTN, lipids, diabetes. Sweating, distressed, pale. Immediate ECG is diagnostic. ECG shows STEMI then primary PCI or thrombolysis if primary PCI not possible. ▶ *Section 11.2*. Treat pain with glyceryl trinitrate (GTN) and/or an opioid (for example IV Diamorphine 2.5–5.0 mg, given slowly over 5 min). Give aspirin 300 mg (unless clear evidence that allergic). Do a 12-lead ECG. NOTE: palpable chest wall tenderness is reported in some cases of ACS and is not a reliable sign to exclude ACS. ▶ *Section 3.8*.
- **Aortic dissection:** History of HTN. Widened mediastinum on CXR. Hypertensive but appears 'shocked'. BP different in arms. Inferior MI on ECG if right coronary artery obstructed at ostia (left main stem obstruction usually fatal). Get urgent CT aortogram or TOE. BP lowering. Proximal lesion move now to cardiothoracic centre for surgery. Treat pain. Avoid ACS management. Lower BP and ▶ *Section 3.17*.
- **Pulmonary embolism:** Clinical context: immobility, cancer, stroke. Sudden pain plus breathlessness. Sometimes with syncope and dyspnoea. Collapse in toilet. Obvious increased RR. Hypoxic ABG. Fall in saturations. Look for risk factors. Look for DVT. Anticoagulate, consider thrombolysis with RV dysfunction or circulatory collapse. IV fluids support RV dysfunction. Needs CTPA/VQ scan. ▶ *Section 4.17*.
- **Pneumothorax:** Sudden breathlessness and chest pain may be seen. Clicking sound heard on auscultation, hyper-resonant, CXR diagnostic but can be subtle. If tension the person's condition is life-threatening: Consider inserting a large-bore cannula through the second intercostal space in the mid-clavicular line, on the side of the PTX, ▶ *Section 4.12*.
- **Pneumonia:** Unwell, toxic, feverish with pyrexia, pleuritic pain, ↑WCC, CXR changes. ▶ *Section 4.14*.
- **Oesophageal spasm:** Central chest pain lasting a few minutes. Can be very intense. Related to eating/drinking. Benign.
- **Oesophagitis:** Food related, reflux symptoms, eased by antacids. History of GORD. Obese.
- **Oesophageal perforation/rupture:** Boerhaave syndrome. Severe chest pain following oesophageal instrumentation or forceful vomiting. Toxic sick patient. Do not pass NG tubes or endoscopy. NBM. IV fluids. Urgent CXR/CT and thoracic surgical discussion.

- **Costochondritis** (Tietze's syndrome): Tenderness over costochondral joints, classically the second costochondral joint. Note that chest wall tenderness can be seen with ACS pain too. Treat with NSAID and determine if there is a physical cause.
- **Chest wall pain/musculoskeletal:** Look for localised defined tenderness. X-ray for fractures of ribs and sternum. May be trauma related. Also consider bone metastases. Check ALP/X-ray. Consider NSAIDs.
- **Takotsubo cardiomyopathy:** Indistinguishable from ACS. Older females classically, chest pain and dyspnoea, palpitations, N&V, syncope, and, rarely, cardiogenic shock have been reported. Reversible. See Cardiomyopathy, ▶ Section 3.23.
- **Acute sickling crisis:** Known sickle cell disease. May be hypoxic with pleuritic type pain. ▶ Section 8.5.
- **Pericarditis:** Younger patient. Possibly viral or recent MI and Dressler's syndrome. Eased by sitting forwards, audible rub, saddle shaped ST elevation. Treat with NSAIDs/Colchicine, ▶ Section 3.19.
- **Shingles:** May be unilateral dermatomal distribution, chest wall pain before the distinctive band of vesicles. Elderly, Immunocompromised.
- **Kawasaki disease:** Young person with chest pain and myocardial ischaemia and an ACS. History of KD with large often calcified coronary artery aneurysms which can thrombose. Take specialist advice.
- **Idiopathic:** Despite investigations cause unknown. Main need is to exclude sinister causes. Manage residual pain with analgesia.
- **Pleurisy/pneumonia:** Can be secondary to infection – viral or bacterial and underlying lung consolidation or possible connective tissue disease, neoplastic or idiopathic. Always consider if the history matches a possible PE and pulmonary infarction. Listen for a pleural rub. Check FBC, ESR, CXR. Consider autoantibodies if suggestion of RA or SLE. Non-sinister causes are managed conservatively with NSAID analgesia. ▶ Section 4.14.

3.4 Palpitations

Red flags to consider admitting to CCU or getting cardiology consult: Palpitations preceding syncope, palpitations with exercise, associated chest pain or dizziness, family history of arrhythmic death, structural heart disease, HCM, poor LV function, abnormal ECG – LBBB, ischaemia, LVH, long QTc, VT, TdP, 2nd/3rd degree heart block.

- **Assessment:** if they use the term find out their definition of "palpitations". Medically it is abnormal awareness of heart beat. Ask patient to tap out the palpitations if possible. How fast and how regular, how frequent. When started. Determine clinical context. Duration. Any obvious precipitants or relieving factors. Caffeine taken, other drugs, e.g. alcohol, cocaine. Antihistamines and other drugs that can alter QTc. Was there any associated dyspnoea, presyncope, polyuria, chest pain or other symptoms? How did it stop – slowly or suddenly? If they can provoke it please attempt it during ECG monitoring. If they have palpitations now then get an ECG or at least feel pulse. A normal pulse and symptoms is reassuring. Some just more aware of normal heart beat.
- **Causes:** if SVT occurs treat it and send home. The commonest marker for a lethal arrhythmia such as VT is the known presence of heart disease, a family history, an episode of syncope or presyncope or other associated symptoms; these patients are 'higher risk' and may need admission or more comprehensive management. Poor LV function. Take expert advice.
- **Investigations:** FBC, U&E, troponin, TFT, 24 h to 7 day tape as available and depending on the frequency of the arrhythmia and likelihood of capture. Patient

should hopefully have an episode with tape on. Infrequent episodes may need a cardio memo device implanted. Advise not to drive. During spell can ask to attend ED for an ECG which may be diagnostic.

- **Risk assessment:** patients must always be assessed in the context of risks for and presence of structural heart disease or abnormal ECG or family history of sudden cardiac death as these are 'higher risk' and may need admission or more comprehensive investigations; speak to cardiology if unsure. Avoid admitting benign ectopics and supraventricular arrhythmias who, once managed acutely, can be given advice and followed up in clinic.
- **Extrasystoles:** atrial and ventricular ectopics cause a strong beat after the compensatory pause which is felt. Treatment not needed if out of the context of ACS or signs of structural heart disease can be reassured and discharged, reduce caffeine. Manage precipitants. Rarely needs treatment. May consider cardiology or ambulatory care; follow up. If severe consider METOPROLOL 25 mg OD or ATENOLOL 25 mg OD as needed. ▶Section 3.11.
- **SVT (AVRT/AVNRT):** often seen in patients. Need to be managed acutely and can be discharged for cardiology follow up for consideration of meds/ablation. Discuss any WPW with cardiologists. Admit WPW and AF. ▶Section 3.14.
- **AF:** if AF is detected then rate/rhythm control and assessment of anticoagulation are needed as outpatient unless compromised and other issues. Take advice. ▶Section 3.16.
- **VT:** admit and assess. See treatment algorithm elsewhere, ▶Sections 3.12–3.13.
- **2nd/3rd degree HB:** admitting – may need pacemaker and stop any rate-slowing drugs. ▶Section 3.15.
- **Pauses:** any pauses >3 sec gets a pacemaker so admit. Lesser degrees may need admitted if history of pre/syncope for monitoring.

3.5   Syncope and transient loss of consciousness (TLOC)

- **Introduction:** Syncope is defined as a sudden transient loss of consciousness and postural tone with spontaneous recovery. Transient loss of consciousness leads to a fall if the patient is upright and unsupported. However, not all falls are due to TLOC and are dealt with elsewhere (Simple falls ▶Section 17.2). Always consider PE, arrhythmias fast and slow, aortic stenosis/HOCM, autonomic dysfunction. Differential includes causes of transient hypotension as well as neurological diagnoses. Transient syncope suggests a global CNS issue such as an episode of cerebral hypoperfusion, a generalised seizure, acute hydrocephalus and others. Some causes remain unknown and are best labelled as a 'funny turn'. This leaves the opportunity for making the correct diagnosis later.
- **Normal physiology of standing:** Standing requires prompt physiological adaptation to gravity. There is an instantaneous descent of about 500 ml of blood from the thorax to the lower abdomen, buttocks, and legs. There can be up to a 25% shift of plasma volume out of the vasculature and into the interstitial tissue, which reduces venous return to the heart. The result is a transient decline in both arterial pressure and cardiac filling. This has the effect of reducing the pressure on the baroreceptors, triggering a compensatory sympathetic mediated increase in heart rate and systemic vasoconstriction. The assumption of upright posture results in a 10–20 bpm increase in heart rate, a negligible change in systolic blood pressure, and approximately 5 mmHg increase in diastolic blood pressure. With age, diuretics, vasodilators, dehydration and any transient obstructive element there is much more likelihood of a simple transient failure of cerebral perfusion pressure. Following gravity to the floor quickly restores cerebral perfusion.
- **Discussion:** Feeling as if about to faint or buzzing ears or vision blurring and constricting, suggests a ↓BP cause with reduced cerebral flow. Bruising to the

face or other injury may suggest severe and sudden loss of consciousness with no time for protective reflexes. Try to get the history from patient and a witness of the episode even if you need to ring them. Was there chest pain, headache (SAH) or breathlessness before? What position – standing, sitting, lying? Doing what – coughing, micturition, and exertion? What was head position – looking up? Patient getting out of a hot bath or standing up in church. Did patient use GTN? Grey colour suggests faint and ↓BP. Vasovagal usually recover quickly. What was BP/pulse in ambulance notes? Vasovagal syncope common and often exacerbated by antihypertensives/antianginals. How long until regain of consciousness – before or after ambulance? Is patient pregnant – a very common cause of fainting. Not all that jerks is a potential seizure. Momentary cerebral hypoperfusion in vasovagal syncope can cause jerks lasting 5–10 sec. Urinary incontinence also seen with vasovagal syncope. Determine real level of consciousness – ask witness if patient was 'like a dead person' and one often finds that an 'unconscious' patient was not so and was even communicating to the witness throughout. Truly syncopal patients will usually go to ground unless held up or supported in some way. Sitting is an active process and patients will fall out of a chair or slump on a sofa. Those who are unable to go to ground to restore perfusion (even simple vasovagals) can end up with more severe presentation with fitting and hypoxic brain injury. Give driving advice. In the UK it is the doctor's responsibility to advise a patient with a potentially recurring cause of syncope not to drive and document it. Take senior advice where unsure. It is the patient's responsibility to inform the DVLA.

- **Secondary trauma:** Exclude ICH, SDH and ruptured spleens and fractures. Non-displaced hip fracture may be missed and so not all will have classical leg shortening and external rotation. Repeated examination may be needed. Pain may not be noted until attempts to mobilise. Initial trauma surveys can miss things so have a low threshold to repeat examination and imaging if there is evidence or suspicion of possible problems. Do not get distracted by the secondary trauma and forget about the primary cause of syncope.

- **Post-syncope clues:** Headache, drowsiness, rapid recovery over minutes (vasovagal), gradual recovery over several hours (seizure). Breathless (PE), weakness (stroke/seizure), abdominal pain (leaking AAA), sore tongue (seizure – bites side of tongue).

- **Note:** The difficulty is often in separating causes of reduced cerebral perfusion and seizure. Potentially malignant causes of reduced cerebral perfusion are rare but need urgent cardiological specialist assessment.

3.6 Differentials of syncope/transient loss of consciousness (TLOC)

- **Acute coronary syndrome:** A potential cause of syncope (elderly and diabetics may not have chest pain). ECG will show ST/T wave changes, ST elevation, CHB, other forms of heart block, LBBB, RBBB, hemiblocks, VT, etc. Paramedics may capture a non-sustained VT, or heart block, or ischaemic changes, or the cause was 'pump failure' and poor LV or even RV. Beware the rush to diagnosing ACS and starting antithrombotics in simple collapses unless there is chest pain and ACS-type ECG changes, or a definite ischaemic arrhythmia. Without these most do not have ACS but may have had head trauma/SAH or hip trauma on falling and they will bleed and develop ICH/SDH, etc. If unclear wait for early troponin. ▶ Section 3.8.

- **Arrhythmia:** Brady- and tachyarrhythmias can cause syncope/presyncope and falls. Ensure ECG checked and any ambulance recordings reviewed. Particularly interested in sinus pauses >3 sec, CHB and VT, non-sustained VT, and ECG evidence of conduction tissue disease. Rarely, but importantly, ECG changes of Brugada syndrome, e.g. RBBB or HCM or RV dysplasia, long QT syndromes precipitating VT, WPW syndrome with short PR and delta wave and SVT or AF,

- ACS, high/low K^+. A 12-lead ECG is mandatory. Most malignant arrhythmias are due to IHD/cardiomyopathy and associated with poor LV function. Ask about chest pain or palpitations prior. If you suspect an arrhythmia then keep for at least 24–48 h of telemetry, Echo and OP 7-day tape and cardiology consult. If there are sufficient concerns (family history of sudden death, poor LV function, Brugada syndrome or cardiac arrest) then patient stays until decision made, e.g. some may need **AICD** insertion. May need 7-day tape or reveal device. If there is conduction disease or ↓HR look to see if it is drug-induced (e.g. beta-blockers, verapamil) and discuss if sufficient evidence for pacemaker with cardiologist. No driving until resolved and DVLA referral. ▶ Section 3.10.
- **Cardiac structural:** Look for murmurs of obstructive lesions (which may disappear with very severe AS and low CO): aortic stenosis severe if mean gradient >40 mmHg or area <1 cm², HCM, mitral stenosis or atrial myxoma, tamponade. Get an Echo and ECG, telemetry and cardiology consult.
- **Pregnancy:** A cause of ↓BP and predisposition to fainting. Always consider in fertile female. Rarely ectopic pregnancy can present with collapse and abdominal pain and shock.
- **Respiratory:** Pulmonary embolism, cough syncope, severe pulmonary hypertension.
- **Vasovagal syncope:** Very common. Vasodepressor (BP falls), cardio-inhibitory (HR falls). Get ECG, consider tilt table if repeated episodes despite simple measures and cause not apparent. Lying/sitting and standing BP. Review medications – GTN spray? Are they hypovolaemic from diuretics? Consider cough syncope, micturition syncope, syncope during/after large meal +/– alcohol. Fasting, fear, heat. Note twitching and jerks and urinary incontinence may be seen and can be misdiagnosed as epilepsy. For a reliable diagnosis look for the 3 'P's – provocation (pain, fright, etc.), prodromal (dimmed vision and hearing for a few seconds) and posture (when standing). If diagnosis is quite clear then driving is allowed, otherwise DVLA referral.
- **Postural hypotension:** Precipitated by dehydration, hypovolaemia, pigmentation (consider Addison's disease), autonomic dysfunction (e.g. diabetes, multiple systems atrophy, amyloid), Parkinson's disease. Check medications for antihypertensives, nitrates, GTN spray, calcium antagonists, levodopa, tricyclic antidepressants, phenothiazine. Telemetry, ECG, look for and stop unneeded drugs. Orthostatic ↓BP can be proven with tilt table.
- **Postural orthostatic tachycardia syndrome (POTS):** Mostly in young females. Orthostatic tachycardia but not hypotension. Complain of symptoms of ↑HR >130 bpm, exercise intolerance, presyncope, disabling fatigue, headache and mental clouding. Heart rate increase ≥30 bpm with prolonged standing, elevated upright plasma noradrenaline, and a low blood volume. Needs tilt table, Echo. Ensure good hydration. Water intake ++. Increase sodium intake – NaCl tablets 1 g/tablet TID with meals. Exercise, propranolol, verapamil, ivabradine, sinus node ablation/modification may be used.
- **Carotid sinus hypersensitivity:** Pressure on neck causes syncope. Tight collars, shaving, head turning. Consider CSM whilst monitored. Looking for symptomatic pauses >3 sec. May need pacemaker. It may be wise to get a doppler before CSM as bilateral internal carotid stenosis can cause syncope and mimic hypersensitivity especially if recent TIA or stroke. CSM should be done 10 sec each side with cardiac monitoring and done when supine and standing.
- **Hypoglycaemia:** A diabetic on insulin or oral hypoglycaemic agents or Addison's disease or insulinoma. Recovered with glucose.
- **Subarachnoid haemorrhage:** worst ever/thunderclap headache and collapse and recovery. Needs CT/LP. ▶ Section 11.23.
- **Pulmonary embolism:** Breathlessness and collapse, ↑HR, hypoxia. Elevated D-dimer. DVT. Risk factors. Consider treatment dose LMWH prior to CT–PA/VQ scan. Mechanism may be a saddle embolus which disintegrates quickly. ▶ Section 4.17.

- **Complex seizure:** Loss of consciousness, tongue biting especially side, slow to wake up, known epilepsy, incontinent, headache after. Get a CT head acutely. No driving and DVLA referral. Seizure advice. Referral to first fit clinic. ▶ Section 11.16.
- **Aortic dissection:** Tearing interscapular/chest pain plus syncope. Consider diagnosis. CXR, CT aorta/chest. ↑ D-dimers. ▶ Section 3.17.
- **Occult haemorrhage:** GI where melena delayed, leaking AAA but pain usually. Hidden bleeding, e.g. retroperitoneal, psoas muscle particularly in those on warfarin. Coagulopathy. PV bleed in pregnancy. Patient ↓BP and syncopal. ▶ Section 2.22.
- **Autonomic dysfunction:** Autonomic dysfunction seen with Guillain–Barré syndrome, acute porphyria or transverse myelitis, amyloid and diabetes and rarer causes. Lose ability to sweat, and suffer bowel and bladder dysfunctions. Bloating, N&V, and abdominal pain and impotence. Constipation will alternate with diarrhoea. HR will be at a fixed rate of 40–50 bpm with inappropriate response. Pupils dilated and poorly reactive to light.
- **Addisonian crisis:** Occasional subtle presentation with syncopal episodes. Systemic ↓BP, pigmentation, ↓Na, autoimmune disease. Some may have had recent abrupt cessation of steroids. Check U&E, cortisol. Short synACTHen test. Give IV HYDROCORTISONE 100 mg ▶ Section 5.1.
- **Colloid cyst:** CT brain generally diagnostic shows a cyst in IIIrd ventricle. Syncope is due to abrupt rises in ICP.
- **Subclavian steal:** Arm movement or exercise precipitates syncope or posterior circulation symptoms. MRA image subclavians to see any stenosis.
- **Somnolescence:** Patients simply falling asleep. Consider sleep apnoea. Epworth sleepiness scale: >10 suggest excessive sleepiness. Sleep studies. Alcohol, sedation, smoking, large neck (obstructive).
- **Pacemaker dysfunction:** Any concerns get check. Pacemaker interrogated and reprogrammed if needed. Often pacing activity only kicks in when needed so absence of activity does not always mean dysfunction.

- **Answering referral:** How is the patient now? BP, HR, pulse, glucose. Unresponsive, no breaths – call arrest team. Are they protecting airway especially if GCS <9. Any injury sustained? Describe the events of syncope – ↓BP, chest pain, breathlessness, confusion (see above).
- **On arrival and thoughts:** The history and witness report are key. Anything sounding like a seizure or cardiac syncope, must advise no driving until full assessment and later discussion. Look for any sign of structural cardiac disease. Run through typical causes. General and cardiovascular and neurological exam. Main worry is malignant arrhythmias and alarm bells should ring if ECG abnormal, history of ACS or poor LV function or long QT syndrome, family history or Brugada. If concerned admit under cardiology and place on CCU for telemetry. Arrange CT head if any concerns of acute seizure, SAH, colloid cyst or any other cause of syncope. Assess any obvious secondary injury. Has there been a hip or other fracture? Is there head or scalp injury? Is intracerebral haemorrhage the cause of the syncope or the result of it? Refer accordingly. Always give driving advice to drivers post-syncope. If unsure acutely of cause and happy to discharge for expectant management then reasonable to advise not to drive until all results back and then you can make an assessment or suggest referral to DVLA. Very definite vasovagal syncope in the standing position is unlikely to occur whilst driving. Eliminate any precipitant. If there is a convincing vasovagal syncope story with precipitant and rapid recovery, limit any causes or precipitants and consider discharge.

Managing symptomatic postural hypotension

- Stop/reduce antihypertensives. Stop/reduce drugs that may lower BP if possible.
- Identify cause – may be a systemic autonomic neuropathy or part of a neurodegenerative illness or neuropathy or amyloid.
- Echo, tilt table, 24-h tape, EST – exaggerated increase in HR with POTS and mild exercise.
- Head up tilt on bed, compression stockings, salt loading.
- Drugs: FLUDROCORTISONE 100 mcg od, MIDODRINE 2.5–10 mg tds (alpha 1 agonist), beta-blockers, PAROXETINE 10–20 mg od.
- PPM: for cardioinhibitory syncope disease and bradyarrhythmias. Pauses >3 sec.

Focused investigations on likely causality

- FBC, U&E, LFT. Short synACTHen, TFT, troponin, D-dimer.
- 12-lead ECG: measure QT, 24-h tape, 7-day tape: NSVT, sinus node disease, bradycardia.
- External loop: if syncope > one attack per week.
- Internal loop: infrequent attacks, useful, expensive.
- ECG with carotid sinus massage: consider in elderly but get ultrasound to exclude severe atheroma which could result in syncope or stroke.
- Tilt table testing for cardio-inhibitory/vasodepressor syncope/POTS: often fails to guide therapy.
- CT brain, MRI brain, LP for SAH, EEG for epilepsy.
- Echocardiogram, electrophysiological studies, cardiac MRI.
- Genetic testing for rare disorder: Brugada, congenital long QT.
- Electrophysiological studies: limited usefulness without IHD or structural disease.

Some guidance on whom to admit, monitor and investigate

- Syncope when supine or exercising, associated palpitations, family history of sudden cardiac death.
- Non-sustained VT, bifascicular block, RBBB + LAFB or RBBB + LPFB, HR <50 bpm.
- QRS >120 msec, long or short QT, pre-excited QRS, RBBB with ST elevation V1–V3 with Brugada.
- Features of ARVC, severe anaemia, electrolyte disturbance.

3.7 ▶ Sudden cardiac death

- **About:** most sudden cardiac deaths (SCDs) are arrhythmogenic and due to ACS/IHD and without early defibrillation (internal or otherwise) survival is poor. Other rare causes are shown below. Divide into those with a normal heart on imaging (echo/MRI/angio) and those without.
- **Management:** if likely acute ACS then see below. Try to determine aetiology. Risk assessment. Echocardiogram. Genetic studies in some. Electrophysiological studies. Selected groups require consideration for an **AICD**. Higher risk: poor LV <35%, cardiac arrest (VF/VT) post-MI especially post-acute phase, family history of sudden cardiac death, inducible VT at EPS, dilated cardiomyopathy.

SCD + macroscopically normal heart

- **Brugada syndrome:** idiopathic VF. 20% of SCD in structurally normal hearts, sudden unexpected nocturnal death (SUND) in SE Asian men, "Coved" ST elevation in V1–V3. ECG changes may be dynamic and concealed. Placing V1 / V2 in the 2nd rather than 4th space can help detect changes. Minority have sodium channel defect. Only **AICD** has been proven to help. May have self-terminating VT/VF, waking up at night after agonal respiration. Drugs used to unmask disease include Amjaline, Flecainide.

- **Long QT syndrome:** congenital and acquired long QT syndrome. Check family history Ca, Mg, drugs and other causes.
- **Pre-excitation syndrome:** WPW with AF and an irregular fast ventricular rate over accessory pathway. ECG may show short PR interval and delta wave of pre-excitation unless the pathway is concealed.
- **Commotio cordis:** young adults with low-impact precordial trauma with a projectile object such as a baseball, hockey puck, fist, rubber bullet, or even a rugby ball. Early CPR and defibrillation.

SCD and a structurally abnormal heart by ECHO/MRI

- **Arrhythmogenic RV cardiomyopathy (ARVC):** see cardiomyopathy ▶ Section 3.23.
- **Ischaemic heart disease:** acute MI setting. May be arrhythmic or asystolic or LV wall rupture and tamponade. Usually due to atherosclerosis but rarely APS, arteritis, coronary embolism, coronary artery anomalies. Ischaemic cardiomyopathy with poor LV function. ▶ Section 3.8.
- **Cardiomyopathy:** DCM, HCM. IHD with poor LV, Hypertrophic cardiomyopathy, LV non-compaction. ▶ Section 3.23.
- **Valve disease:** aortic stenosis. Critical gradient, heart failure, chest pain, syncope. Mitral disease, mitral valve prolapse.
- **Myocarditis:** ventricular arrhythmias. ▶ Section 3.18.
- **Congenital heart disease:** coarctation of the aorta, transposition of great vessels, VSD, Fallot's, anomalous coronary arteries.

3.8 ▶ Acute coronary syndrome

- **Note:** ACS must be considered in all those with chest pain. An ECG is the immediate test to differentiate those with new LBBB and/or ST elevation from those without. The immediate risk is of VF and cardiac arrest and defibrillation must be immediately possible. Those with ST elevation ACS have vessel occlusion and must be assessed urgently for either primary PCI or thrombolysis to enable immediate reperfusion to preserve myocardium. Patients with non-ST elevation ACS are older with more comorbidities. In hospital mortality lower than STEMI, same at 6 months but long term worse. Those at higher risk should be considered for appropriate medical therapy and revascularisation within 72 h of admission.

Classification and pathophysiology

- **ST elevation (or new LBBB) ACS:** plaque rupture/occlusive thrombus: needs 'culprit' vessel opening (PCI/thrombolysis) + antithrombotics. Chest pain or equivalent + ST ↑↑/new LBBB + ↑troponin.
- **Non-ST elevation ACS:** sub-occlusive flow lesion and thrombus: needs antithrombotics and antianginals to maintain patency. Some myocardial damage may be found. Chest pain or equivalent + ECG changes + ↑troponin. Unstable angina – normal troponin.

STEMI classification based on aetiology

- **Type 1:** spontaneous MI due to plaque erosion/rupture, dissection or fissure. Seen in those with atherosclerosis – unstable plaque ruptures releasing thrombogenic material. Causes *in situ* thrombosis +/– vessel occlusion. Type A aortic dissection occluding coronary ostia.
- **Type 2:** MI due to increased demand. Spasm, severe aortic stenosis, embolism into coronary artery, arrhythmias, high and low BP. Arteritis, antiphospholipid syndrome. Vasospasm, abnormal coronary arteries.
- **Type 3/4/5:** MI with sudden cardiac death, post PCI, post CABG.

- **Exacerbating factors:** ↓coronary flow due to ↑wall pressures, e.g. aortic stenosis, HCM, ↑HR, e.g. AF, VT with shortened diastole will ↓coronary blood flow. ↑myocardial work will ↑O_2 demand and ischaemia. Anaemia: ideal Hb is 9–10 g/dL in IHD. Treat severe hypertension. ↑systemic O_2 demands – sepsis, PE, ↓BP, shock.
- **Clinical:** present as cardiac arrest, chest pain, breathlessness. Take careful history of onset of symptoms and relation to exertion. Ischaemic chest pain at rest is ominous. Central chest pain may radiate to arms/jaw. Nausea, vomiting, breathlessness, sweating, palpitations. Signs of LVF – dyspnoea, ↑HR, S3, bibasal crep. Look for murmurs, MR, VSD, aortic stenosis, HOCM. ACS in elderly – falls, delirium and syncope. Epigastric symptoms (inferior MI). No chest pain – MI in elderly and diabetics. Pale, terrified, cold peripheries, pulmonary oedema and cardiogenic shock.
- **Differentials:** pulmonary embolism, aortic dissection, pericarditis, oesophageal spasm/reflux/rupture, biliary tract disease, peptic ulcer disease, pancreatitis, chest wall pain, pleurisy/pneumonia, sickling crisis, herpes zoster, Bornholm disease.
- **Poor prognosis:** on-going and recurrent ischaemia, widespread ECG changes, ↑CK/troponins, low BP. MR with ischaemia, pulmonary oedema, cardiogenic shock. Prognosis for all ACS patients can be assessed using GRACE score (see http://gracescore.co.uk).

Investigations

- **Bloods: FBC:** low Hb exacerbates ACS. **U&E:** renal function. **Glucose:** diabetes. Check lipids.
- **12 lead ECG:** always repeat with new symptoms. Compare with previous ECG. ECG splits patients with a suspicion of ACS in two categories requiring different therapeutic approaches: **STE ACS:** signifies vessel occlusion and need for immediate reperfusion therapy. ST ↑ >2 mm in V1–V6 or >1 mm in any other 2 contiguous limb leads: V1/V2 (septal – LAD), V5, V6, I, aVL (proximal LAD). II, III, aVF (RCA) isolated lateral wall – LCx. Isolated posterior MI: ST ↓V1–V3 with ↑R wave and reciprocal changes. New LBBB may be STEMI in a minority of patients. Take advice. Also see below for analysing LBBB. There is associated ST ↓ in opposing leads as well as T wave changes and later development of Q waves. **NSTE–ACS:** symmetrical T wave changes including inversion (in leads V1–V4 can suggest LAD stenosis). Transient ST elevation +/– but usually dynamic ST depression. **Pseudonormalisation:** T waves which are usually inverted become upright with ischaemia. **Poor R wave progression:** usually transition of ↑R wave height V1 to V6 is lost with anterior wall infarction.
- **CXR:** wide mediastinum consider aortic dissection.
- **BNP:** B-type natriuretic peptide (BNP) and other related tests can give some prognostic information.
- **CKMB:** cardiospecific. May be useful where there are issues with troponin assay.
- **High sensitivity troponin (hsTn) T:** assays being done earlier nowadays with hsTnT at 0 and 3 h, e.g. hsTnT <16–20 ng/L should be interpreted as a negative result. High sensitivity troponins can detect diagnostic changes earlier and allow earlier diagnosis and exclusion and discharge. They are more sensitive but less specific and so must be assessed within clinical context.

High sensitivity troponins (hsTn)

Note troponin can be found in healthy people. The level to diagnose MI has fallen from 0.5 mcg/L to current levels of 0.05–0.1 mcg/L. hsTn assays can measure levels as low as 0.003 mcg/L (3 ng/L). hsTn is positive if >14 ng/L which can be tested at point of admission with a sensitivity of 90–95% which improves to 99% at 3–6 h post-admission. False positives are seen. What is needed is a change to be detected between admission and the 3–6 h sample. Large changes suggest MI. Other causes of elevated levels include sepsis, dissection, PE, myocarditis/pericarditis, cardiac failure, renal failure, stroke. Evaluation should be combined with clinical common sense and with history and risks assessed, ECG, TIMI/GRACE score (*Br J Cardiol* 2013;20(4)).

- **Cardiac troponin T:** at admission and 12 h: <0.01 mcg/L unstable angina, 0.01–1 mcg/L: unstable angina/myocyte necrosis. Some guidelines define this as MI and others (USA) >1 mcg/L: MI.
- **Cardiac troponin I:** at admission, 12 h <0.06 ng/ml: normal; 0.07–0.49 ng/ml: indeterminate, >0.50 ng/ml: consistent with myocardial necrosis. CKMB/AST/LDH are historical biomarkers superseded by troponin. Troponin level is directly proportional to mortality. False positives: tachyarrhythmias, myocarditis, coronary artery spasm from cocaine, severe cardiac failure, cardiac trauma from surgery or road traffic incident, pulmonary embolus, renal failure, acute exacerbation of LVF, Critical illness – ITU, AAA rupture.
- **Echocardiogram:** all should have an assessment of LV function, valves and useful to detect tamponade, cardiomyopathy and effusions. Acutely, echocardiogram can show wall movement abnormalities suggesting ischaemia/infarction. Useful if ECG ambiguous.
- **Cardiac stress tests:** if pain settles and ECG changes equivocal and troponin negative then consider controlled different ways to cause transient measurable myocardial ischaemia. Objective evidence of ischaemia may be displayed on ECG, echo or by scintigraphy. Tests to assess hibernating myocardium whose viability will improve with revascularisation by PCI or CABG. Cardiac MRI or PET scan. Dobutamine stress echo, thallium. Most give a sensitivity of over 90% except stress echo (70%).
- **Angiography in ST elevation ACS / medium to high risk non-ST elevation ACS:** primary PCI is indicated in those with STEMI as it allows opening of culprit vessel and opportunity for angioplasty and stenting or thrombus aspiration. It can help select those for CABG (see below). In non-ST elevation ACS PCI is suggested in higher risk patients to diagnose IHD, to define disease, identify vessels for angioplasty and stenting or patients for CABG.

ECG differentials of ST elevation

- **STEMI:** ST elevation >2 mm in V1–V6 or >1 mm in any other 2 contiguous limb leads. V1/V2 (septal – LAD), V5, V6, I, aVL (proximal LAD). II, III, aVF (RCA), isolated lateral wall – LCx. Isolated posterior – ST dep V1–V3 with tall R wave and reciprocal changes. New LBBB may be STEMI in a minority of patients. Take advice.
- **High take off:** "early repolarization". ST looks elevated in V2, V3. No reciprocal changes elsewhere.
- **Transient apical ballooning syndrome:** Takotsubo cardiomyopathy. Anterior ST elevation. See cardiomyopathy.
- **Myo-/Pericarditis:** saddle-shaped ST elevation all leads except cavity leads (aVr).
- **Prinzmetal's variant angina:** transient ST elevation during angina due to vasospasm settles with antianginals. Can provoke arrhythmias even SCD. Coronary vessels normal/minimal disease. Needs nitrates/CCB.
- **LV aneurysm:** history of previous anterior MI. Diagnose on echo.
- **Brugada syndrome:** see SCD (*Section 3.1*).
- **Hyperkalaemia:** bizarre tall T wave and wide QRS. ▶ Section 5.3.

ECG differentials of non-ST elevation ACS
- Symmetrical T wave inversion (in V1–V4 can suggest LAD stenosis).
- Transient ST ↑ +/– but usually dynamic ST ↓.

LBBB and acute MI (Sgarbossa and Wellen syndrome criteria)
LBBB and chest pain is due to occlusive thrombotic disease in a minority. To avoid inappropriate thrombolysis or PCI, assess and take expert advice if unsure. Try also to review old ECGs. ECG criteria for acute MI in chest pain patients with LBBB or ventricular paced rhythm (VPR) were:
(1) T ↑ >1 mm concordant in leads with a positive QRS complex (+5)
(2) T ↓ >1 mm in lead V1–V3 (+3), and
(3) T ↑ >5 mm that was discordant with the QRS complex (+2) (in the usual opposite direction from the QRS but of heightened amplitude; less specific than 1 & 2 but more useful in VPR). *A total score of ≥3 has a specificity of 90% and sensitivity of 36% for diagnosing MI.*

Use TIMI score to risk assess all non-ST elevation ACS patients

- **TIMI risk score (0–7):** age >65 y +1, >3 risk factors for CAD +1; known CAD (stenosis >50%) +1, ASPIRIN use in past 7 days +1; severe angina (>2 episodes/24 h) +1, ST changes >0.5 mm +1; cardiac marker +1. Use the TIMI score to risk stratify NSTEMI patients for an early angiography strategy: TIMI >4 is associated with 20% risk at 14 days of all-cause mortality, new or recurrent MI, or severe recurrent ischaemia requiring angiography and urgent revascularisation. TIMI 0–2 is low risk and the remainder are higher risk.
- **Look for other markers of high risk:** persistent/recurrent angina, ST depression >2 mm, deep negative T waves. Signs of heart failure or ↓BP EF <0.4, sustained VT, positive stress test, diabetes mellitus, renal impairment, reduced LV function, previous CABG or recent PCI <6/12.

ECG showing STEMI: normal P/QRS/T wave. ST segment is initially isoelectric line. T wave becomes peaked and grown taller. ST elevation starts. T wave inversion is seen. Reciprocal ST depression in opposing leads. After 24 h ST segment elevation reduces and before this is a sign of reperfusion. T wave may remain inverted. ECG develops Q waves. R wave may be reduced in height with poor R wave progression anteriorly.

Acute management of ACS
- **Rapid assessment:** targeted history, good IV access, rapid exam and BP in both arms. Send bloods for troponin, FBC, U&E, glucose, lipids, immediate 12 lead ECG and determine if criteria for ST elevation ACS present. Repeat at 15 min intervals if ongoing symptoms and non-diagnostic. Echocardiogram can be invaluable as it will show wall movement abnormalities suggesting ischaemia/infarction especially if ECG ambiguous. Assess LV function and regional wall abnormalities. May even pick up evidence of a dissection – intimal flap, acute aortic incompetence. Consider differentials – see chest pain, notably PE and aortic dissection, myo-/pericarditis which may have ECG changes. If not ST elevation ACS assess GRACE/TIMI score to direct therapy. There is some variability in anticoagulant or antithrombotic regimens between centres and specialists and so local guidance should be taken and followed.
- **Interpreting biomarkers** (↑ hsTn T): admission and +3 h. If negative consider as low risk chest pain or consider other diagnosis, if both <20 ng/L, likely MI. If change in serial troponins >10 ng/L with one result >20 ng/L, consider alternative diagnoses if both >20 ng/L with change <10 ng/L. **Alternative causes high troponin:** AKI/CKD, CCF/LVF, hypertensive crisis, arrhythmias, PE, severe pulmonary hypertension, myocarditis, stroke/SAH, aortic dissection, aortic valve disease or HCM, cardiac contusion, ablation, pacing, cardioversion, hypothyroidism, apical ballooning

syndrome, infiltrative diseases, e.g. amyloidosis/sarcoidosis, drug toxicity, burns, rhabdomyolysis critically ill patients, especially with respiratory failure, or sepsis.

- **ST elevation ACS:** if ECG criteria then assess eligibility for reperfusion therapy regardless of age, race, sex and unconsciousness. If not eligible then offer medical therapy. If eligible then determine if within 12 h of symptoms onset. If not but there is continuing ischaemia then consider PCI. If local services allow PPCI to be done within 120 min of the time that fibrinolysis could be given then go for PPCI. If not then offer thrombolysis (see agents below). If there is still persisting ST elevation 60–90 min after thrombolysis or evidence of ongoing ischaemia then seek advice on immediate angiography.

- **Non-ST elevation ACS:** use GRACE or TIMI score to assess prognosis. GRACE is a more accurate risk score but more difficult to calculate. Those with more than 3 TIMI risk variables, older than 75 and a positive troponin are at high risk of MI, recurrent ischaemia or death and benefit from intensive medical therapy and coronary angiography/revascularisation within 72 h of admission. Low risk non-ST elevation ACS where pain settles quickly with no or minimal ECG changes and normal troponin and low GRACE/TIMI scores (TIMI 0–2) may be treated with Aspirin, Nitrates, Statin and Beta-Blockers and should have an early EST prior to discharge. If EST positive then consider as higher risk and consider angiography.

- **ABC O$_2$ (BTS)**, no evidence for routine usage. Give 15 L/min if shocked/LVF or hypoxic. Admit to CCU. Monitor for arrhythmias. Ensure access to defibrillation for VF/VT.

- **Aspirin 300 mg PO** stat chew/dispersible within 12 h and then 75 mg/d after (25% mortality reduction). Continued long term in all patients.

- **Chest pain:** give GTN 2 sprays (400–800 mcg) SL or GTN 500 mcg tablet SL or BUCCAL NITRATE 2–5 mg 8 h unless ↓? BP. Watch BP. Ongoing pain or pulmonary oedema consider IV GTN infusion as GTN 50 mg in 50 ml NS IV and run at 2–10 ml/h through syringe driver. Titrate to pain, breathlessness and BP.

- **Ongoing chest pain:** LVF consider DIAMORPHINE 2.5–5 mg IV or MORPHINE 5–10 mg IV with anti-emetic, e.g. METOCLOPRAMIDE 10 mg IV.

- **Additional antiplatelets:** CLOPIDOGREL 300 mg PO stat or if PCI then consider alternatives, e.g. PRASUGREL 60 mg or TICAGRELOR 180 mg may be given unless CABG planned. CLOPIDOGREL 75 mg is continued for at least 3 months in non-ST elevation ACS and 4 weeks in those with ST elevation ACS. Avoid CLOPIDOGREL if CABG imminent. **DUAL ANTIPLATELET** – see below.

- **Beta blockade:** consider METOPROLOL 5 mg IV over 5 min which may be repeated (max 15 mg); stop if SBP <100 mmHg or HR <60 bpm. Later METOPROLOL 50 mg TDS PO for 48 h and then maintenance dose or ATENOLOL 50 mg OD PO or BISOPROLOL 2.5–5 mg OD. Titrate up doses. Avoid if asthmatic, ↓BP, LVF, HR <60, 2nd or 3rd degree heart block. Unable to take beta-blockers try DILTIAZEM 60–90 mg BD PO (up to 360 mg/d). All patients with ACS should be on long term Beta-Blocker.

- **Anticoagulants:** if considered high risk: ENOXAPARIN (LMWH) 1 mg/kg SC BD or FONDAPARINUX (Xa inhibitor) 2.5 mg SC OD for 2–8 days or until revascularisation or discharge. Others may use UFH or BIVALIRUDIN. ACS patient taking warfarin: if warfarin continuation not mandatory (e.g. atrial fibrillation), omit warfarin and start Fondaparinux when INR <2.0. If warfarin continuation mandatory (e.g. mechanical heart valve, recurrent DVT/PE) continue warfarin until cardiology review, DO NOT PRESCRIBE FONDAPARINUX. For patients with renal impairment (SeCr >265 μmol/L or EGFR <20 ml/min OMIT FONDAPARINUX and prescribe ENOXAPARIN 1 mg/kg SC OD.

- **Kawasaki disease:** can present with an ACS and may be STEMI/NSTEMI. Management is usually medical and involves anticoagulation. PCI to aneurysmal arteries usually avoided due to risks of rupture. Use medical therapy including thrombolysis but avoid streptokinase if recent (<6 months) streptococcal pharyngitis. Take early expert help.

Pacing in acute MI
- **Indications:** asystole, CHB + anterior wall MI, alternating BBB, bifascicular block (new RBBB with left anterior fascicular block (LAFB)/left posterior fascicular block (LPFB)) + long PR = trifascicular, Mobitz II block, Mobitz I with anterior or inferior wall MI, with wide QRS escape rhythm (a junctional escape which is narrow QRS and rate 50–60/min and SBP >100 mmHg may be monitored), symptomatic ↓HR despite atropine or chronotropes, new RBBB with anterior wall MI, new LBBB with anterior wall MI. Take expert advice if patient stable. Some may wait and insert a permanent system if haemodynamically stable. Pacing may be used to overdrive VT.

Heart failure: Cardiogenic shock and heart failure, ▶ Section 2.16.
- **Acute pulmonary oedema:** FUROSEMIDE 50–100 mg IV +/– DIAMORPHINE 2.5–5 mg IV or MORPHINE 5–10 mg IV with antiemetic, e.g. METOCLOPRAMIDE 10 mg IV. Consider nitrates, e.g. GTN infusion. Revascularisation.
- **ACE inhibitor:** all patients with ACS and either heart failure, HTN or diabetes should be on long term ACE inhibitor. Consider RAMIPRIL 1.25 mg OD and up-titrate. Those with MI should be commenced on long term ACE inhibitor within the first 36 h. Patients with MI complicated by LV dysfunction or heart failure should be commenced on long term AT2 receptor blocker therapy if intolerant of ACE inhibitor therapy.
- **EPLERENONE 25–50 mg OD.** MI complicated by LV dysfunction (EF <0.40).
- **FUROSEMIDE 50–100 mg IV** and then 20–80 mg/day orally may be considered if severe pulmonary oedema in conjunction with ACE inhibitor and Nitrates and revascularisation. Needs echocardiogram. Closely monitor K. Avoid Low K post MI.
- **NIPPV:** patients with an ACS with acute cardiogenic pulmonary oedema and hypoxia should be considered for NIPPV. Most evidence favours CPAP (2.5–10 cm/H_2O).
- **Beta-blockers:** BISOPROLOL 1.25 mg starting dose is agent of choice in stabilised heart failure.

Hypotension: cardiogenic shock or RV failure
- **Inotropes:** consider if persisting ↓BP and cardiogenic shock. DOBUTAMINE often first line. Consider ENOXIMONE, a phosphodiesterase type-3 inhibitor with inotropic and vasodilator activity.
- **Intra-aortic balloon pump:** ACS complicated by cardiogenic shock, myocardial rupture (VSD and papillary muscle rupture) or refractory ischaemia should be considered for IABP especially when contemplating emergency coronary revascularisation or corrective surgery.
- **Coronary revascularisation:** cardiogenic shock due to LVF within 6 h of MI should be considered for immediate PCI.
- **Cardiac surgery:** mechanical complications of MI (VSD, free wall or papillary muscle rupture) should be considered for corrective surgery within 48 h.
- **RV failure:** IV fluids: can help if evidence clinically, ECG or echo of RV failure due possibly to inferior MI with ↓BP and ↑JVP.

Secondary prevention
- **Dual antiplatelets:** ASPIRIN 75 mg OD long term. CLOPIDOGREL 75 mg or ALTERNATIVE as above, continue for 1 y after STEMI/NSTEMI. Minimum dual antiplatelet: BMS 3 months, DES 12 months. Stopping before 12 months must be discussed with interventional cardiologist.

- **ACE inhibitor:** RAMIPRIL 1.25–5 mg PO 12 hourly or ENALAPRIL 10 mg PO 12 hourly for all non-hypotensive patients can help reduce ventricular remodelling in the first 4–6 weeks. Continue long term if impaired LV function.
- **Nitrates:** for on-going chest pain or pulmonary oedema. IV nitrate or buccal NITRATE 2–5 mg 8 hourly.
- **Beta-blockers:** long term, e.g. METOPROLOL or BISOPROLOL 2.5–5 mg PO OD especially with impaired LV function.
- **Lifestyle modifications:** smoking cessation services and diet/weight management and exercise support.
- **Diabetic control:** HbA1c <7%.
- **Vaccination:** annual influenza and pneumococcal vaccination recommended.
- **Antihypertensive:** aim for BP <140/90 mmHg.
- **Statins:** ATORVASTATIN 80 mg at night for at least 3 months. Reduces cholesterol and mortality. Aim to get total cholesterol <4 mmol/L and LDL-C <2 mmol/L.
- **Warfarin/DOAC** for AF, warfarin for LV thrombus, PE, DVT.
- **AICD:** if VT/VF >48 h after the initial MI then AICD should be inserted before discharge. For those with poor LV then clinical trials support a waiting period of 40 days post MI before AICD insertion. They may need electrophysiology study depending on local guidance.
- **Coronary artery bypass:** those with three vessel complex coronary disease derive a mortality benefit with surgery. Diabetics especially. LIMA to LAD graft is suspected to be superior to saphenous vein to LAD.

Quick review

- **STEMI PCI: pre-angio:** Aspirin + (Clopidogrel or Prasugrel or Ticagrelor) + UFH. At angio: Bivalirudin/UFH and GPIIb-IIIa receptor antagonist.
- **STEMI thrombolysis:** Aspirin + Clopidogrel + Thrombolysis + Enoxaparin/Fondaparinux or UFH.
- **NSTEMI: conservative:** Aspirin/Nitrate/Beta-blocker/Statin/UFH or Enoxaparin or Fondaparinux + Clopidogrel (or alternative).
- **Non-ST elevation ACS: invasive:** Aspirin/Nitrate/Beta-blocker/Statin + Enoxaparin/UFH/Bivalirudin + (Clopidogrel or Ticagrelor) and GPIIbIIIa inhibitor.

Antiplatelets which maybe used post MI as well as aspirin

- **CLOPIDOGREL 300 mg.** Additional 300 mg PO stat if PCI followed by 150 mg OD for a week and then 75 mg OD for 12 months.
- **TICAGRELOR 180 mg** then **90 mg BD** for up to 12 months. Used instead of CLOPIDOGREL in non-ST elevation ACS with ST/T changes and age >60 y, previous MI or CABG, CAD with stenosis >50% in at least two vessels; previous ischaemic stroke/TIA, carotid stenosis of at least 50%, or cerebral revascularisation; diabetes mellitus; peripheral arterial disease; or CKD with creatinine clearance of less than 60 ml/min/1.73 m^2 of body surface area. NICE currently recommend for STEMI as P2Y12 blocker of choice.
- **PRASUGREL 60 mg stat then 10 mg OD for up to 15 months** used instead of CLOPIDOGREL with STEMI, NSTEMI for PCI, stent thrombosis on clopidogrel, ACS with diabetes mellitus, high risk stent thrombosis [NICE 2014, NG317].

Indications for reperfusion strategies

- ST elevation >2 mm in 2 or more precordial leads or 1 mm in limb leads.
- New onset LBBB or ST depression in precordial leads and ST elevation in V7–V9 (posterior MI usually due to LCx occlusion).
- Resuscitated VF arrest.

Not generally advocated beyond 12 h from symptoms onset if asymptomatic or haemodynamically stable. Requires chest pain + ST elevation >2 mm in two or more contiguous chest leads V1–V6, or ST elevation >1 mm in two or more contiguous limb leads, or new LBBB (see above). If there are signs of posterior MI (ST depression and tall R wave V1) take immediate senior advice. Options are mechanical reperfusion by PCI or chemical with thrombolytic agents.

Percutanous coronary intervention

- **Primary PCI:** if it can be done within 120 min of the time that fibrinolysis could be given, or in other terms that the patient can be at the door of the PCI centre within 90 min of the initial call for help. If not, then offer thrombolysis. PPCI is superior to fibrinolysis in reducing death, stroke, and re-infarction where a skilled interventional cardiologist and catheterisation laboratory with surgical backup are available. Perform within 12 h of symptom onset. Allows angioplasty and stenting of culprit lesion with reperfusion and salvage of viable myocardium. PPCI also preferred if contraindication to fibrinolytic therapy, e.g. bleeding risk or older patients (>75 y; increased risk of ICH with fibrinolysis) or those with cardiovascular compromise (LVF/shock) suggesting a high risk of an infarct-related complicated medical course or death. Patients usually receive a combination of antiplatelet and anticoagulants prior to and during PCI as detailed above. Multivessel PCI at the time of PPCI or as a staged procedure is now recommended for ST-elevation myocardial infarction (STEMI); manual aspiration thrombectomy is no longer recommended.
- **Early/delayed PCI:** those with non-ST elevation ACS felt to be at higher risk as assessed by GRACE score can be offered early or delayed PCI.
- **Stenting:** bare metal stents (BMS) use mechanical force to hold open vessel but also induce intimal proliferation. They reduce mortality in acute MI. In those with stable disease they reduce angina but with no effect on death, MI or hospitalisation or costs. They are routinely used and need a minimum 3 months CLOPIDOGREL 75 mg as well as ASPIRIN 75 mg. BMS preferred in those who cannot tolerate long-term dual antiplatelet therapy. Drug-eluting stents (DES) are BMS coated with a drug to suppress intimal proliferation. They need 12 months dual antiplatelet therapy (DAPT). There is a risk of stent thrombosis associated with the use of both DES and BMS, but seemingly more so with DES. *The length of DAPT should be documented by the Interventionalist and depends on the stent type, the lesion/s and the indication – in the setting of ACS or not.* DES have a small reduction in target vessel revascularisation (TVR) rates so only used in higher risk patients (diabetes/high risk lesions) and where the target artery to be treated has less than a 3 mm calibre, or the lesion is longer than 15 mm. DES and BMS show no difference in mortality or MI rates or stent thrombosis. Avoid DES if ↑bleed risk with prolonged DAPT for 12 months. [NICE 2003, TA71: Ischaemic heart disease – coronary artery stents.]
- **PCI protocol:** patients usually receive ASPIRIN 300 mg and CLOPIDOGREL 300–600 mg or alternative acutely as well as an anticoagulant (e.g. heparin or bivalirudin), followed by rapid PCI with stenting. Augmented antiplatelet therapy with a glycoprotein IIb/IIIa (GPIIb–IIIa) inhibitor may be given in selected patients, generally at the time of catheterization.
- **Glycoprotein IIb/IIIa inhibitors** are the most potent antiplatelet agents available and may be used at the time of PCI and for 12–24 h. ABCIXIMAB IV bolus of 0.25 mg/kg, then 0.125 mcg/kg/min IV (max. 10 mcg/min) for 12 h; or EPTIFIBATIDE IV bolus of 180 mcg/kg, then 2.0 mcg/kg/min IV for 18–24 h; or TIROFIBAN 0.4 mcg/kg/min IV for 30 min, then 0.1 mcg/kg/min IV for 12–24 h.
- **PCI after cardiac arrest:** clinical indications are: ST elevation on ECG after resuscitation and chest pain preceding cardiac arrest. About 50% of patients are treated by PCI. Benefit is predominantly confined to those with ST elevation (M Godin, ESC 2012). DAANS scoring for patient selection (non-validated): dyslipidaemia +1, age >70 +2, adrenaline >6 mg +3, time pre-CPR >10 min +4, non-shockable rhythm +5. Score >7 100% in-hospital mortality, score 6–7 mortality 95% (Farhat, A. ESC 2012).

Cardiac thrombolysis (↓mortality by 25–50%)

- Those patients not suitable for PCI (or PCI not available), those who seek medical attention less than 1 h after the onset of symptoms (in whom the therapy may abort the infarction), and those with a history of anaphylaxis due to radiographic contrast material. Door to needle time should be less than 30 min. Offer thrombolysis to those with acute STEMI presenting within 12 h of onset of symptoms. If ST elevation persists for 60–90 min post-fibrinolysis then reconsider PCI. Further administration of fibrinolytic is not recommended.
- **Absolute contraindications to cardiac thrombolysis:** active bleeding or bleeding diathesis (excluding menses), significant closed head or facial trauma within 3 months, suspected aortic dissection, previous intracranial haemorrhage, ischaemic stroke <3 months, structural cerebral vascular lesion, known malignant intracranial tumour.
- **Relative contraindications to cardiac thrombolysis:** current use of anticoagulants, non-compressible vascular puncture, recent major surgery <3 months, traumatic or prolonged CPR >10 min, recent internal bleeding <4 weeks, active peptic ulcer, chronic severe poorly controlled HTN, BP >200/120 mmHg, pregnancy.

Thrombolytic agents (see table below)

- **Post thrombolysis anticoagulation:** Alteplase, Reteplase, Tenecteplase need IV heparin for 24–48 h and then LMWH for 4–8 days or discharge. IV heparin is not needed following Streptokinase.
- **Bleeding on/after thrombolysis:** ▶ Section 8.12. **Advice on agents:** ALTEPLASE/ RETEPLASE/TENECTEPLASE preferred over STREPTOKINASE in anterior MI or new LBBB or those who have previously had Streptokinase where PPCI is not possible. Cerebral haemorrhage risk additional 4 per 1000 patients treated. Bleed risks are 0.5–1.0%.
- Patients with ST elevation ACS should have early coronary angiography and be assessed for revascularisation.

THROMBOLYTIC AGENTS (NS = 0.9% saline)

- **STREPTOKINASE:** 1.5 MU in 100 ml NS over 1 h. S/E ↓BP, fluid challenge but no need to stop. Other agents below preferred for anterior infarction or cardiogenic shock if no PCI. Streptokinase tends not to be reused because antibodies are formed which reduce efficacy. Anaphylaxis (▶ Section 2.18) HYDROCORTISONE 200 mg IV and CHLORPHENAMINE 10 mg IV. ICH 0.4%. Patency 51%.
- **TENECTEPLASE:** 30–50 mg IV push in 10 sec. Dose according to body weight. ICH 0.7%. Patency 80%.
- **ALTEPLASE:** 15 mg IV push, 50 mg over 30 min and then 35 mg over 60 min. ICH 0.7%. Patency 80%.
- **RETEPLASE:** 2 × 10 unit boluses given 30 min apart. ICH 0.8%. Patency 80%.

Risk assessment

- Exercise stress testing is used to risk-stratify patients except in those with severe aortic stenosis, LBBB, on-going typical chest pain, haemodynamic instability, dynamic ST changes, severe LV outflow obstruction and hypertrophic cardiomyopathy, poor mobility.
- Risks of coronary angiography: death 1 in 1000 (0.1%), MI 1 in 1000 (0.1%), stroke 1 in 1000 (0.1%), arterial complications 1 in 500 (0.2%).
- Risk of PCI (angioplasty and stenting): death 0.7%, MI (usually minor) <1%, stroke <1%, emergency CABG 1 in 200 (0.5%), significant arterial complications 1 in 200 (0.5%).

Complications post MI

- **Tachyarrhythmias:** AF, sinus tachycardia, ventricular ectopics, idioventricular rhythm (do not treat if not compromised), VT, VF (particularly VF/VT amendable to early defibrillation, which is key).
- **Idioventricular rhythm:** seen post MI often post reperfusion. Broad complex 'slow VT' <120/min. Monitor and may not need treatment if stable.
- **Bradyarrhythmias:** sinus bradycardia, heart block; may need pacing if haemodynamically compromised and both bundle branches taken out.
- **On-going chest pain:** escalate to look for treatable ischaemia or PCI/thrombolysis if re-infarction or failed reperfusion.
- **LV dysfunction:** heart failure, cardiogenic shock; poor prognosis. Needs echocardiogram. Survival LV function. **Killip score** can give a quick estimation of in-hospital mortality. Killip class I, no CHF (2–5%); Killip class II, S3, rales/creps (10–15%); Killip class III, overt pulmonary oedema (20–30%); Killip class IV, cardiogenic shock (50–60%). Cardiogenic shock and heart failure, ▶ Section 2.16.
- **Venous thromboembolism:** DVT, PE. Prevent with early mobilisation, antiplatelets, LMWH and TED stockings where appropriate.
- **Myocardial rupture:** post MI or traumatic catheter-related perforation due to intervention. Causes tamponade and usually death. In days 3–5 with myocardial softening post STEMI, causes PEA. Recently documented with Takotsubo or regional ventricular ballooning syndrome.
- **Acute mitral regurgitation:** day 2–7 post MI. Partial rupture – loud PSM, S3, low BP and CCF. Complete rupture of papillary muscle can cause rapid death, usually in first week. Surgery is associated with high risk. Echo to confirm. Rupture of free wall causes tamponade and SCD. Discuss with tertiary cardiology centre.
- **Ventricular septal rupture and VSD:** VSD in 3%. Q wave MI affecting septum. Low BP, PSM at the left sternal edge. Less SOB than acute MR and less pulmonary oedema on CXR. Urgent echo and surgical referral, and IABP as a bridge to surgical closure. Discuss with tertiary centre.
- **LV aneurysm:** after 2–3 months presenting with dyspnoea, ↓BP and a dyskinetic parasternal pulsation and ST elevation. Take advice. Echocardiography. Some may need surgery. Rupture is main concern as well as thromboembolism and arrhythmias.
- **Intracardiac thrombus and cardioembolism:** From akinetic cardiac apex, left atrial or LV aneurysm. Causes stroke, ischaemic limb, mesenteric ischaemia. Tends to be acute and needs anticoagulation. Warfarin should be continued for 3 months, unless AF or considered high risk when it may be continued.
- **Psychosocial:** depression, sexual impotence, employment issues.
- **Pericarditis:** early, late (Dressler's syndrome), widespread saddle-shaped ST elevation. Care with anticoagulation as bleeding into pericardial sac is a concern.

3.9   Stable angina

- **Based on NICE guidance (2010). Diagnose stable angina** based on clinical assessment alone or clinical assessment plus diagnostic testing (i.e. anatomical testing for obstructive CAD and/or functional testing for myocardial ischaemia). Take detailed history and risk factors.
- **Anginal pain** is often (1) a constricting discomfort in the front of the chest, or in the neck, shoulders, jaw, or arms, (2) precipitated by physical exertion, and (3) relieved by rest or GTN within about 5 min. If all three features are present the chest pain or discomfort is classified as **TYPICAL ANGINA**. If two of three features are present the chest discomfort is classified as **ATYPICAL ANGINA**. If only one of three features is present the chest discomfort is classified as **NON-ANGINAL CHEST PAIN**.

- **Where angina is controlled the issues are to establish a diagnosis with some certainty in those at 10–90% risk of CAD**. The role of angiography is purely diagnostic and so non-invasive strategies are preferred. Where CAD has >90% likelihood then no further intervention is needed.
- **Estimated likelihood of CAD is <10%**. First consider other causes of chest pain such as gastrointestinal or musculoskeletal pain. Only consider CXR if other diagnoses (e.g. lung tumour) are suspected. Consider other causes of angina (e.g. echo for hypertrophic cardiomyopathy) if there is typical angina-like chest pain.
- **Estimated likelihood of CAD is 10–90%**. Arrange blood tests for conditions which exacerbate angina. Consider aspirin only if chest pain is likely to be stable angina. Do not offer if being taken regularly or the person is allergic. Treat as stable angina while waiting for the results if symptoms are typical of stable angina.
- **Estimated likelihood of CAD is 10–29%**. Offer CT calcium scoring as first line. If score = 0 then investigate other causes. If score 1–400 then offer 64-slice CT angiography and re-estimate risk. If score is >400 then follow pathway for 61–90% CAD.
- **Estimated likelihood of CAD is 30–60%**. Reversible myocardial ischaemia on functional imaging? If uncertain offer angiography. If not then treat as stable angina. If no then look for alternative diagnosis.
- **Estimated likelihood of CAD is 61–90%** and invasive coronary angiography is appropriate and acceptable and coronary revascularisation is being considered then offer coronary angiography. If significant CAD then treat as stable angina. If unsure consider non-invasive functional imaging. If no CAD then look for alternative diagnosis.
- **Estimated risk of CAD >90%**. Features of typical angina. Arrange blood tests for conditions which exacerbate angina and treat as stable angina with no further diagnostic test.

Percentage of people estimated to have CAD according to typicality of symptoms, age, sex and risk factors

Hi = high risk = diabetes, smoking and hyperlipidaemia (total cholesterol >6.47 mmol/litre). Lo = low risk = none of these 3. For men older than 70 with atypical or typical symptoms, assume an estimate >90%. For women older than 70, assume an estimate of 61–90% EXCEPT women at high risk AND with typical symptoms where a risk of >90% should be assumed.

| | Non-anginal chest pain Risk of CAD (%) | | | | Atypical angina Risk of CAD (%) | | | | Typical angina Risk of CAD (%) | | | |
| | Men | | Women | | Men | | Women | | Men | | Women | |
Age (y)	Lo	Hi	Lo	Hi	Lo	Hi	Lo	Hi	Lo	Hi	Lo	Hi
35	3	35	1	19	8	59	2	39	30	88	10	78
45	9	47	2	22	21	70	5	43	51	92	20	79
55	23	59	4	25	45	79	10	47	80	95	38	82
65	49	69	9	29	71	86	20	51	93	97	56	84

 Arrhythmias

ECG interpretation of arrhythmias
- Heart rate = 300/R to R interval squares. ECG is a graph:
  - X axis (horizontal) is time at 25 mm/s; each small square is 40 ms.
  - Y axis (vertical) is millivolts at 1 mV = 1 cm; each small square is 0.1 mV.

- Normal PR interval is 120–200 ms (3–5 small squares); normal QRS is <120 ms (3 small squares).
- QT (measured from the start of the QRS to the end of the T wave); correct for rate (QTc) to 60 beats/min using the equation:

$$QTc = (QT)/(\text{square root of } RR), \text{ where RR is the RR interval in seconds.}$$

- Normal between 0.35 and 0.43 s (9–11 small squares).
- Irregular: measure RR interval and it changes beat to beat. Broad complex QRS >3 small squares.

3.11 Tachyarrhythmias

Rhythm	P wave (leads II and v1)	QRS form and regularity	Onset	Notes
Sinus tachycardia	Normal	Normal width. Regular > 100/min	Gradual onset/ end	Exercise related, hyperthyroid, etc
Atrial fibrillation	Absent	Normal width. Irregular R to R interval. Any rate	Sudden/Chronic, Paroxysmal	See text
Atrial flutter	Saw shaped flutter waves inferior leads seen with CSM	Normal width regular rate is a divisor of 300 e.g. 75/100/150	Sudden/ Paroxysmal	See text
SVT	Variable	Normal width regular. Rate 150–200/min	Sudden stop – CSM, Adenosine	Adenosine, Ablation
Torsades de pointes	Dissociated	Broad changing axis Regular Rate > 120	Sudden	Long QT related
Idioventricular	Dissociated	Broad fixed axis Regular < 120/min	Sudden	Seen post MI usually benign
VT	Dissociated	Broad fixed axis Regular > 100/min	Sudden	See text
Ventricular fibrillation	Dissociated	Random width, Random irregular	Sudden	Cardiac arrest

Risk assessment and management

- **Slow ventricular rate:** look for sinus bradycardia, 2nd degree heart block, slow AF, complete heart block and width of QRS. If rate has caused the associated ↓BP and circulatory collapse consider repeated ATROPINE 0.5–1 mg IV (max 3 mg) and ADRENALINE or ISOPRENALINE infusion or GLUCAGON 2–10 mg IV if on beta-blockers (see beta-blocker toxicity). External pacing as a bridge to transvenous pacing.
- **Irregular broad complex rhythm:** consider fast AF with aberrant conduction. Consider IV AMIODARONE or BETA BLOCKER. If WPW suspected avoid IV DIGOXIN or VERAPAMIL. If unwell consider low voltage DC cardioversion, ▶Section 1.14.
- **Regular broad complex >120/min:** VT or aberrantly conducted SVT/flutter. If unsure always assume and treat as VT. Treat with IV Amiodarone 150–300 mg over 20–60 min. Consider carotid massage if safe (aged <50 and no suggestion of TIA/stroke/bruit) and/or Adenosine if you think it's aberrantly conducted SVT. DC cardiovert if falling BP. **Avoid IV VERAPAMIL**.
- **Narrow complex regular AVRT or AVNRT or atrial flutter 2:1, 3:1 or 4:1 block:** can settle spontaneously. Usually benign unless in context of other cardiac disease.

Consider CSM. IV ADENOSINE or IV METOPROLOL. If unstable consider low voltage DC cardioversion. If AVRT and WPW avoid DIGOXIN or VERAPAMIL.
- **Narrow complex irregular** fast AF: consider IV AMIODARONE or IV METOPROLOL or IV DIGOXIN. If unstable consider low voltage DC cardioversion. Assess need for anticoagulation.

Differential of a narrow complex tachycardia
- **Regular:** sinus tachycardia, paroxysmal SVT, atrial flutter with 2/3/4:1 block, atrial tachycardia with conduction, AVRT (orthodromic) (WPW), AVNRT.
- **Irregular:** atrial fibrillation, atrial flutter with variable block, atrial tachycardia with variable block, multifocal atrial tachycardia.

3.12   Monomorphic ventricular tachycardia

- **About:** all fast unstable rhythms should be considered for urgent DC cardioversion. Most broad complex regular tachycardias are VT especially if IHD/structural heart disease. Some are aberrantly conducted SVT/atrial flutter. VT may be tolerated and then suddenly decompensate. Ensure immediate access to defibrillator. There are some rare benign forms of VT and some aberrantly conducted SVTs that mimic VT but this is for experts in the cold light of day. Assume it's a VT with possible fatal consequences until proven otherwise. A prolonged QT predisposes to both monomorphic and polymorphic VT.
- **Aetiology:** can originate in left or right ventricle. Often due to underlying myocardial damage and development of re-entrant tachycardia as well as some increased automaticity. Electrical waves form 'rotors' that give rise to rapidly rotating spiral waves. Causes also include inherited channelopathies such as Brugada and prolonged QT syndromes. Cardiomyopathies such as arrhythmogenic RV cardiomyopathy are being increasingly identified.
- **Types:** Sustained (> 30 sec) and non-sustained (<30 sec and more benign).
- **ECG:** >3 beats broad regular QRS complex >3 small squares (120 ms) wide and rate over 100/min. There is complete AV dissociation and P waves can be found as atrial activity continues. Idioventricular is a slow VT at 100–120/min seen post MI and usually benign. LBBB and RAD morphology and no other cardiac disease may suggest RV cardiomyopathy.
- **Causes of VT:** cardiac disease: IHD especially with LV dysfunction, dilated or hypertrophic cardiomyopathy, arrhythmogenic RV cardiomyopathy (ARVC), myocarditis, sarcoidosis, haemochromatosis. Drug-induced, e.g. TCA overdose, digoxin, antiarrhythmics, low or high K, Low Mg, Low Ca, cocaine, phaeochromocytoma. Channelopathies: Brugada syndrome, long QT syndromes, drugs causing long QT. Others: chest trauma, idiopathic, structural congenital disorders.
- **Clinical:** some tolerate VT, others develop angina, pulmonary oedema, cardiac arrest. Status depends on LV function, rate and coronary perfusion and comorbidities. Palpitations, breathlessness, pulmonary oedema. ↓BP, chest pain, Cannon 'a' wave in JVP (AV dissociation).
- **Ventricular ectopics:** these are mostly benign and do not need treatment unless severely symptomatic. Reassurance is the usual approach.
- **Investigations:** bloods: check FBC, U&E, cardiac troponin, Mg, Ca. Serial ECGs: ensure capture 12 lead of the arrhythmia if possible. Echocardiogram: for LV systolic

and diastolic function and structural disease. Coronary angiogram to look for treatable coronary artery disease. Electrophysiology studies: provoke arrhythmias, mapping.

- **ECG differential of VT:** (accelerated) idioventricular rhythm (HR 100–120/min) seen post MI, monomorphic VT: regular wide complex, polymorphic VT (torsade de pointes) seen with long QT, SVT/atrial flutter or atrial tachycardia with aberrant conduction, WPW syndrome with retrograde conduction of an AVNRT/atrial flutter, motion artefact, pacemaker syndromes (consider turning off pacemaker with a magnet).
- **Evidence towards an ECG diagnosis of VT rather than SVT with aberrant conduction:** fusion beats, capture (narrow) beats, ischaemic heart disease, structural heart disease, no RS wave in V1–V6, AV dissociation (Cannon 'a' waves), RBBB pattern >140 ms, LBBB pattern >160 ms, extreme LAD, extreme R to R regularity.
- **Management:** if pulseless then ALS algorithm ▶ Section 1.4. If unstable (low BP/chest pain/dyspnoea) then administer synchronised; DC cardioversion, ▶ Section 1.14, ABC, get IV access, Give O$_2$ as per BTS guidelines. Treat any ACS. If STEMI suspected needs PCI/thrombolysis. Monitor. Defibrillator. **Correct electrolytes**. Keep K 4–5 mmol/L. Stop any drugs that prolong QT. Torsade or low Mg suspected (alcohol/diuretics): MAGNESIUM 2 g (8 mmol) IV over 10 min. Persisting VT: commence AMIODARONE 300 mg IV over 10–30 min then 900 mg/24 h. Use large vein or central line. LIDOCAINE IV may also be considered. Most antiarrhythmics are negatively inotropic and even proarrhythmic so use with caution.
- **Prevention:** follow up with a cardiologist specialising in arrhythmias. Needs echocardiogram, angiography and electrophysiological studies and Holter monitoring and cardiac MRI. Treatment of underlying cause, e.g. treat IHD – drugs, PCI, CABG. Consider SOTALOL usually when LV function is good, AMIODARONE when LV function is impaired. Assess for need for AICD implantation.

3.13   Polymorphic ventricular tachycardia (torsades de pointes)

- **About:** Torsades de pointes (TdP) is a polymorphic VT. Axis constantly changes. Due to an acquired or inherited long QT syndrome.
- **Aetiology:** prolonged ventricular repolarisation (QT duration). Some drugs cause a long QTc >500 ms. It does not correlate with risk.
- **Drug causes of long QT** (check all in **BNF**): amiodarone, erythromycin, terfenadine, TCA, quinidine. Methadone, class I and III antiarrhythmics, lithium, phenothiazine. Low K, low Mg, low Ca, congenital syndromes.
- **Congenital long QT syndromes:** genetically driven. Long QT channelopathies. Beta blockade advocated. Some may require AICD.
- **Investigations:** check FBC, U&E, troponin, Mg, Ca. Serial ECGs and ensure capture 12 lead of the arrhythmia if possible. Echocardiogram for LV and valves or structural disease. Electrophysiology studies may be useful.
- **Management:** look for drug causes (see above) and stop any drugs which may be to blame (check *BNF*): avoid amiodarone or other antiarrhythmics because they can lengthen QT. Check and correct electrolytes and K/Ca/Mg. Give MAGNESIUM 2 g (8 mmol) over 10 min IV. Pacing to get a rate of 100/min: temporary atrial or ventricular pacing increases ventricular rate and reduces the episodes of TdP. ISOPRENALINE has been used to increase rate but *not in those with congenital long QT syndromes*. AICD for high risk patients, i.e. QT >500 ms and high risk genotypes with congenital long QT syndromes. If unstable then consider DC cardioversion (▶ Section 1.14).

3.14   Supraventricular tachycardia

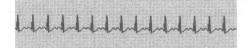

- **About:** SVT (classically excludes AF and flutter). Usually AVNRT or AVRT. A benign but troublesome arrhythmia not typically associated with cardiac death. Hospital admission if there is structural heart disease or severe symptoms. Seen in 3 in 1000, often young females but can occur at any age. The heart is usually structurally normal. The cure is ablation.
- **Differential of fast regular narrow tachycardia:** AVRT, AVNRT, sinus tachycardia, atrial tachycardia. Atrial flutter 2:1 or 3:1 block (vagal stimulation will show flutter waves).
- **AVNRT:** circus re-entry pathways in or around the AV node. Composed of two pathways: one fast conduction but a long refractory period and one slow conduction and shorter refractory period. Usually anterograde (A to V) conduction is through the slow side and retrograde through the fast, then it is a slow–fast AVNRT (90%) and vice versa. Often induced by an ectopic atrial beat when the fast side is still refractory. Captures the slow path and conducts back along the fast pathway. Retrograde activated P waves seen in the QRS. Retrograde ventricular conduction is fast with slow–fast and so this is a short RP form as the atria is stimulated very quickly. Fast–slow are long RP forms. The rarest form is slow–slow.
- **AVRT:** accessory pathway joins atria and ventricles electrically. Seen with WPW syndrome or Lown–Ganong–Levine. Accessory pathways can conduct anterogradely or retrogradely. They are not always evident on the resting ECG and may be 'concealed'. Dangerous when patient develops AF and has an accessory pathway that allows rapid anterograde conduction.
- **Clinical:** palpitations, dizziness, light headed even syncope, mild ↓BP but not cardiac arrest unless coexisting cardiac disease. Post palpitation polyuria due to release of ANP. SVT may cause heart failure if poor LV or other structural heart disease, e.g. mitral stenosis.

Electrocardiogram – record and keep

- **AVRT:** if SR pre-excited delta wave + short PR. Tall R wave in V1 suggests Type A WPW.
- **AVRT:** orthodromic A to V activation via AV node. AVRT 180–220/min. P waves buried in QRS.
- **WPW:** atrial fibrillation in WPW can lead to very rapid conduction down accessory pathway with wide irregular QRS complexes. Dangerous. DC shock.
- **AVRT:** antidromic A to V conduction across accessory pathway and back via AV node. Rate 200–300/min. Wide QRS. Can mimic VT.
- **AVNRT slow–fast:** (common) P waves are often hidden and embedded in the QRS complexes or cause pseudo 'r' (v1) or 's' waves (inf leads).
- **AVNRT fast–slow:** (uncommon) late negative P wave appears between the QRS and T wave.
- **AVNRT slow–slow:** AVNRT can occur with a P wave before the QRS complex looking like sinus tachycardia.
- Abrupt termination occurs retrograde P wave +/– brief asystole or ↓HR.

- **Investigations:** bloods: FBC, U&E, TFTs, CXR, CRP. Echocardiogram: exclude structural disease and show LV function. Troponin only if IHD suspected, e.g. chest pain and ECG changes. Electrophysiology studies as precursor to ablation and other therapies.

- **Management:** ABCs are rarely indicated. If the patient is stable then simply trying some vagal manoeuvres or adenosine is usually successful. Try vagal manoeuvres, e.g. Valsalva, cold water on the face – diving reflex, carotid sinus massage: CSM in a young person is fairly safe, but in an older person aged >50 with a history of TIA or a bruit then best avoided because it may cause TIA/stroke. Consider ADENOSINE 3/6/12 mg IV bolus (use 0.5 mg if on dipyridamole) which is excellent at terminating re-entrant tachycardias, e.g. AVRT and AVNRT, or slowing atrial flutter. Alternatively METOPROLOL 5 mg slow IV over 10 min (up to 15 mg) or other beta-blocker is very reasonable if not asthmatic otherwise VERAPAMIL 10 mg slow IV is useful assuming LV function normal and the rhythm is definitely narrow complex and no WPW. Lastly AMIODARONE 150–300 mg IV over 20–60 min is another possibility but would not be recommended for long term therapy. If unwell as the management for any tachycardia if ↓BP or unwell consider rapid DC cardioversion ▶Section 1.14. Most patients can go home following resumption of sinus rhythm for outpatient cardiology referral to discuss ablation therapy usually of the fast pathway for AVNRT or the accessory pathway in AVRT or drug therapy to prevent further arrhythmias. Exclude thyrotoxicosis.

3.15 Symptomatic bradycardia

	P wave	QRS	QRS regularity	Notes
Sinus bradycardia	Normal rate <60/min	Normal 1:1	Regular/sinus arrhythmia	Intrinsic rate is 100/min. Vagal tone ↓heart rate to 70/min or <50/min when sleeping. High vagal tone, e.g. post vasovagal syncope 'faint', cholestatic jaundice. Excess beta blockade, conduction tissue disease, hypothyroidism, ↑intracranial pressure.
Sinus rhythm	Normal rate 60–100	Normal 1:1	Regular/sinus arrhythmia	Normal
Slow AF	Absent	Normal 1:1	Irregular	Slow AF: irregular QRS complex, absent P wave. Natural rate 100/min. Slower rates are due to digoxin/beta-blockers or AV nodal disease.
Tachy–brady syndrome	AF A flutter Paroxysmal atrial tachy-bradycardia or sinus arrest	Normal 1:1 unless flutter	Regular unless AF	Dysfunction of the sinus node – sinus pauses with AF, flutter or atrial tachycardias. Bradycardia is controlled by pacemaker and drugs (or ablation) NICE (2005) has recommended dual-chamber pacemakers for symptomatic bradycardia due to sick sinus syndrome without AV block.
Sinus arrest	Normal then missing for >3 sec	Normal but may be ectopics	Irregular if recurrent	Sinus pauses/arrest: normal P QRS T wave then no P wave for 3 sec or longer. Stop any exacerbating drugs. May need to be paced if symptomatic.

	P wave	QRS	QRS regularity	Notes
First degree	Normal P wave	Normal but PR is delayed PR >0.2 sec	Normal	1st degree: long PR >200–220 msec; each P wave followed by a delayed QRS complex. Overall ventricular HR unaffected unless other disease. Rarely needs intervention.
Second degree				
Mobitz I	Normal P wave	Lengthening PR until a P wave fails to be followed by a QRS complex	Normal	P wave and lengthening PR until a P wave fails to be followed by a QRS complex: Wenckebach phenomenon is due to a block at AV nodal level. May be physiological or seen at rest or sleeping, or in athletes. Pacing rarely needed.
Mobitz II	Normal P wave	P wave not followed by QRS	Normal	QRS is intermittently dropped. Damage is infranodal and is a more significant arrhythmia with lower threshold to pace than Mobitz I. Pace if permanent or intermittent, regardless of the type or the site of the block, with symptomatic bradycardia. Consider pacing in setting of acute MI. Risk of asystole.
2nd degree with 2:1 or 3:1 AV block	Normal	P wave not followed by QRS every 2nd or 3rd beat	Regular with dropped beat	2nd degree with 2:1 or 3:1 block: every 2nd or 3rd beat does not conduct to ventricles. AV node disease or below. Pace if symptomatic or acute MI.
Third degree				
3rd degree complete heart block	Normal P wave at 60–100/min or no P wave as AF	Wide and slower means lower origin and more unstable QRS rate is 30–40/min depending on the level	Regular but slow	Complete failure of communication between atria and ventricles. Ventricles' intrinsic rate is 30–40/min depending on the level (lower is slower). Cannon 'a' waves are seen with complete heart block. Nearly always requires pacing. Risk of syncope and even asystole.

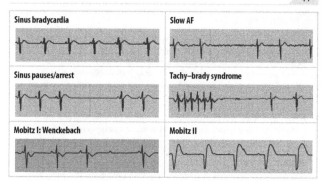

Sinus bradycardia	Slow AF
Sinus pauses/arrest	Tachy–brady syndrome
Mobitz I: Wenckebach	Mobitz II

- **About:** BP more important than HR. An extreme athlete can have a resting HR of 30–40 bpm. Second-degree heart block can suggest impending CHB/asystole.
- **Clinical:** pre/syncope, pale, shocked, low BP, HR <60 bpm. Obtunded. Some patients, e.g. bed-bound elderly, can tolerate CHB quite well. Stokes–Adams attacks are due to short periods of asystole or very slow CHB.
- **Investigations:** U&E, FBC, TFTs, cardiac troponin if ACS suspected. ECG, echocardiogram to assess LV.
- **Management:** ABC O$_2$, IV fluids, IV access, ECG monitor. If BP <90/60 mmHg and HR <60 bpm consider ATROPINE 0.5–1 mg IV (max 3 mg). Persisting ↓BP bradycardia try ADRENALINE infusion. If beta-blocker induced ↓HR ↓BP unresponsive despite atropine consider GLUCAGON 2–10 mg slow IV. Do not give atropine to patients with cardiac transplants. Denervated hearts do not respond to vagal blockade by atropine, which may cause paradoxical sinus arrest or high-grade AV block in these patients.
- **Transvenous cardiac pacing** if ↓BP due to ↓HR despite other measures. **AV block and acute inferior MI:** a branch of the RCA supplies AV node. May cause transient AV block with a high escape rhythm and if patient well no treatment needed. May improve with reperfusion. Can give ATROPINE. If worsens then temporary pacing. AV block tends to resolve in approximately 1 week. AV block in anterior MI suggests significant damage to bundle of His branches, and 2nd or 3rd degree AV block carries risk of asystole and should be paced. Take advice if unsure. Nowadays cardiology services can place a permanent system more quickly and temporary wires avoided.
- **Complications of pacing:** pneumothorax, pericarditis, infection, skin erosion, haematoma, lead dislodgement, venous thrombosis.

Indications for a permanent pacemaker

Absolute: sick sinus syndrome, symptomatic sinus bradycardia, tachy–brady syndrome. AF with sinus node dysfunction, complete AV block (third-degree block). Chronotropic incompetence (inability to increase the heart rate to match a level of exercise). Prolonged QT syndrome, cardiac resynchronization therapy with biventricular pacing.

Relative: cardiomyopathy (hypertrophic or dilated). Severe refractory neurocardiogenic syncope.

3.16   Atrial fibrillation

- **About:** uncoordinated atrial activation with atrial mechanical dysfunction. Major risk of cardioembolism causing ischaemic stroke. Assess with risk score.
- **Aetiology:** atrial fibrosis, loss of atrial muscle mass. Increased automaticity or multiple re-entrant wavelets. Atrial 'rate' of AF is 400–600/min but it is the ventricular response that matters. Ventricular rate held in check by AV node at <200/min slows with age and conduction disease. An accessory bundle (WPW) can allow faster rates to conduct AV causing VF.
- **Haemodynamics:** ↑HR shortens diastole and limits LV filling and coronary perfusion. LV filling already compromised by loss of atrial systole. Rate control with drugs, treat failure and DC shock if needed. Impaired LV function or mitral stenosis makes things much worse.
- **Clinical:** asymptomatic. Palpitations, dyspnoea, chest discomfort. Cardioembolic stroke, mesenteric emboli, limb emboli, dyspnoea. Fatigue and worsening heart failure, syncope, dizziness. ↓BP with fast/slow AF, irregularly irregular pulse. Pulse deficit. Murmurs suggesting valve disease, signs of thyroid disease, hypertension.
- **Causes of atrial fibrillation:** ischaemic, valvular, rheumatic, hypertensive heart disease, cardiomyopathy, post cardiac surgery, thyrotoxicosis, alcohol – acute binge or chronic, sick sinus syndrome, congenital heart disease, pulmonary embolism, pneumonia, sarcoidosis, amyloidosis, haemochromatosis, lone AF (idiopathic), pericarditis, myocarditis.

Classification of atrial fibrillation	
• **Persistent:** lasts >7 days.	• **Permanent:** lasts >1 year and fails to cardiovert.
• **Paroxysmal:** 2+ episodes self-terminating lasting <7 days.	• **Lone AF:** aged <60 years, no HTN, normal echo, no risk factors.

Investigations

- **Bloods:** FBC ↓Hb, ↑WCC with sepsis, U&E, Mg, Ca, K, TFT ?thyrotoxicosis, LFTs, ?alcohol, haemochromatosis.
- **CXR:** cardiomegaly, pulmonary oedema, infection, post cardiac surgery effusion.
- **Troponin:** ↑with ACS or myocarditis and minor rise with DC shock.
- **ECG:** absent 'P' waves – no organised atrial activity, fibrillatory waves that vary in amplitude, shape, and timing, QRS complexes which are irregularly irregular. **Aberrantly conducted AF** – wide complex and fast but irregular. **Pre-excited AF:** QRS 160–300/min and slurred up or down stroke of delta waves seen giving wide complex appearance but very irregular; the irregularity means that it is not VT. Dangerous if it conducts to ventricles at 1:1 and can precipitate VT/VF. This depends on character of the accessory pathway. If there are RR intervals <260 ms this is considered unsafe and needs inpatient cardiology review for ablation. If unstable simply DC cardiovert.
- **Capturing PAF:** 24 h tape in those with suspected asymptomatic episodes or symptomatic episodes less than 24 h apart. Use an event recorder ECG in those with symptomatic episodes more than 24 h apart. Some may use 7 day tape.
- **Transthoracic echocardiogram:** assess LV function, valve disease, LA size. Anticoagulation rarely depends on the echo.
- **Transoesophageal echocardiogram:** closer inspection of valves, mitral disease, ASD, endocarditis, LA appendage thrombus may be seen and can help assess risk of thromboembolism.
- **Coronary angiography:** if IHD suspected.

Atrial fibrillation anticoagulation risk assessment

CHA₂DS₂VaSc score: assess stroke risk in those with AF. **C**CF history (+1), **h**ypertension (+1), **a**ge: 65–74 (+1), >75 (+2), **d**iabetes mellitus (+1), **s**troke/TIA or thromboembolism (+2), **s**ex: female (+1), **vasc**ular disease or CAD, MI, PAD, or aortic plaque (+1). Adjusted annual stroke risk by score: (0) 0%, (1) 1.3%, (2) 2.2%, (3) 3.3%, (4) 4.0%, (5) 6.7%, (6) 9.8%, (7) 9.6%, (8) 6.7%, (9) 15.2%. Recommend anticoagulate if score >0 or 1. Discuss with patient.

HAS-BLED score: assess bleeding risk. **H**ypertension (SBP >160 mmHg) (+1), **a**bnormal renal (+1) and/or liver function (+1), **s**troke in past (+1), **b**leeding (+1), **l**abile INR (+1), **e**lderly age >65 (+1), **d**rugs (+1) or alcohol abuse (+1). A score of 3 or more indicates increased 1 year bleed risk on anticoagulation sufficient to justify caution or more regular review. Risk is for intracranial bleed, bleed requiring hospitalisation or a haemoglobin drop >2 g/L or that needs transfusion.

Management

- **AF and compromised.** Remember AF and fast AF can be a response to an infective, inflammatory or metabolic/toxic cause. Treatment must balance to focus on treating the underlying cause as well as using rate control drugs. Look for causality. If fast AF is causing compromise: ↓BP, LVF, angina then DC cardioversion (▶ Section 1.14) which may be done without anticoagulation but start treatment dose LMWH [NICE 2014]. If not severely compromised consider AMIODARONE 150–300 mg IV 30–60 min via a large bore cannula or preferably a central line. Any deterioration then emergency DC cardioversion. Further amiodarone infusions require a central line. Alternatives include DIGOXIN loading or a BETA-BLOCKER. Consider cardioversion if arrhythmia is less than 48 h, and start rate control if AF duration >48 h or is uncertain. Anticoagulate both. Consider Bisoprolol, Atenolol or Metoprolol (avoid Sotalol) especially if angina or hypertension. Digoxin can be loaded (check not on it already) useful especially if in LVF as DIGOXIN 500 mcg PO/slow IV over 1 h and then DIGOXIN 250–500 mcg PO/slow IV 6 h later. Digoxin slows resting rate and is an inotrope and best for those with CCF or a sedentary life. Reduce dose with renal failure. Rhythm control AF >48 h must wait until anticoagulated for a minimum of 3 weeks.
- **ABC, high flow oxygen** as needed. IV fluids cautiously if at all in LVF or fluid overloaded. Start treatment dose LMWH in all with AF and not anticoagulated with no contraindications. Look for and treat any cause: chest infection, thyrotoxicosis, ACS, PE, sepsis, MI/ACS, pulmonary oedema, PE, alcohol excess or withdrawal.
- **AF and well:** ventricular rate 60–120/min and haemodynamically well. Determine and manage cause. Anticoagulate (as above). Decide rhythm vs rate control strategy as defined below.

Rate control

- Consider oral beta-blocker or rate limiting CCB. Digoxin may be considered if sedentary lifestyle. Avoid Amiodarone long term as side effects significant.

Rhythm control – repeated attempts to regain SR (DC cardioversion, ▶ Section 1.14)

- **Anticoagulation and cardioversion:** you can electrically or chemically cardiovert immediately if you can be certain that AF duration is <48 h or a TOE shows that there is no LA appendage thrombus or it is clinical indicated due to instability. Start LMWH or IV Heparin immediately and continue for at least 3 weeks. If elective cardioversion then anticoagulate for 3 weeks before and at least 3 weeks after, even if successful. Chemical cardioversion – consider IV AMIODARONE infusion or Dronedarone. Flecainide can be used if LV function normal and no significant IHD.

- **Rhythm control preferred:** when patient is unstable and SR would improve haemodynamics, in younger symptomatic patients or those with stroke or cardiomyopathy. Overall prognosis, however, is the same.

Specific scenarios

- **Pre-excited AF and WPW syndrome:** use IV PROCAINAMIDE or IV AMIODARONE (or Sotalol or Flecainide) and if unstable then immediate DC cardioversion. Avoid digoxin, beta-blockers and Verapamil or Diltiazem in pre-excited AF. They may increase risk of VF. Assess for anticoagulation.
- **Prevention and management of postoperative AF:** with cardiothoracic surgery reduce postoperative AF by offering either amiodarone, a standard beta-blocker (not sotalol), a rate-limiting calcium antagonist. DO NOT offer digoxin. Continue any pre-existing beta blockade. Postop offer a rhythm based strategy. For postop AF, use appropriate antithrombotic therapy and correct identifiable precipitants (U&E, low SpO_2) [NICE 2014].
- **Atrial flutter** also needs rate control and risk assessed and anticoagulation. Beta blockade or diltiazem or digoxin for rate control. Cardioversion should be considered with same assessment and anticoagulation as for AF. AMIODARONE is useful for rapid rate control.
- **Anticoagulation:** consider in all with AF, atrial flutter or PAF. Determine **CHA$_2$DS$_2$VaSc score** and **HAS-BLED score** and assess risk/benefits of anticoagulation. Control hypertension, review need for aspirin or NSAIDs, stop/reduce alcohol. Do not avoid anticoagulation purely on 'risk of falls'. Quantify risk and intervene to reduce falls where possible. Anticoagulate CHA$_2$DS$_2$VaSc > 1 in men and >2 in women. If non-valvular AF (those with severe MS or AS or with a metal valve must have warfarin or LMWH) then consider Warfarin or a DOAC (Apixaban, Dabigatran or Rivaroxaban, etc.). High CHA$_2$DS$_2$VaSc score needs urgent commencement on LMWH or a DOAC or Warfarin. If anticoagulation contraindicated or not acceptable then consider cardiology referral for Left atrial appendage occlusion.
- **Bridging anticoagulation:** interruptions in anticoagulation can increase embolic risk. It is common to give LMWH bridging in the perioperative period but this may lead to risk of bleeding. A recent study has looked at this. The study **excluded** those with mechanical heart valves, stroke/TIA/systemic embolization within 12 weeks, major bleeding within 6 weeks, renal insufficiency, low platelets or planned cardiac, brain or spinal surgery. The conclusion was that bridging is not warranted for most AF patients with CHA$_2$DS$_2$VaSc scores of <4, for low-risk procedures. This study must be interpreted along with local expert guidance balancing the risk of peri-procedure bleeding and embolic risk [*N Engl J Med* 2015;373(9):823].

3.17   Aortic dissection

- **Discussion:** aorta consists of the layers intima, media and adventitia. Dissection involves separation of the media and intima often with intramural bleeding with haematoma which can dissect distally or sometimes proximally (into pericardium) powered by the hammering pulsatile force of aortic flow. If dissection suspected then arrange urgent CT aorta and if Type A dissection found you must reduce the BP whilst getting the patient to a cardiothoracic centre immediately. The mortality of untreated Type A dissections is approximately 1% per hour in the first 24 h, peaking with an overall in-hospital mortality of 58%, and 26% for those who undergo surgery. Note: a recent meta-analysis suggests that a negative D-dimer result may be useful to help rule out acute aortic dissection (and PE) in low-risk patients [*Ann Emerg Med* 2015;66:368].
- **Aetiology:** blood tracks under the intima and into the media. Bleeding from lumen or vasa vasorum causes intramural thrombus. The intima can tear distally and on CT

or other imaging there can be a 'true lumen" and 'false lumen'. May be connective tissue disease – cystic medial degeneration, Marfan's and Ehlers–Danlos syndrome. Blunt thoracic trauma causes a tear in the arterial wall. Intima tears within a few centimetres of the aortic valve, usually on the right lateral wall of the aortic arch where shear stresses are high. Distal dissections occur beyond left subclavian artery. Obstruction of RCA more common. Occlusion of LCA usually instantly fatal. Dissection can therefore be accompanied by MI.

- **Causes:** HTN, atherosclerosis, Marfan's syndrome, cystic medial degeneration, Ehlers–Danlos syndrome. Loeys–Dietz aneurysm syndrome, Turner syndrome. Trauma – sudden deceleration, cocaine, phaeochromocytoma, heavy weightlifting. Pregnancy, coarctation of the aorta, bicuspid aortic valves, aortitis – Takayasu's arteritis. Syphilis, aortic valve replacement, familial – autosomal dominant. Iatrogenic aortic manipulation (including angiography and stenting).

- **Stanford classification:** Stanford Type A (60%) – any involvement of ascending aorta. Mortality 80% in first 48 h and related to time to surgery. High risk rupture, tamponade, acute MI, stroke, acute AR and cardiogenic shock, innominate compromised (60–70%): involves proximal aorta and arch. Requires urgent surgery. Most tears are seen in upper right lateral wall of the ascending aorta. Stanford Type B (30–40%): not involving aorta, distal to left subclavian artery and may extend down as far as the iliac vessels and have better outcome; management is medical.

Clinical

- Chest/back pain – sudden anterior (root and ascending aorta) or interscapular (descending aorta) chest wall pain or even abdominal pain. Some pain may radiate into the back. Syncopal or presyncopal episode with tearing/stabbing/sharp interscapular pain. Aortic regurgitation: dissection can shear the aortic valve. Look for new early diastolic murmur suggesting AR and associated with acute LVF. History: Marfan's, bicuspid valve or hypertension. May be shocked if there is blood loss or tamponade. Aortic arch: dissection may shear off vessels in the proximal aorta (right brachiocephalic gives off right subclavian and carotid, left common carotid and left subclavian). Causes stroke. Reduced pulsation or reduced BP because the arm supplied by the subclavian/brachiocephalic artery is obstructed. Coronary artery: left main stem = sudden death with LV infarction; right coronary artery: inferior MI with chest pain. Right brachiocephalic: ischaemia of right subclavian, right common carotid and right vertebral. Devastating if complete with a right TACI with right hemiparesis or posterior circulation signs and right arm ischaemia and low BP. Left subclavian: ataxia (vertebral) and arm ischaemia and low BP left arm and posterior circulation symptoms and signs. Left common carotid: left TACI stroke with right hemiparesis. Anterior spinal artery: paraplegia affecting legs with preserved dorsal columns. Coeliac axis: ischaemic bowel. Renal artery: anuria, haematuria and AKI.

- **Differential:** chest pain (▶Section 3.3) but consider ACS and PE and oesophageal and lung causes.

Investigations

- **Bloods:** U&E, FBC, LFTs, troponin, group and cross-match. ⬆D-dimer with dissection (exclude PE/dissection with urgent CTPA/aorta). CXR: unfolded aorta, wide mediastinum (>6 cm), left pleural effusion may be exudate from an inflamed aorta. Widening mediastinum 80% of acute dissection. ECG: arrhythmias. Inferior MI if RCA involved. Longstanding LVH. Can be normal. CT aorta is diagnostic. Shows false lumen and true lumen of dissection. Defines the operative anatomy and involvement of branch vessels. False lumen can have a greater cross-sectional area. False lumen beaks are often filled with low attenuation thrombus. Outer wall calcification is present in true lumen. It is important to determine the luminal origins of branch vessels before surgery. The beak sign is the cross-sectional imaging manifestation of the wedge of haematoma that cleaves a space for the propagating false lumen and that is present microscopically in all dissections. May be picked up incidentally on CTPA. Transthoracic echo: suprasternal views may be useful. Transoesophageal echo: gives detailed views of aorta and valve. Main advantage is anatomical AND a functional assessment of aortic valve. Where available it is used instead of CT in high-risk patients.

- **Complications:** death from aortic rupture, ischaemic stroke – TACI-like presentation if brachiocephalic occluded. Subclavian obstruction may cause a possible posterior circulation event but collateral opposite vertebral. Cardiac tamponade (blood) – drainage can precipitate more bleeding and death. Acute aortic regurgitation and LVF, spinal cord infarction. Mesenteric/renal ischaemia. Left pleural haemothorax – ominous sign on CXR, sudden death, distal limb ischaemia.

Management

- **ABC resuscitation:** O_2 as per BTS. Good IV access ×2. If haemorrhage or tamponade death is usually imminent. Group and cross-match according to local policy because if cardiothoracic centre is in another hospital they may not accept blood cross-matched elsewhere. Cross-match will be for perioperative blood loss. Acute dissection of the ascending aorta is highly lethal with a cumulative mortality rate of 1–2% per hour so rapid stabilisation and transfer are needed. ECG and CXR to exclude differentials for acute chest pain. Inadvertent anticoagulation or thrombolysis (before PCI not uncommon as mistaken for Inf STEMI) should be avoided as can cause fatal haemorrhage or delay emergency surgery until managed. If suspicious for dissection then discuss now with radiology for CT aortogram which may also diagnose a PE. **Low risk patients:** pain relief: DIAMORPHINE 2.5–5.0 mg IV or MORPHINE 5–10 mg IV for chest pain may help reduce preload and pulmonary oedema. Blood (pulse) pressure: hammering pulsatile driving pressure of dp/dt BP and pulse pressure with NITROPRUSSIDE (lower than normal dose) and LABETALOL IV in Type A. In those with Type B dissection these agents can be used acutely and then patient managed on oral medication. Consider aiming for SBP = 100 mmHg. Cardiac tamponade: emergency pericardiocentesis of an acute Type A aortic dissection complicated by cardiac tamponade can result in sudden deterioration and should be avoided if possible; proceed as urgently as possible to the operative surgical repair of the aorta with intra-operative drainage of the haemopericardium. Cardiothoracic surgery for Type A involves replacement of proximal aorta by a tube graft – may require resection and replacement of the aortic valve and sewing in of coronary vessels and repair of the coronary sinus. Surgery is done using cardiopulmonary bypass and the patient cooled to 22°C. Endovascular treatment involving the insertion of stents is still a research area but is used in some centres. Mortality rate with surgery for Type A dissection is 26% and for those treated medically is 58%. Patients need to move immediately to a cardiothoracic centre. Contact and discuss urgent transfer. Delay increases mortality. Long term management: both Type A and B require long term BP control. Beta-blocker-based therapy is the foundation of long term medical management. ACE inhibitors may be beneficial. Lifelong imaging of the entire aorta at regular intervals for further problems by either CT or MRI is advocated. Uncomplicated Type B dissection has an in-hospital mortality rate of 10%.

Reference: Braverman (2010) Acute aortic dissection: clinician update. *Circulation*, 122:184.

 Acute myocarditis

- **About:** dilated flabby heart with risk of fatal arrhythmias and heart failure. Due to infectious and non-infectious triggers.

- **Aetiology:** inflamed myocardium. Dilated poorly functioning heart. Can result in end-stage cardiac failure, thromboembolism and arrhythmias. Regarded as a precursor of dilated cardiomyopathy (DCM).
- **Causes:** idiopathic: all investigations negative; 50% presumably viral but unproven. Viral infection: parvovirus B19 and HHV6, Coxsackie A (mild), Coxsackie B (severe) and influenza; echovirus; adenovirus; HIV; CMV. Non-viral infection: Chagas disease (*Trypanosoma cruzi*), toxoplasmosis. Rickettsial: Scrub typhus, Rocky Mountain spotted fever, Q fever, Lyme disease causes temporary conduction block. Bacterial: leptospirosis, diphtheria, TB, brucella. Drugs and toxins: doxorubicin, herceptin, cyclophosphamide, penicillin, phenytoin, methyldopa, cocaine abuse. Heavy metals: arsenic, cobalt, mercury exposure. Miscellaneous: radiation, peripartum cardiomyopathy, post cardiac transplant rejection. Inflammatory: sarcoidosis, Kawasaki disease, SLE, Wegener's granulomatosis, thyrotoxicosis, rheumatoid arthritis, rheumatic fever. Giant cell myocarditis: rare usually fatal form of myocarditis. Ventricular arrhythmias and severe cardiac failure.
- **Clinical:** fatigue, dyspnoea, Chest pain, LVF, AF, VT or sudden cardiac death, MR, S4, ask about recent viral illness and drug usage. Coexisting pericarditis, pericardial effusion, tamponade.

Investigation

- **Bloods:** FBC: ↑WCC, ↑CRP ↑ESR. Others: check ANA, dsDNA, ASO titres, TFTs. HIV test. ECG: AF, ST/T wave changes even mimicking STEMI/NSTEMI; those with Q waves or LBBB are a poor prognostic group; ectopics, VT, VF, heart block. **CXR:** cardiomegaly, pulmonary oedema. Cardiac biomarkers: ↑CK and CKMB, ↑troponin in proportion to damage. **Echocardiogram:** assess LV and RV dysfunction, enlarged chambers, thrombus, pericardial effusion, and valve regurgitation. **Cardiac MRI:** non-invasive and valuable clinical tool for the diagnosis of myocarditis. Initial changes in myocardial tissue can be seen on T2-weighted oedema imaging. **Transvenous endomyocardial biopsy:** rarely done but is the gold standard for diagnosis. It may show lymphocytic infiltration and myocyte necrosis. Giant cells in Giant cell myocarditis. **Serology and PCR:** influenza or Coxsackie serology and parvovirus. **Coronary angiography:** if IHD/ACS suspected.
- **Complications:** some develop a dilated cardiomyopathy and end-stage heart failure which may improve. VT / VF. Heart block needing pacing. Sudden cardiac death, thromboembolism.

Management

- **Supportive:** bed-rest, treat heart failure and arrhythmias as usual. Usually in CCU with telemetry depending on presentation and severity. Ensure access to early defibrillation. **Standard heart failure regime** including beta-blockers, diuretics, ACE inhibitors or angiotensin-II receptor blockers (ARBs) should be initiated. **Intraaortic balloon pumping** may be considered to augment cardiac output whilst awaiting improvement, treatment or transplant. VTE prophylaxis and full anticoagulation, especially if AF or LA / LV thrombus. *Steroids have no evidence base.* **IV immunoglobulin** (400 mg/kg per day) for 5 days may help preserve LVEF in adult acute fulminant myocarditis. **Others:** immunosuppression for giant cell myocarditis. Antiprotozoal therapy for Chagas disease. Withdrawal of toxic medications. Avoid exercise during acute period and convalescence. Heart transplant in those with dilated CMP, giant cell myocarditis, end-stage cardiac failure. Cardiogenic shock and heart failure, ▶Section 2.16.

References: Kinderman *et al.* (2012) Update on myocarditis. *J Am Coll Cardiol*, 59:779. Dan-Qing Yu *et al.* (2014) IVIG in the therapy of adult acute fulminant myocarditis: A retrospective study. *Exp Ther Med*, 7:97.

3.19 ▶ Acute pericarditis

- **About:** seen in 5% of CCU chest pain admissions. 90% are idiopathic or viral. May be found in association with acute myocarditis and both have similar aetiologies. Saddle-shaped ST elevation in all leads except aVr is likely to be pericarditis. Avoid anticoagulants as risk of haemopericardium. Also see myocarditis, ▶ Section 3.18.

- **Causes of pericarditis: idiopathic** is commonest (presumably viral). **Viral:** parvovirus B19, echovirus, Coxsackie B, influenza, CMV, EBV, adenovirus, HBV, HCV, H1N1, HIV (may cause *Staph. aureus* effusion). **Bacterial/fungal:** TB may go on to constrictive pericarditis. ↑ESR/JVP, dyspnoea, fever, weight loss. *Coxiella burnetii*, pneumococcus, meningococcal. Pyogenic post-op pericarditis or post pneumonia. Fungal: histoplasmosis. **Inflammatory:** post myocardial injury (Dressler's syndrome), autoimmune disorder (SLE/RA/Behçet's), drug-induced lupus (hydralazine, procainamide), familial Mediterranean fever, rheumatic fever (with associated pancarditis and murmurs, rash, joint aches). **Malignancy:** lymphoma, carcinoma of bronchus or breast cancer, melanoma, leukaemia. **Miscellaneous:** metabolic (uraemia – end-stage kidney disease – needs dialysis), hypothyroid/myxoedema (large chronic effusion but rarely compromising).

- **Clinical:** fever, malaise, myalgia, post-viral syndrome. Pleuritic-type chest pain eased by sitting forwards, worse lying flat and on inspiration. Pain referred to shoulder or scapula. Auscultation friction rub (very useful sign worth looking for) with a systolic (ventricular filling) and atrial systolic component.

- **Diagnostic criteria:** presence of all 4 makes diagnosis probable: (1) typical chest pain associated with pericarditis, (2) pericardial friction rub on auscultation, (3) ECG changes such as diffuse ST elevation, (4) new or increased pericardial effusion.

- **Differential:** ACS, aortic dissection, PE, oesophageal disease, musculoskeletal.

Investigation

- **Bloods:** FBC: ↑WCC, ↑ESR and ↑CRP with infective and inflammatory causes. U&E: AKI or CKD with uraemic pericarditis. TFT: ↑TSH > 10 mU/L and low FT4 diagnoses hypothyroidism. **CXR and tuberculin testing:** if TB suspected. HIV test: where suspected. Other viral studies where indicated. **ECG:** saddle-shaped ST elevation and PR depression in all leads **except aVr** which look into the cavity of the heart where there is therefore an inverted lead, showing ST depression. Eventually ST and PR normalise and there is T wave inversion, which then normalises. May be AF or other atrial arrhythmias. ECG may be low voltage if effusion. **CXR:** usually normal but any cardiac enlargement or globular heart is suggestive of effusion. **Echocardiogram:** to look for pericardial fluid, LV function (as ever very important), tamponade. Pericardial effusion may be classified into 3 groups according to diastolic distance between the pericardium and the ventricle: (1) <10 mm, (2) moderate 10–20 mm, (3) severe >20 mm. The incidence of cardiac tamponade secondary to severe pericardial effusion is about 3%. RV dysfunction seems to be the greatest predictor of mortality and cardiac transplantation. CK and troponin: elevated in 50% if there is an associated myopericarditis. Diagnostic pericardiocentesis: exclude TB and diagnose malignancy where appropriate.

Management

- **Acute treatment:** full dose (consider adding PPI) anti-inflammatories are given, e.g. IBUPROFEN 400–600 mg 8 h (+PPI) until CRP/ESR normalises usually in 10–14 days. Combine this with COLCHICINE 0.5 mg BD for 3 months for patients weighing >70 kg or 0.5 mg OD if weight ≤70 kg reduces symptoms by day 3 and incidence of recurrence from 55% to 24% at 18 months, as well as risk of subsequent hospitalisation. Steroids are associated with an increased risk of recurrence and are usually avoided. Avoid exercise and exertion whilst symptomatic. If systemically unwell or associated myocarditis, significant effusion, arrhythmias, then hospitalise. Most can be managed with ambulatory care. Physical exertion is avoided in the acute phase and in up to 6 months in athletes. Repeat echo where needed. Outpatient management is sufficient in most uncomplicated cases if troponin negative. Therapeutic pericardiocentesis if evidence of tamponade but this is uncommon. Where diagnosis is unclear and pain continues and risk of IHD high then angiography may be required to exclude ACS. Patients should be given clear advice on re-admission if there are new or on-going symptoms.

- **Risk assessment:** admit if fever >38°C, subacute onset, immunosuppression, anticoagulation treatment, traumatic aetiology, myopericarditis, severe pericardial effusion, cardiac tamponade, or no anti-inflammatory response after 1 week. Weigh up risks of low dose VTE and haemorrhage into pericardium. Pericarditis may be seen post pneumonia and may require IV antibiotics depending on the likely organism. Any suggestion of a purulent or malignant effusion will need urgent consideration for drainage following imaging.
- **Recurrent pericarditis:** consider further colchicine and reassessment.
- **Effusion:** any concerns about effusion settled with echocardiogram. The main worry is fluid collection and tamponade. See section below on pericardial effusion; if there is any effusion take expert advice.

Reference: Freixa (2010) Evaluation, management, and treatment of acute pericarditis and myocarditis in the emergency department. *Emergencias*, 22:301.

 ## 3.20 Pericardial effusion/tamponade

Look for tachycardia, ↓BP, narrow pulse pressure, and elevated neck veins, distant heart sounds with recent pericarditis, thoracic malignancy, chest trauma, coagulopathy or recent cardiac procedure. Pericardiocentesis can be lifesaving.

- **About:** see pericarditis above. Reverse all anticoagulants if suspected spontaneous or post interventional/trauma-related bleeding into pericardial space. Tamponade is uncommon even with large pericardial effusions – prevent with elective drainage. Small effusions are often found at routine echocardiogram. Also see Pericarditis, ▶ Section 3.19.
- **Aetiology:** fluid/blood collects in the pericardial space. Normally pericardial space holds less than 50 ml of fluid. Chronic accumulation over months can produce up to 1000 ml without significant compromise as pericardial sac stretches, unless there is chronic scarring or thickening. In cardiac tamponade, the pericardial pressure may reach 15–20 mmHg, leading to an equalisation of pressures into the cardiac chambers and to a huge decrease in the systemic venous return. Acute accumulations of even 100 ml may be enough to cause haemodynamic collapse as increased volume and pressure leads the right atrium and then the right ventricle to collapse in diastole. Beck's triad can be detected with low BP, reduced heart sounds and ↑JVP with prominent *x* descent and absent *y* descent. Slow collections tolerated well. If diastolic cardiac filling compromised then tamponade. Absence of pericardium is not problematic at all.
- **Causes of effusion: (see pericarditis)** idiopathic, viral, hypothyroid, SLE, amyloid, scleroderma, HIV, drugs: isoniazid, phenytoin, hydralazine, procainamide. Causes more likely to produce tamponade are neoplastic disease, idiopathic pericarditis, renal disease, tuberculosis, bleeding – warfarin, DOAC, heparin, DIC, trauma, uraemia, post MI and ventricular rupture, Type A aortic dissection proximally. Post procedure – cardiac catheterisation or pacemaker insertion, transeptal catheter.

- **Clinical** (signs of effusion and likely causes): asymptomatic if small, pericarditis-type symptoms. Cough, fever, malaise and systemic symptoms. Muffled heart sounds. Right heart failure with peripheral oedema and hepatomegaly. Cachexia and weight loss may suggest malignancy, TB or HIV. **Acute tamponade:** ↓HR due to pericardial stretch followed by ↓BP. Pulsus paradoxus: radial pulse impalpable during inspiration (marked fall in BP >10 mmHg). JVP: markedly ↑ (RA pressure ↑) which rises with inspiration. Kussmaul's sign and loss of y descent. Heart sounds are quiet and area of cardiac dullness increases.
- **Differential:** ACS, aortic dissection, PE, oesophageal disease.

Investigation

- **FBC:** ↑WCC, ↑ESR, ↑CRP if inflammatory/infective. **Coagulation screen** if on anticoagulants. **ECG:** low voltage QRS complexes, AF, evidence of pericarditis or recent MI. Electrical alternans. CXR: shows cardiac enlargement (cardiomegaly or effusion need echo to differentiate) or may show underlying neighbouring malignancy. Large effusions present as globular cardiomegaly with sharp margins. If the effusion develops during catheterisation, it may also be identified by the development of lucent lines in the cardiopericardial silhouette or so-called epicardial halo sign or fat pad sign. Straightening and immobility of the left heart border. CXR may show TB or lung malignancy. **Echocardiogram:** pericardial effusion – measure diastolic distance between the pericardium and the ventricle: (1) <10 mm, (2) moderate 10–20 mm, (3) severe >20 mm. The incidence of cardiac tamponade secondary to severe pericardial effusion is about 3%. Tamponade: diastolic collapse of RA and free wall of RV are signs of incipient circulatory compromise. RV collapse is the most specific echo finding. Also look for fall in mitral inflow velocity or aortic velocity by 25% with inspiration. Invasive monitoring would show a fall in aortic pressure and rise in RA pressure. Echo can be used to guide pericardiocentesis. Cardiac MRI is useful for detecting pericardial effusion and loculated pericardial effusion and thickening. **Cardiac troponin I/T:** usually negative except where there is an associated myopericarditis or ACS. Check clotting: if coagulopathy or warfarin and haemopericardium suspected. Diagnostic pericardiocentesis +/– pericardial biopsy if TB or malignancy suspected. Exudate suggests an infective/inflammatory or malignant process. Measure pericardial effusion adenosine deaminase for TB, tumour marker measurement (CEA, cytokeratin 19 fragment) and cytology for neoplasms, and culture and PCR for infections. Protein, LDH, Hb, WCC, viral, bacterial, TB cultures. Others: tuberculin skin test, blood cultures, complement levels, ANA, ESR if SLE suspected.

Management

- **Not compromised** and infection not suspected then diagnosis can be made by other methods and pericardiocentesis not indicated. Treat underlying causes, e.g. Thyroxine for hypothyroid, dialysis for uraemia. Need for anticoagulation should be assessed and balanced with risk of bleeding into pericardial space. Effusions >1 cm depth need repeat echo in 7 days and ongoing follow-up. Elective pericardiocentesis is relatively safe and easy with either echocardiography or fluoroscopy guided pericardiocentesis. Some advocate drainage of large effusions to prevent possible evolution of cardiac tamponade where the effusion >20 mm depth and not responsive to medical therapy after 4–6 weeks. Other indications include evidence of RA or RV collapse, and any significant chronic (>3 months) effusion. Pericardiocentesis often does not aid diagnosis but may prevent tamponade. Not all effusions need to be drained and can be followed by serial echocardiography.
- **Compromised:** ABCs. Resuscitation, O₂. Good IV access. Give 0.5–1.0 L NS to ensure filling pressures. Volume resuscitation and catecholamines are temporary but the only remaining effective treatment in tamponade is urgent needle

pericardiocentesis, except where a Type A proximal aortic dissection is suspected which can cause circulatory collapse – needs cardiothoracic advice. If anticoagulated suspect bleeding into pericardial space – stop and reverse any coagulopathy.

Volume loading: may be beneficial and repeated trials of 250–500 ml of crystalloid should be assessed for improvement of haemodynamics. Catecholamines and IV NITROPRUSSIDE to reduce afterload and/or IV DOBUTAMINE may also be of benefit in some patients. **Emergency pericardiocentesis:** consider transfer to tertiary centre if stable or summon local expertise. If high risk of recurrence consider cardiothoracic referral for pericardial fenestration to prevent any further build-up of fluid. It may be attempted in cardiac arrest in those at risk with PEA [see Emergency Pericardiocentesis Video. *New Engl J Med* 2012;366:e17].

References: Bodson *et al.* (2011) Cardiac tamponade. *Curr Opin Crit Care*, 17:416. Maisch *et al.* (2004) Guidelines on the diagnosis and management of pericardial diseases: executive summary. *Eur Heart J*, 25:587. Imazio *et al.* (2009) *Nat Rev Cardiol*, 6:743.

3.21 Severe (malignant) hypertension

- **About:** less common now as primary care screening and treatment. BP causes end organ damage over years and acute rises should be gradually reduced in most cases. Evidence base for acute hypertensive emergency management is lacking. Malignant hypertension by definition requires fundoscopy to see Grade 3/4 retinal changes.
- **Aetiology:** untreated/undiagnosed essential hypertension; failure to take medication. Phaeochromocytoma or other secondary cause. Acute cocaine, severe anxiety, pain, acute urinary retention, pre-eclampsia. Acute stroke.
- **Clinical:** asymptomatic to mild malaise, mild headache, anxiety, distress. Breathless with pulmonary oedema, microangiopathic haemolytic anaemia. Renal failure, stroke (ischaemic or haemorrhagic). Fundoscopy – retinal haemorrhages and papilloedema, confusion. Delirium – encephalopathy, look for clues in history and examine. Phaeochromocytoma, renal bruits, radiofemoral delay. Renal masses, examine drug chart – NSAID, ciclosporin.
- **Malignant hypertension:** high BP + retinal haemorrhages + papilloedema + nephropathy or chest pain. Beware watershed cerebral infarction with rapid lowering.

Investigations

- FBC, U&E (CKD, low K with Conn's syndrome). ECG: AF, LVH, LAD, LBBB, ST/T wave changes. R plus S greater than 35 mm. CXR: cardiomegaly, rib notching with coarctation of the aorta. Echocardiogram: LVH, diastolic dysfunction, assess LV (exclude coarctation). Renal USS: small kidneys with CKD, polycystic kidneys, difference in size with RAS. Adrenal hyperplasia or tumour mass. Urine for proteinuria, cocaine, amphetamines. Others: urinary catecholamines, dexamethasone suppression, renin/aldosterone levels. CT/MRI head: if new neurology, e.g. haemorrhage or infarct, tumour or posterior reversible encephalopathy syndrome.

Secondary causes of hypertension, clues, investigations and treatment

- **Conn's syndrome:** U&E low K, renin/aldosterone levels. Adrenal imaging. Adenoma or hyperplasia. Consider Aldosterone antagonists.
- **Cushing's syndrome:** ↑urinary free cortisol, dexamethasone suppression, Cushingoid appearance, striae, weight gain, hirsutism. Low ACTH suggests non pituitary source. Needs adrenal/pituitary imaging.
- **Drugs:** OCP, ciclosporin, alcohol, NSAIDs, amphetamines.
- **Cocaine-induced HTN:** use IV nitrates, calcium antagonists and DIAZEPAM. Avoid beta-blockers.

- **Aortic coarctation:** 0.25%. CXR changes, echo, MRA, CT aorta. Hypertension upper body. May need surgery, hypertension often persists.
- **Renal artery stenosis:** 0.5%. USS for size disparity, MRA, flash oedema, renal bruit, AKI with ACE inhibitor.
- **Polycystic kidney disease:** USS, family history, HTN. Risk of Berry aneurysms and SAH.
- **Pre-eclampsia:** pregnancy, proteinuria, etc. (see <u>Eclampsia</u>, ▶ Section 15.5).
- **Phaeochromocytoma:** elevated urine catecholamines, metanephrines and plasma catecholamines. Tumour seen on CT abdomen. 10% are extra-adrenal (in sympathetic chain from neck to bladder) 10% malignant and bilateral. Ensure alpha blockade before beta-blockers for BP control. If acute need to treat then PHENTOLAMINE 2–5 mg IV bolus. If stable then PHENOXYBENZAMINE 20–80 mg/d initially in divided doses followed by PROPRANOLOL 120–240 mg/d. Alternatively start DOXAZOSIN 2–4 mg/d in divided doses. Also consider IV nitrates, calcium antagonists and DIAZEPAM. If perioperative management there can be a huge fall in circulating catecholamines once the tumour is removed and sudden fall in SVR needing rapid volume replacement.

Indications for emergency BP reduction

Acute BP lowering is not risk-free and risks vs. benefits need to be evaluated. Rapid BP drops can cause myocardial and cerebral hypoperfusion. Resist the urge to urgently lower unless there are clear indications. In many 'new' cases, BP has been chronically high for a long time just unmeasured or unrecognised, or recognised but undertreated or non-compliant. Severe hypertension is really a chronic often silent disease causing damage to heart, kidney and small penetrating blood vessels in the brain over years.

- **Acute pulmonary oedema:** lower to level that helps resolves oedema. Preference for starting ACE inhibitor, IV FUROSEMIDE + IV NITRATES.
- **Acute MI:** (↑BP increases myocardial work and ischaemia) preference for IV NITRATES + start small dose ACE inhibitor.
- **Acute aortic dissection:** BP target <120/80 mmHg if tolerated especially for proximal dissection. Use LABETALOL 20–40 mg IV stat then infusion.
- **Acute intracerebral haemorrhage:** gradually lower by 10–20% over several hours, e.g. LABETALOL 20–40 mg IV stat.
- **Hypertensive encephalopathy:** (headache, confusion, seizures, symptoms + papilloedema) use IV LABETALOL though no real preference.
- **Stroke thrombolysis:** lower BP to <185/110 mmHg if safe to do so within the thrombolysis time frame. A rapid drop in BP and cerebral blood flow might cause watershed infarcts and do more harm than thrombolysis benefits. Likely to be more at risk if significant cerebral atherosclerosis.
- **Management:** general measures: a quiet room, good nursing care and a calm bedside manner can help reduce BP, as well as a quiet ward rather than the busy ED. No smoking, no coffee. In an asymptomatic patient with BP >220/120 mmHg then rest, relief of pain, agitation, urinary retention and simple observation and commencing one or more oral agents for a few hours may suffice, and follow-up within days may be reasonable. A higher BP may warrant admission for on-going assessment, especially with evidence of end-organ damage or any symptoms, but ambulatory care should be sufficient. In those without urgent need to reduce BP then lower BP in a slow controlled manner over hours and days to acceptable levels (e.g. to <180/110 mmHg) using slow onset oral agents. Target a gradual reduction to a normal BP over days rather than minutes or hours unless complicated.

Specific cases

- **Urgent reduction:** general measures + oral drugs – lower BP over hours unless urgent indications (see above). No evidence base for which drugs to use. Suggest AMLODIPINE 5 mg PO and/or ATENOLOL 25 mg PO. Avoid beta-blocker if phaeochromocytoma likely (paroxysms of sweating ++, palpitations, headache). Set a target that is perhaps 10–20% lower than the current BP, e.g. 180/110 mmHg. But immediate aim is not to achieve a BP of 140/90 mmHg. If precipitated by stopping usual BP meds and no adverse effects with these then consider re-introduction slowly perhaps one by one until controlled.
- **Emergency BP reduction:** severe cases as described above or, if BP sustained at >220/120 mmHg despite other measures, then consider (if no history of bronchospasm/asthma) LABETALOL 20–40 mg slow IV over 5 min which is easy to give as a bolus or infusion. An alternative, especially if angina or pulmonary oedema, is IV GTN or ISOSORBIDE DINITRATE (ISOKET). The nitric oxide donor NITROPRUSSIDE 0.5–1.5 mcg/kg/min IV can also be considered. No need to treat BP in ischaemic stroke unless sustained BP >220/120 mmHg, or patient is for thrombolysis or acute haemorrhage. Reduce BP slowly.
- **Additional steps:** if agitation or delirium or aggression is a driver to the BP consider DIAZEPAM 2–5 mg PO/IV or HALOPERIDOL 1–2 mg PO/IV which can be given orally or IM/IV. Beta-blockers avoided if phaeochromocytoma suspected. Give FUROSEMIDE 20–50 mg IV or GTN 2 sprays (800 mcg) for pulmonary oedema.
- **Manage AKI and exclude renal causes:** check urine – blood, protein and nephritis and renal parenchymal causes (see AKI, ▶ Section 10.4). Consider a urinary catheter if you really need to assess urine output or exclude obstruction. Always double check (especially in older confused patient) that you haven't missed urinary retention or untreated pain with its usual pressor response. Patients can be significantly volume depleted and may need volume expansion once BP is controlled with IV NS.
- **Ongoing BP management algorithm: age <55** Step 1: ACE or ARB. Step 2: add CCB or Thiazide. Step 3: add CCB and Thiazide. Step 4: low dose Spironolactone/Beta-blocker/Alpha-blocker. **Age >55 or Afro-Caribbean** Step 1: CCB. Step 2: CCB or Thiazide + ACE inhibitor/ARB. Step 3: CCB + Thiazide + ACE inhibitor/ARB. Step 4: add low dose Spironolactone/Beta-blocker/Alpha-blocker.

3.22 Infective endocarditis

- **About:** infection of cardiac valves/endocardium. Underlying structural cardiac defects. Rheumatic heart disease less common so now seen in older patients and those with prosthetic valves. Mortality 15–20%.
- **Pathology:** infective vegetations form on heart valves containing fibrin, platelets, and microorganisms. High pressure jet of blood on endocardium or valve. Vegetations can embolise. Rheumatic heart disease, congenital heart disease or other lesions. Seen with aortic sclerosis, and bicuspid aortic valves. IV drug user has a ×30 greater risk of *Staph. aureus* of tricuspid valve. Mitral valve prolapse ×10 risk and now commonest valve lesion affected.
- **Aetiology: Pacemaker endocarditis:** early cases caused by *Staph. aureus* and late cases by *Staph. epidermidis*. **Native valve endocarditis (NVE):** *Strep. viridans* 40%, *Staph. aureus* 20%, *Enterococcus* spp. 10%, others are streptococci, coagulase-negative staphylococci, Gram-negative bacilli, fungi. **Early onset prosthetic valve endocarditis (PVE)** (<60 days post-op): *Staph. epidermidis* 40%, *Staph. aureus* 9%, *Enterococci* 6%, Gram-negative bacilli 4%, fungi 11%, others. **IV drug users:** tricuspid valve endocarditis with *Staph. aureus/epidermidis*. **Bicuspid aortic valve:** aortic valve endocarditis.

Organisms causing endocarditis

- **Staph. aureus:** most common, more aggressive acute endocarditis-type disease of normal valves or may be post-operative, e.g. post pacemaker. Risks: central IV lines, IV drug users. Causes early and late prosthetic valve endocarditis and pacemaker endocarditis.
- **Strep. viridans:** a low virulence organism seen where there is a history of rheumatic fever. An oral commensal. Causes a subacute clinical picture.
- **Coagulase-negative** staphylococcus: usually causes early PVE. Occasionally pacemaker endocarditis. They may produce a biofilm on prosthetic surfaces, which also promotes adherence.
- **Fungal endocarditis:** prolonged antibiotics or parenteral nutrition. Often immunocompromised. Usually *Candida albicans* or *C. parapsilosis*.
- **HACEK group:** Gram-negative bacteria. Fastidious. *Haemophilus*, *Actinobacillus*, *Cardiobacterium*, *Eikenella*, and *Kingella* species. May be ill for months. Painful embolic lesion to an extremity.
- **Q fever endocarditis:** *Coxiella burnetii* is an example. May be no fever. Valvular heart disease and on immunosuppressive therapy. Vegetations rare on echo. Organism isolated from buffy coat cultures. Serological studies are reasonably specific.

Cardiac disease and risk of endocarditis

- **High risk:** previous endocarditis, aortic valve disease, rheumatic heart disease, prosthetic valves, mitral regurgitation or AR, VSD, ductus arteriosus, aortic coarctation, acyanotic congenital heart disease.
- **Medium risk:** aortic stenosis, mitral valve prolapse with MR (commonest cause), mitral stenosis, tricuspid disease, pulmonary stenosis. HOCM with LV outflow obstruction.
- **Low risk:** secundum ASD, IHD, previous CABG, MVP without MR.

- **Clinical:** fever, malaise, joint pains, stroke/TIA-like episodes if emboli. Peripheral emboli – gangrene/ischaemic bowel, finger clubbing is rare. Osler's nodes – painful, tender nodules on the pulps of fingers. Janeway lesions – small (<5 mm) flat painless red spots seen on palms and soles. Roth's spots – retinal haemorrhage and micro-infarction. New or changing murmurs. Splenomegaly. Splinter haemorrhages hands and feet – also seen in manual workers, labourers on dominant hand.

Investigations

- **FBC:** anaemia, ↑WCC, ESR and CRP. U&E. Urinalysis – microscopic haematuria. ECG: new AV block, increased PR interval suggests aortic valve/root involvement. CXR: evidence of cardiomegaly, mitral stenosis. **Echo (transthoracic) findings:** mobile intracardiac mass (vegetation), root or valve abscess, partial dehiscence of prosthetic valve, new valve regurgitation. **Transoesophageal echo:** TOE indicated if transthoracic echo negative and suspicion or with prosthetic valve. A normal echo does not exclude the diagnosis. **Blood cultures:** at least 6 from multiple sites spaced in time before antibiotics started. Use fastidious care to avoid contaminants. Do not start antibiotics until this has been done unless the organism is known or the infection is proven and severe. Great care especially where common skin contaminants may easily be interpreted as pathogens (e.g. prosthetic heart valves) aids interpretation of cultures showing coagulase-negative *Staph*.
- **Complications:** valve failure with heart failure (and cardiogenic shock), septic emboli, e.g. stroke (avoid anticoagulation), Glomerulonephritis, aortic root abscess, valvular abscess. Pericarditis, death, conduction defects.

Modified Duke criteria for diagnosis: 2 major, or 1 major + 2 minor, or 5 minor criteria (BC = blood culture)

- **2 major criteria are** (1) positive blood culture for typical IE organisms (*Strep. viridans* or *bovis*, HACEK, *Staph. aureus*, enterococcus), from 2 separate BC or 2 positive BC drawn >12 h apart, or 3 or a majority of 4 separate BC (first and last sample drawn 1 h apart) OR *Coxiella burnetii* detected by at least one positive BC or IgG antibody titre for Q fever phase 1 antigen >1:800. (2) Echocardiogram with oscillating intracardiac mass on valve or supporting structures, in the path of regurgitant jets, or on implanted material in the absence of an alternative anatomic explanation, or abscess, or new partial dehiscence of prosthetic valve or new valvular regurgitation.
- **5 minor criteria are** (1) risk: predisposing heart condition or IV drug use. (2) Fever: >38.0°C. (3) Vascular phenomena: major arterial emboli, septic pulmonary infarcts, mycotic aneurysm, intracranial haemorrhage, conjunctival haemorrhages, Janeway lesion. (4) Immunological phenomena: glomerulonephritis, Osler's nodes, Roth spots, +ve RF. (5) Positive blood culture not meeting major criterion.

Management

- Involve cardiology and microbiology for advice. Those with valve destruction and heart failure or abscess formation or vegetations and embolic concerns or failing antibiotics should be urgently discussed with tertiary cardiac surgeons. Vegetations and surface of valves relatively avascular so difficult to treat effectively with antibiotics. See also Cardiogenic shock and heart failure, ▶Section 2.16.
- **Starting antibiotics:** if patient stable and endocarditis uncomplicated can wait 1–2 days to get multiple cultures before starting antibiotics. Complicated endocarditis should receive empirical antibiotic as soon as 3–6 sets of blood cultures taken from different sites over a day if possible. Review antibiotics as soon as aetiological agent is identified. Duration of therapy is usually 4–6 weeks but depends on the organism, microbiology advice and whether native or prosthetic valve.

Antibiotic therapy for endocarditis

- Blind (organism unknown) native valve: AMOXICILLIN +/– low dose GENTAMICIN
- Blind prosthetic: VANCOMYCIN + RIFAMPICIN + low dose GENTAMICIN
- Native valve *Staph*.: FLUCLOXACILLIN IV for 4 weeks; pen. allergy VANCOMYCIN + RIFAMPICIN
- Prosthetic *Staph*.: FLUCLOXACILLIN IV + RIFAMPICIN + low dose GENTAMICIN
- Streptococcal: BENZYLPENICILLIN IV +/– low dose GENTAMICIN OR VANCOMYCIN + GENTAMICIN
- Enterococcal: AMOXICILLIN or BENZYLPENICILLIN IV + low dose GENTAMICIN; pen. allergy VANCOMYCIN + low dose GENTAMICIN
- HACEK group: AMOXICILLIN or CEFTRIAXONE +/– low dose GENTAMICIN

3.23   Cardiomyopathy

- **Aetiology:** a generic term for diseases affecting the myocardium with altered function. Some are inherited (often autosomal dominant), some toxic – alcohol and other drugs and others post infectious and the remainder idiopathic. Ischaemic-induced damage is usually excluded. Can cause issues with contraction (systolic) or filling (diastolic) or both. In some there may be outflow obstruction.

Cardiomyopathies

- **Dilated:** may be post viral myocarditis. Impaired contraction. Heart becomes globular and flabby. Many are idiopathic, some genetic (with muscular dystrophies), some autoimmune. Also seen with HIV. Causes chest pain, embolism, heart failure and SCD. Commoner in males. Needs beta-blockers, ACE inhibitors and consideration for AICD.

- **Restrictive:** impaired filling due to stiff walls. Seen in diseases with deposition of material in myocardium, e.g. amyloid (check for myeloma).

- **Hypertrophic:** inherited defect of cardiac muscle proteins. A minority also have LVOT obstruction (HOCM). ECG shows deep T wave inversion and inferior Q waves can mimic IHD. Heart is stiff with a mainly diastolic dysfunction due to asymmetrical septal hypertrophy (ASH) often with systolic anterior movement of anterior mitral valve leaflet. Jerky pulse, LVH. Systolic murmurs from LVOT and MR. Variants with mainly apical hypertrophy. Exertional chest pain and dyspnoea. SCD is seen often with or after exercise. Rx beta blockade, Verapamil, Disopyramide. Amiodarone for arrhythmias. Myomectomy/septal ablation for LVOT obstruction. Avoid digoxin and vasodilators. High risk need AICD.

- **Takotsubo:** transient anterior and apical ballooning seen on echo. Emotional stress. Post-menopausal women. ECG anterior leads show ST elevation V3–6 then T wave inversion. Normal coronary angiogram. Impaired but reversible LV function resolves in 2 months. Treat with IABP, fluids, beta-blockers or calcium channel blockers.

- **Alcoholic:** chronic alcohol abuse 5–10 years. Usually dilated. Multifactorial. Alcohol and malnutrition. Can entirely resolve with abstention.

- **Arrhythmogenic RV** (ARVC): genetic disorder (AD) of desmosomal proteins. Fibrofatty infiltration of RV. Risk of monomorphic VT with LBBB and RAD or VF and SCD. ECG: precordial T wave inversion in right precordial leads and epsilon waves. Diagnosis/screening by cardiac MRI. Treat with beta-blockers, Amiodarone, AICD.

- **Ventricular non-compaction:** imaging (echo then MRI) shows prominent trabeculae at the apex. In some there is a risk of arrhythmias and thromboembolisms which in some needs an AICD and anticoagulation. In many is benign.

- **Obliterative:** endocardial fibrosis and reduced ventricular cavity. Develops MR/TR. Eosinophilia seen. High mortality. **Diagnosis:** Echo/MRI/biopsy. Associated with Churg–Strauss. Transplantation may be needed.

- **Causes and individual management**. Clinically they present with symptoms of heart failure, thromboembolism (stroke), palpitations, chest pain or arrhythmias – AF, ectopics, VT or even VF and syncope and cardiac arrest. They can be listed as follows. ECG and echocardiography can help identify an abnormality. A cause is often looked for but in many it is idiopathic. Cardiac MRI is the imaging of choice in many. Angiography may be needed to exclude IHD. Management is that of heart failure and arrhythmias. End stage heart failure may require cardiac transplant (see also <u>Cardiogenic shock and heart failure</u>, ▶Section 2.16).

04 Respiratory emergencies

4.1 Pathophysiology

- **Lung anatomy and physiology:** two lungs, one trachea, two main bronchi, 3 lobar and 10 segmental bronchi on right and 2 lobar and 8 segmental bronchi on left. Lungs are covered by visceral pleura which continue as parietal pleura over the lateral surfaces of the mediastinum creating a pleural space. Repeated branching to level of terminal bronchioles, leads to 300 million alveoli. Normal ventilation is driven by external intercostals and diaphragm creating a negative airways pressure. Active process vulnerable to fatigue and neuromuscular weakness. 21% O_2 at atmospheric pressure (760 mmHg or 101.3 kPa) reaches the alveoli. In a perfect system arterial PO_2 = alveolar PO_2 but due to AV shunting in lungs and cardiac venous drainage into pulmonary veins there is a normal 2.5 kPa (20 mmHg) difference. In some pathological states this is increased. Moist atmospheric air at 37°C has a PO_2 of 20 kPa (150 mmHg) and there is an increased A–a gradient. This is seen with impaired diffusion across the alveolar capillary membrane or V/Q shunting. Hypoventilation and Type 2 RF has a normal A–a gradient. PCO_2 is a useful guide of alveolar ventilation and rises with any hypoventilatory state. The alveolar–arterial difference in PCO_2 is only 1 mmHg.

- **Oxygen transport:** blood transports oxygen bound to Hb. O_2 carriage is not directly proportional to partial pressure of O_2. The relationship is sigmoidal (see figure below) due to cooperative sequential binding of four O_2 molecules with Hb. This enables it to load well when O_2 is plentiful and unload well when O_2 is scarce, giving it some advantage over the relationship being completely linear. The flat upper portion is alveoli and shows that the Hb is over 90% saturated even with reduced PO_2 down to 60 mmHg (8 kPa). Giving additional O_2 above 100 mmHg (13 kPa) adds little to O_2 carrying capacity. Where the graph is steepest this reflects the tissues with a PO_2 of 40 mmHg (5 kPa) and shows that increased metabolic demand is met with offloading of O_2 within a very small range of PO_2. It also shows that in giving appropriate O_2 even small increases can improve blood O_2 carriage markedly. Metabolic by-products, e.g. DPG, acidosis and $\uparrow PCO_2$ or temperature move the curve towards the right, which makes Hb release O_2 more readily.

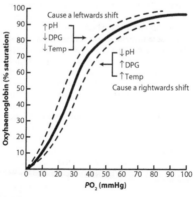

Oxygen dissociation curve.
Reproduced from http://openi.nlm.nih.gov under a Creative Commons License.

Hypoxia and (Alveolar A – arterial a) O_2 gradient = (FiO_2 %/100) * (P_{atm} – 47 mmHg (6.2 kPa) – (PaCO_2/0.8) – PaO_2)

Hypoxia with a normal A–a gradient: hypoventilation, low FiO_2 especially <21% O_2, e.g. at altitude
Hypoxia with increased A–a gradient: diffusion defect or V/Q mismatching or shunting.

 ## Oxygen therapy

- **Note:** BTS guidance on O_2 therapy sets a target SpO_2 of 94–98% and of 88–92% in those with severe COPD.
- **Discussion:** in the acutely ill high concentration oxygen is best given as 15 L/min with a reservoir bag (FiO_2 of over 0.9). The ill patient should receive at least 60% oxygen. However, excessive O_2 may lead to formation of free radicals and cause absorption atelectasis and V/Q mismatches. It may also hide significant deteriorations. Prescribe enough to achieve an O_2 saturation of 94–98% except in those patients with severe COPD where a target of 88–92% would be more appropriate. Adjust FiO_2 to get to that level. Simply giving all patients a high FiO_2 over what is needed can hide significant deteriorations. A patient with pneumonia may be saturating at 98% on 2 L O_2 via nasal route but begins to desaturate to 90%, but the saturation improves to 98% when increased to FiO_2 of 0.4. This suggests a clinical worsening, which would have been hidden if she was on a non-rebreather at 15 L/min from the outset. The patient, however, may have developed a PTX or pulmonary oedema or a PE or had some mucus airway plugging that would have been missed.
- **Prescribe the desired saturation and not the delivery rate or flow or mask** which should be left to ward level policy. Desaturations and increases in FiO_2 to respond to falling desaturations should be escalated to medical staff and acted upon as needed. Where **COPD-related CO_2 retention** is likely it is recommended that treatment should be commenced using a 28% Venturi mask at 4 L/min in prehospital care or a 24% Venturi mask at 2–4 L/min in hospital settings, with an initial target saturation of 88–92% pending urgent blood gas results. This is seen mostly in those with severe COPD, morbid obesity, chest wall deformities or neuromuscular disorders. Monitoring with O_2 saturation probe will detect hypoxia but an ABG is needed to detect hypercapnia (CO_2 retainers). Hypercarbia is multifactorial and involves a mixture of vascular shunting (hypoxia vasoconstricts pulmonary arterioles) and hypoventilation in either or both depth and rate which should be clinically apparent. In chronic hypercarbia, hypoxia may be the main driver to respiration and a high FiO_2 may increase hypoventilation.
- **If peri-arrest and unable to maintain saturations:** BVM ventilation with 100% O_2 and urgently fast bleep anaesthetists or arrest team and consider intubation and ventilation. Consider humidified O_2 for patients who require high-flow O_2 for more than 24 h or in those who report upper airway discomfort due to dryness.
- **Hyperbaric oxygen therapy:** 100% O_2 at greater than atmospheric pressure. Concerns of O_2 toxicity and this must be borne in mind. Indications: CO poisoning, decompression sickness, air embolism, cyanide poisoning, gas gangrene, to improve wound healing (decubitus ulcers), refractory osteomyelitis, thermal burns, improves skin grafting success.

Measuring oxygenation

- Direct by sampling arterial blood – see ABG. Indirect by pulse oximetry – a photodiode uses light to determine the ratio of oxygenated Hb (940 nm) to deoxygenated Hb (660 nm). Measures only the pulsatile flow and subtracts background readings.

- Blood carries 1.3 ml of oxygen per g of Hb. Assuming cardiac output = 5 L/min and Hb is 120 g/L then total carriage = $5 \times 120 \times 1.3$ ml/min = 780 ml oxygen/min.
- **Beware:** carbon monoxide toxicity can show SaO_2 of 98% (falsely high) and ABG shows the true severe hypoxia. On the other hand, IV methylene blue treatment can cause SaO_2 of 70% when ABG shows a true normal reading. The ABG is always the definitive test of blood oxygen carriage.

Oxygen delivery devices: mask types and their applied uses

- **Room air:** FiO_2: room air is 21% O_2 and 78% N_2. Small increases in inspired O_2 produce larger gains in tissue oxygenation.
- **Nasal cannulae:** FiO_2 24–45% at 1–6 L/min: a nasal cannula (NC) is a thin tube with two small nozzles to go into the patient's nostrils. Provides O_2 at low flow rates, 1 L/min = 24%, 2 L/min = 28%, 3 L/min = 32%, 4 L/min = 36%, 5 L/min = 40%, 6 L/min = 44%. Well tolerated – some find this preferable to a facemask. No dead space. High flow rates (>6 L/min) cause nasal mucosal drying and nose bleeds. Indications: SaO_2 85–94% in non-critically ill patient. Reduce to minimum to keep SaO_2 over 94%.
- **Simple facemask:** FiO_2 24–65% at 2–12 L/min: fits over a patient's nose and mouth. Delivers O_2 as the patient breathes. Open side ports allow room air to enter and dilute the O_2 and allow exhaled CO_2 to leave. Connected to O_2 source by a narrow plastic tube. Mask held in place by an adjustable elastic band. Provides O_2 at low flow rates, 24% 1–2 L/min, 28% 2–4 L/min, 35–40% 5–6 L/min, 60% 8–10 L/min, 65% 12 L/min. Indications: SaO_2 85–94% in non-critically ill patient. Reduce to minimum to keep SaO_2 over 94%.
- **Non-rebreather with reservoir bag:** FiO_2 85–90% at 15 L/min: flow should be sufficient to keep reservoir bag inflated on inspiration. Similar to face mask but has 3 one-way valves with the 2 side ports. This prevents room air from entering the mask but allows exhaled air to leave the mask. It has a reservoir bag like a partial rebreather mask. Reservoir bag has a one-way valve preventing exhaled air from entering the reservoir. Allows larger concentrations of O_2 to collect in the reservoir bag for the patient to inhale. High flow delivery systems giving high FiO_2. Flow rate of 15 L/min supplies up to 90% FiO_2, but requires tight fitting mask. Use when very high FiO_2 required and in critically ill patients. Indications: SaO_2 <85% or critically ill. Reduce to minimum to maintain SaO_2 >94%.
- **Venturi mask** [max = 50% FiO_2] indications: COPD + CO_2 retention. Start at 28% mask. Monitor ABG. Variable fixed amounts. High flow delivery system with flow rate between 4 and 12 L/min, FiO_2 can be set specifically with different flow rate and air ports. FiO_2 can be 24% (2–4 L/min), 28% (4–6L/min), 35% (8–10 L/min), 40% (10–12 L/min) and 50% (12–14 L/min). External ports must remain open to entrain room air.
- **Bag–valve mask** (BVM) FiO_2 100% with high flow oxygen with intubation or nasopharyngeal or oropharyngeal airways: Used for emergency ventilation until expected recovery or intubation attempted. BVM ventilation requires a good seal and a patent airway with usual airway opening techniques. It is used with high flow O_2 to an O_2 reservoir and the operator. The O_2 flow rate equals the minute volume of the patient so 100% O_2 is delivered. The BVM can deliver O_2 to a spontaneously breathing patient. Can also be used to manually ventilate a patient via a mask or tube, or with an oral or nasopharyngeal airway. Indications: SaO_2 <85% or critically ill patient. Reduce flow to minimum to maintain BTS guidance.

4.3 Acute breathlessness

- **About:** breathlessness can be due to cardiac or respiratory failure or a metabolic acidosis or be psychogenic.
- **Physiology:** stimulants to breathing are elevated PCO_2 or severe low PO_2, afferents from pulmonary vagal C-fibres.
- **Is breathless new**, e.g. PE, pneumonia or is there chronic dyspnoea, e.g. COPD/asthma/CCF. What are observations: RR, BP and HR, are they hypoxic? Why are they in hospital? Ensure you exclude a metabolic acidosis, e.g. DKA and acidosis.
- **Ask about chest pain, calf pain, haemoptysis.** Have a low threshold for suspecting PE in an inpatient. If the patient is hypoxic or respiratory rate is fast or slow, or nurse is concerned, see immediately. Mildly breathless or *in extremis*? If *in extremis* hurry because it could be pre-arrest.
- **Start O_2 aiming for sats of 94–98%** unless there is chronic COPD (28% O_2). Get ECG especially if chest pain, looking for VT/fast AF/sinus tachycardia or ST changes.
- **Get CXR especially if acute:** LVF, PTX, pneumonia, effusion, PE. Suspected angina or LVF and BP >100 mmHg then give 2 sprays of GTN (2 × 400 mcg) sublingual.
- **If wheeze or known COPD/asthma** advise normal puffer, e.g. SALBUTAMOL 100 mcg/puff progressing to SALBUTAMOL 2.5–5.0 mg nebuliser if needed. Sudden breathlessness, especially if hypoxic or low BP in hospital, consider as PE if there is no obvious better alternative diagnosis.

Diagnostic clues

- **Sudden onset:** pulmonary oedema, PE, acute anaphylaxis and airway oedema, acute PTX, aspiration pneumonia, hyperventilation syndrome, inhaled foreign body.
- **Gradual onset:** pulmonary oedema, non-cardiogenic pulmonary oedema (ARDS), COPD/bronchiectasis, acute asthma, pneumonia, small PTX, lymphangitis carcinomatosis.
- **Exacerbation of known cause:** exacerbation of COPD, bronchiectasis, asthma, CCF, pulmonary fibrosis, cystic fibrosis.
- **Breathlessness with normal CXR:** PE, early pneumonia, PCP, hyperventilation, COPD, small PTX (easily missed), metabolic acidosis with Kussmaul's breathing, e.g. DKA.
- **Post-operative: atelectasis**, hospital-acquired pneumonia, aspiration pneumonia, PE, PTX (esp. if on ventilator), pulmonary oedema. Anaesthesia may reduce normal lung protection and cause atelectasis and predispose to infection. Ensure pain controlled to allow deep breaths. Chest physiotherapy may help expectoration.

Clinical findings

- **Assess:** Check O_2 sats, RR and temperature. Wheeze, pursed lips, prolonged expiration, tripod position of COPD. Is there wheeze (PEFR)? Check HR: ↑HR, fast AF, VT. BP: ↓BP or JVP elevated (pulmonary oedema, PE, tamponade, SVC obstruction).
- **Auscultation:** murmurs, S3, S4, triple rhythm, systolic murmurs. Chest – dull at bases, stony dull effusion. Air entry and breath sounds – is much air moving? Always get patient to breathe through mouth and listen to chest.
- **Chest pain:** ACS, PE, dissection, pericarditis. Legs: pedal oedema or ?DVT.

Differentials for acute breathlessness

- **Acute severe asthma:** known asthmatic with ↑breathlessness, ↑wheeze, ↑cough, ↓PEFR. Infection, pollution are triggers. Ask about previous episodes needing hospitalisation and even ITU. Difficult socioeconomic circumstances, alcohol and drug issues are all associated with poor outcomes (▶ Section 4.11).

- **Upper airway obstruction:** distress, breathless with stridor. Causes include laryngeal oedema, angioedema, inhaled foreign body, chemical burns, physical burns; inspect and remove if possible and consider Heimlich procedure if foreign body suspected. If intubation impossible then a cricothyrotomy may be needed – call ENT and anaesthetic fast bleep. Anaphylaxis or angioneurotic oedema of laryngeal mucosa: stridor or hoarseness may suggest histamine release, oedema and anaphylaxis (▶ Section 2.18).

- **Pneumothorax** (PTX): breathless +/– pain. Look for underlying lung disease or chest trauma. If chest examination shows reduced air entry, hyper-resonant quiet side may be a PTX – CXR diagnostic. Those with underlying lung disease are at higher risk and may need aspiration and a chest drain. 100% O₂ helps resorption but caution if COPD (▶ Section 4.12).

- **Tension pneumothorax:** breathless and BP drops as RA filling compromised and signs and situation suggest tension PTX (ventilated patient or chest trauma). Immediate green/brown Venflon in 2nd intercostal space mid-clavicular line of affected side is called for – do not wait for CXR – should be an immediate hiss and escape of air. Give 100% O₂. Insert chest drain. (▶ Section 4.12).

- **Pleural effusion:** breathless and stony dullness could be fluid. Get CXR. Usually significant size if symptomatic. Controlled drainage of effusion 1–2 L at a time. Risk of pulmonary oedema. Determine cause. (▶ Section 4.13).

- **Pulmonary embolism (PE):** very common in hospital. Medical wards or post-op. Breathless, ↓BP, and increased RR. ↑JVP, RV heave, loud P2, signs of DVT, CXR often normal. Elevated D-dimer and risk factors. Anticoagulate and give IV fluids; thrombolysis in selected severe cases. Vigorous CPR may help. See VTE section. (▶ Section 4.17).

- **Exacerbation of COPD:** pre-existing COPD. Smoking history. Type 2 RF on ABG. Wheezy. Sputum. Consider NIV or if progressively acidotic then discuss ITU admission with intensivists. (▶ Section 4.10).

- **Acute LVF/pulmonary oedema:** acute dyspnoea, bibasal crackles, triple rhythm (S3/S4), worse lying flat. CXR diagnostic. ECG to look for STEMI needing PPCI. Echocardiogram when possible. (▶ Section 2.16).

- **Community-acquired pneumonia:** breathless, sputum, fever, dullness, reduced air entry, pleurisy, fever, ↑WCC/CRP. Consolidation on CXR may not be seen acutely. (▶ Section 4.14).

- **Aspiration pneumonia:** those with poor airways protection, stroke and coma and bulbar paralysis. (▶ Section 4.14).

- **Hospital-acquired pneumonia:** often post-operative atelectasis or debilitated. High mortality. Use local antibiotic protocols. Ensure post-op pain controlled to allow adequate deep breaths. (▶ Section 4.14).

- **Pneumocystis pneumonia:** seen with AIDS and immunocompromised patient, causes a more generalized alveolar shadowing? (▶ Section 4.15).

- **Coronavirus pneumonias:** watch for MERS/SARS, which need immediate isolation. See Index for more information. History of contact or travel in high risk areas with an acute fever and pneumonia. (▶ Section 4.14).

- **Hypoventilating:** COPD, obesity, sedation, CO₂ narcosis, respiratory muscle weakness. May not be breathless. ABG show a Type 2 RF.

- **Respiratory muscle weakness:** high cervical cord lesion, GBS, myopathy, MND, muscular dystrophies. Monitor FVC as well as ABG. Weakness of muscles to shrug shoulders is a sign. An FVC <1.5 L is worrying. Monitor closely. Consider ventilation.

- **Metabolic acidosis:** Kussmaul's breathing seen with DKA, salicylate overdose, etc. Check ABG.

- **Hyperventilation syndrome/panic attack:** setting of stress or anxiety. Examination normal, respiratory alkalosis on ABG. Breathe from bag. Sedation.

Differentials for acute breathlessness

- **Fat embolism:** recent fracture, coma, sickle cell, agitated, skin rash. Hypoxia. (▶ Section 17.3).
- **ARDS:** non-cardiogenic pulmonary oedema. Sepsis, malignancy, lung injury, trauma, obstetric emergency. CXR changes in clinical context. Echo shows normal cardiac function. (▶ Section 4.9).
- **Aspiration pneumonia/pneumonitis:** suspect if NG tube may be misplaced and feed going into bronchus. Recent stroke or neurological disease (MND) or coma. Failure to protect airway due to sedation, alcohol, drugs, anaesthesia. CXR may show usually right middle or lower lobe changes. Mixed bacterial and chemical reaction produces a pneumonitis. A PEG tube does not prevent aspiration. (▶ Section 4.4).
- **Pulmonary haemorrhage:** bleeding within the alveoli and bronchioles. Goodpasture's syndrome, Wegener's granulomatosis, CXR shows alveolar shadowing, renal failure.
- **Cheyne–Stokes breathing:** significant brain damage and brainstem compression. Alternating cycles of slow and then fast respirations in a profoundly comatose patient.

Investigations

- **Bloods:** FBC, U&E, glucose, CRP. **ABG:** look for hypoxia +/− hypercarbia. **Cardiac troponin:** ACS, myocarditis, myocardial injury.
- **D-dimer:** elevated with DVT/PE and other causes (sensitive but non-specific).
- **BNP** >400 pg/ml for decompensated heart failure. BNP <100 pg/ml, heart failure unlikely.
- **ECG:** AF, STEMI, NSTEMI, tachyarrhythmias, S1Q3T3. **CXR:** pulmonary oedema, PTX, consolidation, pleural effusion.
- **Echocardiogram:** MI and poor LV, valve disease, tamponade.
- **CT pulmonary angiogram:** PE, unexpected other pathology.
- **V/Q scan:** for PE if normal CXR and no lung disease.
- **Pulmonary functions tests** – obstruction/restrictive/diffusion defect.

De novo in-hospital acute breathlessness + circulatory collapse without an obvious alternative explanation is usually a PE until proven otherwise, especially if CXR shows no other cause.

Management

- **ABC and give O₂** as per BTS guidelines and reassess after ABG. If *in extremis*, cyanosed or severely hypoxic (SaO₂ <80%) then call cardiac arrest team. If airway obstructed by food or other objects then see choking algorithm. If suspected allergic laryngeal oedema with stridor give IV HYDROCORTISONE 100 mg +/− ADRENALINE 0.5 mg IM and consider urgent cricothyrotomy (fast bleep anaesthetics and ENT).
- **Common causes**, e.g. COPD, LVF, PE, asthma, chest infection. Signs of DVT? Look at hospital notes. Useful signs: ↑JVP (CCF, PE, tamponade), loud systolic murmur, fast AF. New drugs or blood transfusion might suggest anaphylaxis and need for nebulisers, adrenaline and steroids.
- **Look for fever:** ↑CRP, crackles on auscultation suggesting infection. If diagnosis still unclear or needs confirmation then CXR is useful, but may take some time to arrive and get information.
- **Treat as for cause found:** it can be useful to hedge bet and treat several causes at once whilst awaiting confirmatory tests or senior advice, e.g. IV antibiotic, FUROSEMIDE 50 mg IV if pulmonary oedema suspected and SALBUTAMOL 2.5 mg neb. Look for new MI or valve disease.
- **If PE suspected** then follow PE diagnostic pathway. If *in extremis* consider thrombolysis. (▶ Section 4.17).

- **If chest pain and new LBBB or ST elevation** then give GTN 2 sprays (800 mcg) sublingual if SBP >110 mmHg and if pain persists DIAMORPHINE 2.5–5 mg IV and take cardiac advice on urgent revascularisation (PCI/thrombolysis). (▶ Section 3.8).
- **If worsening hypoxia and acidosis** may require NIPPV or intubation and ventilation. Get help early if deteriorating. Consider a chest drain for PTX or massive pleural effusion.

4.4 Acute stridor

- **About:** high pitched upper airway breathing noise due to turbulent airflow through a partially obstructed upper extrathoracic airway. Inspiratory – laryngeal obstruction, Expiratory stridor – tracheobronchial obstruction. Biphasic stridor suggests a subglottic or glottic anomaly.
- **Red flags:** drooling and agitation, tripod position, cyanosis, decreased conscious level. Respiratory distress, silent chest, ↓HR and episodes of apnoea.

Causes

- **Infection:** acute epiglottitis: adults and children, sore throat, drooling, distressed. Peri-tonsilar abscess – pain and swelling. Acute laryngitis – hoarseness.
- **Allergy/inflammatory/other:** acute anaphylaxis or localised inflammatory reaction, pale, ↓BP. Post-extubation laryngeal oedema. Laryngeal tumour, low calcium and tetany, vocal cord dysfunction.
- **Trauma:** oedema and bleeding causing obstruction.
- **Compression:** large goitre or extrinsic tumour mass or haematoma.
- **Partial airway obstruction:** inhaled foreign body, e.g. peanut seen more in children.
- **Childhood:** laryngomalacia, croup, vocal cord dysfunction.

- **Clinical:** cyanosed. Breathlessness. Distressed. Hoarseness of voice and foreign body sensation in throat. Loud stridor, drooling if unable to swallow, feverish, toxic suggests infection. Allergy/inflammatory: rash, ↓BP, urticarial, anaphylaxis, known causative agent. **Extrinsic:** large goitre or mediastinal tumour.
- **Investigations:** delay blood tests if very distressed until airway secure. Mast cell tryptase if allergic. **Lateral soft tissue neck film:** those with epiglottitis exhibit thickening and rounding of the epiglottitis ('thumb sign'), with loss of the vallecular air space. The aryepiglottic folds are thickened, and the hypopharynx is distended. Consider CXR, laryngoscopy, bronchoscopy depending on likely cause.
- **Management: give nil by mouth if compromised as may need surgery:** in acute epiglottitis do not examine throat and summon urgent senior anaesthetic assessment for intubation and ENT for tracheostomy if needed. **Give steroids and antibiotics.** For all close monitoring on ENT/HDU/ITU. ABCDE, ABG and 15 L/min oxygen or a mixture of helium and O_2 (heliox) improves airflow and reduces stridor. **Steroids:** if allergy/local swelling or oedema suspected, then DEXAMETHASONE 10 mg IV and 4 mg IV 6 h or HYDROCORTISONE 200 mg IV stat and then 8 h. Consider ADRENALINE 1 mg of 1 ml diluted in 10 ml 0.9% saline nebulised. If anaphylaxis, then ADRENALINE 1 mg (1 ml) of 1 in 1000 given IM. **Antibiotics:** if infection, e.g. epiglottitis or bacterial tracheitis or abscess antibiotic therapy may be required, e.g. Augmentin, Ceftriaxone. **Airway:** endotracheal intubation may be necessary. If unable then may require cricothyrotomy or tracheostomy to bypass laryngeal obstructions. Oropharyngeal abscess may be incised.

Reference: Mohamad *et al.* (2012) Acute stridor – diagnostic challenges in different age groups presented to the emergency department. *Emergency Med*, 2:125. doi:10.4172/2165-7548.1000125.

4.5 Acute respiratory failure

The breathless patient may not be hypoxic and the patient with severe hypoxia may not appear to be breathless. Check O_2 saturation and ABG.

Definition: respiratory failure is a problem of inadequate arterial oxygenation such that PaO_2 <8 kPa (60 mmHg). Give high FiO_2 if cardiac/respiratory arrest or periarrest, shock, patient *in extremis*, severe Type 1 RF, carbon monoxide poisoning, PTX (speeds resolution), and/or prior to attempting intubation. Give controlled oxygen in longstanding COPD. Respiratory failure is rare in COPD when FEV_1 >1 L and in restrictive diseases when FVC >1 L.

NB: hypercapnia is rarely the result of a loss of drive due to $\downarrow O_2$ but is multifactorial. Involves hypoventilation due to sedation, neuromuscular weakness (GBS/MND/muscular dystrophies), tiredness, pain, mucus plugs, atelectasis with V/Q changes as O_2 is a pulmonary vasodilator and hypoxia a constrictor. True hypoxic drivers usually have severe COPD, polycythaemia/cor pulmonale, FEV_1 <1 L, home O_2, nebulisers, $\uparrow HCO_3$, normal respiratory rate.

Management is to treat hypoxia aiming for a PaO_2 >8 kPa and manage any hypoventilation with pain relief, chest physio, hydration, NIV or invasive ventilation. In the tachypnoeic patient with hypoxia and $\uparrow PaCO_2$ breathing deep and fast then loss of hypoxic drive is not the issue.

Type 1 respiratory failure	Type 2 respiratory failure
PaO_2 <8 kPa (60 mmHg) and normal or low CO_2. • **Ventilation/perfusion** (V/Q) mismatch: increased A–a gradient, e.g. pneumonia. • **Impaired diffusion:** increased A–a gradient, e.g. lung fibrosis/interstitial disease. • **Anatomical right–left AV shunt:** increased A–a gradient, e.g. pulmonary AV malformation. • **Hypoventilation:** normal A–a gradient, e.g. obesity, sedation, neuromuscular weakness. • **Breathing low pressure/FiO$_2$:** normal A–a gradient, e.g. climbing Everest, in aircraft.	PaO_2 <8 kPa (60 mmHg) and PCO_2 >6 kPa (45 mmHg). *(Pulse oximetry will not detect rising CO_2.)* • **Alveolar hypoventilation:** neuromuscular weakness, sedation. • **Lung disease:** emphysema/COPD due to V/Q mismatch. Increased dead space ventilation. • **Increased CO_2 production:** malignant hyperthermia, severe thyrotoxicosis, fever, sepsis, shivering, overfeeding from parenteral nutrition, bicarbonate administration, CO_2 insufflation (laparoscopy).
Causes: pneumonia, cardiogenic oedema, ARDS, pulmonary haemorrhage, acute severe asthma, pulmonary fibrosis, cyanotic congenital lung disease, fat embolism, high altitude.	**Causes:** COPD, central hypoventilation, obesity-related hypoventilation, progressive coma, sedation, GBS, MG, poliomyelitis, muscular dystrophies, chest wall disorders, and all of the causes of Type 1 when tired, hypoventilating with V:Q mismatch.

• **Details:** acute respiratory failure (ARF): defined as PaO_2 <8 kPa (60 mmHg) +/– PCO_2 >6 kPa (45 mmHg). Hypoxia soon leads to death. Respiratory failure usually comes on over hours. It may be on the background of normal respiratory function or chronic RF. Determine pre-exacerbation respiratory and functional status. Patients can move between types of RF. A hypoxic patient with pneumonia, heart failure or even severe asthma can tire and hypoventilate and retain carbon dioxide moving from Type 1 to Type 2.

- **Pathophysiology:** respiration driven by pontine and medullary centres. $\uparrow CO_2$ is a stronger stimulus to ventilation than low PO_2. Response to $\uparrow CO_2$ reduced by chronic hypercapnia and sedation. **Capnography:** reflects alveolar and therefore arterial partial pressures of CO_2 which reflects respiration and circulation. Can help detect tube displacement. During resuscitation, recovery is evident by an abrupt increase in the CO_2 reading. **Clinical effects of hypercarbia:** $\uparrow$confusion, asterixis, peripheral vasodilation, anxiety, obtunded, $\uparrow ICP$, coma, hypoventilation. Compensatory $\uparrow HCO_3$ and $\uparrow K$.
- **Clinical:** typically breathless but not always, especially with hypoventilating Type 2 RF. Cyanosis (increased deoxygenated Hb), reduced cognition, altered behaviour. Comatose and decreased respiratory effort. History – cough, acute onset, smoker. $\uparrow$effort using accessory muscles, intercostal recession, $\uparrow HR$. Tachypnoea. Signs of PTX, consolidation, pulmonary oedema, fibrosis, wheeze.

Investigations

- **FBC:** $\uparrow$Hb suggests chronic hypoxia/smoking, $\downarrow$Hb anaemia. **U&E:** $\uparrow$urea, $\uparrow$creatinine, AKI or pulmonary–renal syndrome.
- **ABG:** arterial hypoxia is seen. If $\uparrow PCO_2$ then Type 2. With acute RF HCO_3 is normal, but with chronic hypercapnic RF with renal compensation the HCO_3 may become elevated. The pH will usually be acidotic. The exception would be early Type 1 failure with hyperventilation.
- **CXR:** pulmonary oedema (cardiogenic or non-cardiogenic), consolidation, alveolar haemorrhage, PTX, pleural effusion, collapse, tumour, bullae, fibrosis, emphysematous change. Often normal in PE.
- **ECG** may suggest a cardiac cause. Look for $\uparrow HR$, AF, ischaemia, RVH.
- **Echocardiography** rarely useful in pure Type 1/2 RF except perhaps to help exclude PE. May suggest pulmonary hypertension.
- **Pulmonary function tests (PFTs):** FVC determines respiratory muscle strength. Reduced FEV/FVC in obstructive lung disease. **CTPA or V/Q scan:** suspected PE.

Management

- **ABC:** airways assessment is the first step in all management of respiratory compromise, followed by breathing and circulation. Look for cause based on clinical assessment, past history, CXR and ECG findings and arterial blood gases. Controlled O_2 therapy: the ward/ITU staff should give the lowest level of O_2 (flow, mask) to hit the saturation of 94–98% or 88–92%. Allow the staff to either increase or reduce the FiO_2 to attain this. An increased O_2 demand to hit the target SaO_2 needs to be escalated and patient reassessed as can signify a deteriorating patient.
- **Treat causes:** reverse or stop sedation, diuresis and nitrates for cardiogenic pulmonary oedema, bronchodilation (antibiotics, steroids, controlled O_2 for COPD), and anticoagulation for acute PE, chest drain for PTX and so on. NIV in COPD with acidosis.
- **NIPPV:** see discussion below. Consider where there is **COPD with progressive CO_2 retention and worsening acidosis (pH <7.25)**. If it fails to oxygenate then mechanical ventilation should be considered and support sought from ITU/HDU.
- **Simple actions:** simple interventions – sitting patients up or out of bed can improve lung ventilation by aiding expectoration of secretions. Chest physiotherapy. Encourage coughing. Basal atelectasis and mucus plugs can all exacerbate ventilation. Occasionally bronchoscopy to remove mucus plugs and other material.
- **Antibiotics:** tailor to the likely pathogen. Is it viral, bacterial, fungal? Is it an exacerbation of COPD or community-acquired pneumonia? Is the patient immunocompromised? Could this be PCP pneumonia with undiagnosed HIV/AIDS?
- **Respiratory stimulants: DOXAPRAM** can be used to stimulate and increase breathing rate/depth and tried if NIV not available or tolerated.

- **Extracorporeal membrane oxygenation** (ECMO) used for potentially reversible RF. It can be lifesaving and considered in patients with persisting RF despite maximal therapy due to a potentially reversible pathology. Talk to local ECMO centre.

Non-invasive ventilation (NIV/NIPPV)

Positive pressure

Normal physiology involves using intercostal muscles and diaphragm to create a negative airways pressure relative to atmospheric pressure, sucking air in to reach the alveoli. Pushing air in which is the most practical way to oxygenate lungs therapeutically alters normal physiology. This can be done invasively by full intubation and ventilation, or non-invasively using face masks or hoods and a ventilator device that provides positive pressure. Positive airway pressure can then be given continuously (CPAP) throughout the respiratory cycle or varied with the cycle (e.g. BiPAP). In some NIV can help to avoid complications of intubation and invasive ventilation, to improve outcomes (e.g. reduce mortality rates, decrease hospital length of stay), and to decrease the cost of care. It is mainly used in those with Type II RF. The machine can automatically detect episodes of inspiration and expiration. NIV is usually used to improve oxygenation and increase minute volume, thus reducing $PaCO_2$.

Continuous positive airway pressure (CPAP): mainly for Type 1 RF/Alveolar oedema

CPAP is the application of continuous positive pressure whilst the patient continues to initiate and generate breaths. Prevents collapse of airways, recruiting more alveoli for gas exchange. The positive pressures are maintained even on expiration. Work of breathing is reduced. Can be accompanied by high FiO_2. Pressures used are 5–20 cmH$_2$0. Adjust FiO_2. Main use is *cardiogenic pulmonary oedema* at typical pressures of 5–15 cmH$_2$0. A trial can be given for 1–2 h to see improvement in O_2 sats, heart rate, etc. Primarily helps hypoxaemia rather than CO_2 retention and can help avoid intubation. Patient wears a tight-fitting mask which is essential to maintain the positive pressure. Outside of the acute setting it is useful for those with obstructive sleep apnoea because it acts as a 'pneumatic splint' maintaining a patent airway throughout the respiratory cycle.

Bi-level positive airway pressure (BiPAP): mainly for Type 2 RF and pH < 7.35

BiPAP usually refers to the application of positive pressure ventilation similar to CPAP except that pressures are changed for inspiration and expiration. Needs a tight fitting face mask and a ventilator that is capable of delivering two levels of pressure: inspiratory (high pressure, e.g. 8 cmH$_2$0) and expiratory (↓pressure, e.g. 4 cmH$_2$0).

- **Advantages of NIV:** ↓risk of infection, ↓length of hospital stay (it can be used at home). NIV and COPD related Type 2 RF: NIV in the ICU/ward has been shown to reduce intubation rate and mortality in COPD patients with decompensated respiratory acidosis (↓pH <7.35 and $PaCO_2$ >6 kPa) following immediate medical therapy. NIV should be considered within 60 min of hospital arrival in all with acute exacerbation of COPD in whom a respiratory acidosis persists despite maximum standard medical treatment, i.e. controlled oxygen to maintain O_2 sats 88–92%, bronchodilators and steroids and antibiotics as per local guidelines.
- **Application:** NIV can be used in both Type I and II RF, e.g. exacerbations of COPD and cardiogenic pulmonary oedema. An effective seal is necessary and the patient needs to be able to tolerate the mask as well as the feeling of breathing out against resistance. Intolerable for some. Positive pressure aids the inspiratory phase of breathing, which is active. Reduces respiratory muscle work, maintains alveoli patency during expiration which improves the ventilatory process. Increased alveolar recruitment and so more air comes into contact with blood in pulmonary

circulation, which reduces V/Q mismatches. NIV is described as trying to breathe with your head out of the window of a speeding car. The flow rate of O_2 is prescribed and administered via the port on the mask or, if available, into the disposable filter attached to the generator. Start at O_2 2–4 L/min depending on the FiO_2 needed. Humidified O_2 is usually given. NIV may be trialled in some conditions, e.g. asthma and pneumonia, but only if the patient is in ITU and can be intubated immediately. It is not for hypoxic asthmatics or pneumonia or those with reversible lung pathology who are tiring and decompensating, unless there is immediate access to invasive ventilation if needed. NIV is not indicated in: impaired consciousness, severe hypoxaemia or patients with copious respiratory secretions.

Indications for using NIV

- COPD + resp. acidosis pH 7.25–7.35 (H^+ 45–56 nmol/L), NIV may be used where ITU not appropriate.
- Hypercapnic RF secondary to chest wall deformity (scoliosis, thoracoplasty) or neuromuscular diseases.
- Cardiogenic pulmonary oedema unresponsive to CPAP, weaning from tracheal intubation.

Contraindications to NIV

- COPD with a pH <7.25 needs consideration for ITU, intubation and ventilation.
- Cardiac/respiratory arrest, haemodynamic instability, moribund, untreated PTX, delirium, GCS <10.
- Vomiting, upper GI bleeding, bowel obstruction, facial trauma, upper airway obstruction.
- Unable to clear sputum, high risk of aspiration.

4.6 NIV protocol and settings

See machine's instruction manual. In Spontaneous/Time (S/T) mode, the ventilator delivers pressure support breaths with PEEP. Patient's spontaneous inspiratory effort triggers the ventilator to deliver inspiratory positive airway pressure (IPAP). It cycles to expiratory positive airway pressure (EPAP) during expiration. If the patient's breathing rate is lower than a prescribed rate, the ventilator triggers a pressure-controlled breath according to the IPAP prescribed. The breath is ventilator-triggered, pressure-limited and time-cycled. The actual level of pressure support is equal to the difference between IPAP and EPAP. The monitor of the ventilator can display expired tidal volume, minute ventilation, peak inspiratory pressure, inspiratory time/total cycle time, and patient peak flow and % patient-triggered breaths.

Suggested protocol for NIV

- Sit patient up. Achieve position of comfort, explain NIV and what to expect and consent verbally. Choose smallest mask providing a proper fit and place over the patient's face.
- Start with IPAP of +10 cmH_2O and EPAP of +5 cmH_2O. IPAP should be gradually be increased over the next 20 min to a target IPAP of 20 cmH_2O.
- Observe respiratory rate and tidal volume (target 5–7 ml/kg). Set back-up breath rate of 10–15 breaths/min.
- Monitor for any distress, coma, vomiting, and secretions ++.
- Adjust FiO_2 to maintain SpO_2 >90%. Repeat ABG at 2 h.
- EPAP may be increased in acute pulmonary oedema.
- Apply strapping to the mask once patient used to NIPPV tight enough to prevent leaks, but allow entry of 1 or 2 fingers.
- Dressing on nasal bridge can help avoid pressure sores.

Settings for NIV

- Pressure settings: broadly, IPAP helps $\downarrow PCO_2$ and EPAP improves PO_2.
- IPAP ranges from 5 to 40 cmH$_2$O (usual max 25) with increments of 2 cm.
- EPAP ranges from 4 to 20 cmH$_2$O (usual max 15) with increments of 2 cm.
- Rate ranges from 4 to 40 breaths/min.
- Timed inspiration ranges from 0.5 to 3 s with increments of 0.1 s.
- IPAP rise time: 0.05, 0.1, 0.2, 0.4 s.
- FiO$_2$ ranges from 21 to 100%. The FiO$_2$ can be adjusted according to the ABG and SpO$_2$.
- Back-up respiratory rate: 12–16 breaths/min.

Parameters for CPAP for cardiogenic pulmonary oedema without hypercapnia: CPAP 5–15 cmH$_2$O via face mask, normal I:E ratio is 1:2 (inspiration: expiration).

- **Measure success:** reduction in $PaCO_2$ or improved pH by +0.06 and/or correction of respiratory acidosis associated with a clinical improvement.
- **Failure:** signs of failing NIV and need for escalation include: worsening acidosis or hypercapnia and/or falling GCS, especially if <9. Determine ceiling of therapy so that escalation if appropriate is rapid.
- **Difficulties:** include copious respiratory secretion with difficulty in clearance may be the issue. Intubation and mechanical ventilation may be necessary depending on the ceiling of therapy which should have been ascertained.
- **Weaning off:** assess on an individual basis for suitability of weaning once there are signs of continued improvement or if NIV is not helping. For COPD a 3-day approach with decreasing time of NIV down to 16 h on day 2 and 12 h on day 3 with 6–8 h overnight adjusted to the patient's condition. Discontinue day 4 as appropriate. Re-check ABG 2 h after discontinuation of therapy. Consider use of NIV overnight if nocturnal hypoventilation is present.

4.7 Invasive ventilation

- **Involves similar concepts to NIV** but requires intubation and ventilation and oxygenation by placing of an endotracheal tube, laryngeal mask or tracheostomy. It can require a mixture of sedation and neuromuscular blockade. The settings usually allow timing to the patient's inspiratory effort. Air is pushed in and increases intra-alveolar pressure or lung tidal volume until a point where the lungs are allowed to deflate passively. Pressures generated can cause a PTX or reduce venous return or cause lung injury. Ventilators can be set basically using either volumes (tidal volume is preset and fixed and pressures vary) or pressure settings. Benefits should be improved gas exchange and a decreased work of breathing.
- **Complications of mechanical ventilation:** lung injury, difficulties in intubation, laryngeal injury, PTX, tension pneumothorax, pneumomediastinum, airway injury, alveolar damage, ventilator-associated pneumonia, weakness and atrophy of the diaphragm, reduced cardiac output, O$_2$ toxicity, acute lung injury (ALI) and acute respiratory distress syndrome (ARDS).
- **Monitoring the effectiveness of mechanical ventilation:** use pulse oximetry, ABG, effort of breathing, tidal volume, respiratory rate, HR and BP, mortality, CXR findings.

Indications for endotracheal intubation and ventilation

- Protection of the airway and/or need to remove secretions.
- GCS <9, airway obstruction, respiratory fatigue or drowsiness.
- Apnoea with cardiac/respiratory arrest.
- Hypoxaemia (PO_2 <8 kPa) despite high FiO_2 +/− NIV.
- SaO_2 <90% despite CPAP with FiO_2 >0.6.
- Control CO_2 (hyperventilate to ↓PCO_2 for ↑ICP).
- Control O_2/CO_2 (Type II RF with acidosis).
- Respiratory rate >35/min or <10/min.
- FVC <15 ml/kg or 1 L or <30% predicted.
- Tidal volume <5 ml/kg or inadequate inspiratory force <25 cmH$_2$O.
- Surgery to head and neck or involving muscular paralysis.

References: British Thoracic Society Standards of Care Committee (2002) Non-invasive ventilation in acute respiratory failure. *Thorax*, 57:192. O'Driscoll *et al.* (2008) BTS guideline for emergency O_2 use in adult patients. *Thorax*, 63(Suppl 6):1. RCP (2008) Non-invasive ventilation in COPD: Management of acute type 2 respiratory failure. London: RCP.

- **Quantitative capnography:** the measurement of CO_2 which is normally present in expired air. End-tidal CO_2 is measured and low levels are detectable even during cardiac arrest. The return of spontaneous circulation is sometimes difficult to assess with other methods, but it is clearly demonstrated on capnography measurements by an abrupt increase in the $PEtCO_2$ (end-tidal PCO_2) value. If $PEtCO_2$ abruptly ↑ to a normal value (35–40 mmHg), it is reasonable to consider that this is an indicator of ROSC. Continuous end-tidal CO_2 monitoring can confirm a tracheal intubation and absence should prompt removal of the tube and face mask ventilation before considering re-attempts at intubation. A good wave form indicating the presence of CO_2 ensures the ET tube is in the trachea. A persistently low level may indicate a poor prognosis.

4.8   Massive haemoptysis

- **About:** massive haemoptysis >600 ml of blood in 24–48 h. Haemoptysis is reasonably common but massive life threatening haemoptysis is rare. Death is from hypoxia, rarely exsanguination, so keep the non-bleeding lung uppermost to protect airway. Sedation and palliation may be more appropriate with advanced lung cancer.
- **Aetiology:** lungs are supplied by the bronchial and pulmonary arteries. Bronchial arteries at 120/80 mmHg, pulmonary arteries at 25/10 mmHg. Severe bleeding more likely from the bronchial arterial vessels which can be embolised in severe haemorrhage.
- **Causes:** primary lung cancer/pulmonary metastases (smoker, weight loss, clubbing). Pneumonia or bronchiectasis (cough + purulent sputum). Aspergillus, lung abscess (with pus). Pulmonary TB (weight loss, CXR changes), pulmonary oedema (bat wing alveolar oedema, Kerley B lines, cardiomegaly). Alveolar haemorrhage (WG/Goodpasture's alveolar shadowing and cavitation, ↑CRP, haematuria). Hereditary haemorrhagic telangiectasia (HHT), pulmonary AV fistula, pulmonary artery aneurysms.
- **Clinical:** distressed, breathless, cyanosed, clubbing and weight loss if underlying tumour. Expectorating bright red frothy blood, hypoxic, ↓BP. Listening over chest may hear gurgling from affected side. Upper zone blood may gravitate to lower lobes depending on position. Consider metastases, e.g. renal, testicular, gastrointestinal. Overseas – HIV/TB more likely oral/facial telangiectasis (HHT).

- **Investigations** (extensive test only if cause not evident): FBC: ↑WCC, ESR, CRP infective, inflammatory or malignancy. U&E, urinalysis (blood and protein): AKI – with WG or Goodpasture's syndrome. Blood cross match: if anaemic or bleeding is significant. Coagulation screen: APTT, prothrombin time (PT), INR, platelets, fibrinogen. ECG: non-specific unless cardiac disease or acute PE. Echocardiogram. Sputum for culture, AFB and cytology. CXR: is valuable because it lateralises the cause and helps diagnose the lesion causing the bleeding. HRCT chest: may provide more information if possible. +/− Lung biopsy. CTPA and/or V/Q: if PE considered. D-dimer likely elevated regardless. Antibodies to c-ANCA (proteinase 3 for WG), anti-GBM (Goodpasture's syndrome), ANA, RF, complement and cryoglobulins. Echocardiogram if cardiac disease or PE suspected. Cardiac troponin if cardiac disease suspected.

- **Management:** ABC FiO$_2$ as per BTS guidelines. Sedation may be useful in a distressed patient. Positioning: lie on side and keep non-bleeding lung uppermost if localised. Get anaesthetic view on protecting airway and if intubation needed. Liaise early with cardiothoracic surgeons in terms of steps needed – they usually dictate care. Supportive: IV fluids, group and cross-match. Transfuse if needed. Treat any coagulopathy. Consider IV TRANEXAMIC ACID. ADRENALINE 5–10 ml (0.5–1 mg) of 1 in 10 000 nebulised may help. Intubation: consider intubation if tiring or there is on-going bleeding and risk of asphyxiation, falling SaO$_2$. Use large bore tube which may be single or double lumen. Flexible bronchoscopy or CT chest is the primary method for diagnosis and localisation of haemoptysis. Bronchoscopy difficult with acute bleeding in visualising the bleeding source. Case by case assessment.

- **Methods to stop bleeding** (after Tranexamic acid/correcting any coagulopathy): bronchial artery angiography and embolisation is indicated from interventional radiology (S/E cord ischaemia/infarction if anterior spinal artery compromised). Bronchial balloon tamponade: where the bronchial balloon of a double lumen tube, or a 4 French 100 cm Fogarty embolectomy catheter, or Arndt endobronchial blocker, inserted via a single lumen tube, can be inflated for 24 h before deflation and observation. There is a theoretical risk of mucosal ischaemia with this approach. Bronchial lavage: use of saline cooled in ice in 50 ml aliquots down the bronchoscope with volumes up to 1 L is well described, and can arrest bleeding.

- **Topical procoagulants:** thrombin and fibrinogen concentrates have been topically instilled, with anecdotal success. Laser, diathermy, or cryocautery: these are possible through a rigid bronchoscope and can be applied to, for example, a bleeding endobronchial tumour.

- **Surgical management** may be applicable in some cases where a more conservative approach is not sufficient. In some cases emergency pulmonary resection provides an effective treatment with acceptable morbidity and mortality in patients with massive haemoptysis. Palliation where the patient has a known terminal lung malignancy and bleeding cannot be stopped is appropriate. Consider MORPHINE and palliative care team.

4.9 Acute respiratory distress syndrome (ARDS)

Berlin modifications to ARDS definition

- Severity increases as the ratio of arterial PO_2/FiO$_2$ falls.
- Acute onset (within 1 week of known clinical insult).
- Bilateral opacities on CXR/CT unexplained by other pathology.
- Pulmonary artery wedge pressure (PAWP) <18 mmHg.
- Ratio PaO_2/FiO$_2$ mild <40 kPa, moderate <26.6 kPa, severe <13.3 kPa.

- **About:** systemic disease with acute hypoxia and multiorgan dysfunction. Complication of trauma, sepsis, tissue damage, other severe illnesses. Mild ARDS was once called acute lung injury.
- **Aetiology:** Type 1 RF without evidence of significant cardiac dysfunction. Loss of Type 2 pneumocytes. Pulmonary inflammation. Proteinaceous alveolar oedema and capillary leakage with flooding and collapse of alveoli. Stiff poorly compliant lungs depleted of surfactant with severely impaired gas exchange.
- **Clinical:** context of other severe illness and worsening PaO_2 and CXR changes. Breathlessness, cyanosis, basal inspiratory crackles. Tachycardia, severe hypoxia in the context of critical illness.
- **Causes:** burns and smoke inhalation, pneumonia, pneumonitis from aspiration, high altitude, fat or air embolism, near drowning, O_2 toxicity. Systemic: sepsis, trauma, eclampsia, acute pancreatitis, heroin, barbiturates, transfusion-associated lung injury, malignancies, cardiopulmonary bypass.
- **Differentials:** congestive cardiac failure, bilateral pneumonia (ventilator associated or community acquired), alveolar haemorrhage (WG/Goodpasture's syndrome), acute interstitial pneumonia, acute eosinophilic pneumonia or hypersensitivity pneumonitis (need steroids).
- **Investigations:** ABG: PaO_2/FiO_2 ≤300 mmHg (40 kPa) consistent with ARDS if obtained on PEEP or CPAP ≥5 cmH_2O. FBC: anaemia, ↑neutrophils. U&E/LFT lactate: AKI may be seen, ↑lactate, deranged LFTs. CXR: bilateral opacities (oedema). Chest CT: not often needed but shows bilateral opacities, ground glass appearance. Echo: normal LV function. Right heart catheter: PAWP <15–18 mmHg. Blood cultures: sepsis. Coagulopathy: DIC may develop with ↑APTT, PT and ↓? platelets. Broncho-alveolar lavage may be useful if undefined infection.
- **Management:** determine and treat cause. Death is primarily due to progressive multiorgan dysfunction. Ventilate if needed, target SaO_2 >88%. Intubation and ventilation (PEEP): for worsening PaO_2/FiO_2. Lung protective ventilation strategies have been developed. The aim is adequate gas exchange with minimal ventilator-induced lung injury. Ventilation and prone positioning may be advocated. Neuromuscular blockade for 48 h may help. Diuretics: consider for oedema to generate a negative fluid balance. Haemofiltration may be used. Inhaled NITRIC OXIDE may be tried as well as aerosolised surfactant and PROSTACYCLIN for refractory hypoxia. Steroids have no evidence base. Antibiotics for sepsis or pneumonia. ECMO may be considered for refractory hypoxia.
- **Complications:** PTX, ventilator-associated pneumonia, multiple organ failure, pulmonary fibrosis, RF. Death 30–50%.

References: de Haro *et al.* (2013) ARDS: prevention and early recognition. *Annals Int Care*, 3:11. Ferguson *et al.* (2005) Development of a clinical definition for ARDS using the Delphi technique. *J Crit Care*, 20:147.

4.10 Acute exacerbation of COPD

- **About:** COPD is a chronic illness punctuated with acute exacerbations, some infective. Community teams can help reduce hospital admissions. Post bronchodilation FEV_1 <80% predicted and FEV_1/FVC <70%. Not all smokers get COPD but unusual if <10 pack years.
- **Causes of worsening:** irritants, e.g. cigarette smoke, noxious particles and SO_2, NO_2, ozone. Viral: 50% rhinoviruses, coronaviruses, influenza, parainfluenza, adenovirus, RSV. Bacterial: *Haemophilus influenzae, Strep. pneumonia, Moraxella catarrhalis, Pseudomonas aeruginosa, Chlamydophila pneumoniae*.
- **Clinical:** ↑dyspnoea, expiratory wheeze, cough, sputum. Malaise, cachexia. Pursed lips breathing, barrel-chested, use of accessory muscles – tripod position. New onset cyanosis, peripheral oedema, nicotine staining and signs of smoking. Bounding

pulse, drowsy, tremor and headache can suggest CO_2 retention. Determine best baseline exercise function – useful guide of overall function and goals. Ask about pets and allergies, occupation, asbestos. Home oxygen.

MRC dyspnoea scale

Grade 0: no breathlessness except with strenuous exercise

Grade 1: breathlessness hurrying on level or walking up a slight hill

Grade 2: walks slower than contemporaries on level ground due to breathlessness or stops for breath

Grade 3: stops for breath after 100 m or a few minutes walking on level ground

Grade 4: too breathless to leave house; breathless dressing/undressing

Disease severity GOLD guideline

Stage 1: mild: FEV >80% FEV_1/FVC <0.7 plus symptoms

Stage 2: moderate: FEV 50–79% FEV_1/FVC <0.7

Stage 3: severe: FEV 30–49% FEV_1/FVC <0.7

Stage 4: very severe: FEV <30% FEV_1/FVC <0.7

Investigations

- **Bloods:** FBC: ↑WCC and ↑CRP suggest infection but steroids increase WCC. U&E: may be dehydrated with ↑urea/creatinine. Low Na. **CXR:** hyper-expanded dark lungs typical of emphysema and may be patchy shadowing. Look for PTX which may be difficult to differentiate from bullae (if unsure CT may be useful). There may be pneumonic changes or possible lung malignancy. Suspect a lung malignancy in all smokers. CT chest helpful to assess emphysema. **ECG:** sinus tachycardia, AF, P pulmonale, RVH, ST/T wave changes. **ABG:** low PO_2 <8 kPa and ↑PCO_2 >6 kPa, pH <7.25. A ↑HCO_3 suggests chronic COPD with compensated respiratory acidosis. Try to find out from past admissions and A&E notes what worst and best ABG was as a guide.
- **Pulmonary function tests:** try to determine FEV_1/FVC <0.7. Carbon monoxide transfer factor low in emphysema. Alpha-1antiproteinase if young and basal emphysema. Consider troponin and risk assess if PE considered for D-dimer: if suspicion this is ACS/PE. Exacerbations of COPD can be LVF or PE and these diagnoses should be sensibly considered.

Management

- **Don't always assume usual exacerbation.** Usually it is the case but this could be PE, heart failure, lung cancer, PTX, pneumonia, upper airway obstruction, pleural effusion, recurrent aspiration. Get patient sitting up supported to allow use of accessory muscles to aid gas exchange. Chest physiotherapy to aid expectoration in those with excess sputum. IV fluids for those too tired/breathless to drink.
- **Controlled O_2** usually 24–28% initially to achieve O_2 saturation of 88–92% and PO_2 >8 kPa with <1.5 kPa rise in PCO_2. Venturi mask initially 28% at 4 L/min O_2 preferred. Repeat ABG 30 min after altering FiO_2. If the PCO_2 is normal then increase target O_2 saturation to 94–98% and repeat ABG after 30 min. Rising PCO_2 and acidosis suggests respiratory support initially NIV.
- **Steroids:** HYDROCORTISONE 100–200 mg IV initially then PREDNISOLONE 30–40 mg OD. Steroids continued for 7–14 days and then stopped.
- **Antibiotics:** AMOXICILLIN 500 mg 8 h PO for 5–10 days or if penicillin allergic DOXYCYCLINE 200 mg day one then 100 mg OD for 5–10 days or CLARITHROMYCIN 500mg 12 h for 5–10 days. Save CO-AMOXICLAV 625 mg 8 h for 5 days for those with known resistance, severe attack or recent antibiotics. Use if infection suspected, e.g. fever, sputum, ↑WCC or CRP. CXR changes suggesting infection. Those with history of bronchiectasis or pseudomonas may need TAZOCIN 4.5 g 8 h IV or

MEROPENEM 1 g 8 h IV if penicillin allergic. There is some evidence that AZITHROMYCIN three times per week long term may reduce frequency of exacerbations and improve quality of life.
- **VTE prophylaxis:** standard LMWH and early mobilisation.
- **Others:** severe cases under expert guidance consider AMINOPHYLLINE 250 mg IV loading dose over 20 min if not on theophylline or else maintenance dose as per formulary.
- **ROFLUMILAST 500 mcg OD** is a once-daily phosphodiesterase type-4 inhibitor licensed for COPD. Some modest improvements in lung function and reduced health care utilization.

Managing acute exacerbation of COPD

- **Initial:** controlled O_2 + sit up + aid expectoration + hydration + antibiotic + VTE prophylaxis and monitor closely. Regular ABG initially.
- **Bronchodilators:** nebulised SALBUTAMOL 2.5–5 mg and IPRATROPIUM BROMIDE 500 mcg every 30 min then 4-6 hourly. Nebs driven by air and not high flow oxygen.
- **Steroids:** HYDROCORTISONE 200 mg IV /PREDNISOLONE 30–40 mg OD.
- **NIV:** consider NIV if pH <7.35 and PCO_2 >6 kPa despite treatment.
- **ITU:** intubation and ventilation appropriate for some.

- **NIV is recommended** (NIV, ▶Section 4.6) in an acute exacerbation of COPD if respiratory acidosis pH <7.35 and PCO_2 >6 kPa despite treatment with controlled O_2: nebulised bronchodilators, oral/parenteral steroids and antibiotics for 1 h. It reduces the need for intubation and ITU admissions, improves blood gases and reduces the work of breathing and also reduces infective complications and hospital stay. Avoid in drowsy uncooperative patients, severe acidosis, unstable haemodynamics. Patients should be conscious and cooperative and able to protect their airway. A full-face mask should be used initially. Start with low pressures to allow patient to get used to the feeling but then escalate to therapeutic pressures. Start with IPAP of 10 cmH$_2$O and EPAP of 5 cmH$_2$O. Increase IPAP by 5 cmH$_2$O every 5–10 min to a target of 20 cmH$_2$O (max 25). Ensure ABG checked 1 h after all changes in settings and this can be reduced once stable to 4 hourly or less if improving. Watch respiratory rate and heart rate. Give nebulisers as needed. NIV can be gradually weaned down to 16 h on day 2 and 12 h on day 3 with 6–8 h overnight adjusted to the patient's condition. Discontinue day 4 as appropriate. If clinically worsening and/or pH falls below 7.25 then senior advice should be sought about ITU. Senior medical staff should discuss with ITU and family and patient if possible. There may be an advance directive. In some cases NIV will be the ceiling of respiratory support. Respiratory stimulant DOXAPRAM IV may be considered in Type 2 RF where H^+ >45 when NIV unavailable or not tolerated or considered inappropriate
- **Discharge:** consider home when patient confident that they can manage, improving generally, pH >7.35 or H^+ <45, alert and orientated, no new focal abnormality on CXR, O_2 sats >88%, ability to cope at home, mobilising to toilet with minimum breathlessness, can attend to own personal ADLs, able to cope with O_2 or nebulisers, no complicating co-morbidities. Early supported discharge may support those who are not self-caring yet needing additional help. **Prior to discharge:** optimise bronchodilator therapy. Check inhaler technique. Consider inhaled corticosteroid/long acting β_2 agonist/Tiotropium. Give Tiotropium at night if early morning symptoms. Avoid Combivent or Ipratropium with Tiotropium – risk of urinary retention in elderly.
- **Prevention:** prompt recognition and treatment of infection/exacerbation. Annual influenza vaccination. One-off pneumococcal vaccination if not given previously. Encouraging smoking cessation and pulmonary rehabilitation (exercise, smoking and nutritional advice). Long term O_2 therapy (LTOT) for COPD if stable post-acute

PO_2 <7.3 kPa or a PO_2 <8 kPa with secondary polycythaemia, pulmonary HTN or peripheral oedema. Requires 15+ h per day. Long-term O_2 therapy: keep SaO_2 >90% and PaO_2 >8 kPa. These patients become accustomed to worsening disease and hospital admissions. Palliation and setting ceilings of care: it is becoming more common to ask patients with end-stage disease to discuss end of life plans with regard to interventions such as ventilation prior to this in the non-acute phase. Patient expectations need to be carefully balanced with the potential futility of some treatments.

References: Soo Hoo (2012) Non-invasive ventilation. *MedScape*, 1–20 (http://emedicine.medscape.com/article/304235-overview [accessed 17 Nov 2016]). RCP (2008) NIV in COPD: Management of acute type 2 respiratory failure. *National Guideline Number 11.*

Acute severe asthma

Severity assessment of acute severe asthma

- **Acute severe:** unable to complete sentence in 1 breath, RR >25/min, HR >110 bpm, PEFR 33–50% best/predicted.
- **Life threatening asthma:** silent chest, cyanosis, confusion, coma, exhaustion, arrhythmia, ↓BP, poor respiratory effort, unrecordable or PEFR or <33% predicted, SaO_2 <92% or PaO_2 <8 kPa, $PaCO_2$ >4.6kPa, pulsus paradoxus is an unreliable sign determining severity.
- **Near fatal asthma:** $PaCO_2$ >6 kPa, needing ventilation with ↑inflation pressures.

- **About:** assess severity, ensure appropriate treatment and rapid escalation. Close observation and early senior input and liaison with ITU are key. No asthmatic patient who gets to hospital breathing should die. If hypoxic give high FiO_2 (over 60%), steroids and nebulisers. Ensure accompanied at all times, e.g. in X-ray dept. Crash team if they are deteriorating. Senior medical and anaesthetic input early. Patients die daily in the UK from asthma.
- **Aetiology:** airway hyperactivity. Reversibility. Diurnal PEFR variation 20%. In some there is a potentially lethal mixture of tiredness and bronchoconstriction. Exacerbated by mucus plugging and V/Q mismatches. In fatal asthma, extensive mucus plugging of the airways is found at autopsy.

Investigations

- **Bloods:** ABG: hypoxia +/− hypercarbia. FBC: ↑WCC, CRP suggests infection. Eosinophilia: consider aspergillus, parasites, drugs, Churg–Strauss syndrome. U&E: ensure normal and check CRP. ECG: sinus tachycardia. BNP, Troponin, D-dimer if diagnosis unclear and needed. **CXR:** is not routinely recommended except suspected pneumomediastinum or PTX, suspected consolidation, life-threatening asthma, failure to respond to treatment satisfactorily, requirement for ventilation. **PEFR:** difficult in acute severe asthma. Compare with baseline. Acute severe 33–50%. Life-threatening <33% or too breathless to blow. Pulmonary function tests: can be done later if diagnosis unclear.

Management (liaise closely with ITU)

- **General:** high FiO_2 via oxygen driven nebuliser. Ensure patient sitting up and comfortable. Start bronchodilators and steroids. Needs support and time. It's the steroids that matter most. Reassurance, hydration, encourage slower and deeper respirations – a positive confident competent attitude from staff can help greatly because patient is working hard and *in extremis* and is often terrified. Ask anaesthetists to review EARLY any patient not rapidly improving.

Antibiotics only if clear evidence of infection. Direct observation: patient must be accompanied and monitored at all times as rapid deterioration is possible, e.g. in X-ray department.

- **OXYGEN:** ABC high FiO_2 15 L/min initially then adjusted to deliver sats of 94–98% and reassess after ABG. If sats <85% then high flow 10–15 L/min with non-rebreather mask and get urgent anaesthetic help (patient is peri-arrest).
- **IV fluids** to avoid dehydration if patient too breathless to drink and dehydrated and tired.
- **BRONCHODILATORS:** SALBUTAMOL 5 mg + IPRATROPIUM BROMIDE 500 mcg neb every 20 min nebulisers driven by high flow O_2 every 20 min then reduce to 4-hourly. SALBUTAMOL IV may be considered if deteriorating, however concerns are Type B lactic acidosis, severe agitation and arrhythmias (monitor). Use with caution.
- **PREDNISOLONE 40 mg stat** PO or **IV HYDROCORTISONE 200 mg stat and 100 mg 6 h IV.** Steroids for at least 5 days.
- **MAGNESIUM SULFATE (1.2–2 g IV infusion over 20 min)** may be considered in persisting acute severe asthma following consult with senior medical staff.
- **AMINOPHYLLINE 250 mg IV over 20 min loading dose:** omit loading dose if on aminophylline. Maintenance dose thereafter. Ensure ECG monitoring if patient not already on theophylline. The therapeutic window is narrow and macrolides and ciprofloxacin can cause toxicity. Watch serum levels.
- **Intubation and ventilation:** early ITU outreach review so intensivists aware in all but mildest. Enables quick escalation if any life-threatening features. 1–3% require intubation. BVM ventilation is very difficult due to severe airway obstruction. Expert rapid sequence induction. NIV only considered following expert review in an ITU setting with a plan for rapid intubation if needed.
- **ANTIBIOTICS:** most exacerbations may be non-infectious or viral so antibiotics not usually needed unless clear evidence of bacterial infection, e.g. consolidation on CXR, fever, purulent sputum, etc.
- **ADRENALINE 0.5–1 mg IM as for anaphylaxis may be used in extremis and under senior supervision**
- **Pregnancy:** see ▶ Section 15.10.
- **Asthma plus syndromes to consider: allergic bronchopulmonary aspergillosis:** 1% of asthma patients, bronchiectasis on CT/CXR, eosinophilia. IgE >1000 ng/ml. Positive IgE RAST. Needs steroids and antifungals. **Churg–Strauss syndrome:** chronic asthma, eosinophils, vasculitis, rash, neuropathy, nephropathy. p-ANCA (MPO). Needs immunosuppressive therapy.
- **Post recovery:** admit: if any feature of a life-threatening or near-fatal asthma attack or any feature of a severe asthma attack persisting after initial treatment.
- **Discharge:** those with PEFR >75% best or predicted within 2 h after initial treatment unless still have significant symptoms. If concerns about adherence, living alone/socially isolated, psychological problems, physical disability or learning difficulties, previous near-fatal asthma attack, asthma attack despite adequate dose steroid tablets pre-presentation, presentation at night, pregnancy, then consider admission. **Discharge medications:** PREDNISOLONE 40 mg for 7 days, give inhaled steroids (double normal dose), advise to return if worsens, see GP within 2 days. Advice: prior to discharge, trained staff should give asthma education on inhaler technique and PEFR record keeping. Records of PEFR and symptoms can allow tailoring of therapy to guidelines. Can reduce morbidity and reduce relapse rates. Household to remove any precipitants, e.g. new pets before return and vacuum clean (high-filtration (HEPA) if possible) to reduce allergen exposure.

Reference: SIGN 2014, 141 British guideline on the management of asthma.

4.12 Pneumothorax

- **About:** air within the pleural cavity. All patients with spontaneous secondary pneumothorax (SSP) should be admitted for inpatient observation. Breathlessness indicates need for active intervention and supportive treatment. Primary pneumothorax occurs in those with normal lungs. Secondary pneumothorax (pre-existing lung disease suspected) are admitted and more cautiously/ aggressively managed as they are higher risk. Severe symptoms and haemodynamic collapse suggests tension PTX.

- **Primary spontaneous PTX:** classically tall thin males age <40 without known lung disease but can be any sex. Increased risk and commoner on right side. Commoner in smokers (possible subclinical lung disease), with higher recurrence if they fail to stop. Increased stresses on the lung apices in tall people cause a predisposition to subpleural bleb formation, which can later cause a PTX. Can recur within 1st year especially in tall adult smokers (40% in 2 years).

- **Secondary spontaneous PTX** (age >50 or traumatic/iatrogenic/chronic lung disease): trauma: especially penetrating chest trauma, iatrogenic trauma – pleural biopsy. Lung biopsy, central line insertion, high PEEP ventilation. Infection: lung abscess, PCP (AIDS), cystic fibrosis. Others: asthma, emphysema, idiopathic pulmonary fibrosis, sarcoidosis. Endometriosis/catamenial PTX – occurs within 72 h of menses. Oesophageal rupture. Lymphangioleiomyomatosis, lung carcinoma, histiocytosis X, eosinophilic granuloma, Marfan's syndrome, and homocystinuria.

- **Tension PTX:** have a high index of suspicion with sudden deterioration in positive pressure ventilated patients on ICU +/– previous PTX – always be prepared for urgent decompression. Trauma patients, resuscitation patients (CPR), lung disease – acute asthma and COPD, chest drain – blocked, clamped or displaced, patients receiving NIV or hyperbaric O_2 treatment.

- **Size:** small PTX rim <2 cm. Large PTX rim >2 cm (suggests >50% lung volume loss). Measure horizontal gap between lung margin and the chest wall at the level of the hilum. Accurate PTX size calculations are best achieved by CT scanning (see *figure* below).

- **Clinical:** <u>small PTX</u>: may be asymptomatic or mild dyspnoea. Symptoms often minimal or absent in primary PTX. <u>Larger PTX</u>: causes mild to severe dyspnoea. Depends on size and lung function. Cyanosis when a large PTX. Localised chest pain and even a click or added sounds. Affected side hyper-resonant with reduced breath sounds. <u>Tension PTX</u>: trachea pushed away, *in extremis*, ↑HR and falling BP. Suspect and decompress immediately if ventilated patient suddenly deteriorates or where there is chest trauma.

Investigations

- **FBC, U&E, CRP:** ↑WCC, infection, anaemia, inflammatory/infectious. **ABG:** if breathless and suspicion of RF. **CXR:** a departmental PA chest (+/– lateral) is the standard and shows an absence of lung markings between the ribs and a line demarcating the edge of the lung. New imaging systems may make it more difficult to see a lung edge than the old X-ray film so care must be taken. Expiratory films no longer advocated. Lateral CXR or even CT may help if PTX suspected and PA chest not definitive. **CXR (PA):** measure and use distance b at level of hilum (see *figure* below). BTS and American guidance interpret PTX rim b >2 cm as large. American guidance defines two markers a and b as large PTX if distance a >3 cm. **Chest CT:** can be useful especially to differentiate bullae from PTX and to determine any underlying parenchymal pathology. Can also aid decisions on drain position in complex cases and detecting small pneumothoraces. **Ultrasound:** has an increasing role and can help identify PTX especially as part of ATLS. **Other:** in selected cases HIV test in at-risk groups, ACE and calcium for sarcoidosis, bronchoscopy and lung biopsy, etc.

Management (small rim <2 cm, big rim >2 cm)

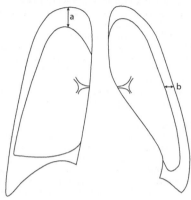

a = apex to cupola distance – American Guidelines
b = interpleural distance at level of the hilum – British Guidelines

- **General points:** O_2 as per BTS guidance; however, there is an argument to giving higher O_2, e.g. 10 L/min because it helps resorb the pleural cavity air and this should be assessed on a case by case basis. PA CXR film should be taken in the department if at all possible. Much better quality than on the ward with a portable machine. Patients with primary or secondary PTX and significant breathlessness associated with any size of PTX should undergo active intervention.
- **Tension PTX:** give high flow O_2. Usually too ill to wait for CXR so proceed on clinical findings. Patient critical then **immediate large gauge IV needle decompression in the 2nd intercostal space in mid-clavicular line on the affected side.** Identify space and mark it. Prepare the area as best one can. If time allows, wash hands, put on sterile gloves, clean area. Get largest Venflon readily available and insert in marked space. There should be a 'hiss' as it decompresses and BP should rise. Remove the inner metal needle and leave it to decompress. Then insert chest drain. A standard cannula may be insufficiently long if used in the second intercostal space and in this case move it to 4th/5th space.
- **Determine if primary or secondary:** if significant smoking history or evidence of underlying chronic lung disease in history, examination or on CXR, then treat as secondary PTX. Symptoms often more pronounced in secondary. Mortality is higher. Patients with pre-existing lung disease tolerate a PTX less well.
- **Primary small PTX:** monitor 4–6 h in A&E. Home if stable and not breathless for follow-up in 2–4 weeks with repeat CXR and assessment. Advise to return if symptoms. Give analgesia as needed.
- **Primary big PTX and/or** breathless, then O_2 10 L/min and aspirate with 16–18 G (grey/green) cannula up to 2.5 L with catheter in 2nd or 3rd ICS at MCL. Repeat CXR. If success (<2 cm and less breathless) then observe for 4–6 h and consider discharge and review in respiratory clinic in 4–6 weeks or sooner. If, however, after aspiration PTX is not <2 cm and breathlessness not improved then a small chest drain is inserted with size 8–14 Fr and admit. Discharged patients should return by calling 999 if new SOB.
- **Secondary PTX (big and small):** All need to be admitted and O_2. If large or symptomatic then chest drain (thoracostomy) with size 8–14 Fr. Smaller 1–2 cm rim of PTX **and** patient not breathless then aspirate with 16–18 G cannula up to 2.5 L and

repeat CXR. If size now <1 cm then high flow O_2 (unless O_2 sensitive) and observe for 24 h. If after aspirating PTX is still >1 cm then chest drain with size 8–14 Fr. Those on positive pressure ventilation require chest drain insertion as positive pressure maintains the air leak. All SSP are admitted.

- **PTX and pregnancy:** PTX recurrence is more common in pregnancy and poses risks to the mother and fetus. Requires close cooperation between chest physicians, obstetricians and thoracic surgeons. PTX during pregnancy can be managed by close observation if not dyspnoeic, no fetal distress and the PTX is small (<2 cm). Otherwise aspiration can be performed, chest drain insertion reserved for those with a persistent air leak. Due to risk of recurrence in subsequent pregnancies, a minimally invasive video-assisted thoracoscopic surgery (VATS) should be considered after convalescence.

- **PTX and AIDS/HIV infection:** the combination of PTX and HIV infection requires early intercostal tube drainage and surgical referral and treatment for PCP and ART. PCP causes necrotising alveolitis and subpleural necrotic thin-walled cysts and pneumatoceles. They have more prolonged air leaks, treatment failure, recurrence and higher hospital mortality. More aggressive intervention indicated.

- **PTX and cystic fibrosis:** this requires early and aggressive treatment with early surgical referral. Pleural procedures, including pleurodesis, do not have a significant adverse effect on the outcome of subsequent lung transplantation.

- **Pleural aspiration for PTX:** infiltrate local anaesthetic down to the pleura, in the 2nd ICS in the mid-clavicular line (the axillary approach is an alternative). Using a cannula (French gauge 14–16), enter the pleural cavity and withdraw the needle. Connect both the cannula and a 50 ml syringe (Luer lock) to a three-way tap, so that aspirated air can be voided. Aspiration should be discontinued if resistance is felt or the patient coughs excessively, or more than 2.5 L (that is, 50 ml removed 50 times) is aspirated. Repeat PA CXR in inspiration (an expiration film is unnecessary) in the X-ray department. If PTX is now only small, or resolved, the procedure has been successful. Note that failure to aspirate further may be due to the cannula being inadvertently withdrawn from the pleural cavity, or becoming kinked. If this is suspected, another attempt at aspiration should be considered; aspiration should not be repeated unless there were technical difficulties. If this fails then a small-bore (<14Fr) chest drain insertion is recommended (see Chest drain, ▶ Section 20.3).

- **Referral to a respiratory physician should be made within 24 h of admission.** Complex drain management is best effected in areas where specialist medical and nursing expertise is available. Failure for lung to expand after chest drain insertion may be due to extrathoracic placement, placed within a major fissure, obstructed or kinked tube. Other causes are ipsilateral bronchial obstruction, absence of suction, or 'trapped lung' due to pleural fibrosis. Occasionally if large PTX >72 h re-expansion can cause pulmonary oedema which usually resolves within 48 h.

- **Pleurodesis:** to prevent recurrence. Incite inflammatory response by mechanical abrasion of the pleura or chemically instilling substance into the pleural space leading to visceral and parietal pleura adhering.

- **Discharge:** patients should be advised to return to hospital if increasing breathlessness develops. All patients should be followed up by respiratory physicians until full resolution. No flying until CXR shows complete resolution – take specialist advice. Most airlines suggest flying acceptable after 6 weeks of full resolution or a definitive surgical procedure. Risk is significant for a year and some may prefer to wait. Never scuba dive unless bilateral pleurectomies and given specialist approval.

- **Smoking cessation** reduces recurrence rate and is an important part of PTX management and prevention.

Reference: Management of spontaneous pneumothorax: BTS pleural disease guideline. *Thorax*, 2010;65(Suppl 2):ii18. doi:10.1136/thx.2010.136986.

4.13 Pleural effusion

- **About:** pleural effusions may be signs of local or systemic pathology. When very large they can impair respiratory function. May become infected and if so need to be drained. Check a drug history.
- **Aetiology:** collection of fluid within the pleural space can restrict lung function.
- **Clinical:** signs of RA, SLE, heart failure, clubbing, malignancy. Assess symptoms. Depends on size, rate of accumulation and underlying cardiorespiratory function. Increased SOB, pleuritic chest pain, reduced wall movement, vocal resonance, and breath sounds. Stony dull to percussion, deviation of the trachea/mediastinum away if large.

Investigations

- **FBC:** anaemia, ↑WCC infective or inflammatory, malignant cause. U&E CRP: ↑AKI. ↑LFTs: albumin, ↑CRP/ESR, ↑ALP, ALT (metastases), PT. CXR **(preferably a PA):** needs 300 ml to be detectable. Hilar enlargement, cardiomegaly, pulmonary oedema, malignancy, TB, breast shadowing. **Echocardiogram or BNP** is useful to exclude heart failure as cause. **Chest CT:** for pleural effusion should be performed with contrast enhancement of the pleura and before complete drainage of pleural fluid. CT scans should be performed in all undiagnosed exudative pleural effusions. It can be useful in distinguishing malignant from benign pleural thickening. Useful for complicated pleural infection when initial tube drainage has been unsuccessful and surgery is to be considered. **Pleural USS:** should be used at the bedside to select a pleural aspiration site with safety. Helpful if fluid loculated. A lateral site is preferred.
- **Further investigations:** send **30 ml pleural aspirate:** protein, glucose, LDH, Gram stain, cytology and culture. This can be done with a fine bore (21 G) needle and a 50 ml syringe. Inspect appearance and send aspirate for cytology: protein, lactate, glucose, LDH. A low glucose (<3.3 mmol/L) suggests infection, tumour, RA, mesothelioma. Aspiration should be avoided for bilateral effusions in a clinical setting strongly suggestive of a transudate and CCF, unless there are atypical features or they fail to respond to therapy. Aspiration can be done on mechanical ventilation but with increased risk of a tension PTX if the lung is punctured. **Pleural fluid inspection:** bloody fluid can be confirmed by measuring haematocrit. Grossly bloody pleural fluid is usually due to malignancy, PE with infarction, trauma, benign asbestos effusions or post-cardiac injury syndrome. Milky fluid suggests a chylothorax which may be due to damage to the thoracic duct. In this situation measure pleural fluid triglyceride and cholesterol levels. **Cytology:** malignant effusions show pleural fluid cytology in about 60% of cases. Immunocytochemistry should be used to differentiate between malignant cell types and can be very important in guiding oncological therapy. Others test on pleural fluid: amylase – only useful for oesophageal rupture or pancreatic disease suspected. pH useful where infection suspected; a pH <7.2 with a suspected parapneumonic effusion indicates the need for tube drainage. Glucose: <1.6 mmol/L in RA. Adenosine deaminase (ADA) to rule out TB. It is significantly raised in most tuberculous pleural effusions. **Percutaneous pleural biopsy** under image guidance for pleural thickening on CT. **Thoracoscopy:** considered for an exudative pleural effusion where a diagnostic pleural aspiration is inconclusive and malignancy is suspected.

Causes of pleural effusion by Light's criteria

- **Criteria:** exudate if pleural protein >50% serum protein, pleural LDH >60% serum LDH, pleural LDH >66% ULN for serum **Transudate:** (↓protein, ↓LDH). Failures: cardiac failure, nephrotic syndrome, liver failure. Others: myxoedema, hypo-albuminaemia, Meigs's syndrome with ovarian tumour and right pleural effusion.

Exudate: (↑protein, ↑LDH). Infection: pneumonia; tuberculosis; empyema. Cancer: (blood stained) bronchogenic, mesothelioma, lung metastases, ovarian tumours. Cardiac/vascular: pulmonary infarct (bloody), post-MI; constrictive pericarditis. Gastro: pancreatitis, oesophageal rupture (both ↑amylase). Connective tissue disease: SLE, RA, FMF. Drugs: methysergide, nitrofurantoin. Miscellaneous: radiotherapy; trauma; post-cardiac surgery; asbestosis (blood stained); yellow nail syndrome.

Management

* **ABC and FiO₂** adjusted to deliver sats of 94–98% or 88–92% if severe COPD. Depends on determining the likely cause and managing that through simple investigations. If the effusion is large and causing compromise or associated with PTX then drainage required. Caution should be taken if removing >1.5 L on a single occasion. Otherwise a diagnostic tap can be performed as suggested above. In a parapneumonic effusion, a pH of <7.2 indicates the need for tube drainage. **Outpatients:** if stable, not breathless on minimal exertion or at rest, and mobile, consider referral of selected patients to a pleural effusion clinic. Advise to return if worse. Some can have on-going investigations, e.g. CT chest and investigation for secondary causes as an outpatient.

References: British Thoracic Society Pleural Disease Guideline Group (2010) BTS Pleural Disease Guideline. Kearon *et al.* (2016) Antithrombotic therapy for VTE disease: CHEST guideline and expert panel report. *Chest* [e-pub: doi.org/10.1016/j.chest.2015.11.026].

4.14   Pneumonia

* **About:** infection and acute inflammation of the air spaces and substance of the lung, which are normally sterile. Lobar is restricted to the whole of one lobe, exclude a bronchostenotic lesion. Bronchopneumonia affects lobules and bronchi. CURB-65 scoring for community-acquired pneumonias.
* **Types: community-acquired (CAP):** symptoms + signs of consolidation. Often healthy young patients. At-risk groups: aspiration (stroke/MND), alcohol, diabetes, steroids and immunosuppression, smokers, COPD, nursing home residents. **Hospital (HAP) or institutional:** onset >2–3 days after admission. Acquired following admission. Often post-op or debilitated. High mortality. Excludes ventilator associated pneumonia. These patients have significant co-morbidities. Difficulty swallowing. Poor nutrition. More likely to have aerobic Gram-negative infections, e.g. *Klebsiella, Pseudomonas, E. coli,* anaerobes and *Staph. aureus.* Elderly, immunosuppressed, respiratory disease, post-operative, ITU. **Aspiration pneumonia:** gastric acid pH <2.5 into lungs + foodstuff; a chemical pneumonitis. Often to right mid zone or apex of right lower lobe. May be a more subtle micro-aspiration syndrome especially where there is bulbar weakness. **Atypical pneumonias** due to *Mycoplasma pneumoniae, Chlamydophila pneumoniae,* or *Legionella pneumophila.* Dry cough. Headache, diarrhoea, vomiting, abdominal pain, myalgia and the chest symptoms may take time to appear clinically and radiologically. **Viral pneumonia:** influenza, adenovirus, RSV with secondary bacterial infection.
* **Risks:** young and elderly. Co-morbidities – renal disease, HIV, diabetes, heart disease. Lung disease: COPD, cystic fibrosis, bronchiectasis, old TB, bronchostenotic lesion. Others: smoker, alcohol excess, IV drugs, steroids, dementia, stroke. Causative organisms: vary by study, age, location, co-morbidities, exposure (see *table* below).
* **Pathology stages:** (1) congestion and vascular engorgement and alveolar bacteria;
  (2) red hepatisation – alveolar spaces full of polymorphs and fibrin and red cells;
  (3) grey hepatisation – RBC breakdown, fibrin and suppurative inflammation;
  (4) resolution – exudate removed by macrophages.

- **Clinical:** fever, sweats, rigors, dry cough initially, malaise, delirium (elderly and *Legionella*). Breathlessness, cyanosis, ↑HR, ↓BP, pleuritic-type chest pain. Rusty sputum (*Pneumococcus*), yellow/green sputum, haemoptysis. Flare-up of herpes simplex (*Pneumococcus*), atypical diarrhoea. Myalgia, headache, reduced air entry and expansion and dullness to percussion. ↑vocal resonance, stony dull if effusion/empyema.
- **Complications:** lung abscess, exudative pleural effusion, parapneumonic effusion. Empyema, bacteraemia, sepsis, cerebral abscess, meningitis. ARDS, respiratory failure, cardiac failure, multi-organ failure, death.

Investigations

- **Send sputum/blood cultures:** help expectoration and send sputum samples for culture and sensitivity and blood cultures if pyrexial. Bloods: FBC: ↑WCC. Low or mild ↑with *Legionella* and atypicals. U&E: AKI. ↓Na *Legionella*. LFT: ↑*Legionella*. Blood film: red cell agglutination suggests cold agglutinins and *Mycoplasma*. Procalcitonin levels ↑with bacterial infection. ESR/CRP ↑with pneumonia and fails to fall with abscess/empyema or wrong antibiotics.
- **Serology:** sputum/throat gargle (20 ml saline) for virology and mycoplasma PCR. Send **urine (universal container/white top)** for *Legionella* antigen and pneumococcal antigen and serum for *Legionella* antibody. If psittacosis suspected discuss with microbiology for appropriate investigation.
- **CXR (PA +/– lateral):** patchy consolidation with bronchopneumonia. Look for consolidation (Lobar), masses, cavitation, parapneumonic effusion, PTX, bullae. Changes often lag behind clinical changes. CXR within 4 h of presentation to hospital. Consider Differentials of consolidation: alveolar blood, aspiration, lung infarction.
- **ABG:** Type 1 or Type 2 RF with V/Q mismatch and coexisting COPD.
- **Bronchoscopy:** in some cases to look for any bronchostenotic lesions or remove foreign bodies or mucus plugging or for sampling, e.g. PCP.
- **HRCT chest:** to look for and exclude other related pathology or complications – abscess, empyema. Others: always consider HIV test and ask about risk factors. Slow resolution – consider empyema, underlying neoplasm or antibiotic resistance, or is it the wrong diagnosis?
- **Differentials of pneumonia:** PE, pulmonary oedema, ARDS, pulmonary haemorrhage. Cryptogenic organising pneumonia, lung cancer, acute extrinsic allergic alveolitis. Rare infections – anthrax, plague, tularaemia.

CURB-65 scoring defines severity and aids clinical management	
• Confusion: MTS <8 = +1 • Urea (BUN) >7 mmol/L = +1 • RR >30/min = +1 • BP (<90/60 mmHg) = +1 • Age >65 = +1	**Risk score and response:** 0/1: low (<3% mortality risk), consider home-based care; **2:** intermediate (3–15% mortality risk), consider hospital-based care; **3–5:** high (>15% mortality risk), consider ITU outreach and HDU/ITU or defining level of care. CRB-65 (urea omitted) may be used in primary care to assess. Hospital assessment CRB-65 >0 especially >2. CURB-65 should only be used to assess severity in CAP. **Additional evidence of severity: WCC** >20 or <4 or 10% band forms. **CXR:** multilobe involvement. **Albumin** <35 g/L. **Microbiology:** positive blood culture. **Others:** stroke, COPD, cardiac disease, diabetes.

Microbial causes of CAP

- **Strep. pneumoniae** (39%): cold sore, rusty sputum, consolidation/cavities (serotype 3). Antigen in urine/serum.
- **Chlamydophila pneumoniae:** epidemics, ↑AST.
- **Viral pneumonia** (20%): influenza A and B, parainfluenza, measles, RSV in infants. Varicella can cause severe pneumonia with miliary nodular shadows, which may calcify. Direct fluorescent antibody stain sputum for viruses.
- **Mycoplasma pneumoniae** (10%): children and young adults. Autumnal, erythema nodosum and multiforme, myocarditis, pericarditis, meningoencephalitis, GBS, haemolytic anaemia, bullous myringitis, cold agglutinins in 50%, headache, otalgia, transverse myelitis, pancreatitis, lymphadenopathy, splenomegaly. Check IgM.
- **Legionella pneumoniae:** age >50 usually. Showers/air conditioning. Headache, malaise, myalgia, ↑fever, dry cough, NV, diarrhoea, confusion, hepatitis, ↓sodium, ↓albumin, ↑LFTs, ↑CK. Delayed diagnosis worsens outcomes. Macrolides or fluoroquinolones. It is not passed person to person. *Legionella* antigen in urine. Direct fluorescent antibody stain sputum.
- **Moraxella catarrhalis:** (COPD) 2%.
- **Haemophilus influenzae** (5%): bronchopneumonia.
- **Staph. aureus:** winter. Post-influenza/viral pneumonia. CXR cavitation and abscess. Needs Flucloxacillin.
- **Chlamydophila psittaci** (3%): sick bird. Malaise, low-grade fever, hepatosplenomegaly.
- **Coxiella burnetii** (1%): animal contact. Chronic influenzal illness with dry cough, conjunctivitis, hepatosplenomegaly, endocarditis. CXR: multiple segmental shadows.
- **Klebsiella** pneumonia: widespread consolidation and cavitation (upper lobes). High mortality. Bloody viscous sputum.
- **Pneumocystis** pneumonia: immunosuppressed, e.g. HIV, drug therapy.
- **Tuberculosis** not usually included as a cause of CAP but is a cause of pulmonary infection.

Management

- **ABC and O$_2$** to deliver sats of 94–98% or 88–92% if severe COPD. Check ABG.
  IV fluids: hydration important. Mobilise as tolerated. Sit out of bed if able.
  Antibiotics: give as shown below within 4 h for CAP patients who are admitted.
  Those with atypical pneumonias need a macrolide or doxycycline and can often
  be managed as outpatients. **Resp failure:** Type 1 (and Type 2) requires O$_2$. Usual
  care in COPD. Severe hypoxaemia needs ITU and invasive ventilation. Role for CPAP
  and NIV without COPD/pulmonary oedema undefined. Trials of NIV/CPAP in this
  situation should be short (1–2 h), and if no improvement admit to ITU if pH <7.26
  or PO_2 <8 kPa or rising PCO_2 or breathless tiring patient. **Steroids:** a 7-day course,
  e.g. Prednisolone 20–60 mg/d for hospitalised CAP patients may reduce adverse
  outcomes and costs. **Others:** aspirate pleural effusions. Chest drain for empyema.
  Chest physiotherapy. VTE prophylaxis. Nutrition. Prevention: influenza and
  pneumococcal vaccination should be considered. **Discharge:** not if in past 24 h they
  have had 2 or more of temp. >37.5°C, RR >24/min, HR >100/min, SBP <90 mmHg, O$_2$
  sats <90% on room air, abnormal mental status, inability to eat without assistance.
  Patient advice: symptoms reduced by: 1 week for fever, 4 weeks for chest pain
  and sputum production, 6 weeks for cough and breathlessness, 3 months for all but
  fatigue, and by 6 months most people will feel back to normal. Persisting symptoms
  beyond these should seek advice.
- **Differentials:** lung cancer: lobar pneumonia due to underlying bronchostenotic
  lesion. Repeat CXR at 6 weeks. Fails to resolve needs CT/bronchoscopy. Suspect
  more so in smokers. **Tuberculosis:** if considered avoid drugs with anti-TB activity,
  e.g. fluoroquinolones. Send 3 sputum samples for smear and culture. Atypical
  presentation in HIV, immunocompromised and diabetics. Isolate especially if smear
  positive. **Heart failure:** ↑BNP and abnormal echo. **HIV:** low threshold to testing.

Could this be PCP (▶Section 4.15)? **Asthma/exacerbation of COPD:** dyspnoea, cough, wheeze, smoking. **Fungal pneumonia:** histoplasmosis, cocc/oidioides, blastomycosis. Animal exposure, endemic areas, immunocompromised. Southwest USA or Mexico. **Organising pneumonia:** diagnosis of exclusion – usually diffuse bilateral patchy changes. May need lung biopsy and steroids.

- **Antimicrobial management of CAP:** mild (CURB-65 = 0/1): AMOXICILLIN PO or CLARITHROMYCIN PO for 7 days. **Moderate** (CURB-65 >2): AMOXICILLIN IV/ PO plus CLARITHROMYCIN PO/IV for 7–10 d. De-escalate IV to PO when suitable. **Severe:** CO-AMOXICLAV IV plus CLARITHROMYCIN IV for 7–10 d. Alternatives include CEFUROXIME IV or MEROPENEM IV. Suspect *Staph. aureus* (measles, flu, immunocompromised, alcohol abuse, IVDU): FLUCLOXACILLIN IV for 14–21 d. In all de-escalate IV to PO when suitable. If MRSA suspected give VANCOMYCIN IV.
- **Hospital-acquired pneumonia:** mild/moderate consider CO-AMOXICLAV PO or IV. Alternatively, TAZOCIN IV, or MEROPENEM IV if penicillin allergic (severe/ anaphylaxis). If evidence of aspiration, consider adding METRONIDAZOLE. Contact microbiology if MRSA-positive or if no improvement in 24 h. Palliation: more than half of pneumonia-related deaths occur in people older than 84. Support end of life care where appropriate.

Reference: NICE 2014, CG191: Diagnosis and management of community and hospital-acquired pneumonia in adults.

4.15 *Pneumocystis* pneumonia

- **About:** infection by opportunistic fungus *P. jirovecii* (formerly *P. carinii*). Seen in untreated HIV infection (CD4 <200/mm^3) or in those on immunosuppression. Post-transplantation, methotrexate, long-term steroids. Slow insidious onset of an AIDS defining illness.
- **Aetiology:** infection damages alveolar epithelium, impedes gas exchange and leads to Type 1 RF.
- **Clinical:** progressive breathlessness, PTX, fever, dry cough, fine crackles. Desaturates on mild exertion. Look for signs of AIDS, e.g. oral candida, Kaposi's sarcoma, hairy leukoplakia, herpes zoster, etc.
- **Investigations:** bloods: **FBC and U&E:** low WCC. Elevation of LDH >500 mg/dL is common but non-specific. *ABG:* PaO$_2$ <8 kPa on air defined as severe PCP. Increased A–a oxygen gradient. Desaturation with exercise is useful but nonspecific. **Rapid HIV test:** CD4 cell counts (usually <200/mm^3) and HIV viral load measurements. **CXR:** diffuse, bilateral, symmetrical interstitial infiltrates emanating from the hila in a butterfly pattern, cavitation, cysts, TB in AIDs, nodules or PTX. **HRCT:** characteristic ground-glass appearance, cysts, nodules, PTX. CT scan of the chest will usually show filtrates when the CXR is normal. Diagnosis requires histopathologic or cytopathologic evidence of organisms in tissue from bronchoalveolar lavage (BAL) fluid, or induced sputum samples.
- **Management** (O$_2$, antibiotics, steroids, HAART): take advice from HIV team/ infectious diseases. ABC + high FiO$_2$ to deliver sats of 94–98%. **ITU referral:** if severe hypoxaemia. Watch out for PTX which is seen with PCP. Current guidelines recommend high-dose CO-TRIMOXAZOLE (see *formulary*) for 2–3 weeks. Newer evidence suggests a lower dose may be preferred in lower risk patients. Take expert advice. Adjust dose to renal function. Alternatives include DAPSONE 100 mg OD for 21d. CLINDAMYCIN also used in severe disease. SpO$_2$ may fall in the first few days after treatment commences and does not signify clinical failure. **Steroids:** give following PCP therapy if room air SaO$_2$ <8 kPa (some quote 9.3 kPa) or ↑A–a O$_2$ gradient and within 72 h of therapy. PREDNISOLONE 40 mg BD for 5 days, tapering off over the next 2–3 weeks. **HAART:** should be initiated by local specialists within 2 weeks of diagnosis of PCP irrespective of CD4 count. Risk of immune reconstitution inflammatory syndrome which can be life-threatening. **Stop smoking:** smoking

cessation is advocated. PCP prevention: CO-TRIMOXAZOLE 960 mg PO daily. **In pregnancy: diagnostics the same.** Preferred initial therapy during pregnancy is TMP-SMX plus folic acid first trimester.

Reference: Guidelines for Prevention and Treatment of Opportunistic Infections in HIV-Infected Adults and Adolescent (last updated October 28, 2014, see http://aidsinfo.nih.gov/guidelines).

4.16 Empyema

- **About:** pus in the pleural space usually post-bacterial pneumonia. It requires effective drainage and systemic antibiotics.
- **Aetiology:** parapneumonic effusion after bacterial pneumonia becomes infected. Associated with diabetes, alcohol abuse, IV drug use, GORD. Post trauma or a complicated lung abscess or thoracic surgery or infected draining catheter.
- **Clinical:** purulent cough, pyrexia, dyspnoea after recent pneumonia. Weight loss, pleurisy and fever, night sweats, clubbing.
- **Investigations:** bloods: FBC: ↑WCC, ↑CRP. U&E: AKI. CXR: pleural effusion, consolidation, mass, bronchiectasis. Pleural aspiration: shows a purulent or turbid/cloudy pleural fluid exudate which may be neutrophil-rich and viscous with ↑protein, ↑white cells. **Empyema:** glucose <2.2 mmol/L, pH <7.2. A pH >7.8 suggests *Proteus*. Ensure all pleural fluid analysed in blood gas machine has been heparinised. LDH: >1000 IU/L. Low pH (<7.30) causes an empyema, RA, malignancy, tuberculosis, lupus, oesophageal rupture. Blood cultures for aerobic and anaerobic bacteria performed. **Enhanced chest CT:** to help locate drain optimally because the cavities may become loculated. CT is ideal to define the anatomy. Gas usually suggests an empyema.
- **Management:** ABC O$_2$ as per BTS guidelines. Ensure adequate nutrition in patients with pleural infection. Abstain from alcohol/smoking. Identify any immunocompromise. Ensure VTE prophylaxis as high risk and give LMWH. **Chest drain:** if diagnosis confirmed by aspiration then insert a drain large enough to drain the fluid. A small bore catheter 10–14 Fr will be adequate for most cases of pleural infection. Occasionally viscid and difficult to drain but in many cases a small tube inserted by Seldinger method is adequate. The small catheters can be placed using either ultrasound or CT scans. Previously streptokinase to cause localised fibrinolysis has been used but less so now as data have not been positive. If parapneumonic effusion not confirmed by aspirate then do not drain but continue antibiotics and watch CRP and reassess and take advice. *Pleural procedures should not take place out of hours except in an emergency.* **IV antibiotics:** take microbiology advice – usually same antibiotics as pneumonia. Aminoglycosides are inactivated by low pH. May need to cover anaerobes and pseudomonas. Get results of culture and adjust accordingly. Involve chest team and they may need to involve thoracic surgery (thoracotomy and decortication) in difficult cases. Decortication involves the removal of all fibrous tissue from the visceral pleura and parietal pleura, and the evacuation of all pus and debris from the pleural space.

Reference: British Thoracic Society Pleural Disease Guideline Group (2010).

4.17 Pulmonary embolism and deep vein thrombosis

- **About:** deep vein thrombosis (DVT) and pulmonary embolism (PE) are all part of same disease. Reduce by early mobilisation and low dose LMWH or equivalent in those at increased risk. Untreated mortality is 30% (not all PEs are the same), which falls to 3–8% with treatment. However, data come from a time when only larger PEs were detectable. Can expect 500 per DGH per year. 65–90% emboli from legs. Several DOACs now licensed to treat DVT/PE. Many small DVTs and even PEs are potentially benign. Anticoagulation has risks and these need to be balanced. Need better algorithms to select those in whom risk of VTE exceeds that of anticoagulation.

- **Aetiology:** most thrombi originate in the proximal veins of the lower leg and pelvis. Consider a thrombophilia disorder in those under 45 without a clear precipitant. DVT can embolise across a right/left shunt (e.g. PFO/ASD) and cause an embolic stroke. Most emboli are multiple to lower lobes and 10% cause infarction. Autopsies show high incidence of undiagnosed VTE as a cause of death.

- **Clinical DVT:** pain, redness, swelling, dilated veins, increased circumference, can extend to the calf or the whole leg swollen in large proximal thrombosis. Thrombus usually starts distally and extends proximally even to pelvic veins. Proximal clots are most likely to embolise. **Upper limb DVT:** comprises 10% of DVT: risk are local cancer, pacemakers, central lines, thrombophilias or Paget-Schroetter syndrome involving dominant arm. PE is less likely. May be clinically silent post ITU.

- **Clinical PE:** <u>small PE</u>: single small emboli may be silent or subtle and non-specific, e.g. causing confusion especially in elderly. PE with severe pleuritic chest pain as the dominant symptom tends to be peripheral with infarction and anatomically small. <u>Chronic PE</u>: may over time lead to progressive ↑SOB and pulmonary hypertension. <u>Medium sized PE</u>: ↑RR, ↑HR, haemoptysis, pleuritic chest pain, pleural rub, collapse, ↓BP, syncope or presyncope. <u>Large PE</u>: there is acute right heart failure with marked dyspnoea, tachypnoea, presyncope or syncope. Urge to defecate (often collapse in toilet), chest pain, ↑HR, ↑JVP and loud P2 on auscultation, ↓↓BP. <u>Massive PE/saddle embolism</u>: embolism to one or both pulmonary arteries – sudden cardiac death, obstructive shock ↓↓BP.

- **Complications:** sudden death, pulmonary hypertension in PE survivors mean pulmonary artery pressure >25 mmHg more than 6 months after PE is diagnosed. Death is usually due to progressive pulmonary hypertension culminating in RVF. Post-thrombotic syndrome of the legs: chronic venous insufficiency seen in 50% of those who experience DVT or PE. Can lead to leg ulcers and oedema. Paradoxical embolism: those with right to left shunts and stroke.

- **High risks:** previous DVT/PE, systemic malignancy, hospital immobility, perioperative event, stroke, severe illness, spinal injury, GBS, trauma, HHS, localised trauma. Varicose veins +/− phlebitis, post-MI, pregnancy and postpartum, pelvic tumour.

- **Medium/low risks:** thrombophilias, smoking, combined OCP, HRT, recent long haul travel >6 h, obesity, blood transfusion, antiphospholipid syndrome, nephrotic syndrome, polycythaemia, sickle cell disease. Steroids are associated with increase in VTE occurrence.

Wells clinical model for assessing probability of DVT

- **Predisposing factors:** active cancer (treatment <6 months or palliative) = +1, paralysis, paresis, recent cast immobilisation of leg = +1, recently bedridden >3 days, or major surgery requiring regional or general anaesthetic in the previous 12 weeks = +1, previously documented DVT = +1.

- **Clinical:** calf swelling >3 cm compared to asymptomatic calf (measured 10 cm below tibia tuberosity) = +1, collateral superficial veins (non-varicose) = +1, pitting oedema (confined to symptomatic leg) = +1, swelling of entire leg = +1, localised tenderness along deep venous system = +1. Clinical assessment: alternative diagnosis at least as likely as DVT = −2.

- **Pretest probability:** clinical probability of DVT: score of 2 or higher – DVT is 'likely'; score of less than 2 – DVT is 'unlikely'.

- **Wells** >2 (don't do D-dimer) do compression ultrasound. If positive treat DVT. If negative consider repeating USS in 1 week.

- **Wells** <2 then check D-dimer and if negative DVT excluded. If positive do compression ultrasound: if positive treat DVT; if negative consider repeating in 1 week.

Wells clinical scoring systems for predicting pretest probability of a PE

- Note these scores are validated in those who develop a PE/DVT in an outpatient setting. They have less validity in inpatient events where risks are skewed by being in a different risk group and patients may be on VTE prophylaxis and so traditional assessment is needed on a case by case basis [JAMA Intern Med. 2015;175:1112].
- **Predisposing factors:** previous PE/DVT = +1.5, recent surgery or immobilization (<30 days) = +1.5, malignancy (treated <6/12 ago) = +1.
- **Clinical:** HR >100/min = +1.5, clinical signs of DVT = +3, haemoptysis = +1. Clinical assessment: alternative diagnosis less likely than PE = +3.
- **Pretest probability of PE:** 'unlikely' <4 (do D-dimer) and 'likely' >4 (don't do D-dimer).
- **Probability score:** PE unlikely then check D-dimer and if normal then PE excluded. If elevated do CTPA or V/Q.
- **Probability score:** PE likely (D-dimer not needed), all need CTPA or V/Q.

Assessment

- **Differential diagnosis for DVT:** leg trauma +/− haematoma, internal derangement of the knee, muscle tear and damage, ruptured Baker's (popliteal) cyst, cellulitis, obstructive lymphadenopathy, lymphoedema, drug-induced oedema (amlodipine, etc.).
- **Investigations:** bloods: FBC, U&E, LFTs, CRP, ESR typically normal unless reflecting underlying cause, e.g. malignancy. **ABG:** medium to large PE can cause a reduced PO_2 and reduced/normal PCO_2 (Type 1 RF). *In extremis* may be acidotic and ↑lactate. **D-dimer by ELISA:** high negative predictive value. A normal D-dimer excludes PE/DVT in patients with a low or intermediate/moderate pretest likelihood to the extent that no further testing needed. In those at high risk D-dimer does not come into play and all need second step diagnostic imaging: V/Q or CTPA. A D-dimer level >500 ng/ml is seen in nearly all patients with DVT/PE, and false positives in others. D-dimer elevated in pregnancy, infections, sepsis, anticoagulated, post-op. It is a degradation product of cross-linked fibrin. Don't bother if high probability. **ECG findings:** sinus tachycardia, new AF. Others include S1Q3T3 pattern. RV strain and right access deviation. New incomplete RBBB. ECG may be normal. **CXR: done in all including pregnant,** a normal CXR is entirely compatible with a large PE. Segmental wedge collapse, pleural effusion, area of lung infarction, ↑hemidiaphragm, prominent pulmonary artery and a localised absence of vascular markings (Westermark sign), dilated pulmonary arteries. **Cardiac troponin** ↑ and **BNP** ↑ or **N-terminal (NT)-proBNP** ↑ in large PEs and associated with a worse outcome. **Echocardiogram:** RA and RV dilated, TR, right heart strain, pulmonary hypertension. Diagnostic in massive PE but less helpful in sub-massive PE. RV hypokinesis has been shown to be associated with double the 30-day mortality.
- **Diagnostic imaging for DVT:** contrast venography: largely superseded by compression USS and rarely done. Considered gold standard. **NB.** The superficial femoral vein is a deep vein and thrombosis requires treatment. To avoid confusion it has been renamed the distal femoral vein. Compression ultrasonography of lower or upper limb veins if upper limb DVT suspected is the preferred diagnostic test. It is non-invasive, relatively inexpensive and readily available. It has replaced contrast venography as the modality of choice. It is particularly useful for pelvic and iliofemoral clots.

Diagnostic imaging for PE

- **Ventilation–perfusion (V/Q)** scanning using single photon emission computed tomography (SPECT) is the preferred initial imaging, especially in pregnancy or young with a normal CXR or renal failure or allergy to IV contrast. False positives in those with asthma and bronchospasm. Follow local guidance. Ventilation scan by inhaling radioactive xenon gas. Perfusion using injected radiolabelled albumin macro-aggregates. Look for areas of 'mismatch' with ventilation but low perfusion. Intermediate results will require CTPA or USS to risk assess.

- **CT pulmonary angiography (CTPA):** multislice helical involves giving IV contrast. Identifies if PE or other pathologies, e.g. pneumonia or aortic dissection or tamponade. It is quick (a whole lung scanned within a 10 sec breath hold) and can be done out of hours. Current fear of overdiagnosis as scanners can image sixth-order vessels and visualise thrombi so small that clinical importance is uncertain. Subsegmental PE may not be clinically significant and may not need treatment – take advice. **Pulmonary angiography** is the gold standard but rarely done nowadays. When PE is the diagnosis but CTPA or V/Q scan not desired, e.g. pregnant or not possible, then the finding of thrombus on USS legs may be used as a surrogate marker for PE, when there is DVT and appropriate chest symptoms and a decision to anticoagulate is straightforward. Magnetic resonance angiography: in PIOPED III (Prospective Investigation of PE Diagnosis III) study, MRA showed poor sensitivity for detection of PE and cannot be recommended.
- **General comments:** CTPA is sensitive and easy to obtain, but for clinically stable patients alternative tests reduce exposure radiation, cost less, and are less likely to lead to overdiagnosis. V/Q scans may be preferable in younger patients (less radiation), patients with normal lungs (a definitive result is more likely), and patients with renal dysfunction (no nephrotoxic contrast). Detection of DVT by ultrasonography of the legs when PE is suspected makes subsequent lung imaging unnecessary because patients need anticoagulation anyway. There is no single pathway. Depends on access to tests and availability of ambulatory testing – this is a complex and difficult area so take advice.

Other tests
- **Thrombophilia testing:** consider testing for APL antibodies in patients who have had an unprovoked DVT/PE or if it is planned to stop anticoagulation at the end of treatment. Consider testing for hereditary thrombophilia in patients who have had unprovoked DVT or PE and who have a first-degree relative who has had DVT or PE. **Do not** offer thrombophilia testing to patients who have had a provoked DVT or PE. **Do** offer thrombophilia testing to first-degree relatives of people with a history of DVT or PE and thrombophilia. Factor V Leiden mutation is the commonest thrombophilia and seen in 5% of European descent. Present in 11–21% of patients with a venous thromboembolic event.
- **Occult malignancy:** NICE recommend follow-up for all those over 40 with a first unprovoked DVT or PE: should have a general exam and CXR, FBC, Ca, LFTs, urinalysis. In those over 40 perform further investigation with an outpatient CT abdomen and pelvis and a mammogram for women.

Prognosis scoring
Allows early discharge or outpatient care for low risk patients. There are two: sPESI and MBOVA:
- **Simplified pulmonary embolism severity index (sPESI score):** PESI score: age >80 = +1, history of cancer = +1, chronic lung/heart disease = +1, HR >110/min, SBP <100 mmHg = +1, SaO_2 <90% = +1. Combining results of the hsTn T assay with the simplified PESI appears to yield additive prognostic information. Those with a low PESI score can be considered for outpatient management. Score 0: low risk 30 d mortality of 1%; score of 1 or more: 30 d mortality of 10.9%.
- **Modified BOVA score:** classifies the risk for PE-related complications, e.g. lung infarction, death and pneumonia within 30 days after diagnosis using four variables assessed at the time of PE diagnosis: HR >110/min = +1, SBP <100 mmHg = + 2, cardiac troponin (cardiac cTnI >0.4 ng/ml) = +2, echo shows RV dysfunction = +2. Worse prognosis in those with a score >4. It helps to identify those at intermediate to high risk of complications and may be used with sPESI [*Neth J Med*, 2015;73:410].

Management

- **Primary prevention is best:** risk assessment and LMWH, early mobilisation in medical patients. Perioperative LMWH or use of anticoagulants, e.g. DOACs. Early mobilization post-op. Hydration. Use of LMWH in higher risk pregnancies and those with APLS or thrombophilia up to 6 weeks after. Use of LMWH in oncology patients.
- **Acute PE:** ABC high FiO_2 as per BTS guidelines. ALS algorithm if collapsed and unresponsive, give prolonged CPR. Cardiac monitoring of BP, HR, O_2 sats. Commence 1 L IV crystalloid to ensure adequate RV filling, especially if ↓BP. **Thrombolysis** is considered in a compromised patient – those who are shocked, have severe RV dysfunction and elevated biomarkers. Assess for bleeding risks as co-morbidities may exist. Major bleeding risk – 9.24% with thrombolysis vs. 3.4% rate in the anticoagulation cohort. Intracranial haemorrhage: thrombolysed 1.46% vs. 0.19% placebo. Benefits of lower mortality (1.39% vs. 2.92%) with thrombolytic compared to anticoagulation extended to intermediate risk group [*JAMA*, 2014;311:2414]. See *formulary* for ALTEPLASE dosing. **Pulmonary Surgical embolectomy** may be available in local cardiothoracic centres if there is a large central thrombus refractory to lysis. In the moribund there is little to lose. Discuss with surgeons according to local pathways. Some research has been done on extending use to those with anatomically extensive PE and concomitant moderate to severe RV dysfunction, despite preserved systemic BP; requires cardiac bypass and heparinisation [*Circulation*, 2002;105:1416].

DVT management

- **Acute massive DVT:** discuss with vascular team or interventional radiologists. Catheter-directed thrombolytic therapy for patients with symptomatic iliofemoral DVT who have symptoms <2 weeks, good functional status, a life expectancy of 1 year or more, and a low risk of bleeding. There is risk of limb ischaemia and postphlebitic syndrome.
- **Below knee DVT:** repeat USS after 7 days to see if there is extension above the knee. The management of isolated calf DVT is controversial. Those undergoing orthopaedic procedures, malignancy, and the immobile had a higher risk of propagation. Risk of PE and other complications seems low. Most (90%) PEs arise from above the knee thrombus. Mortality rate of proximal DVT > distal DVT. No consensus on whether to treat, observe or not treat. Full dose anticoagulation is not risk free. Follow local expert guidance. Consider the choice between anticoagulation and serial ultrasound at 1–2 weeks and risk for thrombus extension, bleeding, and patient preference.
- **Upper limb DVT:** treat cause or risks. Anticoagulate for 3 months. SVC filters are available for those where anticoagulation is contraindicated, but efficacy data is limited. Investigate – some have occult malignancy, most commonly lung cancer or lymphoma.

Anticoagulation for DVT/PE

- Anticoagulation with LMWH (ENOXAPARIN/TINZAPARIN) or FONDAPARINUX or IV HEPARIN (much less so). Treat on the basis of clinical suspicion and balance bleeding risk whilst awaiting CTPA, V/Q, USS. Stop if tests are negative. If a PE/DVT is identified then risk/benefit analysis and start a DOAC or Warfarin or continue long term LMWH. See *formulary* for doses. New guidance for 2016 states that for low-risk, isolated, subsegmental PE, clinical surveillance is an option and recommended, rather than anticoagulation. **Warfarin (INR 2–3) 3–6 months** for a first idiopathic PE/DVT is routine. **Provoked DVT/PE:** a 3 month course where the precipitant has been removed. Warfarin and heparin overlap for 5 days because a transient pro-coagulant condition can exist. 5 year risks of recurrence is 10%. **Unprovoked proximal DVT or PE** treat and continue for 3–6 months. At 3 months, assess the risks and benefits of continuing treatment with DOAC/Warfarin/LMWH for a full 6 months or longer. They have a ↑baseline risk and a ↑D-dimer 1 month after stopping may suggest greater risk. Unprovoked 5 year recurrence is 30%. At this stage do thrombophilia testing in the young or those with a family history. **Direct oral anticoagulants** (DOACs) are now recommended [NICE 2013, TA287] for the acute treatment of PE/DVT to preventing recurrence. It is recommended to continue LMWH for the first 5 days with Dabigatran but not Apixaban or Rivaroxaban. See *formulary* for dosages.

- **IVC filters** may be used where there is a DVT/PE and bleeding such that anticoagulation is not possible. They appear to reduce PE but increase DVT risk but no clear mortality benefit. No benefit in using them as well as anticoagulation in high risk patients [*JAMA*, 2015;313:1627]. Attractive in concept but robust evidence is lacking and deaths purely due to IVC filter insertion have occurred. Patients should eventually be anticoagulated when safe to do so. Remove them as early as is possible, e.g. after 2–6 weeks when it is anticipated that anticoagulation can be started in short term or the risk of VTE/PE is short term. Complications include vessel wall erosion and haemorrhage, IVC occlusion because of thrombus, recurrent DVT, and post-thrombotic syndrome with ulcers and leg oedema.

- **PE and known cancer:** standard practice is to offer LMWH to patients with active cancer and confirmed proximal DVT or PE, and to continue the LMWH for 6 months or indefinitely if there is active cancer or active treatment of cancer. At 6 months, assess the risks and benefits of continuing anticoagulation. No useful data on IVC filter usage.

- **Anticoagulation is not harmless:** CTPA can detect isolated small subsegmental pulmonary emboli which are not clinically important and so where the real risks of anticoagulation may outweigh benefits – take expert advice. Interestingly, the higher resolution of CTPA versus V/Q scan diagnosis increases the number of PEs diagnosed, but detecting small PEs may not alter overall outcome.

- **Ambulatory care of suspected PE:** exclusion criteria as follows: studies have shown that for selected low risk patients with acute symptomatic PE, outpatient treatment with LMWH is not inferior to inpatient treatment in terms of effectiveness and safety. Those who are sent home must be a very well, stable, independent group who can readily seek help. Check low sPESI score.

- **Admission and not ambulatory care if breathless at rest**, O_2 sats <97%, PO_2 <10 kPa on air, HR >100 bpm or SBP <100 mmHg, CKD or other need for IV heparin therapy. Other illnesses requiring admission: ↓platelets <70 × 10^9/L precluding heparin therapy, active bleeding or high bleeding risk, acute anaemia. History of heparin-induced thrombocytopenia, suspected PE on anticoagulation. Current alcohol/illicit drug abuse, psychosis, dementia. Homelessness or difficult social circumstances. Pregnancy, ECG RV strain, pain-requiring IV opiates.

References: NICE (2012) CG144: Venous thromboembolic diseases. Task Force for the Diagnosis and Management of Acute Pulmonary Embolism of the European Society of Cardiology (2008) Guidelines on the diagnosis and management of acute pulmonary embolism. *Eur Heart J*, 29:2276. Wiener *et al.* (2013) When a test is too good: how CT pulmonary angiograms find pulmonary emboli that do not need to be found. *BMJ*, 347:f3368. RCOG Green-top Guideline No. 37a (www.rcog.org.uk).

4.18 Lung 'white out'

- **About:** complete opacification usually of one lung field. Position of the mediastinum/trachea is key. Do not insert a chest drain to remove fluid without confirming effusion using ultrasound/CT.
- **Differential using tracheal/mediastinal shift: collapse (atelectasis)** of an entire lung: volume loss resulting in mediastinal shift towards the opacification. **Pleural**

effusion: large pleural effusion pushes the trachea away from the affected side. **Consolidation:** no mediastinal shift, air bronchogram may be seen against the consolidated lung. **Mesothelioma:** there is typically no mediastinal shift. **Post-pneumonectomy/thoracoplasty:** when an entire lung is surgically removed, there is volume loss with fluid accumulation and fibrotic opacification of the pleural space. A resected rib may be absent. Thoracoplasty for TB prior to 1944. **Congenital absence or hypoplasia of lung:** trachea pulled towards affected side. **Mixed:** both an effusion and lung collapse. The tracheal position will tell you which of these is greater in terms of volume loss and gain using the above.

- **Clinical:** smoker, cough, weight loss, asbestos exposure, asthma, COPD, old TB. Pyrexia, sputum, haemoptysis, recent pneumonia, previous lung surgery.
- **Investigations:** bloods: FBC, U&E, LFT, CRP/ESR, ABG, calcium. **CXR** (PA +/– lateral): position of the trachea is key to see if it is pulled towards the affected side (volume loss) or pushed away (extra volume) or central. Look for other pathology. Absent breast shadow (cancer), Hilar mass. **CT chest:** for confirmation and to look for underlying pathology. **Local ultrasound** can distinguish consolidated lung from effusion and can be essential prior to performing a thoracentesis.
- **Management:** ABC, O_2 as per BTS guidelines. Bronchodilators may aid expectoration and help bronchospasm. Supportive: manage respiratory failure and infection. Chest physio may help if endobronchial mucus. Determine likely causation and treat. Severe hypoxaemia with RF should lead to intubation and mechanical support. **Old pneumonectomy:** old CXR will show lesion. Signs of old surgery. Optimise ventilation if compromised. **Total lung collapse/atelectasis:** post pneumonia, asthma, COPD. Foreign body inhalation. Consider intrabronchial lesion. If acute may be a sputum plug and chest physio and hydration and mucolytic may help. Bronchial stenosis which may be endobronchial or extra bronchial should be considered. Smoker. Cachexic. Clubbed. May need a fibreoptic bronchoscopy with suction. Consider CT chest. Urgency depending on ABC, O_2 and ABG +/– antibiotics if infection. Position involved side uppermost (opposite to haemoptysis) to promote increased drainage of the affected area, vigorous chest physio, and encourage the patient to cough and to breathe deeply. CPAP may help lung expansion. **Consolidation:** needs assessment and appropriate antibiotics. May need HDU/ITU if RF. See *Pneumonia* (▶Section 4.14). **Pleural effusion:** consider ultrasound to confirm fluid if unsure and then remove. Urgency depending on clinical picture. See *Pleural effusion* (▶Section 4.13). Heart failure unusual to be unilateral unless patient recumbent on one side. If signs of empyema needs antibiotics and drainage. **Diaphragmatic hernia/pulmonary agenesis:** respiratory support as needed.

4.19 Lung abscess

- **About:** formation of an infected pus-filled cavity within the lung parenchyma.
- **Aetiology:** post pneumonia usually *Staph. aureus*, *Klebsiella*, Gram negatives, anaerobes. Infected cavity, TB, aspiration pneumonia, bronchiectasis. Trans-diaphragmatic spreads from amoebic abscess. Distal to endobronchial obstruction, e.g. inhaled foreign body or tumour.
- **Clinical:** fever, malaise, weight loss, breathlessness, pain, foul breath. Clubbing may be seen with chronic untreated suppurative disease.
- **Investigation:** FBC: ↑WCC, ↑ESR, ↑CRP. Sputum/blood cultures. CXR and HRCT: infected cavity or tumour, and lymph nodes and lung parenchyma.
- **Management:** ABC. Prolonged IV antibiotics and surgical or percutaneous drainage. Bronchoscopy to remove any foreign body or biopsy endobronchial lesion.

05 Endocrine and diabetic emergencies

Introduction

Endocrinology testing usually involves a snapshot picture of function. Some hormone secretion is pulsatile, other hormones have diurnal variation and increase with sickness, protein binding can all make results less reliable. Dynamic testing provokes suspected underactive glands and suppresses suspected overactive glands and gives a better assessment of true function.

5.1 Primary hypoadrenalism (Addisonian crisis)

- **About:** acutely reduced adrenocortical function (glucocorticoids, mineralocorticoids). Insidious and subtle or acute and life threatening, provoked by illness, e.g. infection. Iatrogenic due to cessation of medically prescribed steroids. Adrenal cortex provides cortisol, sex hormones and mineralocorticoids. Increased demand during stresses (infection, trauma, illness). Never stop long-term steroids acutely. Ill patients need them even more.
- **Types: primary:** adrenal destruction or dysfunction. Low cortisol, high ACTH. Needs 90% adrenal destruction before detectable. **Secondary:** pituitary disease and ACTH insufficiency. Low ACTH and cortisol. **Tertiary:** impaired hypothalamic CRH release. Low CRH and ACTH and cortisol.

Causes of hypoadrenalism

- **Iatrogenic:** exogenous steroid suppresses adrenal production. Abrupt cessation of medically prescribed steroids +/− physiological stress (sepsis or surgery). Needs only 3 weeks of steroids to suppress intrinsic production. Taper off steroid doses slowly.
- **Autoimmune adrenalitis:** 70% (lymphocytic infiltration) often with autoimmune disease (Graves' disease, Hashimoto's thyroiditis, pernicious anaemia, hypoparathyroidism or Type I diabetes or vitiligo and primary ovarian failure).
- **Infections:** 5% of those with TB get adrenal destruction (may calcify on AXR), HIV, CMV, adrenalitis. Progressive disseminated histoplasmosis.
- **Haemorrhage:** Waterhouse–Friderichsen syndrome associated with meningococcaemia. Also sepsis, coagulopathy and antiphospholipid syndrome.
- **Malignancy:** bilateral adrenal metastases from breast and lung and melanoma and lymphoma.
- **Genetic:** adrenoleukodystrophy, congenital adrenal hyperplasia – 21-hydroxylase (*CYP21A2*) or 11β-hydroxylase (*CYP11B1*) genes.
- **Miscellaneous:** amyloidosis, post-bilateral adrenalectomy, polyglandular autoimmune syndromes.
- **Secondary adrenocortical insufficiency:** pituitary haemorrhage, Sheehan's syndrome.
- **Relative adrenal insufficiency:** is suspected in some critical care patients but is controversial.

- **Aetiology:** adrenals produce 15–30 mg/day of cortisol and more when under stress. Endogenous production falls with chronic steroid therapy. 8–9 am normal is 110–520 nmol/L (4–19 mcg/dL), but midnight <140 nmol/L (5 mcg/dL). Cortisol – wound healing, BP, immune function, stress response. Adrenal failure causes low glucocorticoids and aldosterone. Failure to retain salt and water causes ↓BP. Pituitary releases increased ACTH/MSH with pigmentation.
- **Clinical:** subacute with fatigue, anorexia, weight loss, tiredness, diarrhoea, vomiting. Easily misattributed to virus, chronic fatigue or anorexia or depression. Abdominal pain, generalised weakness, precipitated by sepsis, surgery. Postural ↓BP, ↑HR, shocked, confusion, hypoglycaemia. In secondary disease (pituitary) K

normal and no pigmentation and BP less affected. Loss of axillary and pubic body
hair in females (loss of adrenal androgens). Pigmentation in gums, buccal mucosa,
skin, pressure points, skin creases, scars (not in those with corticosteroid therapy).
Hypoglycaemia is more common in secondary adrenal insufficiency. May also see
Type 1 DM, RA, vitiligo, Hashimoto's thyroiditis, coeliac, pernicious anaemia.

Investigations

- **FBC:** ↑eosinophils. **U&E:** low Na, high K, low HCO_3, low Cl, low glucose, low or high
  urea, high Ca. K normal if due to pituitary hypofunction. **ABG or venous gas:** low
  HCO_3 mild metabolic acidosis.
- **Random plasma cortisol:** at 8–9 am value >276 nmol/L is normal and >400 nmol/L
  makes adrenal insufficiency unlikely. Random cortisol <80–100 nmol/L makes
  diagnosis very likely unless patient on oral/inhaled steroids. If level between
  100 and 400 nmol/L then perform a short synACTHen test.
- **Short synACTHen test:** give Synacthen 250 mcg IV or IM (1 vial). Check 30 min
  cortisol. Diagnosis excluded if cortisol at 30–60 min >500 nmol/L. Usually a flat
  response is seen. Treat on clinical evidence if result delayed. Some have relative adrenal
  insufficiency which manifests with acute illness, infection, bleed, surgery/trauma. A
  short synACTHen may show a muted response. They may need steroids in their acute
  phase when unwell and re-evaluate later. In a sick patient testing should never delay
  steroid replacement. The diagnosis can always be confirmed later post the acute phase.
- **ACTH:** (normal 4.4–22 pmol/L or 20–100 pg/ml) if cortisol low then check ACTH.
  ACTH >80 ng/L at 9 am with low cortisol confirms diagnosis.
- **Renin/aldosterone:** low aldosterone and renin is high. Plasma
  dehydroepiandrosterone (DHEA) and DHEA sulphate are low.
- **Adrenal antibodies to 21-hydroxylase** seen in 80% autoimmune disease.
- **CXR/AXR:** to look for active TB disease and classically small heart. Calcification.
- **CT abdomen:** may show enlarged necrotic glands with calcification. Small adrenals
  in autoimmune disease. Large with infection or metastases. Haemorrhage may be
  seen. **Adrenal biopsy** in selected cases.
- **Plasma C26:0 fatty acids** will detect adrenoleukodystrophy.

Differential

- **Hypopituitarism:** see ▶Section 5.9 for pituitary assessment.
- **Anorexia nervosa:** normal/high cortisol, low LH, FSH. Fear of weight gain.

Management

- **ABC and O_2** as per BTS guidelines. 1 L NS over 30–60 min. Check for and manage
  any hypoglycaemia. Send random cortisol 10 ml in a heparinised tube. **Do not** delay
  glucocorticoids while awaiting laboratory results or attempt endocrine stimulation
  testing in acutely ill patients. Treat with suspicion alone and confirm later.
- **Immediate: give** HYDROCORTISONE 50–100 mg IV then IM every 6 h. Alternatively
  DEXAMETHASONE 4 mg IV OD. Once stable and able to take oral then start
  HYDROCORTISONE 20 mg 8 h and gradually wean down to 30 mg per day in divided
  doses, usually with a larger morning dose.
- **Long term for life:** HYDROCORTISONE (20–30 mg/day) 10 mg at 8 am, 5 mg at
  1 pm, 5 mg at 4pm (avoid late as may cause insomnia). Later add FLUDROCORTISONE
  50–200 mcg/day if postural ↓BP. Alternatives to hydrocortisone are PREDNISOLONE
  2.5–5 mg OD. Double dose in times of stress/infection, see below.
- **Relative adrenal insufficiency:** suspected incidence in critical care patients
  as high as 77%. Management controversial. Trials conflicting. Has been shown
  that **HYDROCORTISONE 50 mg IV 6 h** may be beneficial for severe septic shock
  refractory to fluid resuscitation and vasopressors if given early (<8 h).
- **Determine cause:** investigate and treat for TB or HIV, malignancy, adrenal imaging,
  etc. Endocrine consult and follow up for advice and monitoring.

- **Patient advice on sick day rules:** double steroid dose if minor illness or unwell or physiological stress. Family should be aware. Patients should carry a steroid card to alert staff. Ensure know to never stop steroid. Aware that nausea and vomiting may be signs of a crisis and to seek help. Recommended to have an ampoule of HYDROCORTISONE for IM administration in the event of being unable to take oral.
- **Prior to operative procedures** patients should be given HYDROCORTISONE 100 mg IM then 50–100 mg IM 6 h until back on oral therapy.

5.2 Hypoglycaemia

Starvation in those not on insulin or oral hypoglycaemics or with acute alcohol rarely, if ever, causes significant hypoglycaemia. Be sceptical about diagnosing light-headedness and funny spells as hypoglycaemia unless there is clear evidence, e.g. a laboratory glucose reading.

- **About:** prolonged hypoglycaemia causes brain injury and death. Check capillary blood glucose and send lab sample in any confused or comatose patient. Treat any symptomatic blood glucose <4.0 mmol/L.
- **Aetiology:** causes neuroglycopaenia and neuronal dysfunction and increased sympathetic drive. Neurons do not need insulin to allow glucose to enter cells. High metabolising brain is dependent on a steady supply of glucose/ketones. Any shortfall in supply quickly leads to neuronal dysfunction.
- **Clinical:** sweating, trembling, palpitations, anxiety, blurred vision, hunger, headache. Lack of coordination, ataxia, stroke mimic – hemiparesis, confusion, aggression. Loss of inhibitions, convulsions, coma, brain damage, death, violence, agitation. Morning headache, night sweats, vivid dreams suggest nocturnal hypoglycaemia or nocturnal seizures.
- **Causes:** drugs: insulin, sulphonylurea, meglitinides (not metformin), pentamidine, quinine, salicylates, acute alcohol, propranolol. Endocrine: Addison's disease, growth hormone (GH) deficiency, hypopituitarism. Liver failure, insulinoma, chronic pancreatitis with a loss of glucagon activity. Worsening renal function increases insulin sensitivity.
- **Not usually caused by:** metformin, glitazones, thiazolidinediones, DPP-4 inhibitors, GLP-1 analogues. Starvation: those in fasts or famines or hunger-strikes do not usually succumb to acute hypoglycaemia.
- **Impaired awareness of hypoglycaemia** (IAH): acquired syndrome with insulin treatment. Diminished warning symptoms of hypoglycaemia. Increases vulnerability to severe hypoglycaemia. Prevalence increases with duration of diabetes and seen T1DM > T2DM.
- **Investigations:** high morning glucose may suggest overnight hypoglycaemia with stress response. Measure overnight 16 h fast levels of glucose and insulin to look for low glucose and high insulin suggestive of insulinoma. U&E, LFTs, cortisol, C-peptide which mirrors endogenous insulin production. Test if overnight blood glucose <4 mmol/L. Urine sulphonylurea screen in rare unexplained cases.

Management

- **Hypoglycaemic symptoms:** blood glucose <4 mmol/L treat with 10–20 g GLUCOSE as sugary soft drink or sugary tea or juice (not diet drink) or small carbohydrate snack only. Adults who are conscious but uncooperative but can swallow can give a small snack or 1.5–2 tubes Glucogel/Dextrogel squeezed into the mouth. **If ineffective or oral intake unsafe** consider GLUCAGON 1 mg IM/SC but if no response within minutes then 20–50 ml 50% GLUCOSE IV or equivalent must be given. **Note:** there may be a marked disparity between arterial and venous blood glucose which can lead to misdiagnosis of hypoglycaemia based on symptoms and misleadingly low venous levels when arterial levels are actually normal.

- **Adults with suspected hypoglycaemia (check CBG and send venous blood sample) who are unconscious or fitting** then check ABC + O₂ and give 20–50 ml IV 50% GLUCOSE through a large vein and place in recovery position and manage as for status epilepticus (▶ Section 11.16). If no venous access or no IV GLUCOSE then GLUCAGON 1 mg IM/SC. Glucagon may take up to 15 min to take effect because it mobilises glycogen from the liver and so it will be less effective in those who are chronically malnourished (e.g. alcoholics) or in patients who have had a prolonged period of starvation and have depleted liver glycogen stores, or in those with severe liver disease. In this situation, or if prolonged treatment is required, IV GLUCOSE is better. Once normoglycaemic, assess cause and make changes to diabetic regimen if needed. If there is any suspicion of adrenocortical insufficiency then HYDROCORTISONE 50–100 mg IV 8 h should be given and later investigated for hypoadrenalism. An insulin and C-peptide assay can be done where hypoglycaemia is unexplained and deliberate or accidental misuse of insulin suspected. Exogenous insulin causes a rise in insulin but not C-peptide. Endogenous insulin release is accompanied by C-peptide release. If hypoglycaemia confirmed with no obvious cause, then one should consider admission for further tests, e.g. a prolonged fast and other assessments of endocrine function.

Hyperkalaemia

Medical emergency if K >6.5 mmol/L or ECG changes then give 10–20 ml of 10% CALCIUM GLUCONATE slow IV.

- **Clinical:** asymptomatic, arrhythmias, muscle weakness, cramps, paraesthesia. ↓BP, ↓HR, cardiac arrest.
- **Severity: mild** (K 5.5–6.0 mmol/L) or **moderate** (K 6.1–6.5 mmol/L). **Severe** (K >6.5 mmol/L) or if **ECG changes** or symptoms.
- **Investigations:** U&E: repeat sample in case it is false, especially if ECG normal and high K inexplicable. AKI. FBC/LDH: haemolysis. CK: rhabdomyolysis. Venous/arterial blood gases: metabolic acidosis. ECG signs: peaked 'tented' T waves, widened QRS, sine waves, agonal rhythm and VT/VF.
- **Causes** (most commonly drugs – check drug chart) [can get falsely high result: haemolysed sample, laboratory or sampling error]: AKI, CKD, digoxin poisoning (poor prognostic sign). Rhabdomyolysis, tumour lysis syndrome, vigorous exercise, haemolysis, blood transfusion. **Drugs:** ACE inhibitors, AT2 blockers, spironolactone, eplerenone, amiloride, NSAIDs, ciclosporin, depolarising muscle relaxants, trimethoprim. Metabolic acidosis, Addison's disease (pigmented, ↓BP, fatigue), Type 4 RTA (diabetes), hyperkalaemic periodic paralysis (AD familial).

Further management
- **ABC. Assess ECG changes.** Stop all potentially offending drugs or infusions immediately. This is easily overlooked. Ensure IV access, repeat any sample if surprise result. Start IV fluids. K >6.0 mmol/L or ECG changes needs telemetry and defibrillator available.
- **Severe** (K >6.5 mmol/L and/or ECG changes) then cardioprotect with CALCIUM GLUCONATE 10 ml 10%. Next give 50 ml of 50% GLUCOSE with 10 units of SOLUBLE INSULIN (moves K into cells) and consider SALBUTAMOL 10–20 mg in 4 ml saline nebulised with caution in those with IHD/arrhythmias. FUROSEMIDE 10–20 mg IV may be considered if not dehydrated. U&E needs to be repeated every 2 h and blood gas, capillary blood glucose for 6–12 h. The remainder need ECG and underlying cause to be found and close monitoring. These actions only lower K for 4 hours. If metabolic acidosis (low HCO₃) consider either IV 500 ml 1.26% solution (75 mmol)

over 60 min but caution with volume overload. Alternatively 50–100 ml 8.4% $NaHCO_3$ by central line. Do not give calcium if likelihood of digoxin toxicity.
- **Cation exchange resins,** e.g. CALCIUM RESONIUM 30 g initially and then 15 g QDS PR/PO. PR route is possibly more effective than PO. When given rectally the calcium resonium must be retained for 9 h followed by irrigation to remove resin from the colon to prevent faecal impaction. Bowel perforation can be a rare complication.
- **AKI assess and manage cause:** renal referral needed. If AKI/CKD and refractory/ severe hyperkalaemia despite treatment, then discuss suitability for haemodialysis/ haemoperfusion. Adopt a 'low potassium diet', e.g. avoid chocolate, fruit juices. Ensure that any amiloride, spironolactone, ACE inhibitor, ARB or similar has been stopped. See AKI, ▶ Section 10.4.

Reference: Clinical Resource Efficiency Support Team (2005) Guidelines for the treatment of hyperkalaemia in adults (www.crestni.org.uk).

5.4 Hypokalaemia

- **About:** major intracellular cation. In cardiac patients aim for a K of 4.0–5.0 mmol/L. Beware rapid administration of IV potassium can cause lethal arrhythmias. The IV rate of KCl administration should not exceed 20 mmol/h.
- **Aetiology:** the daily intake of potassium in the western diet is between 80 and 120 mmol. Low K reduces muscle and nerve excitability and enhances digoxin toxicity. Hypokalaemia and hypomagnesaemia often coexist, and treatment of hypokalaemia is unlikely to be successful without reversal of hypomagnesaemia.
- **Causes:** thiazides and loop diuretics, Conn syndrome, Cushing syndrome. Severe diarrhoea (villous adenoma, fistulas, laxatives or a VIPoma). Alcohol abuse and Magnesium depletion. Renal tubular acidosis 1 and 2, nephrotoxic drugs, severe vomiting with metabolic alkalosis. Insulin therapy in setting of DKA, giving sodium bicarbonate, IV/nebulised salbutamol. Familial (low K) periodic paralysis, amphotericin B, gentamicin, levodopa. Congenital adrenogenital syndromes, Liddle, Bartter (alkalosis, hypocalciuria) and Gitelman syndromes.
- **Clinical:** mild: lethargy, weakness, paralysis, diarrhoea (as a cause). More severe hypokalaemia: muscle pains, rhabdomyolysis, paralytic ileus, palpitations (ectopics). Look for hypertension (Conn or Cushing syndrome). Check drugs: loop diuretics, thiazides.
- **Investigations: U&E:** K <3.5 mmol/L (severe K <2.5 mmol/L) with normal K 3.5–5.0 mmol/L. Look for a low magnesium. **ECG:** atrial/ventricular ectopics, arrhythmias, ST changes, U wave, T wave flattening. **TFT:** ↑FT_4 and low TSH if hyperthyroid. **HCO_3** is low in RTA. **Endocrine testing** for Cushing or Conn syndrome. **Blood gases** may show a metabolic alkalosis.

Management (aim to keep K 4–5 mmol/L on CCU)

- **Mild (3.0–3.4 mmol/L):** give 50–100 mmol KCl over 24 h as oral/NG or IV replacement. Treat any hypomagnesaemia.
- **Moderate (2.5–2.9 mmol/L):** give 100 mmol KCl over 24 h as oral/NG or IV replacement. Treat any hypomagnesaemia.
- **Severe (<2.5 mmol/L):** replace in total 100–200 mmol KCl over 24 h. Give 40 mmol KCl in 0.5–1 L by infusion pump over 4 h. Max 10 mmol/h in ward area. May be repeated 2–3 times per day with twice daily monitoring. Treat any low Mg. Higher rates e.g. 20 mmol/h only given by infusion pump in critical care areas with close ECG/K monitoring.
- **Cardiac arrest:** if hypokalaemia is suspected to be a contributory factor then 10 mmol KCl over 5–10 mins and then commence infusion 40 mmol over 1 h. Treat any hypomagnesaemia.

- **Oral/NG and IV replacement:** one Sando-K tablet = 12 mmol KCl; 25 ml Kay-Cee-L = 25 mmol KCl. Avoid solutions more concentrated than 40 mmol in 1 L as they can cause phlebitis and pain. Use the largest peripheral vein available. Given by central line with close monitoring. K solutions should be given by infusion pump to avoid accidental high flow rates. Treat any hypomagnesaemia.
- **NPSA recommends:** a second practitioner should always check for correct product, dosage dilution, mixing and KCl concentrate and other strong potassium solutions.

References: Rastergar & Soleimani (2001) Hypokalaemia and hyperkalaemia. *Postgrad Med J*, 77:759. NPSA (2002) Potassium chloride concentrate solution. *Patient Safety Alert.*

5.5   Hypercalcaemia

- **About:** severe high Ca is a corrected calcium of >3.5 mmol/L or severe symptoms. 90% of hypercalcaemia is due to primary hyperparathyroidism (HPTHM) or malignancy. Severity of corrected calcium = measured [Ca] + ((40 − [albumin]) × 0.02). If <3.0 mmol/L: often asymptomatic and does not usually require urgent correction; 3.0–3.5 mmol/L: can be well tolerated but if symptomatic then prompt treatment is usually indicated; >3.5 mmol/L: requires urgent correction due to risk of dysrhythmia and coma.
- **Aetiology:** body contains 1–2 kg calcium, almost all of which is in bone. Total Ca (2.1–2.6 mmol/L) = free ionized (1.1–1.4 mmol/L) (active) + BOUND Ca. Calcium is bound to albumin, citrate and phosphate (inactive). A fall in serum albumin leads to a fall in measured total serum calcium.

Causes

- **1° HPTHM:** ↑PTH and calcium often in an otherwise well patient. Symptoms may be minimal and patients otherwise appear well.
- **Malignancy (low PTH):** if undiagnosed often unwell with weight loss and other malignancy symptoms. Due to bone metastases (lung, breast, renal, thyroid and myeloma) or PTH-related peptide (squamous cell lung). Needs CXR. Symptoms usually marked. Myeloma screen.
- **Sarcoidosis, TB, Lymphoma:** ↑ectopic 1,25(OH)$_2$D$_3$.
- **Drugs:** thiazides, calcium, vitamin D, and lithium.
- **Endocrine:** Addison's disease, hyperthyroid, phaeochromocytoma, acromegaly, MEN I / II.
- **Familial hypercalcaemic hypocalciuria:** autosomal dominant with increased PTH – it is important to identify patients with familial hypocalciuric hypercalcaemia to prevent a wrong diagnosis of 1° HPTHM.
- **Milk-alkali syndrome:** was seen with milk + excess antacids.
- **Paget's disease:** with immobilisation. Usually calcium normal in Paget's disease.
- **3° HPTHM:** 2° HPTHM which becomes autonomous usually with CKD.

Clinical

- Constipation, N&V, confusion, depression, delirium even psychosis and coma. Polyuria and/or polydipsia, hypotonia, hyporeflexia, weakness +/− hyperreflexia and tongue fasciculation.
- Long-standing high Ca may cause band keratopathy. Peptic ulcer disease. Renal stones, pancreatitis. Can cause seizures and arrhythmias.
- Look for malignancy: weight loss, neck, respiratory, abdomen, breasts, lymph nodes, finger clubbing, chest signs.

Investigations

- **FBC and U&E:** ↑urea, **ESR** (myeloma/malignancy). TFT: hyperthyroid. Corrected calcium: measured [Ca] + ((40 − [albumin]) × 0.02). Phosphate: ↑in 3° HPTHM.

- **ECG:** a short QT interval, prolonged PR and risk of dysrhythmias. **CXR:** squamous cell carcinoma, sarcoidosis, TB.
- **PTH level:** a normal or high PTH in the setting of an ↑calcium is suggestive of 1° HPTHM. A low PTH suggests malignancy or sarcoid or other cause. Measure PTH-related peptide in malignancy.

Management (G5 = 5% glucose, NS = 0.9% saline)

- **Emergency:** if corrected calcium level >3.2 mmol/L and/or dehydrated start 3–6 L NS IV (125–250 ml/h) per day titrated to degree of fluid depletion (HR/BP).
- It may require HDU admission and central line insertion to avoid fluid overload and the risks of oedema in the elderly.
- In some patients with mild to moderate high Ca (corrected calcium <3.2 mmol/L) then admission may not be needed and if no heart or renal issues advise the person, provided there are no contraindications, to maintain good hydration by drinking 3–4 L of fluid per day. Encourage mobilisation and return if symptoms worsen. Monitor closely via next day ambulatory care clinic.
- **BISPHOSPHONATES:** *after rehydration* if the corrected calcium is >3.0 mmol/L and renal function is normal (rehydrate first for 12 h and repeat calcium) then IV PAMIDRONATE 30–60 mg at 40 mg/h. Lower dose in renal failure and GFR <20 ml/min. Alternatives, e.g. ZOLEDRONATE 4 mg IV infusion in NS over 15 min.
- **Other steps:** drugs: stop any calcium/vitamin D medication (this is often forgotten). FUROSEMIDE: should not be used until the patient is fully volume replaced if at all. Consider CALCITONIN 200 units every 6–12 h until calcium falls. Used rarely nowadays. PREDNISOLONE: useful if cause is lymphoma, myeloma, 25(OH)D₃ toxicity or sarcoidosis. Steroids inhibit 1,25(OH)D₃ production. Start at PREDNISOLONE 40 mg daily responding after 2–4 days. Parathyroidectomy: for 1° and 3° HPTHM. Indications in primary disease is for those with stones, renal impairment, bone disease, Ca >3.0 mmol/L and in younger patients. Monitoring may be appropriate for older patients with Ca 2.65–3.00 mmol/L.

References: NICE (2010) Hypercalcaemia, CKS. Society for Endocrinology (2013) Acute hypercalcaemia (www.endocrinology.org/policy).

5.6 Hypocalcaemia

Tetany is caused by hypocalcaemia but also by alkalosis due to hyperventilation, vomiting, and excessive antacids.

- **About:** normal Ca 2.1–2.6 mmol/L. Total (bound + free) Ca <2.05 mmol/L. Check for and correct any hypomagnesaemia first. See *Hypercalcaemia* for pathophysiology.
- **Aetiology:** acidosis reduces protein binding sites and increases the amount of ionised Ca. Alkalosis increases protein binding sites and ionised Ca is lower, causing tetany.

Causes

- **Low PTH:** most common cause is post thyroidectomy with resultant low PTH which can be transient or permanent. Radiation or autoimmune damage.
- **Low albumin:** liver disease or the nephrotic syndrome.
- **Renal failure:** CKD-5 usually (failure of renal hydroxylation).
- **Acute pancreatitis:** seen with moderate to severe pancreatitis.
- **PTH resistance:** pseudohypoparathyroidism. *GNAS1* mutation. Short stature, short metacarpals.
- **High phosphate:** phosphate binds calcium, which precipitates.
- **Malabsorption:** coeliac disease, Crohn's disease, short bowel syndrome, CF or chronic pancreatic insufficiency.
- **DiGeorge syndrome:** hypoparathyroid with thymic aplasia.

- **Miscellaneous:** low Mg (diuretics, alcohol abuse), cinacalcet, tumour lysis syndrome, multiple blood transfusions, rhabdomyolysis, sepsis/toxic shock syndrome, hungry bone syndrome post correction of primary hypoparathyroidism; bisphosphonates, foscarnet.

Clinical

- **Mild:** asymptomatic. **Chronic:** cataracts, basal ganglia calcification, dry skin, pruritus.
- **Moderate:** numbness, paraesthesia, mild muscle weakness, wheezing. Positive **Chvostek sign** – tapping over facial nerve causes facial muscles to contract. Positive **Trousseau sign** – inflate BP cuff to 20 mmHg above SBP for 3–5 min – causes muscle spasm, and flexion of the wrist and metacarpal phalangeal joints can be observed with extension of the interphalangeal joints and adduction of the thumb (carpal spasm). More specific but less sensitive than the Chvostek sign.
- **Severe:** delirium, seizures, papilloedema, movement disorders, tetany, refractory ↓BP, or arrhythmias (needs IV calcium + magnesium).

Investigations

- **FBC, U&E, LFTS:** AKI, CKD. Determine estimated glomerular filtration rate (GFR). **Ca, phosphate, PTH, 25(OH)D₃, 1,25(OH)₂D₃:** $hypoparathyroidism:$ low calcium, high phosphate, low PTH. **Pseudohypoparathyroidism:** low calcium, high phosphate and PTH. **Osteomalacia:** calcium/phosphate low, ALP/PTH high, $25(OH)D_3$ low. **CKD:** high phosphate, ALP, creatinine, PTH high. $25(OH)D_3$ normal, $1,25(OH)_2D_3$ low. In critically ill patients measure uncuffed sample.
- **Parathyroid antibodies** – autoimmune hypoparathyroidism.
- **Magnesium** <0.5 mmol/L typically results in symptomatic low Ca.
- **Radiographs** for Looser zone and osteomalacia and short 4th metacarpals in pseudohypoparathyroidism. **ECG:** a long QT interval. **Amylase** if pancreatitis considered.

Management (G5 = 5% glucose, NS = 0.9% saline)

- **Mild/moderate:** oral replacement, e.g. ADCAL D3 3 tablets BD or CALCICHEW Forte 2 tablets BD. **Severe** (<1.9 mmol/L and/or symptomatic at any level below reference range): give 10–20 ml of CALCIUM GLUCONATE over 15 min in 50–100 ml NS/G5. Then dilute 100 ml of 10% CALCIUM GLUCONATE (10 vials) in 1 L of NS or G5 and infuse at 50–100 ml/h. Monitor calcium.
- **Treat any** low Mg: IV MgSO₄ 2 g (8 mmol in 100 ml) over 20 min until symptoms have cleared. Mg avoided in CKD. PPI can cause a low Mg.
- **Vitamin D:** replace as required. Monitor calcium levels. Referral to endocrinology for complex patients, e.g. PTH resistance should be managed by specialists.

References: Hannan & Thakker (2013) Investigating hypocalcaemia. *BMJ*, 346:f2213. Acute Emergency Hypocalcaemia (2013) (www.endocrinology.com).

5.7   Myxoedema coma

Consider hypothyroidism in every older patient with low Na, hypothermia, ↓HR and delirium. Mortality can exceed 20% even with optimal treatment.

- **About:** may complicate long-standing often undiagnosed/untreated hypothyroidism. May be precipitated by an acute physiological stress event.
- **Risk factors:** mostly older females (mean age = 75) usually during winter. Usually long-standing primary thyroid failure but rarely pituitary failure.
- **Causes:** Hashimoto's disease, post-thyroidectomy, radioactive iodine, antithyroid drugs. Drugs: lithium, amiodarone, iodine deficiency, thalidomide. Congenital, Infiltration of thyroid – haemochromatosis, amyloid, Riedel's.

- **Precipitants:** look for infection/sepsis (chest/urine/encephalitis), GI bleed. Drugs (slow metabolism): alcohol, sedatives, tranquilisers, narcotics, amiodarone, lithium, beta-blockers. Lung disease, stroke, CCF, ACS, upper GI bleed, acute trauma/surgery/burns. Hypothermia, hypoglycaemia, noncompliance with thyroid replacement.
- **Clinical:** fatigue, increased weight, constipation and cold intolerance. Psychosis with delusions and hallucinations ('myxoedema madness'). Hypothermia, generalised oedema, cool dry rough skin, sparse hair, macroglossia. Seizures, coma, ↓HR, ↓BP, hypoventilation. Abdominal distension/pain. Paralytic ileus, megacolon, old thyroidectomy scar. Goitre with Hashimoto's disease, iodine deficiency.

Investigations

- **FBC U&E:** macrocytic anaemia, leukopenia, low Na, decreased GFR.
- **Glucose:** may be low, elevated **CK/LDH**, hyperlipidaemia. Short SynACTHen test if coexisting hypoadrenalism suspected.
- **TFT:** TSH >10 mU/L (low if pituitary disease), low FT_4. TSH can be unreliable generally in acute illnesses and should at least be accompanied by a FT_4. TFTs should be rechecked when patient is better. Sickness can cause deranged TFTs and this must always be considered.
- **Thyroid autoantibodies** (TPO Ab) in Hashimoto's disease. CSF: ↓pressure, ↑protein.
- **ABG:** Type 2 RF may be seen. ECG: ↓HR, flattened T-waves, low QRS. TdP.
- **CXR:** cardiomegaly, pericardial and pleural effusion.
- **Abdominal X-ray:** ileus and distended bowel and faeces.

Management

- **Supportive:** look for precipitant. Admit to ITU to manage hypoventilation, ↓O_2, ↓BP, hypoadrenalism and hypothermia. Give O_2 and fluids/inotropes. Gradually rewarm if hypothermic. Overactive warming may vasodilate and drop the BP. Watch for arrhythmias and monitor electrolytes and ABG. Interpretation impaired if hypothermic. Avoid any sedatives or sedating analgesics. Metabolism and drug excretion reduced.
- **Sepsis:** have a low threshold for IV antibiotics as signs of sepsis may be concealed by hypothyroidism, e.g. fever and ↑HR.
- **LEVOTHYROXINE** (T_4) loading dose 100–500 mcg IV once followed by 50–100 mcg OD IV until tolerating PO or via NG tube. T_4 (a prodrug converted to T_3) may provide a smoother and more gradual though slower onset of action than T_3. Lower doses of T_4, e.g. 25–50 mcg OD, may be advocated in elderly or those with cardiac disease.
- **LIOTHYRONINE** T_3 is available and may be the choice of some. Recommended doses range from LIOTHYRONINE 2.5 to 20 mcg 8 hourly. Give T_3 10 mcg bolus IV and then 10 mcg 8–12 hourly for 24–48 h and then start oral T_4. Lower doses may be advocated in elderly or those with cardiac disease.
- **HYDROCORTISONE 100 mg IV** and then IM 8 h given for first few days and then tapered off. The rationale being possible hypopituitarism and adrenal insufficiency.
- **Hypoglycaemia:** glycogen is often depleted so hypoglycaemia may be seen and so glucose should be monitored. A glucose infusion should be considered.
- **Poor prognosis** associated with hypothermia, advanced age, ↓HR, ↓BP, MI/CCF. No indication for prescribing T4 or any preparation containing thyroid hormones to patients with thyroid blood tests within the reference ranges.

Reference: Wall (2000) Myxoedema coma: diagnosis and treatment. *Am Fam Physician*, 62:2485.

5.8 Thyroid storm/thyrotoxic crisis

- **About:** rare and life-threatening condition due to excess T_3/T_4. 2% of those with hyperthyroidism. Mortality is quoted as 10–20%.

- **Aetiology of T4/T3 excess:** untreated or inadequately treated Graves' disease is the commonest pathology. Toxic adenoma or multinodular goitre, thyroiditis, post-partum thyroiditis. Excessive T_4 ingestion – deliberate or accidental. Recent amiodarone or intravenous iodinated contrast.
- **Precipitant:** recent minor/major illness or post radioactive iodine treatment. Post thyroid surgery or stopping treatment, e.g. carbimazole or propylthiouracil.
- **Clinical:** ↑HR, palpitations, AF, heart failure, weight loss, tremor, lethargic. Sweating and agitation, fever, hypo- or hyperactive delirium. Apathetic (more like hypothyroidism) in elderly, abdominal pain. Graves' eye disease: proptosis, lid lag, chemosis, acropachy. Pretibial myxoedema, tender gland suggests thyroiditis. Goitre may be seen with Graves' (bruit) or thyroiditis (tender).
- **Differential:** hyperactive or any form of delirium, septic shock, anticholinergic toxicity. Delirium tremens, acute pulmonary oedema, apathetic cases can be subtle.
- **Investigations:** bloods: FBC, U&E, ESR/CRP: ↑Ca. ECG: SR, sinus tachycardia, AF, ST/T wave changes, especially if IHD. TFT: ↑FT$_3$ and FT$_4$ and TSH <0.05 mU/L. Antibodies: thyroid peroxidase (TPO), thyroglobulin antibodies and TSH receptor antibodies (TRAb) in Graves' disease whose level parallels disease activity. CXR if infection suspected. Blood cultures and CSF if obtunded. Echo: may show a transient rate-induced cardiomyopathy and reduced LV function. Increased ^{123}I uptake in Graves' compared with Hashimoto's thyroiditis.

Management

- **Start ABC.** O$_2$ as per BTS guidelines. Consider ITU/HDU. Start IV fluids and correct electrolytes. **Antipyretics:** use Paracetamol. Avoid ASPIRIN (displaces protein bound T_4). Look/treat any sepsis: blood/urine/CSF (if indicated). **Sedation:** if very agitated then HALOPERIDOL 1–5 mg or LORAZEPAM 1–2 mg IV/IM or DIAZEPAM as needed. PROPRANOLOL 40–80 mg 12 h PO to rate control tachycardia/AF. Cardioversion futile until rendered euthyroid.
- **Anticoagulate** any AF as cardioembolic risk using LMWH acutely.
- **Antithyroid drugs:** CARBIMAZOLE 20 mg BD/TDS. PO/NG often with THYROXINE 75–100 mcg as block and replacement therapy. A smaller dose CARBIMAZOLE 15–40 mg may also be given and titrated against TSH. Alternative PROPYLTHIOURACIL 200 mg BD is an alternative and often preferred in pregnancy. PTU reduces T_4 to T_3 conversion.
- **POTASSIUM IODIDE** 15 mg 6 h PO or LUGOL's iodine (8 mg iodine/drop): 10 drops (0.1–0.3 ml) PO/NGT every 8 h. Blocks organification of iodine. Reduces T_4 to T_3 conversion. Give after Carbimazole. This is the Wolff–Chaikoff effect.
- **HYDROCORTISONE 100 mg 6 h IM/IV to prevent** T_4 to T_3 also suppresses the autoimmune process.
- **Plasmapheresis (PLEX):** has been used to treat thyroid storm in adults.
- **Thyroid eye disease** (Graves' orbitopathy) in 15%. Presents with proptosis (Grade 3), redness, pain, diplopia (Grade 4), swelling and oedema. Emergency – those unable to close eyes fully have high risk of corneal ulceration (Grade 5), reduced acuity (Grade 6). Need urgent specialist ophthalmic/thyroid referral. The rest need surveillance, smoking cessation and Sodium SELENITE 100 mcg 12 h and management of thyroid disease. Tape eyes closed overnight, artificial tears/lubricants for gritty eyes. High dose steroids: PREDNISOLONE 1 mg/kg/day and decompression surgery if sight is at risk. Once controlled refer for radioiodine or subtotal thyroidectomy. Radioiodine avoided if active eye disease as can worsen situation but prophylactic steroids may be given.
- **Heart failure:** chronic tachycardia causes a cardiomyopathy and so ECHO may be needed and anti-failure medications.
- **Thyroiditis:** usually self-limiting 1–2 months. Symptoms control with PROPRANOLOL 40 mg TDS. Malaise, fever, pain settles. PREDNISOLONE 20–40 mg/day

may be given. May be transient hypothyroidism after. A post-partum thyroiditis may be seen in some women <6/12 post-delivery and associated with anti-TPO antibodies in half.

References: Perros *et al.* (2015) Management of patients with Graves' orbitopathy: initial assessment, management outside specialised centres and referral pathways. *Clinical Medicine*, 15:173. Marcocci *et al.* (2011) Selenium and the course of mild Graves' orbitopathy. *N Engl J Med*, 364:1920 (doi: 10.1056/NEJMoa1012985).

5.9 Pituitary apoplexy

- **About:** pituitary macroadenoma (>1 cm) undergoes infarction +/− haemorrhage. Get urgent CT head. Seen in 1% of pituitary tumours. Apoplexy may be precipitated by anticoagulants or surgery. Rare in pregnancy. The pituitary is shaped like a 6 and releases at least 6 important hormones: ACTH, (MSH), GH, Prolactin, TSH, LH, FSH. May need urgent neurosurgical referral to preserve vision and steroids for any secondary adrenal insufficiency.
- **Aetiology:** rapidly growing tumour outgrows blood supply or compresses its own blood supply. Expanding mass arising from the sella turcica can compress optic nerve and chiasma. Pituitary vascular supply from the inferior hypophyseal branch of the internal carotid artery. Result is hypopituitarism with secondary hypoadrenalism, hypothyroid, hypogonadism, etc. Secretory pituitary tumour has 3 effects: hormone excess, space occupying (headache), hypofunction of other hormones.
- **Clinical:** pre-existing adenoma and severe headache +/− eye signs, coma. ↓BP with secondary hypoadrenalism. Ophthalmoplegia, bitemporal superior quadrantanopia and loss/reduced visual acuity. Horner's syndrome. Palsy of II, III, IV and VI and V1 (lateral wall cavernous sinuses). Look for signs of prolactinoma, acromegaly and Cushing's syndrome.
- **Differentials:** SAH, bacterial/viral meningitis, brainstem infarction (eye signs/ Horner's), cavernous sinus thrombosis.

Investigations

- **Bloods:** FBC, U&E, LFT, clotting screen. **Hormones:** prolactin, GH (can be zero between pulses in normals so also check IGF-1), TSH and FT_4, ACTH and cortisol, LH/ FSH and testosterone or oestradiol. Commonest tumours secrete prolactin/GH. However, most pituitary tumours that undergo apoplexy are endocrinologically silent. If suspected hypopituitary and ACTH and GH low these can be stimulated with hypoglycaemia induced by an insulin tolerance test. If GH high and acromegaly suspected attempt to suppress with OGTT. These tests and results are assessed in the post-acute phase.
- **CT head:** acutely, haemorrhage in an existing pituitary tumour, subarachnoid bleed or ischaemic with no haemorrhage.
- **MRI/A pituitary:** more sensitive after 24 h showing blood, tumour, pituitary ring sign from central necrosis. MRA shows close vascular anatomy.
- **Formal visual fields** assessment as early as possible (when clinically possible) looking for a bitemporal superior hemianopia suggesting optic chiasmal compression from below.

Management

- **HYDROCORTISONE 200 mg IV bolus and then 100 mg IM/IV 6 h** to manage acute period. Adequate IV fluid replacement with NS.
- **Urgent MRI/A (or CT/A if MRI not possible)** and discussion with local neurosurgical and endocrine team.
- **CABERGOLINE** or other dopamine agonist *may be sufficient* in non-visually impaired prolactinoma and suffices in 80% and can rapidly reduce tumour size. Need for

urgent surgery decided by a neurosurgeon with endocrinologist. Stop and reverse any coincidental anticoagulation.

- **Neurosurgery:** If vision is at risk or cranial nerve or other pressure effects then consider urgent trans-sphenoidal surgical decompression to reduce pressure on local structures. Complications include damage to local structures, especially the carotid arteries laterally. GH secreting tumours are less common than prolactinoma and more likely to need surgery / Octreotide / Pegvisomant / Radiotherapy.
- **Endocrine review:** long-term pituitary hormone replacement may be needed with Thyroxine, Hydrocortisone, etc. Remember to titrate to the T_4 not the TSH. Posterior pituitary function rarely affected with even a large macroadenoma so if diabetes insipidus is seen consider inflammatory cause or metastases. Long term imaging shows an empty sella.

Reference: Rajasekaran *et al.* (2011) UK guidelines for the management of pituitary apoplexy. *Clinical Endocrinology*, 74:9.

5.10 Hyponatraemia

- **About:** low serum Na with ↓serum osmolality causes intracellular movement of water and cerebral oedema, progressive coma and seizures. Rapid uncontrolled normalisation can lead to permanent neurological deficits.
- **Pathophysiology:** normal Na 135–145 mmol/L. Plasma osmolality is 275–295 mOsm/kg. Any rise in osmolality leads to ADH release and free water retention. ADH causes free water retention and lowers serum osmolality. ADH acts on renal V2 receptors.

Different scenarios

- **Salt level fixed and water excess:** ↑ADH release (SIADH) fails to excrete water, excess IV Dextrose/Glucose, potomania, water from prostate irrigation, ADH release to pain, opiates, surgery.
- **Excess salt loss and water loss:** diuretics, tubular disorders, surgical drains, Addison's disease.
- **Salt loss but water level constant:** compensated diuresis, Addison's disease.

Assessment

- **Severity:** mild: 125–130 mmol/L: no symptoms or mild lethargy. Not uncommon in elderly. Moderate: 115–125 mmol/L: headache, nausea, cramps, confusion. Severe: <115 mmol/L: confusion, seizure, delirium, coma, cerebral oedema and brain herniation.
- **Clinical:** assessment: is patient hypervolaemic, euvolaemic or hypovolaemic/dehydrated? **Dehydrated:** oliguria, low lying/standing BP, heart rate, thirst, poor skin turgor, weight. **Fluid overloaded:** peripheral and/or pulmonary oedema, basal crepitations, S3, ↑JVP. Fluid balance shows water taken orally or IV Glucose suggests water overload. Salt losses: surgical drains and NG tube may suggest shows excessive salt losses +/– water losses. **Euvolaemic:** meningitis, brain injury or small cell lung tumour or pneumonia suggests SIADH.

Types

- **Hypovolaemic hyponatraemia:** reduced ECF with low BP, dehydrated, renal or GI or burns or other losses or overdiuresis. **Divide into renal losses** (urine Na >20 mmol/L): diuretics (renal salt loss + ADH stimulation and free water retention), salt-losing nephropathy, RTA, cerebral salt wasting (SAH), Addison's disease, and **non-renal losses** (urine Na <10 mmol/L: gastrointestinal losses, burns, pancreatitis, 3rd space losses. Avoid Na retention and so urine Na <10 mmol/L, and the urine may be low volume and hyperosmolar. **Needs fluid and Na replacement** if normal renal function then salt retention possible so correction should be simpler. Manage underlying cause of losses. Well patient: increase salt intake with slow sodium 80 mmol/day or slow IV NS. If vomiting then simply match losses with IV NS with 20 mmol KCl per litre. If slow to respond or encephalopathic then consider 500 ml of 3% over 6–12 h depending on urgency and response to replacement. Test and treat for any concerns of adrenal insufficiency. Try to limit increases <10–12 mmol/day.

- **Euvolaemic hyponatraemia** (increased ICF and ECF no oedema): causes include thiazide diuretics, SIADH, hypothyroidism, acute porphyria, adrenal insufficiency, Guillain–Barré syndrome. Dilutional hyponatraemia. Avoid excessive hyponatraemic water intake (runners, ecstasy users, potomania). Correct cause. Increase salt intake with slow sodium 80 mmol/day. Consider IV NS. Give 3% NS if urgent correction needed but bring levels up slowly. IV HYDROCORTISONE if hypoadrenalism. Stop thiazides. Try to limit improvements to less than 10 mmol/day.
- **Hypervolaemic hyponatraemia** (increased ICF and ECF, oedema): ascites, ↑JVP, CCF, cirrhosis, nephrotic syndrome, renal disease: hyperaldosteronism, diuretic-induced renal salt loss. Dilutional hyponatraemia so the key is fluid restriction to 500–1000 ml per day and diuresis of free water by inducing diabetes insipidus or blocking ADH. In exceptions 3% saline 500 ml over 6–12 h may be given. Saline may be given with FUROSEMIDE to aid water loss. DEMECLOCYCLINE 300 mg BD or TOLVAPTAN 15 mg OD for several days may be used to get rid of free water by inducing a nephrogenic diabetes insipidus.
- **Spurious hyponatraemia** (normal osmolality) may be due to high triglyceride, protein or glucose.

Investigations

- FBC, U&E, urine Na excretion, glucose, urine and plasma osmolality. In acute correction the U&E should be checked every 2–4 h. TFT: check TSH and cortisol levels. CXR: infection/tumour. Short synACTHen if adrenal failure considered (low BP, ↓BP, pigmentation).
- **SIADH:** urine inappropriately concentrated when dilute serum and often >100 mOsm/L with hyponatraemic plasma osmolarity. Osmolality = 2 Na + glucose + urea (all in mmol/L).

Management

- **Rises in Na should be actively managed not to exceed 12 mmol/24 h or 18 mmol/48 h.** Acute hyponatraemia can be corrected more quickly and more safely than chronic hyponatraemia.
- **ABC + supportive:** if fitting or low GCS and cerebral oedema then ITU with full support and consider urgent management with hypertonic saline. Manage seizures as per status epilepticus. CT scan if any concern as to cause of coma. General principles depend on likely cause. **Principles:** what is the volume status? If severe low Na been present for less than 48 h then can be reversed more quickly and vice versa. Aim for improvement of 12 mmol/day and not immediate normality. Assess fluid balance, osmolality and urinary osmolality, volume and salt loss. Monitor Na closely and frequently and clinical state. Try to break it down into hypo-, eu-, hyper-volaemia, though some have mixed. Chronic hyponatraemia (>48 h) should have the sodium corrected much more slowly. A target of 120 mmol/L attained over 24–48 h depending on baseline should resolve acute symptoms.
- **SIADH:** excessive free water retention. Low serum osmolality and ↑urine osmolality (>100 mOsm/kg) and urine Na >30 mmol/L where hypopituitarism, hypoadrenalism, hypothyroidism, renal insufficiency and diuretic use have been excluded. Check and stop any causative drugs and look for other causes (malignancy, ecstasy (MDMA often combined with excess water), CNS disorders, drugs, lung disease, nausea, postoperative pain, HIV, infections, Guillain–Barré syndrome, acute porphyria). Fluid restriction to 800 ml/day is needed. See above for managing severe hyponatraemia.

- **Drug treatments:** Demeclocycline, Conivaptan and Tolvaptan antagonize effects of ADH by different mechanisms to cause free water loss. If euvolaemic: DEMECLOCYLINE 150–300 mg 6 h can be given to induce NDI and lose free water. Conivaptan or Tolvaptan may also be used. They may also be used with hypervolaemic/euvolaemic hyponatraemia, e.g. TOLVAPTAN 15 mg (up to 60 mg/day) for short periods. Need to watch for rapid rises in Na which can result in neurology. Specialist use. Fluid status should be monitored frequently and the patient should be encouraged to drink freely.
- **Adrenal insufficiency** should be treated as per Addisonian crisis with IV NS and steroids. See ▶ Section 5.1.
- **Rapid correction can lead to central pontine demyelination** now called osmotic demyelination syndrome: manifests after 2–3 days as brainstem symptoms of dysarthria, dysphagia, seizures, coma, quadriparesis and can be seen on MRI. Classically seen in malnourished alcoholic with rapid correction. Exact treatment regimens are difficult because multiple factors are involved, but an effort to increase serum osmolality with either NS, or hypertonic saline if volume must be restricted, must be done carefully and cautiously with regular checking of status and bloods; if seizures and coma then more urgency may be applied. Comatose or fitting hyponatraemic patients are best managed in an HDU/ITU setting. It is certainly a time to enlist expert experienced help.

5.11 Hypernatraemia

- **About:** most often free water loss or no access to water. Occasionally excessive salt. Mild hypernatraemia Na >145 mmol/L; severe hypernatraemia >160 mmol/L. Mortality can be up to 50% in elderly patients. Correct slowly at <12 mmol/day. Most often due to an impaired access to water or loss of free water greater than can be replaced by drinking or other routes.
- **Aetiology:** ↑serum osmolality causes water to leave cells and cells to shrink. A small rise in osmolality detected by osmoreceptors causes desire to drink. Hypernatraemia occurs where there is limited access to water, e.g. lost in the desert or stuck in a side room and too confused or comatose to drink, or water not to hand.
- **Causes:** water/hypotonic fluid loss or impaired water intake. Polyuria with excess free water loss unmatched by water intake: high Ca, low K, cranial and nephrogenic diabetes insipidus, diabetic ketoacidosis, HONK. Simple dehydration + fever especially older people + impaired access to water. Water losses due to burns, sweat, vomiting, severe diarrhoea. Renal fluid losses: nephropathy, myeloma, obstructive uropathy, adult polycystic kidney disease. Excessive sodium intake: mild hypernatraemia with Conn or Cushing syndrome. Salt poisoning, ingestion of seawater, salt tablets, IV $NaHCO_3$, hypertonic saline.
- **Clinical:** dehydration, thirsty, agitation, ataxia, progressively obtunded and comatose. ↓BP, thready pulse, sunken eyes, low BP, coma and seizures.
- **Investigations:** FBC, U&E, Ca, K, glucose: exclude AKI, high glucose, high Ca, low K. ↑serum and urine osmolality (>600 mOsmol/kg) unless renal concentrating issue or diabetes insipidus. CT/MRI head if suspect cranial diabetes insipidus. Urine volume and osmolality: diabetes insipidus > 3 L/day of a dilute urine despite dehydration.
- **Management:** determine cause: this is fundamental and key. Investigate for free water loss. Assess renal concentrating function and serum and urine osmolality and look for high glucose and calcium or low K which can cause polyuria. May just be failure to match normal losses as listed above in *Causes*.
- **Fluid replacement:** no definite treatment plan. Cautious rehydration if cardiac disease or elderly. Treat and look for a cause if not obvious. Encourage oral fluids. Consider IV G5 slowly with administration guided by plasma Na and urine output. This can be alternated with NS, to avoid too rapid a fall in plasma osmolality which

can cause cerebral oedema. Can use a mixture of both. Volume replacement may be up to 4 L/day. Titrate to clinical response. Do not change [Na] by more than 12 mmol/day. Oral fluids may be given as long as losses are replaced and fluid balance maintained.

- **Risk of VTE:** administer VTE prophylaxis with Enoxaparin or equivalent.
- **Diabetes insipidus** (> 3 L/day of dilute urine despite dehydration) with thirst, headache: nephrogenic: fluid replacement, look for cause, e.g. lithium, correct electrolytes and paradoxically may need to give thiazide diuretics. Cranial: look for cause, replace losses. Consider DESMOPRESSIN 5–20 mcg nasal spray or tablets. Watch for hyponatraemia and fluid retention. Endocrine review.

5.12 Hypophosphataemia

- **About:** phosphate <0.8 mmol/L. Severe if phosphate <0.4 mmol/L.
- **Causes:** critically ill, DKA (insulin moves phosphate into cells), refeeding syndrome, malabsorption, vomiting or renal loss.
- **Clinical:** muscle weakness, ileus, cardiac failure, rhabdomyolysis.
- **Management:** for mild loss replace orally with Phosphate-Sandoz tablets up to 6 tablets per day. More severe deficiency then replace with IV PHOSPHATE 10–12 mmol given in 250 ml NS or G5 over 12 h. Watch serum calcium. Treat any vitamin D deficiency. May precipitate low Ca.

5.13 Hyperphosphataemia

- **Aetiology:** renal reuptake inhibited by PTH. Retained in renal failure.
- **Investigations:** U&E, phosphate > 1.4 mmol/L.
- **Causes:** AKI/CKD, (pseudo+) hypoparathyroidism, tumour lysis syndrome, rhabdomyolysis. Usually causes calcium deposition.
- **Management:** volume expansion, with IV NS if renal function normal, and gut phosphate binders such as calcium carbonate.

5.14 Hypomagnesaemia

- **Causes:** Mg <0.75 mmol/L. Malnourished patients or (loop) diuretics, alcoholism, diarrhoea, laxative abuse, malabsorption, pancreatitis, Gitelman's syndrome, DKA, severe burns, PPI. Mild Mg <0.7, moderate Mg <0.5, severe Mg <0.3 mmol/L.
- **Clinical:** weakness, tremor, carpopedal spasm, ataxia, hyperreflexia, adrenal insufficiency, confusion, fits, TdP. Daily intake is 15 mmol.
- **Investigations:** U&E: low Mg, low K often, ECG: 1st degree heart block, T wave flattened, widened QRS, ventricular arrhythmias, TdP. [1 g MgSO$_4$ = 4 mmol MgSO$_4$.] High urine Mg suggests renal problem (Gitelman's syndrome).
- **Management:** severe symptomatic give IV MAGNESIUM SULFATE 2 g (8 mmol) over 15–30 min. Replace with IV Mg 50 mmol (12 g) in 1 L of NS or G5 in the first 24 h. Mild/asymptomatic moderate can have up to 50 mmol/L day given as Maalox 10–20 ml qds (10 ml Maalox = 6.8 mmol Mg) but may cause diarrhoea. Also replace other electrolytes K/Ca if low. Amiloride can reduce Mg urine loss in some.

5.15 Hypermagnesaemia

- **Causes:** Mg >1 mmol/L. Cause is large MgSO$_4$ doses mistakenly given, e.g. pre-eclampsia or with impaired renal excretion.
- **Clinical:** reduced reflexes, weakness, cardiac arrest. May be seen in obstetric practice when Mg given as tocolytic or pre-eclampsia.
- **Investigations:** U&E, Mg symptomatic >2 mmol/L.

- **Management:** STOP Mg infusion. Give 10–20 ml of 10% CALCIUM GLUCONATE as per hypocalcaemia. Haemodialysis for renal failure. IV FUROSEMIDE + IV fluids can aid excretion. GLUCOSE and insulin can also be given (as for high K). Cardiac arrest – maintain CPR whilst giving calcium/IV fluids.

5.16 Lactic acidosis

- **About:** increased lactic acid due to tissue hypoperfusion or drugs or mitochondrial toxicity from NRTIs /other causes.
- **Aetiology:** impaired glycolytic metabolism increases lactate and reduces pH. L-lactate is endogenous; D-lactate from gut bacteria.
- **Type A lactic acidosis** (tissue hypoxia): severe sepsis, diabetes, pancreatitis, malignancy, shock, LVF, renal and liver failure, respiratory failure, carbon monoxide, severe anaemia, local hypoperfusion, e.g. limb ischaemia or bowel ischaemia.
- **Type B lactic acidosis** (no tissue hypoxia): alcohol, iron, salicylates, isoniazid, metformin, zidovudine. Inborn errors of metabolism, thiamine deficiency, pyruvate dehydrogenase dysfunction, cyanide, exercise, seizures.
- **Clinical:** Kussmaul's breathing, ↓BP, sepsis, shock, hypoxia. Do they have AIDS and on NRTIs, e.g. fatigue, nausea, aches, weight loss?
- **Investigations:** FBC, U&E: anaemia, AKI, lactate >4 mmol/L with sepsis/metabolic acidosis. **ABG:** hypoxia, hypercarbia may be seen. With mitochondrial dysfunction, e.g. cyanide, oxygen not extracted and so venous oxygen levels maintained. **Metabolic acidosis:** low HCO_3 may not be seen even with a modest rise in lactate. **Anion gap:** is increased $[Na+K] - [Cl+HCO_3] >12$ mmol/L.
- **Management:** ABCs, oxygen, resuscitate, supportive. Determine and treat cause. Stop causative drugs. Lactate is a useful marker of poor prognosis requiring expert and rapid intervention. Manage as per shock guidance or sepsis guidance. Dialysis can be considered in severe cases. Get expert help before considering an infusion of 500 ml isotonic 1.26% bicarbonate.

5.17 Acute porphyria

- **About:** deficiency of an enzyme in the haem biosynthesis pathway with overproduction of porphyrin precursors. Haem made from succinyl-coA + glycine by 8 enzymic steps in cytoplasm and mitochondria. Drugs can induce some of the initial steps in the pathway precipitating acute attacks. Acute attacks may occur with: acute intermittent porphyria, variegate porphyria, hereditary coproporphyria.
- **Clinical:** diagnosis often known. Often a family history is available. Episodes of neuropathic abdominal pain, back pain, constipation. ↑HR, hypertension. Women > men aged 20–40. **Look for precipitants:** fasting, infection, surgery, drugs.
- **Drug precipitants:** sulphonamides, rifampicin, OCP, anaesthetic agents, barbiturates, alcohol, some ACE inhibitors, carbamazepine, dapsone, furosemide, methyldopa, theophylline, some NSAIDs. Check any new drug in *BNF*.
- **Investigations:** FBC, U&E: urea, ↑LFTs: bloods as indicated with signs. **Increased porphobilinogen (PBG) and ALA:** urine darkens to port wine on standing and goes pink with Ehrlich's reagent, which remains despite chloroform. Urine PBG analysis to confirm an acute attack of porphyria or for monitoring known patients can be carried out at UK Porphyria centres. Collect a random 10 ml urine sample in a plain tube, check the tube is labelled with patient details, and protect from light by wrapping in foil or a brown envelope. Sample request card should state 'urine for porphobilinogen quantitation' for a patient with known porphyria, or 'urine for porphobilinogen screening test' for a patient without a previous diagnosis of porphyria. Refrigerate the sample prior to analysis. Follow local laboratory guidance.

- **Management:** supportive: hydration, pain relief, rest, increased carbohydrate intake oral or IV dextrose. Referral to specialist for individual enzyme assays and further tests. If conservative management not effective then consider administering an IV haem infusion. Recommend HAEM ARGINATE 3 mg/kg (to a maximum of 250 mg) once daily for four consecutive days which shortens attacks with less risk of complications. Haem arginate replenishes the body's haem stores. Through negative feedback this inhibits ALA synthase, thus reducing the production of porphyrins and their precursors, ALA and PBG.

Drugs which can be used with acute porphyria	
Analgesics	Aspirin, Diamorphine, Dihydrocodeine, Ibuprofen, Morphine, Paracetamol, Pethidine.
Anti-emetics	Chlorpromazine, Ondansetron, Prochlorperazine, Promazine.
Hypertension and tachycardia	Atenolol, Labetalol, Propranolol.
Sedation, seizures	Chlorpromazine, Clonazepam, Lorazepam, Promazine.
Constipation	Bulk-forming (ispaghula), Lactulose, Senna.
Prevention	Avoid precipitating drugs and alcohol, stopping smoking, stress, fasting or dieting.

Reference: NAPS section for Medical Professionals (www.cardiffandvaleuhb.wales.nhs.uk/national-acute-porphyria-service-naps); also www.porphyria.org.uk.

5.18 Diabetic ketoacidosis

Priorities are switching off ketone production with fixed rate insulin to normalize pH, to replace volume lost and lastly to correct blood glucose.

- **About:** manage with a defined well-documented and communicated plan. 10% of DKA is with new diabetes, 15% from known diabetes, often provoked. Seen in Type 1 diabetics with intercurrent illness who reduce/stop insulin. Severe deficit of water, insulin and potassium.
- **Note of caution:** DKA typically most commonly seen with T1DM but can be seen with 'ketosis-prone T2DM' especially in the non-white population. Treat as DKA but ketosis-prone T2DM may not need insulin long term. Treat all with insulin initially and arrange expert outpatient follow-up and measurement of C-peptide which is preserved with T2DM.
- **Differential of ketoacidosis:** alcohol ketoacidosis – ↑ketones, normal glucose, alcohol misuse. Starvation ketosis – ↑ketones, normal glucose.

Definition – following can be seen with T1DM and T2DM

- Ketonaemia ≥3 mmol/L or significant ketonuria (>2+ on urine sticks).
- Hyperglycaemia: blood glucose >11 mmol/L, or known DM.
- Metabolic acidosis: bicarbonate <15 mmol/L and/or venous pH <7.3.
- Diabetic pregnant patients can develop DKA with normal blood sugars.

- **Aetiology:** glucose (and K) enters cells by the actions of insulin on the insulin receptor. Insulin deficit leads to cell starvation despite being surrounded by a sea of excess glucose. Switch to burning fatty acids and beta-oxidation of fats creates acidic products which lower the pH. Ketone bodies include acetone, 3-beta-hydroxybutyrate (main one) and acetoacetate. Dehydration due to profound osmotic diuresis as a result of severe hyperglycaemia. Increased cortisol, adrenaline, glucagon, and GH cause hepatic gluconeogenesis and glycogenolysis. Vomiting can compound the fluid losses. All adds to a perfect storm leading to spiralling metabolic derangement. Rhinocerebral mucormycosis due to increased iron availability as a result of a change in tissue pH.

- **Recent key recommendations:** (1) IV NS is the recommended fluid of choice. (2) Cautious replacement in young adults to avoid cerebral oedema. (3) Measure venous HCO_3 and pH, use blood ketone meters for near patient testing. (4) Continue any long-acting analogue insulin, e.g. Levemir or Lantus. (5) In DKA, insulin is given at a fixed rate IV infusion calculated on body weight. (6) Avoid priming dose (bolus) of insulin. (7) HCO_3 or phosphate administration is not recommended routinely.
- **Clinical:** progressive polyuria, polydipsia, tachypnoea, Kussmaul's respiration to blow off CO_2. Acetone 'nail varnish' smell on the breath (not all of us can smell it), dehydration. Cold peripheries, delayed capillary return, sunken eyes, ↓BP, vomiting, ↑HR, oliguria. Look for sepsis, chest and urine and other acute illness, e.g. ACS, meningitis, acute abdomen.
- **Other precipitants:** MI, pancreatitis, alcohol excess, poor control.

Investigations

- **FBC** ↑WCC, ↑CRP may suggest infection.
- **U&E:** ↑urea, ↑creatinine, ↑Na. ↑K due to acidosis but potassium levels fall with insulin administration. This can lead to severe and potentially dangerous hypokalaemia.
- **Glucose:** usually >20 mmol/L at presentation. ↑↑Urine, glycosuria. ↑Ketonuria 3+. Treat to suppress ketonaemia. Measure blood ketones to monitor the response to treatment.
- **Venous blood gas:** metabolic acidosis with raised anion gap: VBG preferred over ABG unless suspect hypoxia or hypercarbia. HCO_3 (<15 mmol/L) indicates metabolic acidosis with pH <7.30. It can be <7.10 in severe cases.
- **Anion gap:** $[Na+K] - [Cl+HCO_3]$ >16.
- **Cardiac troponin** if suspected ACS.
- **CXR** if chest disease, e.g. breathless, fever, coughs.
- **CT head** scan if comatose to exclude other diagnoses.
- **Assess severity:** mild: blood pH 7.25–7.30, HCO_3 15–18 mmol/L; the patient is alert. Moderate: pH 7.00–7.25, HCO_3 10–15 mmol/L, mild drowsiness may be present. Severe: pH <7.00, HCO_3 <10 mmol/L; stupor or coma may occur.
- **Treatment goals** (see table below): the key aims are restoration of circulatory volume, clearance of ketones and correction of electrolyte imbalance, particularly potassium, and insulin replacement. Set clear goals and expectations of therapy. Ensure treatment plans are well documented. Ensure good handover between doctors on shifts.

Immediate assessment

- Check ABC, get good IV access and start IV NS. Assess basic RR, HR, BP, O_2 sats aim for 94–98%, and temperature and GCS.
- Examine for infection: urine, chest, CNS, skin and soft tissue. Monitor oximetry. Establish if pregnant.
- Send: blood ketones, capillary blood glucose, venous plasma glucose, U&E, VBG, FBC, blood cultures, ECG, CXR, urinalysis and culture.
- Insulin causes a marked drop in K which must be managed. Clinical and biochemical review.

Markers of severe DKA

- Needs HDU level 2 bed and CVP/intra-arterial line if any of: ketones >6 mmol/L, pH <7.0 or HCO_3 <5 mmol/L, initial K <3.5 mmol/L, anion gap >16, GCS <12, abnormal AVPU score, O_2 sats on air <92%, SBP <90 mmHg, HR <60 bpm or HR >100 bpm.

0–1 h: treatment goals
- Reduce ketones by 0.5 mmol/L/h and increase venous HCO_3 by 3 mmol/L/h.
- Reduce capillary blood glucose by 3 mmol/L/h.
- Maintain K 4.0–5.0 mmol/L.
- Lower glucose cautiously and start 10% glucose if CBG <14 mmol/L.

Assess patient
- **RR:** temp, BP, pulse, O_2 sats, GCS, full clinical exam. Capillary blood glucose (CBG) and laboratory glucose, venous BG, U&E, FBC, blood cultures, ECG, CXR, MSU.
- **Establish monitoring regimen.** Check hourly CBG, capillary ketone measurement if available.
- **Venous HCO_3/K** at 60 min, 2 h and 2-hourly thereafter, 4-hourly plasma electrolytes.
- **Continuous cardiac monitoring and pulse oximetry if required.** Find and treat any precipitating causes.
- **Commence insulin:** start a FIXED rate IV insulin infusion (IVII) (0.1 unit/kg/h, e.g. 7 units/h for 70 kg). Give as infusion: 50 units soluble insulin (Actrapid or Humulin S) in 50 ml NS. Continue any long-acting insulin analogues (Glargine, Detemir, Degludec) at usual dose and time.
- **Initial fluid needs are determined by BP:** start NS infusion (use large bore cannula) via infusion pump. If SBP <90 mmHg give (cautions if history of heart failure) 500 ml of NS over 10–15 min. If SBP remains <90 mmHg give further 500 ml of NS and get senior input or ITU/critical care team. Most need 0.5–1.0 L. Once SBP >90 mmHg give 1 L NS over next 60 min, usually with potassium in this second litre of fluid as below. If **SBP on admission >90 mmHg give 1 L NS over first 60 min.**
- **Potassium level (mmol/L):** replacement mmol/L of infusion solution: If K >5.5: give none; if K 3.5–5.5: give 40 mmol/L; if K <3.5 senior review – additional K required.

1–6 h (see treatment goals above)
- **Re-assess patient, monitor vital signs:** hourly blood glucose (lab blood glucose if meter reading 'HI'), hourly blood ketones if meter available. VBG for pH, bicarbonate and potassium at 60 min, 2 h and 2-hourly thereafter.
- **Potassium:** insulin will shift K into the intracellular space causing low K. Add 20 mmol K per litre from the 2nd bag. Check U&E regularly: hourly initially then every 2–4 h when stabilised or more if needed. K >5.5 mmol/L: add none; K 3.5–5.5 mmol/L: give 40 mmol/L; K <3.5 mmol/L: senior review as increased K needed.
- **Fluid replacement:** *risk of cerebral oedema so recommend more cautious fluid replacement in young people aged 18–25 years, elderly, pregnant, heart or renal failure (consider HDU and/or central line).* 1 L NS + KCl over next 2 h, then another 1 L NS + KCl over next 2 h. 1 L NS + KCl over next 4 h. Add 10% glucose 125 ml/h if blood glucose falls below 14 mmol/L.
- **Insulin infusion rate may need review if:** ketones not falling by at least 0.5 mmol/L/h. Venous HCO_3 not rising by at least 3 mmol/L/h. Plasma glucose not falling by at least 3 mmol/L/h. Continue fixed rate IVII until ketones less than 0.3 mmol/L, venous pH over 7.3 and/or venous bicarbonate over 18 mmol/L.
- **Treatment not working:** *if ketones/glucose not falling as expected always check the insulin infusion pump is working and connected and that the correct insulin residual volume is present (to check for pump malfunction). If equipment working but response to treatment inadequate, increase insulin infusion rate by 1 unit/h increments hourly until targets achieved.*
- **Additional measures:** regular obs and Early Warning Score (EWS). Accurate fluid balance chart. Target minimum urine output 0.5 ml/kg/h. Consider urinary catheterisation if incontinent or anuric (not passed urine by 60 min). NG tube with airway protection if patient obtunded or persistent.

Other considerations

- **Acidosis:** adequate fluid and insulin therapy will resolve the acidosis in DKA and the use of HCO_3 is not indicated, though some consider treatment with a pH <7.0 and give 500 ml of sodium bicarbonate 1.26% plus 10 mmol KCl – take local expert advice if considered.
- **Urinary catheter:** if anuric or oliguric and concerns about renal function or fluid balance. Oxygen as per BTS guidance. **Consider NG tube** if vomiting. Give **VTE prophylaxis** usually LMWH as high risk.
- **Exclude sepsis:** CXR and urinalysis, soft tissue (look for boils, abscesses), consider meningitis. Always ask why DKA occurred in this patient.
- **Note:** An acute abdomen or even meningitis could also present as DKA. DKA can present with abdominal pain. Surgical consult if you suspect acute abdomen. Amylase can also go up × 4 in DKA.

6–12 h

- At 6 h check venous pH, HCO_3, K, capillary ketones and glucose. Ensure clinical and biochemical parameters improving. Continue IV fluid replacement. Avoid low glucose and start 10% glucose if BG <14 mmol/L.
- Continue IV fluid at reduced rate of 1 L NS + KCl over 4 h and then 1 L NS + KCl over 6 h.
- Monitor GCS for cerebral oedema. Review all bloods at 6 h. Resolution is suggested by pH >7.3 or ketones <0.3 mmol/L.
- If not improving (see treatment goals above) then repeat review and check insulin infusion is working and line is not blocked and that it contains insulin and no errors with making it up.

12–24 h

- Check venous pH, HCO_3, K, capillary ketones and glucose. Resolution is defined as ketones <0.3 mmol/L, venous pH >7.3. Ensure targets are hit and progressive improvement. Ketonaemia and acidosis should have resolved.
- Request senior review if not improving. Continue IV fluid replacement if not eating and drinking. If ketonaemia cleared but not eating and drinking move to a variable rate IVII as per local guidelines.
- Look for complications of treatment, e.g. fluid overload, cerebral oedema and continue to treat precipitating factors. Transfer to SC insulin if patient is eating and drinking normally.

After 24 h and discharge planning and follow up

- **If DKA not resolved determine why.** It suggests possible failure to get enough insulin or fluids. Are the IV lines working? Does the insulin infusion contain insulin? Get expert review. Transfer to SC insulin when biochemical resolution (capillary ketones <0.3 mmol/L, pH >7.3) and the patient is ready and able to eat. Give subcutaneous insulin and then after 30 min stop IV insulin as there should be some overlap. Conversion to SC insulin should be managed by the Specialist Diabetes Team. If the team is not available use local guidelines. If the patient is newly diagnosed it is essential they are seen by a member of the specialist team prior to discharge. Arrange follow up with specialist team.
- **Complications:** cerebral oedema (suspect if fall in GCS – more common in young so go easy on the fluids). Arrhythmias (potassium), circulatory collapse/shock, AKI. Hypoglycaemia with over-treatment, aspiration pneumonia. ARDS, myocardial infarction. Rhinocerebral mucormycosis – destructive lesions affecting face and nose.
- **Education and prevention: structured education is a key component and NICE recommend DESMOND** (diabetes education and self-management for ongoing and newly diagnosed) **for those with T2DM. For T1DM, DAFNE** (dose adjustment for normal eating) is recommended and learning how to manage insulin. Ensure patient educated about 'sick day rules': patients need strict advice to never

stop their insulin even if ill. If unable to eat/drink then they must come to hospital immediately. Diabetic team should reinforce this message.
- **Pregnancy:** an inherently ketosis-prone state and is a high-risk time for DKA in women with T1DM.

Reference: Joint British Diabetes Societies Inpatient Care Group (2013) *The Management of Diabetic Ketoacidosis in Adults*, 2nd edition.

5.19 Hyperosmolar hyperglycaemic state (HHS)

- **About:** previously called hyperglycaemic hyperosmolar nonketotic coma (HONK). Mortality 10–20% compared with 3–10% for DKA. Seen in the elderly. Minimal ketosis or acidosis. Increased risk of VTE so give LMWH.
- **Definition and diagnosis:** hypovolaemia (HR >100, SBP <100 mmHg) + BG >30 mmol/L + ketones <3 mmol/L. pH >7.3 and HCO_3 >15 mmol/L and osmolality >320 mOsm/kg.
- **Precipitated by:** *de novo* presentation of T2DM or T2DM + stress, steroids, surgery, thiazides, infection. Pancreatitis, non-compliance with treatment, alcohol, drug abuse, stroke, inadequate insulin.
- **Clinical:** thirst, polydipsia, polyuria, and mental clouding, seizures, and delirium and coma. Usually known T2 diabetic. Exacerbated by high sugar drinks or water restriction.
- **Investigations:** FBC: ↑WCC **U&E:** ↑Na often >150 mmol/L, AKI. ↑↑Glucose: >30 mmol/L *without significant ketonaemia/acidosis*. Measure and calculate serum osmolality: >320 mOsm/kg, 2 × [Na] + urea + glucose. **Ketones:** usually <3 mmol/L. ↑**Lactate:** may see. **ABG/VBG:** pH >7.3 and HCO_3 >15 mmol unless lactic acidosis.
- **Management:** ABC, good venous access × 2. May need ITU/HDU if in coma/moribund and airway protection needed. Indications for HDU/ITU include serum osmolality >350 mOsm/kg, Na >160 mmol/L, GCS <12, K >6.0 or <3.5, O_2 sats <92%, SBP <90 mmHg, pulse <60 or >100, urine output <0.5 ml/kg/h, hypothermia.
- **Start fluid replacement:** significant fluid losses with osmotic diuresis due to glycosuria. Fluid replacement alone will lower glucose. Losses, e.g. 100–200 ml/kg. Isotonic solutions result in fewer changes in osmolality than hypotonic solutions. Start 1 L NS aiming for 3–6 L over the first 12 h and then replacing rest within 24 h. Losses can be huge: 10–15 L.
- **Potassium:** give added K if serum level <5.0. Suggest 20 mmol/L when K 3.5–5 mmol/L and 40 mmol/L when K <3.5 mmol/L.
- **Hypernatraemia:** a rise in Na is usually seen as water shifts out of the vascular space as glucose levels fall. Consider 0.45% saline if osmolality fails to fall. Rising sodium is only a concern if the osmolality is NOT declining concurrently. Try to keep changes in Na concentration to less than 12 mol/L per day. Complete normalisation of electrolytes and osmolality may take up to 72 h.
- **INSULIN:** start an insulin infusion if ketosis (urine ketones >2 or blood ketones >1 mmol/L). Aim for a blood glucose of 10–15 mmol/L. Lower glucose by less than 5 mmol/h. Patients need lower doses in HHS than DKA and may be sensitive to large doses. Consider insulin if glucose and acidosis fail to improve with hydration. Use a fixed rate insulin infusion of 0.05 units/kg/h, e.g. 4 units/h in 80 kg person. IV insulin can usually be discontinued once they are eating and drinking but IV fluids may be required for longer if intake is inadequate. Most can be transferred to SC insulin. Those with previously undiagnosed diabetes or well controlled on oral agents, can be switched to the appropriate oral hypoglycaemic agent after a period of stability (weeks or months). Long-term insulin usually not needed and can be discontinued but review diabetes.

Management
- **VTE:** give at least prophylactic dose of LMWH as high risk of VTE. Consider looking for and treat cause, e.g. sepsis, MI, pneumonia. Observe for cerebral oedema.

- **Sepsis:** treat if any detected – urine, chest, blood cultures, CXR. Remove urinary catheter when possible.
- **Anticoagulation:** encourage early mobility, all should receive weight-adjusted LMWH prophylaxis for VTE.
- **Hypophosphataemia** (▶ Section 5.12)

Reference: Joint British Diabetes Societies Inpatient Care Group (2012) The management of the hyperosmolar hyperglycaemic state (HHS) in adults with diabetes.

5.20 Diabetic foot infections

- **About:** neuropathy and vascular compromise can lead to significant soft tissue damage. Infection can extend through to bone. Beware because pain perception impaired.
- **Clinical:** may be painless, ulceration, necrosis, loss of pulses, claudication. Inspect foot, toes and soles of feet, peripheral neuropathy, Charcot's joint. Neuropathy: painless, high arch, clawed toes, warm good pulses, painless plantar ulcers. Vascular: cold feet, poor pulses, rest pain, hair loss over shin, ulcerated heels and toes. Probe ulcers to see if bone involved.
- **Investigations:** bloods: FBC, U&E, glucose, **CRP.** Swabs as available. HbA1c, albumin. **Plain X-ray:** may show bony involvement, foreign bodies and fractures. **MRI scan:** show early osteomyelitis and marrow oedema early. Vascular studies: **Ankle-brachial** pressures may be required. **Femoral angiography:** if considered for vascular surgery.
- **Management:** multidisciplinary care involving specialist podiatrist, diabetic team, vascular surgery, microbiology. Debridement and removal of dead tissue and appropriate dressings and good glycaemic control. Ulceration but no infection: uninfected/colonisation: no antibiotics needed. Monitor and dress. Smoking cessation.
- **Mild:** check previous MRSA status, if negative CO-AMOXICLAV PO. In penicillin-allergic CLINDAMYCIN PO. Duration: 7–10 days.
- **Moderate:** check previous MRSA status, if negative CO-AMOXICLAV IV. For penicillin allergy, contact consultant microbiologist.
- **Severe:** blood cultures, swabs from wound. Check previous MRSA status. If MRSA negative TAZOCIN IV + GENTAMICIN IV stat (if ↓BP). If MRSA positive or penicillin allergy TEICOPLANIN IV (adjust dose to renal function).

5.21 Diabetes and surgery

Non-insulin treated diabetics and minor surgery

- **Preoperatively:** random blood sugar on admission <10 mmol/L – give normal medication until day of op. However, if random glucose >10 mmol/L follow as for major surgery (see below).
- **On day of operation:** omit oral hypoglycaemics. Check blood glucose: 1 h pre-op and at least once during op (hourly if op >1 h long) and post-op 2-hourly until eating.
- **Postoperatively:** restart oral hypoglycaemics with first meal.

Insulin-treated diabetics and minor surgery

- This regime only suitable for patients whose random sugar is <10 mmol/L on admission, will only miss one meal pre-op and are first on the list for very minor surgery, e.g. cystoscopy.
- **Pre-op:** normal medication. **Day of operation:** no breakfast, no insulin, place first on list. Blood glucose: 1 h pre-op and at least once during op (hourly if op >1 h long) post-op 2-hourly until eating then 4-hourly. **Post-op:** restart normal SC insulin regime with first meal.

Diabetes and major surgery or critical illness

- Applies to all diabetics who are poorly controlled (blood glucose >10 mmol/L) irrespective of whether on insulin or not at baseline. **Pre-op:** give normal medication until day of operation. **Day of operation:** omit oral hypoglycaemics and normal SC insulin.
- Check capillary blood glucose (and potassium) 1 h pre-op then 2-hourly from start of infusion at least once during operation (hourly if op >1 h long) at least once in recovery area, and 2-hourly post-op.
- One combination is 16 U of soluble insulin + 10 mmol of KCl in 500 ml of 10% glucose. Infusion rate of 100 ml/h with glucose checked every 2 h.
- Alternatively, a variable rate insulin infusion is used, especially in emergency setting and allows insulin to be administered IV and titrated to the CBG.

5.22 Variable rate intravenous insulin infusion

- The term variable rate intravenous insulin infusion (VRIII) replaces the term sliding scale. No one size fits all VRIII; they must be tailored to a patient and they are an attempt to mimic endogenous insulin production. Insulin response to a particular blood glucose depends on many physiological factors. A VRIII is an attempt to plan and direct glucose control when insulin demand is unpredictable and varying. Use only as long as is necessary. Convert to an insulin regimen as soon as requirements stable. Before stopping a VRIII prescribe appropriate insulin therapy. In comatose patients, e.g. stroke, very tight control may lead to hypoglycaemia and coma with few symptoms and signs and further damage may occur.
- **Indications for VRIII are** hyperglycaemia in patients with known diabetes or with hospital-related hyperglycaemia unable to take oral fluid/food and for whom adjustment of their own insulin regime is not possible, e.g. vomiting (exclude DKA), nil by mouth and will miss more than one meal, severe illness with need to achieve good glycaemic control, e.g. sepsis. Other indications are ACS (follow local guidelines), TPN/enteral feeding, steroid use, pregnancy. **NB.** Withhold usual diabetes treatment during the VRIII BUT CONTINUE any basal (long-acting) insulin.
- **Aims of VRIII are** a CBG in range 6.0–10.0 mmol/L (4.0–12.0 mmol/L acceptable), avoid hypoglycaemia (CBG <4.0 mmol/L), limit use to <24 h where possible, try to avoid using in those patients able to eat and drink. **Those on VRIII need:** hourly monitoring of CBG with regular review of insulin infusion rate to achieve target range of glucose, at least daily review of the need for the VRIII, at least daily clinical review of patient including fluid status and daily urea and electrolytes.

CBG check every 1–2 h (mmol/L)	50 U ACTRAPID in 50 ml 0.9% NS and run as below (use larger dose if insulin resistance suspected, e.g. obese)
<4.0	None; treat hypoglycaemia
4.1–8.0	1–2 U/h (0.5 U/h insulin sensitive)
8.1–12.0	2–4 U/h (1 U/h insulin sensitive)
12.1–16.0	4–6 U/h (2 U/h insulin sensitive)
16.1–20.00	5–7 U/h (3 U/h insulin sensitive)
20.1–24.0	6–8 U/h (4 U/h insulin sensitive)
>20	8–10 U/h check line (6 U/h insulin sensitive). Ensure insulin was added. Seek medical review.

VRIII must also be accompanied by IV fluids at 125 ml/h (adjust for patient size, cardiac/fluid status) containing at least 5% glucose, e.g. 1 L 0.45% NaCl with 5% glucose and 40 mmol/L KCl or 5% glucose with 40 mmol/L KCl. If K is >5.5 mmol/L do not add K. If K is <3.5 mmol/L senior review needed as extra K needs to be given.

- **Preparation:** use an insulin syringe/pen to draw up 50 U of a short-acting insulin, e.g. Actrapid. Add to a 50 ml syringe containing 49.5 ml of NS giving 1 U/ml. Always ensure lines and IV access working. Some patients need 100 U/day and others 30 U/day so the VRIII doses need to reflect this. Basal insulin needed will escalate with physiological stress, surgery, sepsis and insulin resistance.
- The insulin is given alongside IV fluid, which must be administered using a **volumetric infusion pump.** This should be 0.45% saline with G5 and 0.15% **or** 0.3% KCl. Omit KCl if K >4.5 mmol/L. The amount of KCl depends on the most recent U&E. For patients with renal impairment and high K, 0.45% saline with 5% glucose **without** KCl should be used. In low Na IV NS may be used.
- Set the fluid replacement rate to deliver the hourly fluid requirements of the individual patient. The rate must not be altered thereafter without senior advice. Insulin must be infused at a variable rate to keep the blood glucose 6–10 mmol/L (acceptable range 4–12 mmol/L).
- Stopping the VRIII: for T2DM **oral hypoglycaemics:** restart when oral intake possible at normal pre-op doses. Reduce or stop sulphonylurea if oral intake likely to be reduced. Metformin avoided if eGFR <50 ml/min. **Restarting insulin:** wait until normal oral intake possible. Restart normal dose but adjust down if oral intake reduced or increase if on-going sepsis or infection or post-op stress. Aim for a level of 4–12 mmol/L. Involve diabetic specialist team for optimising control. Ensure that the VRIII / IVII overlaps the giving of SC insulin by 30–60 min.

Reference: Joint British Diabetes Societies (2014) The use of variable rate intravenous insulin infusion (VRIII) in medical inpatients (www.diabetologists-abcd.org.uk/jbds/JBDS_IP_VRIII.pdf).

General rules for acute control in known diabetic

- If blood glucose >12 mmol/L then check capillary ketone levels using an appropriate bedside monitor if available. If capillary blood ketones are greater than 3 mmol/L or urinary ketones greater than +++ then follow DKA guidelines (▶ Section 5.18) and contact the on-call medical/diabetes specialist team for advice. For all others with known diabetes see as follows.
- **T1DM: always need insulin.** Give SC rapid acting analogue insulin (i.e. Novorapid, Humalog) and assume that 1 U of insulin will drop glucose by 3 mmol/L BUT wherever possible determine baseline needs. Recheck the blood glucose 1 h later to ensure it is falling. If control is still unsatisfactory discuss with medical/diabetic team. Consider VRIII.
- **T2DM:** use SC rapid acting analogue insulin (i.e. Novorapid, Humalog). Assess using CBG measurement. Always recheck blood glucose 1 h later to ensure it is falling. If worsening or unsatisfactory then contact medical/diabetic team and consider VRIII.
- **New diabetes:** determine if T1DM (young, thin, may be ketotic), will usually need insulin therapy and a VRIII is reasonable initially and an estimate of insulin needed can be made. Involve diabetic team. At earliest reasonable opportunity commence insulin regimen. Older, obese diabetics will usually be T2DM and dietary advice and oral medication can be considered.
- It is advisable to use your own hospital's protocol where available. The important level is to ensure enough insulin to render normoglycaemic without any ketones. If this is for DKA, continue insulin at all times (to switch off ketone production, and so reduce acidosis). If for other reasons (e.g. control peri-operatively) <4 mmol/L should stop insulin. Hypoglycaemia should be treated as usual.

5.23 Diabetes care in emergencies

Increasing numbers of diabetic patients. Increased risks with critical illness and surgery. These risks are heightened if patient has had diabetes for an extended period of time, there is poor control or brittle (have difficulty controlling glucose level) diabetes. Diabetic patients often have co-morbidities.

- **Introduction:** best management policy for diabetic emergencies is prevention. Many are due to issues with less than satisfactory self or medical care. Need to know and understand management of hypoglycaemia, DKA and HHS.

Diagnosis of diabetes

Diagnosis	Fasting sugar	GTT (75 g in 2 h)
Normal	<6.1 mmol/L	<7.8 mmol/L
Impaired fasting glucose	5.6–6.9 mmol/L	
Impaired glucose tolerance		7.8–11 mmol/L
Diabetes	>7.0 mmol/L	Random or 2 h post GTT >11.1 mmol/L

General principles of acute diabetic glycaemic control

- Insulin (from endogenous pancreatic B cells or exogenous IV/SC/IM) allows glucose to enter cells for ATP generation and lowers blood glucose. Excess insulin or sulphonylurea or meglitinides can cause hypoglycaemia which, if prolonged or severe, can cause brain injury and death.
- Absence of insulin, e.g. T1DM, leads to hyperglycaemia. Cells starved of glucose which leads them to burn fats causing acidosis and ketonaemia/ketonuria which can be measured. Those with T2DM have insulin but not enough insulin to manage their blood glucose but enough to prevent ketosis. DKA very rarely occurs, but hyperglycaemia and severe fluid loss can, which can cause HHS.
- Physiological stress, e.g. illness, surgery, physical trauma or even pregnancy can cause a state of hyperglycaemia which causes polyuria, dehydration and volume loss. This is controlled by insulin release normally, but the diabetic patient needs to have their insulin dose increased. If there is an absence of insulin + stress then the result will be a rapid development of DKA.
- In diabetic patients you must supply the correct amount of insulin to match the physiological needs, ideally maintaining blood glucose, but this can be difficult as physiological demands vary as well as calorific intake and other factors. The primary aim is to avoid severe hypoglycaemia and severe hyperglycaemia (>20 mmol/L). **If the blood glucose is high you must give more insulin. If low you give less.** Insulins come in various formats to change the half-life, but the active molecule is the same. The formulation just alters the half-life so that it can be short acting or long acting. Hospital is the safest place to adjust insulin if monitoring is frequent and hyperglycaemia and hypoglycaemia can be quickly detected and treated. Hypoglycaemia can develop silently in comatose or obtunded patients, e.g. stroke, and so monitoring must be frequent if patients are on insulin or oral hypoglycaemic drugs.

Types of commercial insulin

- **Fast acting short half-life:** Actrapid or Humulin S (soluble/short). These act within a half hour and peak at 2–4 h and last about 6 h in total. They are used to make up sliding scales now called VRIIIs.

- **Intermediate acting:** Humulin I or Insulatard, which are normally given in BD doses pre-breakfast and pre-evening meal.
- **Long acting:** Glargine or Detemir. These have a much longer period of activity and can be given either once or twice daily. They can mimic the basal level of insulin.
- **Combined insulins:** fast and intermediate acting insulins can be combined and so can mimic the basal level and there is a short acting insulin which can deal with mealtime hyperglycaemia. Twice daily and three times daily insulins are prescribed, usually before meals.
- In most cases the potential problems can be discussed and control improved pre-operatively and discussed at the pre-operative assessment. There is no such opportunity to optimise diabetic control prior to emergency surgery. Before, during and post-op the aim is to keep the blood glucose level within the range 6–10 mmol/L at all times.

06 Gastroenterology emergencies

6.1 Acute diarrhoea

Answering bleep/taking referral

- Diarrhoea: is there known IBD? Is or was the patient on antibiotics? Pyrexial, tachycardia, unwell, dehydrated? How many times have bowels opened today and is stool bloody?
- Use the Bristol stool chart to characterise diarrhoea (Type 6/7). Suspected infective causes need isolation and stool culture. Wash hands with soap and water. Alcohol hand washes are insufficient.
- Why are they in hospital? When did it start? Frequency? Bristol stool chart scale.
- Abdominal pain or vomiting, recent antibiotics, excessive laxatives. Known bowel disease. Pain, guarding, tenderness – is this an acute abdomen?

Causes of diarrhoea defined as stool weight >250 g/day

- **Bacterial infective:** *Salmonella* and *E. coli* usually cause a sudden onset gastroenteritis which can be bloody with a toxic patient. Usually with fever and abdominal pain. *Shigella* – bloody diarrhoea. ▶ Section 9.40.
- **Clostridium difficile:** caused by enterotoxins A and B. Associated with antibiotic usage that alters gut flora. Can lead to pseudomembranous colitis, megacolon and perforation and even death. Stop any antibiotic. Needs urgent METRONIDAZOLE 500 mg 8 h PO or VANCOMYCIN 125 mg 6 h PO and surgical consult if abdominal pain. ▶ Section 6.11.
- **Viral infective:** norovirus must be isolated quickly. N&V. Spreads quickly. Isolate and infection control and watch for patient/staff in proximity complaining of same.
- **Acute colitis:** known IBD may be on treatment. Bloody stools, fever. Needs stool chart and gastroenterology review and steroids. ▶ Section 6.10.
- **Ischaemic colitis:** abdominal pain, vascular risks, AF, diarrhoea (bloody). ▶ Section 6.14.
- **Amoebic:** caused by invasive infection by *Entamoeba histolytica*. Foreign travel. Acute colitis. Check stools. ▶ Section 9.48.
- **Laxatives:** overuse and sometimes abuse.
- **Autonomic:** stasis and small bowel bacterial overgrowth.
- **Constipation with overflow:** rectum full of hard stools with liquid stool emerging. PR is helpful and AXR shows faeces. Needs enema and laxatives and medication review.
- **Osmotic diarrhoea:** in hospital commonly seen starting NG or PEG feeding regimens; can cause an osmotic diarrhoea which can be reduced by slowing feed temporarily and stopping laxatives.
- **Neoplastic disease:** colorectal malignancy is certainly a cause of on-going altered bowel function. However, more altered bowel habit than diarrhoea. Needs colonoscopy.
- **Carcinoid syndrome:** causes flushing, diarrhoea, wheezing. Measure urine 5-hydroxyindoleacetic acid (5-HIAA), plasma chromogranin A. Liver USS for metastases. Octreoscan, Rx: Octreotide.
- **Malabsorption:** pancreatic insufficiency, pale bulky stools or an osmotic diarrhoea with lactose intolerance. Need lactose hydrogen breath test. Low B12/folate/Fe.
- **VIPoma:** severe watery diarrhoea and low K due to vasoactive intestinal peptide.
- **Thyrotoxicosis:** increased frequency rather than diarrhoea. ↑T_4, low TSH and look for signs of Graves' disease. ▶ Section 5.8.
- **Toxic shock syndrome:** diarrhoea, rash in patient who may have an infective source, e.g. simple skin wound or tampon. Rapid deterioration with ↓BP and shock. ▶ Section 2.19.

On arrival

- **Review early warning score.** Review notes and drug chart particularly antibiotics and laxatives and stop them if possible. Discuss with microbiology if need for antimicrobials.
- Abdominal examination including PR – may be hard stools with overflow.
- Check basic bloods if concerned about dehydration. If severe diarrhoea or poor oral intake then IV fluids.
- Caution with loperamide if any suggestion of infective cause. Hand washing. Isolate patient and send stool cultures if infected cause suspected.

Investigations

- **Bloods:** FBC, U&E, TFT, CRP.
- **Request stool culture:** cysts, ova and parasites and *C. difficile* toxins A and B.
- **AXR:** features of IBD, toxic megacolon if pseudomembranous colitis.
- **Sigmoidoscopy:** look for inflamed mucosa, rectal biopsy if diarrhoea persists.
- **Colonoscopy:** if colitis or polyps/tumour suspected. Colonoscopy is best investigation to diagnose colonic cancer in those without significant co-morbidities. If there are such issues then CT colonography may be considered or flexible sigmoidoscopy and barium enema.
- **CT/MRI:** rarely needed. Get if suspected intra-abdominal pathology. MRI best for pelvic Crohn's disease or other inflammatory bowel disease.
- **Rare:** look for carcinoid syndrome, VIPoma, etc.

General management

- Isolation if an infective cause suspected. Gown up and wear gloves, which should be placed in bin in patient's room. Ensure hands washed with soap and water to remove any *C. difficile* spores.
- See individual cases above, but all patients need to maintain adequate hydration either orally or IV depending on losses. Monitor fluid balance and U&E and general observations.
- Use codeine/loperamide sparingly in lowest dose for short period if severe symptomatic diarrhoea if infective causes suspected. Use with caution, concern is that they may delay resolution. Avoid if suspected *C. difficile* and pseudomembranous colitis. Surgical review if acute abdomen.

6.2 Constipation

Answering bleep (is the patient a bowel obstruction/ileus or simple constipation?)

- Has there been dietary intake? When did bowels last open? Is patient in pain or discomfort?
- Patient taking opiates or dehydrated or bed bound or Parkinson's disease or hypothyroid?
- Rarely an acute issue unless nil PR is a sign of obstruction with pain and abdominal distension and abnormal bowel sounds.

On arrival

- Review notes, observations and drug chart. Assess patient and usual bowel frequency. Once a week may be normal for some. Is it physical/psychological, e.g. having to use bed pan or commode?
- Pain, e.g. anal fissure or haemorrhoids will make patient avoid defecation. Needs stool softeners.

- If there are signs of bowel obstruction then nil by mouth, bloods and AXR and surgical consult.
- If not obstructed and mild may simply require improved hydration, high fibre diet and oral laxatives.
- If constipated (AXR may show stool ++) with watery diarrhoea and an enema, e.g. Microlax enema or a Picolax (sodium picosulphate) enema, can be very effective in emptying the rectum.
- **Examination:** tenderness, bowel sounds, peritonism, masses. PR examination: anal pain or discomfort, rectal tumour or impacted faeces. Spinal cord disease or multiple sclerosis usually already known. Hirschsprung's disease usually from childhood. Myxoedema: look for clinical signs, ↑TSH.

Causes of constipation

- A poor dietary intake or lack of dietary fibre, immobility or dehydration.
- **Drugs:** opiates, anticholinergic, diuretics, CCBs, e.g. verapamil, iron, ondansetron.
- **Metabolic:** low K or Mg. High Ca, hyperglycaemia, dehydration, hypothyroid.
- **Physical:** volvulus, stricture, ileus, colorectal tumour, anal pain, difficulty toileting.
- **Others:** acute porphyria, spinal cord disease, Hirschsprung's disease, Parkinson's disease, depression, dementia.

Management

- Hydrate orally if possible and high fibre diet and early mobility and provide time and access to optimal toileting conditions with as much privacy as can be provided. Make use of gastrocolic reflex – toileting patient after eating.
- On-going or new constipation for several weeks warrants consideration to exclude a colorectal malignancy. Try stool softeners (e.g. SODIUM DOCUSATE 200 mg tds), bulking agents (e.g. FYBOGEL one sachet BD), stimulants (e.g. SENNA 1 tab BD is useful especially if stools are large, soft and bulky).
- Osmotic laxatives (e.g. LACTULOSE 10–20 ml BD) really are to be avoided if possible, except to improve stool output with hepatic encephalopathy. Movicol (e.g. contains polyethylene glycol or codanthramer). Enemas (e.g. glycerin suppository or Picolax enema) are useful for distal stool.
- Occasionally all fails and you may be asked to perform a manual evacuation, which is digital removal of rectal faeces. Be sure to wear two pairs of gloves and have lots of pads. Constipation is common but significant complications are very rare, but include faecal impaction where the rectum fills with 'rocks' of hard stool with soft stool leaking around sides and overflow diarrhoea.
- Can even cause intestinal obstruction and perforation and megacolon leading to sigmoid volvulus. Rectal prolapse can be seen. It may provoke urinary retention and UTI.

Laxatives and bowel preparation

- **Stimulant laxative:** SENNA 15 mg (2 tabs) BD SE: cramps, diarrhoea and low K. Avoid if bowel obstruction. BISACODYL 5–10 mg nocte.
- **Osmotic laxative:** LACTULOSE 10–30 ml 12 h, higher doses in hepatic encephalopathy (30–50 ml TDS) to have 2+ soft stools/day.
- **Bulk forming laxative:** ISPAGHULA HUSK 3.5 g BD or one sachet BD.
- **Bowel cleansing for severe cases:** SODIUM PICOSULPHATE 10 mg single dose and review.
- **Enema:** MICROLAX one PR and the more potent PHOSPHATE enema.

6.3 Dyspepsia

Definitions: recurrent epigastric pain, burning, fullness, early satiety or discomfort. Symptoms often poorly localising and several tests may be needed. Symptoms are defined to be present for at least 4 or 12 weeks depending on definitions. Red flags needing endoscopy – age >55, bleeding, anaemia, vomiting, dysphagia, abdominal mass, early satiety. Finding gallstones does not mean that this is the cause and often find those with continuing symptoms post-cholecystectomy.

Causes of dyspepsia

- **Peptic ulcer disease:** epigastric discomfort with eating. OGD – gastritis or erosions mucosal breaks <5mm are erosions, otherwise ulcers. Gastric and duodenal. Presents: iron deficiency anaemia. Outflow obstruction. Haematemesis. GU epigastric pain. DU pain to back – patient points to epigastrium. Risks: NSAIDs, steroids, aspirin and combinations of same. *Helicobacter pylori*. Prevention: MISOPROSTOL reduces NSAID ulcers or PPI for those on long term aspirin/steroids/NSAIDs aged over 60 or with symptoms. Stop smoking. Needs OGD. FBC, haematinics, test for *H. pylori* and treat.
- **Oesophageal cancer:** weight loss, progressive dysphagia to solids then fluids, regurgitation. Needs endoscopy +/− stenting, biopsy and staging.
- **Gastric cancer:** weight loss, bleeding, anaemia, early satiety, vomiting. Needs endoscopy +/− stenting, biopsy and staging.
- **GORD:** reflux causes heartburn and waterbrash. Worse on lying or bending. OGD may show oesophagitis or erosions.
- **Gastroparesis:** impaired gastric motility. Type 1/2 DM. OGD shows food still present.
- **Biliary colic/gallstones:** RUQ pain. Stone in gallbladder or cystic duct. Needs USS and LFTs. May need ERCP.
- **Irritable bowel:** abdominal pain and bloating and intermittent diarrhoea or constipation or mucus. Feeling of incomplete evacuation. Bloods should be normal. No red flags – bleeding, anaemia, no weight loss or family history and age <60, no abdominal mass or rectal mass and negative CA125 where ovarian cancer is possible. Normal faecal calprotectin can help distinguish from inflammatory disease and avoid colonoscopy when cancer is not suspected.
- **Non ulcer dyspepsia:** OGD normal. Functional. Reassurance.
- **Pancreatic cancer:** weight loss, pain, anaemia, early satiety, vomiting. Needs ERCP +/− stenting, biopsy and staging.
- **Pancreatitis:** elevated lipase/amylase. Epigastric pain. Gallstones and alcohol. See below.
- **Coeliac disease:** check FBC, duodenal biopsies, antibody testing for coeliac disease (endomysial antibodies (EMA) or tissue transglutaminase (TTG)).
- **Medication:** most drugs in BNF cause dyspepsia. Ask about all medication given. Steroids, aspirin, NSAIDs, L-Dopa-containing meds, macrolides, bisphosphonates, nitrates, calcium channel blockers, codeine, theophylline, etc.
- **Chronic alcohol abuse:** dyspepsia is common.
- **Metabolic:** uraemia and renal failure, hypercalcaemia.
- **Cardiac:** ACS as inferior MI can classically cause epigastric discomfort. Needs ECG and troponin. Myocarditis and pericarditis.
- **Aortic disease:** dissection or aneurysm. Chest pain into back. Needs CT aortogram.
- **Ischaemic bowel:** uncommon but should be considered.
- **Pulmonary:** embolism, pneumonia, malignancy. Get CXR and other tests as needed.
- **Lactose intolerance:** ingestion of lactose (milk) increases symptoms. Try without. Need lactose hydrogen breath test.

- **Investigations:** diagnostics can help where cause not evident. Send FBC. U&E, LFT, Ca, amylase/lipase, CRP, troponin (if needed), ECG, USS biliary tracts and pancreas, endoscopy, urea breath test for HP. HP serology identifies only prior exposure.
- **Management:** treatment can be with **SUCRALFATE 2 g BD PO, RANITIDINE** or **PPI**. *H. pylori* eradication – see BNF for latest regimen. Transfuse if anaemia Hb <80 g/L or bleeding. Iron replacement. See below for acute upper GI bleed and for gallstones. Always ask if this could be an ACS.

 ## Upper gastrointestinal bleeding

About: bleeding from above the ligament of Treitz. Nasopharynx, oesophagus, stomach, duodenum. Multiple causes may co-exist – varices and gastritis and a duodenal ulcer. Epistaxis and swallowed blood can mimic GI bleed. If physicians can't stop life-threatening bleeding it's a surgical problem. 90% of non-variceal bleeds (VBs) and 50% of VBs stop spontaneously. Mortality is 10%, rising to 26% in patients who bleed when in hospital for other reasons. Use the Blatchford and Rockall score to assess patients.

NB. With a suspect GI bleed first make sure there are at least two good wide bore IV lines before all peripheral venous access disappears.

Causes of upper GI bleeding

- **Peptic ulcer disease (38%):** usually lesser curve of stomach or duodenal bulb where an ulcer can erode into a large vessel. *H. pylori* +ve, NSAIDs. Multiple ulcers with Zollinger–Ellison syndrome. Needs OGD and endoscopic therapy and PPI and *H. pylori* eradication. Rarely surgery.
- **Oesophageal ulcer/severe oesophagitis (13%):** pain on swallowing, dysphagia, GORD symptoms. In HIV, infections with candida, CMV, HSV. Local ulceration with bisphosphonates and NSAIDs.
- **Oesophageal/gastric cancer (7%):** progressive dysphagia to solids then liquids. Weight loss, bleeding, adenocarcinoma.
- **Gastric:** chronic blood loss more usual. Early satiation and weight loss.
- **Coagulopathy:** patient on warfarin or liver disease or severe thrombocytopenia with any other gastric pathology.
- **Gastric oesophageal varices (16%):** needs OGD + Terlipressin 2 mg QDS + endoscopic management + antibiotics, Sengstaken tube and TIPS. VB due to portal HTN due to: cirrhosis (alcohol, NAFLD, viral hepatitis, haem, PBC, PSC, idiopathic, etc.), schistosomiasis (commonest worldwide), extrahepatic portal vein thrombosis, idiopathic portal hypertension, cardiac fibrosis. Assess cirrhosis mortality with Child–Pugh score below. Useful prognostic marker of cirrhosis and varices. Has been used to aid selection of those for further interventions. Cirrhosis causes portal pressure >12 mmHg and so blood redirected to lower oesophagus and small vessels become distended and thinned walled. Alcohol history, signs of chronic liver failure and caput medusae. Splenomegaly suggests portal hypertension. Look for causes of cirrhosis and portal hypertension.
- **Aorto-enteric fistula:** previous AAA surgery with fistula with 3rd part of duodenum causing severe GI bleeding.
- **Mallory–Weiss tear (4%):** history of retching and often alcohol misuse. Linear mucosal tear found near the oesophagogastric junction. Mucosal tear can be injected with ADRENALINE. If this fails haemoclips or band ligation.
- **Peptic ulcer:** ASPIRIN/NSAIDs/STEROID make this more likely. Alcohol. Epigastric discomfort.
- **Gastric vascular ectasias (6%):** may be found and also seen with hereditary haemorrhagic telangiectasia, arteriovenous malformation and other vascular lesions. Angiodysplasia with CKD.
- **Dieulafoy's lesion (2%):** a large calibre arteriole, which lies just below the mucosa and causes an arterial bleed through a pinpoint mucosal lesion. Most commonly on the lesser curve.
- **Spurious:** swallowed epistaxis blood or from nasopharynx can cause haematemesis and melena. Ask about these. Epistaxis can be severe with swallowed blood but the history should be clear if asked.
- **Right colonic bleed:** may cause melena-type stools but this is rare.

- **Clinical history/risk factors:** most of the time the story is difficult with dark material passed orally or rectally and the usual 'coffee grounds', which may be bile. Ask about liver disease, peptic ulcer disease, alcohol intake, aspirin usage, NSAIDs, warfarin, steroids. Ask about a history of bleeding problems – dental extractions, etc. Bright red haematemesis implies active bleeding from the oesophagus, stomach or duodenum. This can lead to circulatory collapse and constitutes a medical emergency. Coffee ground vomitus refers to the vomiting of black material assumed to be blood. Its presence implies that bleeding has stopped or has been relatively modest. It may simply be bile. Often over-reported. Melena is the passage of tarry black stool usually due to acute upper GI bleeding but occasionally from bleeding within the small bowel or right colon. Iron preparations will cause some black faeces. Haemochezia is the passage of fresh blood per rectum usually due to colonic bleeding but occasionally due to profuse upper GI bleeding.

- **Examination:** look for signs of liver disease and portal hypertension suggests varices but bleeding may be other pathology. Liver disease – ascites, jaundice, gynaecomastia, Dupuytren's contracture, clubbing, spider naevi, caput medusae, palmar erythema, etc. Liver decompensation, e.g. jaundice, encephalopathy, asterixis. Liver flap. Evidence of significant blood loss: postural fall in SBP >20 mmHg, postural HR increase >30 bpm (lying/sitting when too ill to stand). Signs of shock and haemodynamic compromise. Thready pulse, thirst, poor skin turgor, cold nose. Increased capillary refill time. Oliguria – measure urine output. Rectal exam for melena. Facial telangiectasias (HHT).

- **Look for evidence for bleeding:** upper GI bleeding manifests as either vomited bright red or altered blood 'coffee grounds' called haematemesis, or altered blood products passed PR as melena. Normal dark bile often mistaken for coffee grounds. 'Coffee grounds' and melena show bleeding that occurred minutes to hours before. Huge amounts of GI bleed will pass quickly and cause bright red blood passing within minutes. The GI protein load of blood and the anaemia and ↓BP can cause agitation and delirium. Bleeding may, however, be occult with just progressive signs of anaemia.

Investigations

- **FBC:** initially often normal and misleading because haemodilution yet to take place. Check platelets. Target Hb 80 g/dL. Recent evidence suggests that higher Hb targets associated with increased mortality.
- **U&E:** ↑urea may suggest GI blood loss and protein load in gut. May see AKI.
- **LFT and coagulation screen:** at baseline and repeat as needed.
- **Blood group and cross-match** 2–4 units depending on estimated losses.

Management (see also <u>Haemorrhagic shock ▶ Section 2.22</u>)

- **Risk assess:** use Glasgow Blatchford score to assess on admission and full Rockall post-endoscopy to guide management. Escalate high score or unstable patients. Resuscitate those who are actively bleeding and discuss need for urgent endoscopy. In suspected GI bleeding, consider the patient for non-admission or early discharge if before endoscopy the Blatchford score is 0, i.e. no melena and no haemodynamic disturbance, no significant co-morbidity and normal FBC and normal urea. Low score patients may be managed as outpatients on a next day list.
- **Get good IV access and protect it:** if ↓BP and ↑HR or melena or witnessed haematemesis then need good venous access with **2 GREY VENFLONS in each antecubital fossa**. If difficult IV access get immediate help from registrar or anaesthetist. A central line is too long and fine bore for good flow and not good for giving volume quickly. Once access gained send bloods FBC, U&E, LFT, clotting,

and group and cross-match 4 units or more if needed. Upper GI endoscopy: usually within 24 h or sooner.

- **Give crystalloids:** start 1 L NS, use Dextrose and transfuse if Liver failure (avoid or caution against saline if liver disease) over 20–60 min and high flow O_2 if shocked.
Transfuse: if actively bleeding and Hb <9, or the patient is shocked. In stable non-actively bleeding patients, transfuse if Hb <7, or if <8 and there is significant co-morbidity. See massive transfusion protocol. Early effective resuscitation reduces mortality. If patient dying in front of you from obvious active witnessed bleeding consider **universal donor O negative blood** and send someone to fetch it.
- **Nil by mouth:** keep patients who are actively bleeding, or are shocked at presentation, NBM. Unless actively bleeding, patients should be NBM for 4 h before endoscopy. Otherwise stable non-bleeding patients should be allowed to eat.
- **PPI:** start oral PPI and give IV only if cannot take PO.
- **Coagulopathy:** offer FFP if actively bleeding and INR >1.5. If a patient's fibrinogen level remains less than 1.5 g/L despite FFP use, offer cryoprecipitate as well. Consider platelet transfusion in those actively bleeding with count <50 × 10^9/L. Those on warfarin and bleeding need prothrombin complex concentrate and vitamin K. Those on dabigatran need Praxbind. Give FFP at 15 ml/kg (each unit is about 150–200 ml). Give cryoprecipitate (2 units) as per transfusion policy. Patients with critical CAD or new or drug-eluting stents should be discussed with cardiology prior to next dose. Uncontrolled bleeding and anaemia exacerbates IHD.
- **Endoscopy:** most arteries go into spasm and stop bleeding after the initial rupture. In patients who continue to bleed or re-bleed following admission, endoscopic therapy or surgery may be necessary. The decision on the timing of endoscopy is individualised for patients depending on the severity of the bleed and their co-morbidities. If endoscopy is required out of hours contact the on-call consultant endoscopist. All other patients with upper GI bleeding should have endoscopy within 24 h of admission.
- **Interpretation of endoscopic findings:** risks of rebleeding – active bleeding 90%, non-bleeding visible vessel 25%, adherent clot 25–30%, oozing without visible vessel 10–20%, flat spot 7–10%, clean ulcer base 3–5%
- **Drugs:** stop all antiplatelets if possible. Patients with critical CAD or stents <1 year should probably continue these drugs except in the most severe bleeding episodes. Consider seeking advice from a cardiologist.
- **Observations:** repeat frequent assessments of BP, HR and JVP and titrate volume and blood replacement with these. Take care not to volume overload the frail and elderly and those with poor cardiac function. A urinary catheter can be the poor man's central line because it can give some measure as a surrogate marker of renal and general perfusion. If you can get the patient to an HDU/ITU bed then that is ideal for the shocked bleeder.
- **Starting PPI:** IV PANTOPRAZOLE 40 mg BD is used only in patients with severe active bleeding from ulcers after endoscopy. Otherwise give OMEPRAZOLE 20 mg PO after endoscopy, unless endoscopy is likely to be delayed. NICE recommends that PPI treatment is not started before endoscopy. Although it is logical to begin treating bleeding peptic ulcers with PPIs as soon as possible, there is no evidence that treatment before endoscopy alters outcome. Treatment with PPIs makes testing for *H. pylori* less reliable.
- **Recurrent bleeding:** patients with one episode of recurrent bleeding following initially successful endoscopic therapy are typically treated with a second attempt at endoscopic therapy. Surgery or angiography-guided intervention is indicated for patients who fail endoscopic therapy (persistent bleeding or recurrent bleeding after two therapeutic endoscopies).

- **Surgical liaison:** if bleeding continues despite endoscopy then surgeons and anaesthetists will be involved, as laparotomy may be the only way to stop the bleeding. The patient becomes a surgical rather than a medical emergency.
- **ITU/HDU:** patients may be best on HDU/ITU, especially if need for intubation or ventilation or inotropic support or multi-organ failure. Speak to ITU team and involve them early in a deteriorating patient.

PRE-ENDOSCOPY Blatchford score at admission	POST-ENDOSCOPY Rockall score (*Gut*, 1999;44:331)
- **Blood urea:** 6.5–7.9 (**+2**), 8.0–9.9 (**+3**), 10–25 (**+4**), >25 (**+6**) - **Hb** (men g/L): 120–129 (**+1**), 100–119 (**+3**), <100 (**+6**) - **Hb** (women g/L): 100–119 (**+1**), <100 (**+6**) - **Systolic BP:** 100–109 (**+1**), 90–99 (**+2**), <90 (**+3**) - **Pulse:** >100 (**+1**), melena (**+1**), syncope (**+2**) - **Hepatic disease** (+2), **cardiac failure** (+2) Score >6 suggests need for intervention	- **Age:** <60 (+0), 60–79 (+1), >80 (+2) - **Shock:** HR <100 SBP >100 mmHg (+0), HR >100 SBP >100 mmHg (+1), SBP <100 mmHg (+2) - **Co-morbidities:** none significant (+0), IHD/CCF or other major co-morbidity (+2), liver failure/kidney failure/metastatic cancer (+3) - **Post-endoscopy findings** - **Endoscopic diagnosis:** Mallory–Weiss tear (+0), all other diagnosis (+1), gastrointestinal malignancy (+2) - **Bleeding at endoscopy:** none or dark spots only (+0), blood, spurting vessel, adherent clot (+2)

Calculate total: Pre-endoscopy score used to risk assess. Helps gastroenterologists to select those for urgent endoscopy.

Post-endoscopy score. Those with an additional low score may not require urgent endoscopy and some may be managed as outpatient. **Score: very low risk: 1–2** can be considered for instant discharge and OP OGD and PPI and follow up. **Low risk <3:** 0% expected mortality and 5% rebleed – good prognosis; consider discharge, outpatient endoscopy on PPI. **Intermediate 3–8:** monitor as inpatient. **High risk >8:** high (41%) mortality and (42%) rebleed – consider urgent endoscopy.

- **Warnings:** elderly patients decompensate early; healthy younger patients (under 50) decompensate late and quickly so take care and don't be lulled into a false sense of security. Alleged GI blood loss by its nature is occult initially and management is expectant – it will appear PR eventually. There are those with spurious unconfirmed bleeding and alleged witnessed 'coffee grounds' or 'dark stool' with no definite physiological or clinical or lab evidence and those with clear evidence of active GI bleeding. Need to have risk assessed and monitored and managed accordingly. Be careful with those on beta-blockers where normal ↑HR response may be muted. Steroids can mask perforation and acute abdominal pathology.
- **Coagulopathy: warfarin-induced bleed:** needs IV VITAMIN K 5–10 mg and prothrombin complex concentrates, e.g. Octaplex/Beriplex. Target INR <1.5. REVERSE WARFARIN EVEN IN THOSE WITH METAL HEART VALVES WITH MAJOR BLEED. Risk of harm from temporary reversal of anticoagulation for several days is likely much less than the risk of exsanguination in those with genuine signs of significant haemorrhage. **Upper GI bleeding and stent or metal valves:** risk of proven bleeding usually is the more pressing and anticoagulation/antiplatelets should be stopped and reversed acutely. Stent thrombosis is a concern if bleeding occurs soon after PCI and stenting, however, so is anaemia-induced cardiac ischaemia and exsanguination. Liaise closely with cardiologists and gastroenterologists to manage risk.
- **Severe oesophagitis:** OMEPRAZOLE 40 mg OD PO. Manage blood loss. Consider also SUCRALFATE 2 g BD PO.

Oesophageal variceal bleed

- **Resuscitate.** Consider ITU and intubation: failure to control severe bleeding, encephalopathy, hypoxia, aspiration. Terlipressin and antibiotics may be started pre-endoscopy if varices likely.
- **Antibiotics:** give a broad spectrum antibiotic usually parenteraly when acutely unwell, e.g. IV CO-AMOXICLAV or IV TAZOCIN (unless penicillin allergy) or CEFTRIAXONE to any patient with cirrhosis who presents with an upper GI bleed. Other antibiotics include NORFLOXACIN PO and QUINOLONES.
- **Bleeding:** treat any coagulopathy with FFP. Transfuse platelets if there is continued bleeding and platelet count is <50 000/μL. Consider IV VITAMIN K 10 mg. Consider TRANEXAMIC ACID 1 g tds PO. Give blood products as needed. Target Hb >80 g/L and INR 1.3 with FFP. Platelets >50. Fibrinogen >2 with cryoprecipitate. Consider IV VITAMIN K 5–10 mg slow IV if prolonged PT.
- **Active management:** 40% will not settle conservatively and need active treatment to control bleed. Admit HDU. **Target Hb 80 g/L**. Over transfusion may increase bleeding. Endoscopic bleeding risk factors: severity of cirrhosis, ↑hepatic vein pressure, variceal size, tense ascites, endoscopic appearance, e.g. haematocystic spots, diffuse erythema, bluish colour, cherry red spots, or white-nipple spots. Large varices >5 mm diameter. Prophylactic treatment to prevent variceal bleeding is recommended with large oesophageal varices irrespective of the presence or absence of red colour signs.
- **TERLIPRESSIN (GLYPRESSIN)** 2 mg IV followed by 1–2 mg 4-hourly for 3 d (C/I if severe IHD or stroke or peripheral vascular disease); mesenteric/splanchnic vasoconstrictor decreases portal venous inflow. 34% reduction in mortality for VB. Give immediately prior to endoscopy if varices likely. Alternative is OCTREOTIDE 50 mcg/h infusion for 3–5 days (can be used in those with IHD) but evidence base poorer.
- **Laxatives:** reduce risk of encephalopathy: LACTULOSE 30–50 ml TDS and PHOSPHATE ENEMAS to get 2+ or more soft bowel motions per day.
- **Endoscopic management: variceal band ligation:** is first choice option for oesophageal varices where a rubber band placed around varix. **Sclerotherapy:** first choice for gastric varices and may also be used for bleeding from oesophageal varices.
- **Balloon tamponade:** Sengstaken tube with gastric and oesophageal balloons. Placed in intubated patient in Level 3 care by experienced operator. Gastric balloon placed in stomach via mouth and filled with 200–300 ml of water as per instructions. AXR to check position. Gentle retraction pressure on balloon can stop bleeding – usually the weight of a 500 ml or 1 L bag of fluids. Oesophageal balloon rarely needs filling. Sedation, intubation and ventilation will aid airway protection and tolerance of the procedure.
- **Transjugular intrahepatic porto-systemic shunt** (TIPS): if persistent bleeding. Radiological guidance. Guide wire inserted into internal jugular to IVC to hepatic vein into liver. Stent passed over wire to create communication, allows high-pressure portal veins to shunt into systemic veins. This drops portal pressure, reducing bleeding and shunts portal venous blood bypassing liver to IVC, but can worsen encephalopathy. Local gastroenterologists will suggest when appropriate. Usually done at tertiary centre for uncontrolled VB.
- **Long term:** beta-blockers for varices decrease rebleed by 40%. Re-banding for varices until obliterated. Liver transplantation.

Peptic ulcer disease

- **Adequately resuscitate and correct clotting and platelets before endoscopy.** High risk patients have melena, haemodynamic instability, anaemia and co-morbidities and should be considered for endoscopic therapy once resuscitated.

- **Urgent endoscopic therapy:** visible clot removed and bleeding vessel injected with ADRENALINE which tamponades and vasoconstricts vessels with a second endoscopic treatment such as thermal coagulation or clips improving outcome in high risk bleeding ulcers. Failure to stem bleeding consider angiography or surgery if unstable.
- **Rebleeding** is from large GU over 2 cm and lesser curve and posterior wall DU. Visible clot and visible bleeding increase bleed risk. The risk of rebleeding from a peptic ulcer decreases significantly 72 h after the initial episode of bleeding. Start IV PPI if signs of risk of rebleeding. If there is evidence of high risk ulcers with active bleeding, adherent clot, visible vessel start OMEPRAZOLE 80 mg IV bolus and 8 mg/h for 72 h. PPI raises gastric pH and aids clot stability and haemostasis. Continue for 3 days when rebleeding most common. Reduces bleeding and need for transfusion. For the remainder start an oral PPI, post-endoscopy, which should be used for at least 4 weeks to heal ulcers, e.g. OMEPRAZOLE 20–40 mg OD. *H. pylori* should be eradicated if present (biopsy result or CLO test). Some consider this to be unnecessary if the patient is going to be on long-term PPI treatment.
- **Angiography** combined with selective vessel embolisation or selective intra-arterial VASOPRESSIN may be used where available if bleeding persists.
- **Surgery:** when endoscopic measures fail and bleeding persists then direct ligation of bleeding vessel needed. Uncommon event nowadays. Declining surgical experience. Liaise quickly if deteriorating. Perforation is rare (rigid abdomen, toxic, masked in those on steroids) but commoner with DU than GU. Needs surgical closure and abdominal drainage.
- ***H. pylori* eradication:** all should have CLO test and *H. pylori* eradication if positive. Early pre-endoscopy PPI can reduce sensitivity of *H. pylori* detection at endoscopy. Eradication is OMEPRAZOLE 20 mg + (METRONIDAZOLE 400 mg OR AMOXICILLIN 1 g) + CLARITHROMYCIN 500 mg ALL given 12 h for 7 days. **Follow up: all *H. pylori* +ve** need testing for successful eradication. All gastric ulcers need to be rescoped at 4–6 weeks to ensure healed and no gastric malignancy.
- **Additional:** SSRIs should be used with caution in those at risk of upper GI bleed particularly if on NSAID, clopidogrel or aspirin, Consider switching to non-SSRI.
- **Repeat OGD for patients with a gastric ulcer at 6–8 weeks.** This is because occasionally gastric ulcers are malignant even though at first presentation they appear benign.

Other causes
- **Gastritis/duodenitis:** oral PPI therapy and *H. pylori* eradication if CLO test positive.
- **Gastric/oesophageal cancer:** treat much the same as peptic ulcer disease. Argon laser or other comparable interventions may be tried. Some may need surgery.
- **Dieulafoy's lesion:** cautery or angiographic embolisation. Surgical over-sewing if other management fails.

Reference: NICE (2012) CG141: Acute upper gastrointestinal bleeding: management issued.

6.5 Lower gastrointestinal bleeding

- **About:** bleeding from beyond the ligament of Treitz. May be from small bowel or colorectal. If source unclear do OGD. A torrential upper GI bleed can cause fresh PR bleeding. Always exclude a colorectal cancer.
- **Causes:** diverticular disease (blood, mucus), haemorrhoids (fresh bright blood on toilet paper), colorectal cancer (anaemia, bowel habit, weight loss), ulcerative/Crohn's colitis (known IBD), ischaemic colitis (AF, atherosclerosis, smoker), pseudomembranous colitis (recent antibiotics + *C. difficile*). Angiodysplasia, colorectal polyps, Meckel's diverticulum. Radiation enteropathy, e.g. for gynaecological malignancies. Use of

NSAIDs, anticoagulants, antiplatelets. Localised trauma – foreign bodies, sexual assault with anal fissure (severe pain on defecation, tear can be seen).

- **Clinical:** look for signs of shock and volume loss/anaemia. A history of pain and weight loss and altered bowel habit suggests cancer. Check if patient on warfarin, antiplatelet or a DOAC. Evidence of coagulopathy – liver failure. Gynaecological malignancies and bowel irradiation (radiation proctitis). Perform digital rectal examination and proctoscopy. Any local trauma.

Investigation

- **FBC, U&E, coagulation** if coagulopathy suspected or warfarin. **Group and cross-match** 2–4 units or more as needed.
- **Colonoscopy:** usually with good bowel can visualise entire colon. Often difficult to see source when bleeding acutely and often deferred to allow bleeding to settle.
- **OGD:** if source unclear. A torrential upper GI bleed can cause fresh PR bleeding. May be multiple sources.
- **Flexible sigmoidoscopy:** for the rectum and left side of the colon. Can be done without full bowel preparation. Proctoscopy to examine anal canal and useful to identify haemorrhoids.
- **Mesenteric angiography:** for angiodysplasia and occult bleeding lesion. The yield is low and therefore usefulness in question. Needs an arterial bleeding rate of at least 0.5 ml/min. It may allow for embolisation to take place.
- **Technetium-labelled red cell scan:** for occult and active bleeding.
- **CT and CT angiography** may localise pathology. CT colonography being used increasingly to look for colonic polyps and cancer.

Markers of poor prognosis

- **Age:** acute lower GI bleeding occurs most often in the elderly.
- **Acute haemodynamic disturbance:** ↑HR, ↓BP, shock.
- **Gross rectal bleeding** on initial examination (× 2.3–3).
- **Co-morbidity:** 2+ conditions double the chance of a severe bleed.
- **ASPIRIN or NSAIDs:** increased risk of severe lower GI bleeding × 1.8–2.7.
- **Inpatients:** (any cause) who bleed after admission have a mortality rate of 23% compared with 3.6% in those admitted to hospital because of rectal bleeding.

Management

- **Supportive:** ABC, high flow O_2 if shocked and resuscitate. See Haemorrhagic shock, ▶ Section 2.22. Correct any coagulopathy and transfuse and replace fluids as required. Most cases settle conservatively. In the acute stage, colonoscopy can be difficult and the usual first lower GI investigation will be a flexible sigmoidoscopy following an enema bowel preparation. If no bleeding cause then consider colonoscopy which may help haemostasis as an effective means of controlling haemorrhage from active diverticular bleeding or post-polypectomy bleeding, when appropriately skilled expertise is available. Other options include CT abdomen, technetium-labelled red cell scanning, angiography and emergency surgery.
- **Surgery:** rarely needed as most bleeding self-limiting and can be managed medically/endoscopically. The exceptions would be massive on-going bleeding (>5 units in 24 h). Involve surgeons early if bleeding does not settle, especially if there is a suspected underlying malignancy, failed medical therapy for ulcerative colitis or ischaemic colitis or ongoing recurrent bleeding from a diverticulum. Localised segmental intestinal resection or subtotal colectomy is recommended.
- **Catheter mesenteric angiography** and embolisation may be attempted (evidence on which this practice is based is limited).

Reference: SIGN (2008) 105: Management of acute upper and lower gastrointestinal bleeding: a national clinical guideline.

6.6 Acute abdomen

- **About:** rapid onset of abdominal pain, vomiting, pyrexia and possibly ↓BP. This is a surgical emergency potentially requiring operative management. However, may be admitted mistakenly under medical teams or *de novo* presentation in medical patients.
- **Atypical 'understated' presentations** seen in: elderly, immunocompromised, high dose steroids which mask symptoms and signs when gravely ill and septic. Get urgent help if ↑HR, low BP, peritonism, bleeding, pregnant or high NEWS.
- **Frequency of causes:** acute appendicitis 30%, acute cholecystitis 10%, small bowel obstruction 5%, perforated peptic ulcer 3%, pancreatitis 3%, diverticular disease 2%.
- **Urgent senior review needing resuscitation and possible surgery: (1)** severe haemorrhage (↓BP, ↑HR, ↓Hb appears late with bleeding due to AAA or ectopic pregnancy or splenic rupture). **(2) Perforation or rupture of a viscus** (toxic appearance, rigid abdomen, absent bowel sounds, *in extremis*, air under diaphragm), ascending cholangitis (jaundice, rigors, RUQ pain). **(3) Viscus necrosis**, e.g. ischaemic bowel from atherosclerosis, embolism or strangulated hernia, pancreatitis, intussusception, volvulus. **(4) Missed ectopic pregnancy** can lead to death; is she pregnant?
- **Historical clues:** previous surgery – adhesions suggest causes of obstruction. Known IBD. Peptic ulcer disease and perforation: use of NSAIDs, steroids. Previous appendectomy excludes appendicitis. Warfarin – psoas/retroperitoneal haematoma. Known AAA. Immunosuppression.
- **Volume status:** look for ↑HR, ↓BP on sitting or standing suggests significant hypovolaemia, e.g. acute haemorrhage and blood loss (GI bleed, leaking AAA) or volume loss into obstructed bowel.
- **Abdominal pain:** examine abdomen carefully looking for area of maximum tenderness. Pain tends to come on suddenly or sub-acutely. Mechanism is either peritonitis with well-localised pain that is painful on coughing and movement and patient lies still with guarding and a rigid abdomen. Pain may also be colicky in nature and patient moves about and suggests a more obstructive luminal mechanism, e.g. intestinal obstruction. Associated N&V.
- **Position:** sitting bending forward – chronic pancreatitis; lying still – perforation; restless – renal colic.
- **Visible peristalsis and distension:** suggests obstruction.
- **Radiation of pain:** to shoulder – diaphragmatic irritation; to the back – consider AAA or acute pancreatitis or posterior perforation; to umbilicus – acute appendicitis.
- **Guarding:** reflex contraction of abdominal muscles and discomfort on light abdominal palpation.
- **Rebound tenderness:** increase in severe pain and discomfort when the examining hand abruptly stops pressing on a localised region of the abdomen or on percussion suggests peritonitis (25% don't have it).
- **Rigid abdomen:** contraction of abdominal muscles. Abdomen feels hard like a wooden board. Suggests perforation.
- **Fever:** >38°C suggests infective or inflammatory process.
- **Jaundice:** common bile duct obstruction, liver failure, gallstones, haemolysis.
- **Dehydration:** peritonitis, small bowel obstruction, DKA, high Ca.
- **Ascites:** bulging flanks, abdominal distension with shifting dullness. Bowel floats and ascites gravitates to lowest point. Consider spontaneous bacterial peritonitis and diagnostic paracentesis in liver disease.
- **Murphy's sign:** palpation over RUQ causes acute severe pain stopping inspiration. Acute cholecystitis.
- **Don't forget:** check groin and all hernial orifices as well as scrotal sac and contents.

- **Per rectum examination** – tenderness, induration, mass, frank blood.
- **Per vaginum examination** where indicated – bleeding, discharge, cervical motion tenderness, adnexal masses, and tenderness, uterine size.
- **Bowel sounds:** listen for 2 min to ensure absent. May be high pitched and tinkling.
- **Check hernial orifices**, e.g. strangulated femoral hernia, and the testes of men for a testicular torsion or hernia. Can identify cause of bowel obstruction.

6.7 Acute abdomen – surgical causes

- **Cholecystitis:** gallstones, RIF pain, Murphy's sign, fever, jaundice if stone in common bile duct.
- **Acute appendicitis:** pain begins peri-umbilical and moves to RIF as becomes more peritonitis.
- **Leaking abdominal aortic aneurysm (AAA):** midline pulsatile expansile mass, low BP, may have lost a femoral pulse.
- **Acute pancreatitis:** history of gallstones or alcohol and ↑amylase.
- **Bowel ischaemia:** older, ↑lactate, abdominal pain, melena, AF. May need resection of necrotic bowel.
- **Adhesions causing bowel obstruction:** previous surgery, abdominal scars and old incisional wounds.
- **Incarcerated or strangulated hernia:** bowel obstruction and tender hernial orifices.
- **Pelvic inflammatory pain:** may have similar history, vaginal discharge, history of STIs.
- **Acute diverticulitis:** left iliac fossa pain, older patient.
- **Abdominal wall haematoma:** on warfarin or antithrombotics. Coughing. Localised tender.
- **Gastrointestinal malignancy:** stomach, pancreas, small bowel, colonic.
- **Budd–Chiari:** prothrombotic, RIF pain, jaundice.
- **Inflammatory bowel disease:** Crohn's disease predominantly a small bowel obstruction picture. Ulcerative colitis mainly a colitis picture. Watch for toxic megacolon.
- **Testicular torsion:** acute severe testicular pain.
- **Ureteric colic/renal stones:** renal angle to loin pain, restless, paroxysmal. Stone on CT KUB
- **Meckel's diverticulum:** pain in RIF. May perforate. Seen in adolescents and young adults. Can mimic appendicitis.
- **Gynaecological: endometriosis:** recurrent pain. Ectopic pregnancy: positive pregnancy test and abdominal pain. Acute salpingitis: on right can mimic appendicitis. Ovarian torsion: on right can mimic appendicitis. Mittelschmerz: ovulation mid-cycle pain. May need urgent gynaecological consult and urgent surgery.

6.8 Acute abdomen – medical causes

- **Gastroenteritis:** vomiting and diarrhoea predominate with vague pain and tenderness; gradually settles.
- **Myocardial infarction** (diaphragmatic/inferior): ECG – ST/T changes and troponin.
- **Lower lobe pneumonia:** fever, breathless, chest signs, CXR signs may be delayed.
- **Pyelonephritis:** positive urinalysis, tender renal angle, female.
- **Addisonian crisis:** pale, pigmented creases and scars, ↓BP.
- **Diabetic ketoacidosis:** hyperglycaemic, ketotic.
- **Sickle cell crisis:** Afro-Caribbean origin, similar past history, anaemia. Hyposplenism.

- **Herpes zoster:** rash may not be seen early on – pain affecting abdominal dermatome does not cross midline.
- **Acute porphyria:** variegate and acute intermittent porphyria, hereditary coproporphyria.
- **Familial Mediterranean fever:** Turkish/Middle Eastern. Mesenteric adenitis: viral type illness – younger patients. Mimics appendicitis.
- **Tabes dorsalis:** as part of tertiary syphilis.

Pain and localisation

- Localisation is not an exact science and there is much variability, e.g. late pregnancy.
- **RUQ:** cholecystitis, gallbladder empyema, hepatitis, liver abscess, duodenal ulcer, pneumonia, subphrenic abscess, hepatic flexure of colon.
- **LUQ:** gastroenteritis, splenic disease (infarction/rupture), splenic flexure of colon, subphrenic abscess, perinephritis, acute pancreatitis.
- **Epigastrium:** oesophageal/gastric disease (perforation, gastric ulcer or duodenal ulcer), ruptured AAA, acute pancreatitis, myocardial infarction, PE, pancreatic cancer.
- **Right flank:** ureteric colic (loin to groin), pyelonephritis (renal angle), retrocaecal appendix, muscle strain, perinephric abscess.
- **Periumbilical:** early appendicitis, small bowel disease – obstruction and inflammatory bowel disease, gastroenteritis, pancreatitis, ruptured AAA, ischaemic bowel.
- **Left flank:** ureteric colic (loin to groin), pyelonephritis (renal angle), muscle strain, perinephric abscess.
- **RIF:** appendicitis, mesenteric lymphadenitis, perforated duodenal ulcer, caecal obstruction, Meckel's diverticulum, ectopic pregnancy, ovarian pathology, terminal ileal disease (Crohn's/*Yersinia* pseudotuberculosis) or very rarely RLQ diverticulitis, biliary colic with low lying gallbladder, acute salpingitis.
- **LIF:** sigmoidal diverticulitis, constipation, ectopic pregnancy, ovarian pathology, ischaemic colitis, rectal cancer, IBS, ulcerative colitis.
- **Suprapubic:** cystitis, UTI, acute urinary retention, testicular torsion, pelvic inflammatory disease, ectopic pregnancy, uterine disease, diverticulitis.

Investigations

- **Bloods:** FBC, CRP, U&E, pancreatic amylase/lipase. LFT and INR if any suggestion of liver disease or gallstones. Group and cross-match if suspected AAA, ectopic pregnancy or laparotomy or frank bleeding. Consider ABG and lactate.
- **Erect CXR** and **erect AXR** can help exclude pathology. Perforation of viscus with free air visible under the diaphragm or between viscera and subcutaneous tissue on lateral decubitus. Distended small bowel proximal to small bowel obstruction with air–fluid levels. Small bowel more central. Thickened oedematous valvulae conniventes span entire wall of small bowel unlike colonic haustra. Renal stones may be seen best with AXR or CT. Normal AXR does not exclude ileus or many other pathologies. Toxic megacolon if diameter >7 cm in midtransverse colon. Pancreatic calcification may suggest acute or chronic pancreatitis. 'Thumb printing' with ischaemic bowel.
- **CT abdomen:** imaging important but does not substitute for good clinical assessment – appendicitis shows inflamed appendix fluid-filled with fat stranding and a hyper attenuated wall with IV contrast. Uncomplicated sigmoid diverticulitis can show fat stranding and focal thickening of the colonic wall in an area with diverticula. Abscess formation or fistulas may or may not be seen. Colonic cancers may be seen. Renal stones. Obstruction with transition zone showing level of blockage.
- **USS:** imaging of choice for cholecystitis with gallstones and thickened wall hydropic gallbladder. A stone may be seen blocking cystic duct. Sludge or stone material may

be seen in the gallbladder. Gallstones may also suggest pancreatitis. Collections in the pelvis or subdiaphragmatic. Abscesses.
- **Urinalysis:** blood, protein, stones. **Pregnancy test** in all fertile women.

General management

- **Supportive:** ABC, O_2 as per BTS guidance. Get good IV access and protect it. Start IV crystalloid fluids with good IV access and monitor physiology. Give 1 L Hartmann's or IV NS over 1–2 h as needed. Most patients are dry. Analgesia: MORPHINE 5–10 mg IV + CYCLIZINE 50 mg IV. If tachycardic, ↓BP or bleeding then get senior help urgently. Fertile female consider ectopic pregnancy for all acute abdominal pain and/or ↓BP. Full monitoring BP, HR, temperature and urinary output. Catheterise. FBC, U&E, clotting if liver disease, amylase, group and hold/cross-match if haemorrhage or laparotomy. Severe haemorrhage – give O-negative blood. Suspect sepsis then start TAZOCIN 4.5 g 8 h IV and fluid resuscitation (see Sepsis, ▶ Section 2.21). Maintain NBM until senior review decides otherwise. Normal important meds can sometimes be given with sip of water. Diabetic patients need to be started on a VRIII and keep CBG 4–12 mmol/L. AXR is helpful and depending on findings may need abdominal CT. Laparoscopy may reduce rate of unnecessary laparotomy and improve diagnostic accuracy.

6.9   Gastric outlet obstruction/pyloric stenosis

- **About:** weight loss, food regurgitation.
- **Causes:** pancreatic cancer (10–20%) or gastric malignancy. Peptic ulcer disease with scarring and oedema of pylorus. Gastric polyps, duodenal malignancy, cholangiocarcinoma.
- **Clinical:** fullness and vomiting (HCl loss) postprandial which is non-bilious. Weight loss, succussion splash if NBM for 2–3 h. Palpable abdominal mass and gastric dilation. Malnutrition is seen late. Aspiration pneumonia. Supraclavicular lymph nodes. Hepatomegaly and jaundice if liver metastases.
- **Investigations: FBC, U&E,** ↑urea and creatinine, low K develops later after 2–3 weeks. **LFT:** ↑ALP or bilirubin may suggest malignancy. **Venous blood gas:** vomits HCl loss, increased HCO_3 and low Cl. Alkalosis increases serum K. K excreted to preserve Na. Results in hypochloraemic (hypokalaemic) metabolic alkalosis.
- **Plain AXR:** calcification, masses, perforation.
- **Barium upper GI studies:** can be helpful to identify the gastric silhouette and site of obstruction.
- **USS abdomen:** liver metastases, obstructive jaundice. CT abdomen with oral contrast: will define and stage any masses or mets.
- **Upper GI endoscopy:** may still be food residue in stomach and difficulty passing probe. A lesion may be seen and biopsies taken. A stent may be passable.
- **Management:** IV rehydration and fluid and electrolyte replacement and nutrition. Prolonged vomiting causes loss of hydrochloric (HCl) acid and produces an increase of bicarbonate in the plasma to compensate for the lost chloride and sodium. The result is a hypokalaemic hypochloraemic metabolic alkalosis. Alkalosis shifts the intracellular potassium to the extracellular compartment, and the serum potassium is increased factitiously. With continued vomiting, the renal excretion of potassium increases in order to preserve sodium. The adrenocortical response to hypovolaemia intensifies the exchange of potassium for sodium at the distal tubule, with subsequent aggravation of the hypokalaemia. Manage electrolytes and acid–base disturbances. Specific management depends on cause. Stenting may be possible depending on circumstances. Surgical referral in appropriate cases. (Hypovolaemia, ▶ Section 2.20).

6.10 Acute severe colitis

Stools >8/d or ↑CRP >45 on day 3 of admission predicts an 85% likelihood of requiring a colectomy during that admission.

- **About:** combined medical/surgical approach is best. Always exclude *Clostridium difficile* even in those with known ulcerative colitis.
- **Causes:** IBD: ulcerative colitis, Crohn's disease, colitis of undetermined type and aetiology (CUTE) infection, e.g. *Shigella* and certain *E. coli* (risk of HUS). *C. difficile*: recent antibiotics. Amoebiasis or CMV colitis can mimic ulcerative colitis. Others: radiation colitis, ischaemic colitis (older, AF, vascular disease).
- **Clinical:** diarrhoea, mucus, tenesmus, bloody often 10–20/day and urgency. IBD flare up can be provoked by infection, stress, NSAIDs, antibiotics. Crampy abdominal pain, weight loss, fevers, ↑HR. Silent rigid abdomen suggests perforation but steroids mask signs and perforation may not be dramatic. Rebound suggests peritonism. Distension, vomiting suggests obstruction. Look for signs of sepsis and volume depletion. Enquire if infective source – chicken, contact with livestock, salads.
- **Findings suggesting IBD (most will have a known diagnosis):** mouth ulcers, eye disease – conjunctivitis, iritis, episcleritis. Erythema nodosum – painful red lesions usually over the lower legs. Joint pain – large joints, migratory, asymmetrical. Ankylosing spondylitis seen with Crohn's disease, sacroiliitis – low back pain. Pyoderma gangrenosum pustule, expands as a large ulcer with violaceous margins. Pleuritis, primary sclerosing cholangitis.

Different presentations

- **Distal ulcerative colitis:** starts distally and confined to sigmoid colon and rectum (proctitis). Contact bleeding. Left sided cramps, diarrhoea, mucus and bleeding, tenesmus and pain. Ulcerative colitis affecting only the rectum tends to have a better prognosis than other forms.
- **Ulcerative colitis:** pancolitis: where the whole colon is affected from caecum to rectum. Risk of megacolon. Severe diarrhoea fluid loss, bleeding. Abdominal distension, fever.
- **Crohn's disease:** anywhere mouth to anus, skip lesions, often affects terminal ileum, can be perianal involvement, colitis/proctitis, transmural and often penetrating and fistula with abscess forming inflammation.
- **Differential: pseudomembranous colitis:** adherent surface membrane, *C. difficile* toxin. If suspected then take urgent advice whether to hold steroids until toxin results known. Manage supportively with METRONIDAZOLE 400 mg 8 h PO and/or VANCOMYCIN 125 mg 6 h PO. *Campylobacter* and other bacterial infections. Check stool samples. CMV colitis mimics ulcerative colitis but biopsies show inclusion bodies and PCR CMV DNA is positive and needs IV GANCICLOVIR. Ischaemic colitis causes bloody diarrhoea with abdominal pain in older patients, with AXR appearance and ↓BP and AF and atherosclerosis. Surgical consult is needed.

Severity (modified Truelove and Witt's criteria)

- **Mild:** bloody stool <4/day and at least one of temp <37.5°C, HR <90/min, ESR <20 mm/h, CRP <5 mg/dL, Hb >115 g/L.
- **Moderate:** bloody stool 4–6/day and at least one of temp ≤37.8°C, HR ≤90/min, ESR ≤30 mm/h, CRP <30 mg/dL, Hb >105 g/L.
- **Severe:** bloody stool >6/day and at least one of temp >37.8°C, HR >90/min, ESR >30 mm/h, CRP >30 mg/dL, Hb <105 g/L.

• **Fulminant:** 10 stools/d, continuous bleeding, toxicity, abdomen tender or distension, transfusion requirement, colonic dilation on AXR.

Investigations

• **FBC:** ↓Hb. ↓MCV if ↓Fe, ↑MCV if ↓B12/folate. CRP, ↑ESR ↑ferritin: acute phase response. **U&E:** ↑urea, ↑creatinine. **LFTs:** low albumin. ↑ALP and AST with liver disease. **Serology:** antineutrophil cytoplasmic antibodies **pANCA** positive in ulcerative colitis, anti-*Saccharomyces cerevisiae* antibodies (ASCA).

• **Stool:** culture and sensitivity × 3, ova cysts and parasites **and C. difficile toxin testing** if suspected. Exclude an infective cause.

• **Plain AXR:** look for megacolon with colonic diameter >6 cm, perforation, no faeces, mucosal oedema, mucosal islands, thumb printing. Extent of disease can be assessed with reasonable accuracy by the distal extent of faecal residue visible on a plain abdominal radiograph. Should be repeated daily whilst the patient fulfils the criteria for severe colitis and with any evidence of worsening such as an increase in pulse rate, temperature or stool frequency.

• **Small bowel imaging:** is needed with suspected Crohn's disease and abdominal symptoms.

• **Flexible unprepared sigmoidoscopy with air insufflation:** can be considered in the absence of colonic dilation. It confirms diagnosis and shows erythematous inflamed, even haemorrhagic, mucosa with contact bleeding and allows biopsies. Ulcerative colitis shows continuous areas of inflamed mucosa.

• **Colonoscopy:** can also be done but not in the acute phase. It can show extent of disease and used to exclude malignancy in longstanding colitis.

• **Barium enema:** may show loss of haustral pattern and featureless colon. Avoided during acute flare-up. Biopsies – goblet cell depletion, inflammatory, mucosal ulcers, crypt abscesses.

• **Abdominal CT or MRI:** if intra-abdominal infection, e.g. abscess suspected or an acute abdomen or perforation suspected. MRI preferred for pelvic Crohn's disease.

Management of severe disease
Needs frequent senior gastroenterology/colorectal surgical review

• **General:** severe cases admitted with daily senior review at least. AXR to exclude toxic megacolon (>6 cm), stool for culture and *C. difficile* toxin, frequent CRP. Fluid and electrolyte (K) balance. Stool chart. Often dehydrated then ensure IV access and volume replacement. Transfusion as required to match losses to maintain Hb >100 g/L. Potassium replacement at up to 60–100 mmol/day. Stop any antidiarrhoeals, anticholinergics, NSAIDs, opiates which could precipitate megacolon.

• **Aminosalicylates:** mild–moderate: acute attack MESALAZINE up to 4.8 g PO daily in divided doses until remission (or 12 weeks) then 2.4 g/day or BALSALAZIDE 2.25 g TDS until remission. Distal disease: MESALAZINE FOAM enemas 1–2 g daily for 4–6 weeks or MESALAZINE suppository 1 g daily or SULFASALAZINE 1–2 g QDS PO +/– steroids until remission.

• **Steroids severe:** HYDROCORTISONE 100 mg IV 6 h × 5 days – convert to oral when improves. PREDNISOLONE 0.5 mg/kg/day PO for 4 weeks then reduce by 5 mg/week. **Distal disease** PREDNISOLONE FOAM 20 mg PR or SUPPOSITORY 5 mg or RETENTION ENEMA 20 mg/100 ml. Oral and local applied steroids may be combined in moderate to severe disease. If ongoing steroid needs, consider OMEPRAZOLE 40 mg OD and calcium and cholecalciferol (current formulary preparation is Calceos 1 tablet bd). A failure to respond, perforation or toxic megacolon all demand urgent surgical review. Typical clinical signs of perforation may be minimal, because patients are being treated with steroids. Response rate to IV steroids in acute severe colitis is 40%. Oral steroids, e.g. prednisolone, can be used and continued as an outpatient.

- **Treatment failure** after 4 days may lead to a decision to treat with CICLOSPORIN 2 mg/kg/day or INFLIXIMAB the antibody to TNF administered as a single dose IV infusion of 5 mg/kg under specialist care or COLECTOMY. Side-effects of Infliximab are a risk of infection and disseminated TB. This is for specialist use only.
- **Surgery:** a colorectal surgeon should review those with acute severe ulcerative colitis early in their stay. IBD may be complicated by either toxic megacolon, uncontrolled colonic bleeding or failure to settle with optimal medical therapy. Surgery can be lifesaving. Early review can help prepare the patient for possible colectomy and introduce them to a stoma therapist. Surgery is either total colectomy with ileo-anal anastomosis and pouch or panproctocolectomy with ileostomy.
- **Enteral feeding:** should be continued as long as tolerated, often in conjunction with other agents including biologicals. Nutrition is fundamental to a good outcome.
- **VTE prophylaxis: LMWH** should be given because this is a prothrombotic period even with mild–moderate bloody stool but watch Hb.

Crohn's disease

- Can develop a severe colitis but in 'unwell patients' exclude any co-existing complex transmural penetrating disease with localised abscess/fistula formation which needs to be treated first where steroids alone could be harmful. Get early expert review. Collections may be seen on USS/CT/MRI.
- Management is with antibiotics, abscess drainage (surgical or USS guidance) and liquid formula diet. Complications of Crohn's include stricture and abscess, fistula formation, perianal disease, infection, colorectal cancer with long term Crohn's colitis. MRI is best imaging modality for perianal disease. Antibiotics, e.g. METRONIDAZOLE or CIPROFLOXACIN. Smoking cessation helps.

Management of mild–moderate disease

- **Mild–moderate colitis:** treated with oral steroids (PREDNISOLONE 30 mg reducing dose for 8–10 weeks) and/or an aminosalicylate with telephone or direct advice from IBD specialist nurses, and regular consultant review as needed.
- **Distal disease affecting rectosigmoid:** steroid and mesalazine enemas and suppositories. Mild and moderate cases may go home on steroids if sensible, coping and knowing to return if worsens. Direct telephone access to IBD nurse specialists. Senior assessment if unwell.

Reference: Jakobovits & Travis (2006) Management of acute severe colitis. *Br Med Bull*, 131:75.

6.11 Clostridium difficile colitis

- **About:** avoid or minimise use/duration of broad spectrum antibiotics, e.g. cephalosporin, clindamycin and ampicillin.
- **Aetiology:** large Gram +ve anaerobic spore-forming bacteria. Found in the soil, bowel or environment as spores. Found in 5–15% of healthy adults. Rib type 027 causes a virulent form of infection with higher toxin production and quinolone resistance.
- **Risks:** exposure to organism + broad spectrum antibiotics, elderly, PPI usage, antidepressants. Co-morbidities, IBD.
- **Pathophysiology:** toxin A: enterotoxin inactivates Rho-GTPase; toxin B: cytotoxin. Toxins cause hypersecretion, disruption of tight junctions and death of colonic luminal cells. Together these cause ulceration and diarrhoea.
- **Clinical:** diarrhoea 4 days to 6 weeks after antibiotic treatment. Mild diarrhoea to severe colitis with bloody diarrhoea. Copious liquid stool with fever, malaise,

abdominal pain and distension and toxic megacolon. Acute abdomen, peritonitis and perforation and death.

- **Investigations:** FBC: ↑WCC, ↑CRP. U&E: prerenal AKI failure. Stool culture, colonoscopy/sigmoidoscopy may show yellow adherent plaques. Anaerobic culture on cycloserine, cefoxitin and fructose (CCFA) media. EIA for detecting toxins A and B has sensitivity of 80% and specificity of 98%. AXR/CXR exclude perforation, ileus, megacolon. CT abdomen and pelvis is recommended in patients with complicated *C. difficile*. Immunosuppression increases the risk of *C. difficile*. Low threshold for testing if diarrhoeal illness. Only stools from patients with diarrhoea should be tested for *C. difficile*. Nucleic acid amplification tests (NAAT) such as PCR for *C. difficile* toxin genes are superior to toxins A + B EIA testing.
- **Complications:** prerenal AKI, toxic megacolon, colonic perforation.
- **Severe:** serum albumin <3 g/dL plus ONE of the following: WCC >15, abdominal tenderness, temp >38.5°C, ↑creatinine, severe colitis.
- **Severe and complicated:** ITU if severe + ↓BP, fever ≥38.5°C, ileus or significant abdominal distention, mental status changes, WCC >35 or <2, serum lactate levels >2.2 mmol/L. End organ failure.
- **Management:** supportive. IV fluids, VTE prophylaxis. Prevention: transmission can be reduced by good hand washing using alcohol hand gels in most infections, but not with *C. difficile* spores. Soap and water is advised. Antimicrobial advice + surgical review. Assess severe or complicated from above.
- **Mild–moderate:** METRONIDAZOLE 500 mg PO TDS for 10 days. **Severe:** VANCOMYCIN 125 mg QDS PO for 10 days.
- **Severe/complicated:** no significant abdominal distension: VANCOMYCIN 125 mg PO QDS plus IV METRONIDAZOLE 500 mg 8 h.
- **Severe/complicated disease with ileus, toxic colon or abdominal distension:** VANCOMYCIN 500 mg QDS PO and PR (500 mg in 500 ml QDS) plus IV METRONIDAZOLE 500 mg TDS. Keep antibiotics going even if for surgery.
- **Hartmann's pouch, ileostomy, or colon diversion**, VANCOMYCIN enema given until the patient improves.
- Alternative is FIDAXOMICIN 200 mg BD PO for 10 days, which is non-inferior to vancomycin in curing patients with mild to severe *C. difficile* infection.
- Avoid loperamide or any drug which slows GI transit. Involve gastroenterologists and surgeons in management if abdominal signs worsen (see below). Important to continue antibiotics even if NBM. Acute surgical management especially with toxic megacolon or perforation requiring subtotal colectomy with ileostomy.
- **Indications for surgical consult** are low BP needing vasopressors, age >65, ↑WCC >20 × 10⁹/L, ↑lactate >5 mmol/L, peritonism, severe ileus, perforation or toxic megacolon, failure to improve after 5 days of medical therapy. Prognosis is poor in elderly patients. About 25% can have a relapse.

Reference: Surawicz *et al.* (2013) Guidelines for diagnosis, treatment, and prevention of *Clostridium difficile* infections. *Am J Gastroenterol*, 108:478.

6.12 Intestinal obstruction

- **About:** can cause bowel ischaemia, infarction, and perforation, peritonitis, sepsis and death. How severe is the obstruction, what level is it at and what is the likely aetiology? Is strangulation present?
- **Aetiology:** strictures, scars, hernias and adhesions from old surgery. Luminal obstruction – tumour, strictures. Extrinsic masses, volvulus, malignancies. Intussusception. Pseudo-obstruction – see before.
- **Clinical:** nausea, vomiting seen the more proximal the blockage, crampy abdominal pain, distension and gas-filled abdomen. Constipation/diarrhoea, pyrexia, ↑HR. Late leads to absolute constipation and no flatus PR. High pitched bowel sounds, silent abdomen. Look for a hernia with bowel loops – inguinal, femoral.

- **Investigations:** FBC: ↑WCC. U&E: ↑AKI, Ca, LFTs, ↑CRP, ↑INR if on warfarin, erect CXR, ECG. **Erect CXR and AXR** – determine level of small or large bowel obstruction. Small bowel obstruction: plain AXR shows multiple air-fluid levels. **CT abdomen:** small bowel obstruction shows dilated small bowel loops (diameter >2.5 cm from outer wall to outer wall) proximally to normal calibre or collapsed loops distally.
- **Management:** ABC, NG suction, involve surgeons/ITU early. Rehydration with IV fluids with strict monitoring of Input//Output, antiemetics (avoid METOCLOPRAMIDE). Adequate analgesia, NBM. IV antibiotics if sepsis or ischaemic bowel. Monitor CRP, WCC, lactate. Exclude medical functional 'pseudo-obstruction'.

6.13 Acute colonic pseudo-obstruction

- **About:** colonic obstruction and severe dilation usually in elderly without an obstructive lesion. If any doubt needs gastroenterology/surgical review to ensure no physical cause.
- **Complications:** colonic dilatation, perforation (caecal), peritonitis, death. Risks of perforation higher with caecal diameter >14 cm, delayed compression, and elderly.
- **Clinical:** abdominal distension (measure abdominal circumference at umbilicus), pain, vomiting, constipation, acute abdomen if perforation.
- **Causes/precipitants:** co-morbidities, e.g. CCF, sepsis, renal and respiratory failure, spinal injury. Recent trauma, surgery, burns. Diabetes. Opiates, antimuscarinics, calcium channel blockers, TCA, electrolyte abnormalities.
- **Investigations:** FBC: ↓Hb, ↑WCC. U&E: ↑Creatinine – AKI/dry. Ca, Mg, TSH? hypothyroid. **AXR:** massive colonic dilation most pronounced at caecum so repeat and measure diameter daily if needed. Look for free gas and evidence of perforation. **Abdominal CT scan:** contrast enema or colonoscopy to exclude a physical cause of colonic obstruction. **Water-soluble contrast enema:** can exclude lesion and break up hard faeces. **Colonoscopy:** can exclude obstructive lesion and aid decompression.
- **Management:** supportive: daily review. Exclude a physical obstructive cause. Treat/remove any identifiable cause. Review medications. Correct electrolytes and hydration. **Treat infection.** If vomiting NBM and NG tube to decompress from above. Encourage mobilisation as tolerated, e.g. sit out. **Nutrition:** if prolonged may even need total parenteral nutrition (TPN). Consider PRUCALOPRIDE 1–2 mg PO OD (unlicensed). Anticholinesterase NEOSTIGMINE 1–2 mg IV over 5 min (treats 85–90% of cases; may be repeated after 3 h). May cause ↓HR (give ATROPINE if significant). **Decompression:** flexible sigmoidoscopy/colonoscopy and/or insertion of a rectal tube considered if caecal diameter >8–9 cm. Repeated until condition settles. **Surgical caecostomy** if not settling conservatively.

6.14 Acute bowel ischaemia

- **About:** seen in older population at risk of atherosclerosis and thromboembolism particularly with AF. Can be small or large bowel, be segmental or diffuse, acute or chronic.
- **Aetiology:** occlusion of vascular supply to gut or ↓BP causes ischaemia and sepsis. AF, IHD, HTN, smoker, cholesterol, AAA, shock, dissecting aorta, embolism to superior mesenteric artery (SMA). Mechanical – twisting of the blood supply, rarely venous or vasculitis. Very rare – antiphospholipid syndrome, PAN, etc.
- **Anatomy:** coeliac axis supplies distal oesophagus to the descending duodenum. SMA: the transverse and ascending duodenum, the jejunum and ileum, and the large bowel to the splenic flexure. Inferior mesenteric artery (IMA): left colon from the splenic flexure to the rectum.

- **Clinical:** crampy diffuse abdominal pain, vomiting, diarrhoea (bloody), lower GI bleeding, atrial fibrillation, murmurs, chest pain if ACS, ↓BP and septic or cardiogenic shock, pyrexia, absent or altered bowel sounds, incarcerated hernias.
- **Investigation:** FBC: ↑WCC, CRP. Elevated lactate, glucose. Metabolic acidosis. U&Es: AKI. Amylase: exclude pancreatitis. **Erect CXR:** exclude perforation. **AXR:** thumb printing due to mucosal oedema, sentinel loop, distended bowel due to ileus, gas due to dilatation caused by ileus, intramural gas from necrotic bowel. **CT abdomen:** thickened bowel loop, oedema, embolism in SMA. ECG: AF, ACS, troponin, TFT, exclude MI. May need echocardiogram.
- **Differential:** AAA, pancreatitis, renal colic, biliary disease, dissection.
- **Management:** ABC, NBM, IV fluids. Analgesia. Manage nutrition – may need TPN post-op. Suspicion of ischaemic bowel warrants laparotomy and resection of compromised section. Percutaneous interventional vascular radiology in acute mesenteric artery occlusion may be considered to aspirate thrombus, thrombolyse or stent. Manage any AKI – good volume support, treat infection. Ongoing AF – assess for later anticoagulation.

6.15   Acute diverticulitis

- **About:** diverticulae are protrusions of mucosa and submucosa through muscular wall of large bowel.
- **Aetiology:** pouches of mucosa and submucosa herniate through the muscular wall of the bowel at points of weakness. Tends to affect sigmoid colon. Possibly high intraluminal pressures. There may be a local neural problem. Low fibre Western diets may play a role.
- **Clinical:** diverticulae are clinically silent in 90% and very common. Diverticulitis classically causes left-sided iliac fossa pain. Fever, N&V, constipation or diarrhoea. Frank bleeding PR which can be significant. Fistula to bladder or vagina with subsequent UTI and foul discharge.
- **Investigations: FBC:** ↑WCC. U&E: AKI. ↑ESR, ↑CRP. **Abdominal USS:** show mucosal thickness, excludes an abscess and pericolic fluid. **Barium enema:** presence of diverticulae. **Flexible sigmoidoscopy and colonoscopy** can show diverticulae but acutely risk of perforation. **Spiral CT of abdomen or CT colonograpy:** can show diseased sections, narrowing of lumen and thickening of bowel wall and lack of clarity of pericolic fat.
- **Management:** supportive: ABC. If unwell start IV fluids, e.g. 1 L NS. Associated haemorrhage usually managed conservatively. Surgical involvement especially if any signs of bowel perforation or peritonitis. Perforation can lead to fistula formation. If markers of infection consider TAZOCIN 4.5 g 8 h IV. Mild attacks may be managed with oral antibiotics as an outpatient. Laparoscopic surgery may be considered. An open Hartmann's procedure may be needed.
- **Complications:** diverticulitis, pericolic abscess. Perforation and peritonitis and/or fistula formation to bladder, uterus, small intestine. Local narrowing and stricture formation and intestinal obstruction.

6.16   Re-feeding syndrome

- **About:** restarting nutrition after a period of starvation. Need to manage low potassium, phosphate, magnesium and give thiamine. Re-feeding (whether it's oral, enteral or parenteral nutrition) triggers a switch from fat to carbohydrate metabolism, with consequent insulin release, and uptake of potassium, phosphate, magnesium and water into cells.

- **Screening for those at risk – any 2 of:** (1) MI <18.5 kg/m^2, (2) unintentional weight loss >10% in past 3–6 months, (3) little or no nutritional intake for over 5 days, (4) history of alcohol excess or chemotherapy.
- **Clinical:** Wernicke's encephalopathy – encephalopathy, ataxic gait, oculomotor dysfunction, ophthalmoplegia. Look for cardiac or respiratory failure, arrhythmias, rhabdomyolysis, seizures, coma, death.
- **Investigations:** FBC: ↓Hb. U&E: ↓K, ↓Mg, ↓phosphate. Check lactate and VBG.
- **Management:** prevent by monitoring phosphate and starting re-feeding slowly at 25% normal requirement to minimise rise in insulin. Close involvement of dietitian. Watch potassium, phosphate, magnesium prior to and for the first few days of feeding. Give IV fluids as required. **Potassium:** K 3.0–3.5 mmol/L give Sando K (12 mmol each) – 2 tds, K 2.5–2.9 mmol/L IV KCl 40 mmol in 1 L NS or G5 over 8 h (at 125 ml/h). Concentration must not exceed 40 mmol/L peripherally. Maximum infusion rate is 20 mmol/h unless via a central line with ECG monitoring. **Phosphate:** level 0.5–0.8 mmol/L give Phosphate Sandoz (16 mmol each) – 2 tds, level 0.3–0.49 mmol/L give 25 mmol PO$_4$ Polyfusor (250 ml) over 12 h peripherally, level <0.3 mmol/L give 50 mmol PO$_4$ Polyfusor (500 ml) over 24 h peripherally, measuring PO$_4$ at 12 h. **PABRINEX** IV paired vials (vitamin B and C) TDS for 1–2 days before giving any carbohydrate. **Magnesium:** level: 0.5–0.7 mmol/L give Magnaspartate – 1 sachet bd (10 mmol/sachet), level: <0.5 mmol/L give IV MgSO$_4$ 35–50 mmol in 1 L NS or G5 over 12–24 h peripherally.

6.17 Ingested foreign bodies and food impactions

- **About:** foreign body and food impactions are seen mainly in children but do occur in adults with learning difficulties and in those who are self-harming. In most cases the risk of harm is minimal and objects pass harmlessly but there are exceptions, which must be noted for early escalation as needed. The need and urgency of intervention depend on patient age and clinical condition. Also depends on size, shape, content, anatomic location and orientation of the ingested object, and the time since ingestion.
- **Clinical:** there may be no symptoms, ranging up to severe chest discomfort and difficulty swallowing or breathing and inability to swallow even saliva. With distal perforation, abdominal pain and symptoms of bowel obstruction or perforation or GI bleeding.
- **Investigations:** lateral and AP radiographs of neck, chest and abdomen can help locate object as well as exclude any mediastinal or peritoneal air. CT scan is possibly more useful. Some materials – small chicken and fish bones or plastics may be difficult to see radiologically.
- **Management:** ABCs. Initially keep NBM and avoid emetics. Avoid oral contrast as this may make endoscopic removal more difficult.

Urgency of endoscopy

- **Emergency:** complete oesophageal obstruction (i.e., unable to manage secretions), disk batteries in the oesophagus, Sharp-pointed objects in the oesophagus.
- **Urgent:** oesophageal foreign objects that are not sharp-pointed, oesophageal food impaction in patients without complete obstruction, Sharp-pointed objects in the stomach or duodenum, Objects >6 cm in length at or above the proximal duodenum, magnets within endoscopic reach.
- **Non-urgent:** coins in the oesophagus may be observed for 12–24 h before endoscopic removal in an asymptomatic patient. Objects in the stomach with diameter <2.5 cm. Disk batteries and cylindrical batteries that are in the stomach of patients without signs of GI injury may be observed for as long as 48 h. Batteries remaining in the stomach longer than 48 h should be removed.

Management of ingested substances

Urgency	Indications for endoscopy
Disk batteries	The current generates NaOH causing localised alkali burns and perforation even within 2 h of ingestion, particularly in the oesophagus. Symptoms can, however, be late up to 28 days. Batteries greater than 2 cm diameter are particularly dangerous. The negative smaller side is more harmful if opposed against mucosa. Batteries only retrieved if signs of injury to the GI tract. A large-diameter battery (>2 cm) in the stomach longer than 48 h, shown by AXR, should be removed. Once past the duodenum, 85% pass out of the body within 72 h. AXR every 3–4 days is adequate to assess progress through the GI tract.
Food bolus impaction	Meat or other materials can become stuck in the oesophagus and endoscopy is needed to either extract piecemeal/advance the bolus. Stricture dilation can be attempted if present. Caution with advancing food if distal oesophagus may be ulcerated particularly with a bolus present for a period of time or a history of eosinophilic oesophagitis.
Miscellaneous	Objects longer than 6 cm are likely to have difficulty passing the duodenum and should be removed.
Magnets	More than one magnet or combined with any metallic object needs to be removed as the adhesion between bowel can cause obstruction and perforation. Consider urgent removal of all magnets within endoscopic reach and for the rest close observation and surgical consultation for non-progression through the GI tract.
Body packers	See ▶ Chapter 14: Toxicology emergencies for management. Reference: ASGE Standards of Practice Committee (2011) Management of ingested foreign bodies and food impactions. *Gastrointestinal Endoscopy* 73:1091.

07 Hepatobiliary emergencies

7.1 Jaundice

Pathophysiology: jaundice is caused by excess circulating bilirubin, a breakdown product of haem with levels >50 μmol/L when it becomes detectable clinically (normal <17 μmol/L). Seen most easily in pale skin in good light or in the scleral part of the eye. It may be seen in 3% of population as Gilbert's syndrome. It must be viewed in clinical context. It is included here as a sign of liver function. Is the patient toxic and unwell, is there pale stool and dark urine, wasting, cachexia and likely cancer? Bilirubin is conjugated with glucuronate within the liver so pre-hepatic is excess unconjugated form. Excreted in urine and faeces and gives them their distinctive yellow and brown colours, respectively. Look for IV drug use, alcohol, toxins, all drugs, history of gallstones, pregnancy. Most commonly the question is whether it is hepatic or post-hepatic and the most critical test is abdominal USS. Severe liver damage causes loss of synthetic function making procoagulant: fibrinogen, prothrombin, factors V, VII, IX, X and XIII. Anticoagulant proteins C and S. NOT gammaglobulins. Antithrombin, transferrin and caeruloplasmin. Albumin $t_{1/2}$ about 20 days. Glucose homeostasis – controlling blood sugar.

Causes	Details and notes
Pre-hepatic	Haemolysis with increased (unconjugated = indirect) bilirubin formation, ↑reticulocytes, anaemia, high LDH. Gilbert's syndrome. LFTs are normal.
Hepatic	Alcoholic/non-alcoholic and other causes of cirrhosis, hepatitis A/B/C, toxins, drugs, anaesthetic agents, paracetamol, ALF, ischaemia, malignancy, severe right heart failure. Needs liver USS and usual work up. Viral studies, cirrhosis work up. Defined by aetiology. ↑ALT/AST, bilirubin. ALP may be elevated.
Post-hepatic	Pale stool, dark urine, abdominal pain, fever. Gallstones/worms/strictures/tumour/pancreatic cancer occluding CBD. Cholangitis. Elevated GGT and ALP. AST/ALT may also be ↑. Obstruction seen on USS or MRCP. Needs mechanical release – ERCP/surgery.

7.2 Acute liver failure

About: Fulminant hepatic failure is where encephalopathy develops in under 2 weeks with a previously normal liver. Prothrombin time is a useful marker of synthetic function. Take an accurate drug history including over the counter and herbal remedies. Classification based on time from appearance of jaundice to developing encephalopathy. **Hyperacute <1 week:** usually paracetamol or viral. There is massive necrosis and loss of function. **Acute <4 weeks:** viral, drugs, others. **Subacute 12 weeks:** viral, drugs, others.

Causes	Details and notes
Infectious	**Viral hepatitis:** see below. **Bacterial:** leptospirosis, severe bacterial infections. **Protozoal:** amoebic infection.
Paracetamol overdose (1/2 of UK cases)	Within 4 h of presentation give activated charcoal just prior to starting *N*-acetyl cysteine. NAC should be used promptly in all patients where paracetamol-induced liver injury is anticipated or there is concern of such and may be given acutely even if cause is unclear. ▶ Section 14.28 for paracetamol overdose protocol.
Other drugs and toxins	MAOIs, halothane, isoniazid, phenytoin, sulphonamides, amiodarone, propylthiouracil, Ecstasy, herbal remedies. *Amanita phylloides* mushroom, carbon tetrachloride. Enquire about all drugs taken, environmental toxins, herbal and natural remedies. Tetracycline, valproate and nucleoside reverse-transcriptase inhibitors can cause fatal liver disease. Many others so check all.
Inherited	**Wilson's disease:** autosomal recessive. ↓Serum Cu, ↓caeruloplasmin. Haemolysis. ↑Urinary Cu. Treat with penicillamine. **Haemochromatosis:** AR. Iron overload, ↑ferritin. Transferrin saturation >50%. HFE gene mutation positive >95%. MRI ferriscan or liver biopsy. **Alpha-1 antitrypsin deficiency,** ↓alpha-1 antitrypsin.
Ischaemic	Circulatory failure and shock. ↑AST. Manage underlying cause.
Venous	**Venous thrombosis: Budd–Chiari syndrome:** acute ascites, USS diagnostic with thrombosed hepatic vein. Consider thrombolysis and TIPS. Hepatic failure is an indication for liver transplantation, provided underlying malignancy is excluded.
Pregnancy	Acute fatty liver of pregnancy, HELLP syndrome with haemolysis, ↑AST/ALT and ↓platelet count. Expeditious delivery needed.
Reye's syndrome	Inhibition of beta-oxidation and uncoupling of oxidative phosphorylation in mitochondria. Acute encephalopathy with fatty infiltration of the liver. Precipitated by aspirin ingestion and viral infections.
Mushroom poisoning	ALF patients with known or suspected mushroom poisoning. Consider administration of PENICILLIN G and SILYMARIN (III) and should be considered for urgent orthoptic transplantation, the only lifesaving option.
Autoimmune hepatitis	Patients with ALF (usually a biopsy is done) due to autoimmune hepatitis should be treated with corticosteroids (PREDNISOLONE 40–60 mg/d). In ALF patients with evidence of ischaemic injury, cardiovascular support is the treatment of choice.
Malignancy	Hepatoma: check USS and alpha-fetoprotein.
Miscellaneous	**Others:** idiopathic: viral, ischaemia: severe RHF, non-alcoholic steatohepatitis.

- **Clinical:** history of drug/toxin exposure key. Encephalopathy: flapping tremor, poor concentration. Reversal of day/night cycle, jaundice usually but not always – date when first appeared, bleeding and coagulopathy. Hypoglycaemia, fetor hepaticus, look for Kayser–Fleischer rings. RUQ tenderness, NO splenomegaly or ascites, exception is Budd–Chiari syndrome.
- **Identify likely precipitants of acute on chronic decompensation:** sepsis, spontaneous bacterial peritonitis, fluid overload, albumin. Transjugular intrahepatic porto-systemic shunt, renal failure, CNS suppressants. Electrolyte abnormalities, diuretic overuse, GI bleeding.
- **Clinical:** reversal of day/night sleeping, psychomotor dysfunction, impaired memory. Sensory abnormalities, poor concentration, disorientation, tremor,

shuffling gait. Melena, haematemesis. Fetor hepaticus, flapping tremor, asterixis. See Encephalopathy ▶ Section 7.11.

- **Investigations:** FBC: ↑WCC, ↑ESR, ↑CRP, ↓platelets (alcohol, HELLP). Haemolysis in Wilson's disease: ↓Hb, ↑reticulocytes, ↑LDH. ↑Prothrombin time. ↑Bilirubin: elevated unconjugated. LFT: ↑AST, ↑ALT often >1000 (transaminases fall eventually). U&E: ↑creatinine. Check paracetamol levels and salicylates. **VBG:** metabolic acidosis and ↑arterial lactate and arterial ammonia. **Viral serology:** anti-HAV IgM, HBsAg, anti-HBc IgM, anti-HEV, EBV, CMV, HSV, HIV, anti-HCV(rare cause). **Others:** paracetamol level, caeruloplasmin and 24 h urine copper, ammonia levels. Autoimmune: ANA, anti-smooth muscle actin, anti-liver/kidney microsomal antibodies and immunoglobulins. **USS doppler:** liver size and pathology, and hepatic veins for Budd–Chiari syndrome. **Miscellaneous:** pregnancy test. ANA, anti-smooth muscle, immunoglobulin, HIV status. **NB.** Focal neurology not typical and suggests need for CT brain.
- **Management:** stop all potentially implicated drugs. Regard all as potentially hepatotoxic if no other evident cause. Consider N-acetyl cysteine (NAC) infusion – possibly useful in both paracetamol and non-paracetamol ALF. **Supportive:** ABCs and O$_2$ to get and maintain sats >92% and admit to an HDU/ITU environment.
- **Hypovolaemia/↓BP:** cross-match blood and transfuse if bleeding or anaemia. 4.5% human albumin solution is the colloid of choice to elevate CVP to 10 cmH$_2$O or until clinically euvolaemic. G5 if fluids needed (but can worsen hyponatraemia). Give 100 ml 20% human albumin solution per 2.5 L of ascites during paracentesis, or if SBP. Avoid NS (worsens fluid overload).
- **Hypoglycaemia:** stat dose 20 ml 50% IV GLUCOSE and then 10% GLUCOSE infusion as needed. GLUCAGON 1 mg has limited effectiveness if no liver glycogen. ▶ Section 5.2.
- **Low K, phosphate, magnesium:** replace as needed (▶ Sections 5.4, 5.12, 5.14).
- **Hyponatraemia:** may need hypertonic 3% saline. ▶ Section 5.10.
- **PABRINEX IV ×2 TDS for 1–2 days.** Provide thiamine if alcoholic or malnourished. If suspected Wernicke's syndrome give for 7 days to prevent Korsakoff psychosis. Give before any nutrition/IV glucose. Long term THIAMINE 100 mg TDS PO.
- **Cerebral oedema:** nurse at 20° head elevation. Consider intubation and hyperventilation to reduce PCO_2. MANNITOL 200 ml of 20% (20 g/100 ml) IV over 20–30 min and can be repeated.
- **Stress ulcer prevention:** start IV PPI or RANITIDINE 150 mg BD PO.
- **Antivirals:** ACICLOVIR for HSV or VZV and GANCICLOVIR for CMV.
- **Antibiotics:** low threshold to treat any infection. Bacterial and fungal. Impaired immunity. Treat if encephalopathy. TAZOCIN IV is often first line.
- **Coagulopathy:** VITAMIN K 2–5 mg slow IV, 2–4 units FFP, platelets if <50 × 10^9/L and bleeding. VITAMIN K replaces any deficit so any resulting coagulopathy is entirely due to reduced liver function.
- **Hepatic encephalopathy:** avoid the use of FFP unless actively bleeding. FFP renders the PTT (a vital prognostic marker) less useful. Give LACTULOSE 20 ml BD +/– enemas to ensure three bowel movements per day. Use phosphate enemas if unsuccessful. ▶ Section 7.11.
- **Ascites and spontaneous bacterial peritonitis,** ▶ Section 7.9.
- **Acidosis:** take expert advice and consider IV NaHCO$_3$. A pH <7.3 at >24 h after paracetamol overdose is a poor prognostic indicator.
- **Renal failure** and AKI common with ALF and may require haemofiltration or haemodialysis. ▶ Section 10.4.

King's College criteria for liver transplant (discuss before these levels reached)	
Discuss when	INR >3.0, hepatic encephalopathy, ↓BP despite resuscitation. Metabolic acidosis. Prothrombin time (seconds) > time from overdose (hours).
Transplant ALF due to paracetamol	pH <7.30 OR (INR >6.5 (PT >100 s) and serum creatinine >300 μmol/L (>3.4 mg/dL) in patients with grade 3 or 4 hepatic encephalopathy).
Transplant ALF due to Other cause	INR >6.5 (PT >100 s), OR any 3 of the following: age <10 or >40 y; aetiology non-A, non-B hepatitis, or idiosyncratic drug reaction; duration of jaundice before hepatic encephalopathy >7 days; INR >3.5 (PT >50 s); serum bilirubin >300 μmol/L (>17.6 mg/dL).

7.3 ▶ Viral hepatitis

Causes	Details and management
A	Faeco-oral spread. Incubation 2–6 weeks. Malaise, jaundice. Usually self-limiting. 10% hospitalised. Prevent with vaccination. No chronicity. Check anti-HAV IgM.
B	Commonest viral cause of fulminant hepatitis. Sexual and maternal transmission (90% chronic). Blood, HBsAg, anti-HBcIgM. Incubation 6 weeks to 6 months. Currently no antiviral improves clinical outcome, some may advocate Lamivudine. Infants born to HBsAg-positive mothers must receive hepatitis B immunoglobulin and be vaccinated within 12 h of birth. Fulminant hepatitis 1 in 1000.
C	Mild to severe illness. Sharing needles or from maternal route (6 out of 100), sexually rare. Malaise, fever, jaundice. Elevated ALT. Anti-HCV antibodies, HCV RNA. Nearly 10% prevalence in Egypt. Fulminant hepatic failure rare but is seen in HIV-positive men who have sex with men and has been reported sporadically in Asia. Acute infection treated with pegylated interferon.
D	Seen in those with hepatitis B. Prevent by hepatitis B vaccination.
E	Hepatitis E is generally mild unless pre-existing liver disease or pregnant. Causes acute and chronic disease. 4 genotypes. Faeco-oral transfer so need good hand hygiene. Flu-like illness, malaise, jaundice. Send anti-HEV IgM antibodies. Usually self-limiting. 1 in 20 may develop GBS.
Non A/E	Acute hepatitis of presumed viral cause with negative serology. Due to unknown viruses or variants of hepatitis B.
Others	CMV, EBV, VZV, yellow fever, adenovirus, parvovirus. Patients with known or suspected HSV or VZV as the cause of ALF should be treated with ACICLOVIR. GANCICLOVIR for CMV.
General	Consider virus-specific therapy for HCV, all with acute viral hepatitis should avoid alcohol consumption and paracetamol. Sexual contact should be avoided if the partner is not immune. Those with sub-fulminant or fulminant hepatitis should be referred early for possible liver transplantation and supported in an ITU setting. The ALT level is not prognostic, but PT and bilirubin and lactate are prognostic.

7.4 Alcoholic hepatitis

- **About:** the aim of the liver clinician is to keep the patient alive long enough to allow them to benefit from alcohol cessation (Hazeldine, *et al.*, 2015).
- **Acute liver dysfunction** with jaundice in known alcoholic. Poor prognosis. Discriminant function >32 implies >50% mortality at 1 month. Reversible if patients are non-cirrhotic. The term hepatitis is a misnomer as transaminases (AST and ALT) are marginally elevated.
- **Causes:** acute exacerbation in known alcohol abuser. Look out for SBP. Quantity of alcohol ingested is not always directly proportional to risk of liver disease. Steato-hepatitis (fat + hepatocellular injury + inflammation +/– fibrosis). Loss of liver function.
- **Clinical:** pyrexia, ↑HR, jaundice, encephalopathy, anorexia. Hepatomegaly (tender), abdominal discomfort, nausea, worsening ascites. Alcoholic neuropathy, cerebellar degeneration, cardiomyopathy, AF. Evidence of hepatitis B/C/HIV infection.
- **Aetiology:** polymorphs + necrosis in zone 3. Mallory bodies seen but non-specific.
- **Investigations: FBC, U&E, LFT:** ↑WCC, ↑reticulocytes (haemolysis suggests Zieve's syndrome), ↑CRP, ↑bilirubin, AST, ALT (usually <200 and rarely ever >400 U so not a severe biochemical 'hepatitis').
- **Abdominal USS:** hepatomegaly, coarse edge, increased echogenicity, free fluid.
- **Ascitic tap:** if spontaneous bacterial peritonitis suspected – neutrophil count >250 cells/mm³. Infection seen in 10%. Transudate total protein <30 g/L, e.g. cirrhosis, CCF/RHF, nephrotic syndrome. Exudate has a total protein >30 g/L, e.g. cancer, infection, TB.
- **Specialist tests:** 'Hepatic screen': immunoglobulins, anti-mitochondrial antibody, anti-smooth muscle antibody; ANA/dsDNA; ferritin (↑ in acute illness, check iron studies and transferrin saturation), caeruloplasmin (if <45 y); αFP; anti-HA IgM, HBsAg, anti-HCV ± EBV, CMV ± tumour markers (CA125, CA15-3, CA19-9, CEA, AFP) ± haptoglobin/LDH (haemolysis).
- **Liver biopsy:** histological confirmation is required where there is uncertainty about the diagnosis. 25% of presumed alcoholic hepatitis not confirmed on histology. Trans-jugular biopsy is required if coagulopathy.

Severity scorings to determine prognosis and need for abstention

- Several prognostic scores are available but the most practical one to assess severity is the Glasgow Alcoholic Hepatitis score (GAHS, see table below). This predicts 28 day and 3 month mortality and can be used as a guide for treatment with corticosteroids or Pentoxifylline. It has an overall accuracy of 81% in predicting 28 day mortality.

Glasgow alcoholic hepatitis score (poor prognosis if score >9)			
Score	1	2	3
Age (y)	<50	≥50	
WCC (× 10⁹/L)	<15	≥15	
Urea (mmol/L)	<5	≥5	
Prothrombin ratio	<1.5	1.5–2.0	≥2
Bilirubin (µmol/L)	<125	125–250	>250

- **Management:** supportive. Long-term abstinence from alcohol – refer to appropriate support on discharge. Management is supportive care to allow liver regeneration without additional 'toxin' exposure. Nutrition must be maintained with enteral feeding if required. Manage alcohol withdrawal, complications of portal hypertension, ascites, encephalopathy, variceal haemorrhage. PABRINEX IV paired vials TDS for 1–2 days + IV VITAMIN K. Commence and continue THIAMINE 200 mg PO OD. Signs of agitation of alcohol withdrawal consider CHLORDIAZEPOXIDE PO or DIAZEPAM PO.

- **Active treatment:** the role of steroids has been questioned by the STOPAH trial. However, some may consider in those with GAHS ≥9 (severe alcoholic hepatitis) either PREDNISOLONE 40 mg od for 28 days (reassess at 7 days) or PENTOXIFYLLINE 400 mg PO TDS for 28 days. Take local expert advice as some continue to use. If advice is to give steroids ensure all infection is excluded/treated. NAC has also failed to improve 6 month survival. Reassess at day 7 to decide on continuing steroid/Pentoxifylline therapy.
- **Severe liver dysfunction: liver failure (INR >2, albumin <30, encephalopathy)** discuss with local or regional liver centre. In those with decompensated cirrhosis or alcoholic hepatitis then any rise in creatinine by 50% must be met with stopping diuretics and nephrotoxins with plasma expansion with albumin (see *Section 7.11* on hepatorenal syndrome) and renal advice. If signs of encephalopathy give LACTULOSE 20 ml 12 h +/– enemas to ensure two bowel movements per day. ▶ Section 7.11.
- **Best supportive care** involves access to 24 h endoscopy, expert fluid management, variceal banding and TERLIPRESSIN 2 mg 4 h for bleeding and early active management of sepsis – the commonest cause of death.
- **Antibiotics:** broad spectrum antibiotics indicated for variceal bleeding. Prophylactic antibiotics after SBP such as NORFLOXACIN or CIPROFLOXACIN should be considered.
- **Early transplantation:** consider with severe alcoholic hepatitis because it reduces mortality, though some will go back to alcohol.

References: European Association for the Study of the Liver (2010) EASL clinical practice guidelines. *J Hepatol*, 533:97. Hazeldine *et al*. (2015) Alcoholic liver disease – the extent of the problem and what you can do about it. *Clinical Medicine*, 15:179. O'Shea *et al*. (2010) Alcoholic Liver Disease. *Am J Gastroenterol*, 105:14.

7.5 Alcoholic ketoacidosis

- **About:** seen with severe alcoholic liver dysfunction + alcohol and/or starvation.
- **Causes:** acute exacerbation in known alcohol abuser due to sepsis, starvation. Look out for spontaneous bacterial peritonitis.
- **Clinical:** signs of advanced alcoholic liver disease, ↑HR, dehydration. Jaundice, alcoholic hepatitis, ascites, coagulopathy, encephalopathy. Anorexia, N&V may be prominent. May follow 2–3 days after a binge. Ketones detectable in breath, Kussmaul's respiration.
- **Investigations:** FBC, U&E, LFT: low urea or AKI. ↑LFTs. Anaemia. Measure Mg, Ca, phosphate. **Glucose:** hypoglycaemia. Urine: ketones. **Venous blood gas:** ↑AG **metabolic acidosis** with ↑ketones (beta-hydroxybutyrate). Metabolic alkalosis if vomiting. **Ascites:** test as may have SBP – always aspirate.
- **Management:** supportive as for advanced alcoholic liver disease: IV fluids and IV GLUCOSE and IV PABRINEX paired vials TDS for 1–2 days. Replace electrolytes and phosphate and magnesium as needed. Long-term abstinence from alcohol and refer to appropriate support on discharge. Alcoholic hepatitis, ▶ Section 7.4.

7.6 Alcohol abuse

- Alcohol is a colourless odourless liquid and liver toxin. Additives give the associated smell. CNS depressant and sudden withdrawal can cause hyperexcitability, delirium and seizures. Alcohol misuse is common. Take an alcohol history from all patients. Recommended limit of 14 units/week (males and females). 1 unit = 8 g alcohol = small glass of wine or half pint of beer. The liver effect of alcoholism is one facet compared to its effects on relationships, children, violence, unemployment, drink driving, hypertension, mental health issues.

- **Screening for those at risk:** assess intake per week. What is told to the doctor is often an underestimate. Family estimate useful. Empty bottles per week. When is first drink taken – mornings, drinking all day or binging? Does person have responsibilities, e.g. to children, then it may become a social services issue of child safety and care. Is patient drink driving? What role does alcohol play in their life?
- **Alcohol cessation:** sudden acute alcohol withdrawal can lead to DTs 1–3 days later and is potentially lethal. Patients should be encouraged to gradually reduce their alcohol intake over time.

CAGE questionnaire is recommended
- **Alcohol problem very likely if 2 or more positive answers to the following:**
  (1) Have you felt you should CUT down on drinking? (2) Have you been ANGERED by suggestions you cut down? (3) Have you felt GUILTY about drinking? (4) Have you used alcohol as an EYE opener in the morning?

Clinical presentations of alcohol abuse
- **Alcoholic hepatitis:** jaundiced, toxic, unwell, elevated ALT. (▶Section 7.4).
- **Progressive liver failure:** jaundiced, coagulopathy, encephalopathy, ascites. (▶Section 7.2).
- **Delirium tremens:** agitated, fever, sweating, picking at bedclothes (now is the time to treat), hallucinations, e.g. rats, terrified – can progress to acute seizure. (▶Section 7.8).
- **Suicide:** often seen combined with alcohol abuse. High rate of suicide and needs psychiatric review.
- **Trauma:** involved in violent assaults, head injuries as well as road traffic accidents and simple falls.
- **Alcoholic cerebellar ataxia:** chronic cerebellar disease with ataxia.
- **Social:** spending one's life focused on obtaining and consuming alcohol leads to unemployment, divorce, homelessness, malnutrition, violence.
- **Cancer risk:** hepatoma, pancreatic cancer, various other cancers, e.g. of oesophagus, head and neck.
- **Medical and social costs of alcoholism:** head injury, falls, assaults, road traffic accidents, seizures, overdoses, suicidal attempts, self-harm. Cerebral haemorrhage, hypothermia, meningitis and chest infections, cardiomyopathy. Ketoacidosis, pneumococcal infections, low potassium, magnesium and calcium. Renal failure, Wernicke's and Korsakoff's psychosis and B_1 deficiency. Variceal haemorrhage and liver disease, peptic ulcer disease. Peripheral neuropathy, cerebellar degeneration, atrial fibrillation. Social and family break up, abuse, divorce, poverty, violence.
- **Management:** alcohol-induced liver damage is silent often until a late stage when it presents in 80% as decompensated cirrhosis or alcoholic hepatitis. Long-term abstinence from alcohol is needed to allow liver regeneration. All attempts should be made to identify and change harmful behaviour early with information and coping strategies. A coordinated approach from primary and secondary care is needed as well as governmental and societal changes and attitudes to alcohol. Screening tools involve questionnaires in those at risk, GGT has a high predictive value in terms of liver disease and death. **Liver elastography** can assess fibrosis and is helpful. Various blood markers of fibrosis are being examined. See *Section 7.4* on alcoholic hepatitis for further information on acute presentation.

7.7 Zieve's syndrome

- **About:** rare, but failure to recognise can be misunderstood as anaemia due to bleeding in alcoholic liver disease.

- **Clinical:** jaundice, RUQ pain due to alcoholic hepatitis, alcohol related issues.
- **Investigations:** FBC: low Hb, ↑reticulocytes, ↑LDH, low haptoglobins. U&E/ LFTs: ↑bilirubin. **Blood film:** anaemia, spherocytosis due to haemolysis. Raised triglycerides.
- **Management:** supportive. Alcohol avoidance. Haematinics as needed.

7.8 ▶ Delirium tremens/alcohol withdrawal

- **About:** a cause of seizures and coma. Exclude SDH, pneumococcal bacterial meningitis, drugs. Best predictor is a past history of alcohol-related delirium tremens.
- **Aetiology:** withdrawal symptoms 1–3 days after last drink. Mortality from DTs is about 15%. Alcohol is a central depressant. Withdrawal leads to a hyperadrenergic state. Complications are seizures, aspiration, respiratory failure, arrhythmias.
- **Clinical:** nausea, indigestion, coarse tremor and hyperactive delirium within 24 h. Fever, visual hallucinations and seizures occur after 24 h peaking at 50 h. Signs of advanced alcoholic liver disease, ↑HR, dehydration. Jaundice, alcoholic hepatitis, ascites, coagulopathy, encephalopathy.
- **Differential:** opiate or cocaine use, hypoglycaemia, head injury (SDH/stroke/ skull fracture). Sepsis, hepatic encephalopathy, psychotic illness. Encephalitis, non-convulsive status.
- **Investigations:** FBC, U&E and LFT. CRP: exclude infection and liver failure. **CXR:** exclude tumour, infection, TB, aspiration, perforation. **Sepsis screen:** chest, urine, aspirate ascites to exclude spontaneous bacterial peritonitis. ECG: exclude MI, AF. **Coagulation screen** if possible liver failure. **CT head:** if concerned about head injury or stroke or sub-dural haematoma, or some other pathology. Have a low threshold to scan if concerned. LP: if suspected meningitis (pneumococcal seen in alcoholics).
- **Management:** supportive: ABC, O₂ as per BTS guidelines. Manage in a well-lit area; involve family or known trusted carers to reduce anxiety. If significant sedation is needed then consider HDU/ITU environment for ABC. Monitor glucose, Mg and K and dehydration and treat accordingly. Agitated confused patient: start a reducing dose regimen of CHLORDIAZEPOXIDE or DIAZEPAM. Determine when was last drink. Fits tend to classically occur about 48–96 h later. Titrate the dose to the level of agitation. Fixed dose schedule: (consider higher doses in very agitated and those with high body weight; watch for over-sedation): Days 1–2: CHLORDIAZEPOXIDE 10–30 mg 6 h. Days 3–4: CHLORDIAZEPOXIDE 10 mg 8 h. Days 5–6: CHLORDIAZEPOXIDE 10 mg 12 h and stop. Early discharge (>48 h) possible if asymptomatic and 24/7 supervision until Days 5–6.
- **Seizures:** manage as status epilepticus. Monitor GCS and ABCs. May need nasopharyngeal airway, recovery position and HDU bed or even ITU. Take advice if GCS <9. Low threshold to CT head if any concerns about head injury, SDH, meningitis, delirium, stroke. In the case that you are unable to convince the patient to take medications then LORAZEPAM 1–2 mg IV/IM or DIAZEPAM IV/PO could be considered. **Avoid haloperidol.** Identify early and sedate patients likely to 'go off' when they are compliant. Consider the fixed dose schedule below. Start as soon as any hyperactive features appear or high risk, e.g. a patient with previous delirium tremens and now off alcohol. Watch for over-sedation and precipitating encephalopathy. Consider HDU/ITU. Prophylactic anticonvulsants not usually recommended.
- **Wernicke–Korsakoff syndrome:** ataxia, ophthalmoplegia, nystagmus, low BP, memory disturbance, comatose, confusion, hypothermia Give IV PABRINEX two sets of paired ampoules TDS for 3–5 days and then THIAMINE 200 mg PO OD.

7.9 Decompensated cirrhosis, ascites and spontaneous bacterial peritonitis

- **About:** decompensated cirrhosis is a medical emergency with a high mortality. Effective early interventions can save lives and reduce hospital stay. Complete checklist in all with decompensated cirrhosis within the first 6 h of admission.
- **Clinical:** jaundice, increasing ascites, hepatic encephalopathy, renal impairment, GI bleeding, signs of sepsis/hypovolaemia, occasionally signs may be minimal. May be mild to severe abdominal pain, ascites and generalised tenderness and signs of liver disease. Document current alcohol intake and other drugs.
- **Ascites grading:** Grade 1 (mild) – detectable only by USS. Grade 2 (moderate) – moderate symmetrical distension of the abdomen. Grade 3 (large) – marked abdominal distension.
- **Precipitants:** GI bleeding (variceal and non-variceal), infection/sepsis (spontaneous bacterial peritonitis, urine, chest, cholangitis, etc.), alcoholic hepatitis, acute portal vein thrombosis, development of hepatocellular carcinoma, drugs (alcohol, opiates, NSAIDs, etc.), ischaemic liver injury (sepsis or ↓BP), dehydration, constipation.

Investigations

- FBC, U&E, LFT, coag. screen, glucose, Ca/Mg/phosphate, blood cultures, urine dip/MSU and CXR for infection, CRP.
- **Liver USS:** liver size, coarse edge, increased echogenicity, free fluid throughout abdomen, hepatocellular carcinoma, portal vein or hepatic vein thrombosis, renal tract abnormalities.
- **Aspirate of ascites:** in all within 24 h (SBP can be clinically silent): a 10 ml aspirate with a blue/green needle in all unwell patients with ascites to exclude SBP: ↑WCC and CRP. Neutrophil count >250 cells/mm^3 and low pH of ascitic fluid. Gram stain and aerobic and anaerobic culture. Measure ascitic protein because SBP more common with ascitic albumin <15 g/L and may need antibiotic prophylaxis. Secondary peritonitis is likely if ascitic fluid shows >1200 cells/mm^3. Serum/ascites albumin gradient: >11 g/L suggests portal hypertension. Cirrhotic patients with low ascitic fluid protein concentration (<10–15 g/L) and/or high serum bilirubin levels are at high risk of SBP so consider prophylactic antibiotics.
- **Management: ABC, HDU** if worsening EWS and liver failure. **Sodium restriction:** moderate restriction of salt intake to sodium of 80–120 mmol/day, which corresponds to 4.6–6.9 g of salt/day. No added salt diet. Avoid pre-prepared meals. Avoid IV NS. Alcohol ingestion then give IV PABRINEX 2 pairs of vials TDS for 1–2 days.

Managing ascites

- **Spontaneous bacterial peritonitis:** diagnostic paracentesis >250 polymorphs/mm^3 (0.25 × 10^9)/L. Treat with antibiotics, e.g. IV TAZOCIN or CEFTRIAXONE 0.5–2 g IV BD for at least 5 days or as per local policy. EASL guidelines recommend HUMAN ALBUMIN (HAS) (day 1 give 1.5 g/kg and day 3 give 1 g/kg) reduced the incidence of hepatorenal syndrome from 30% to 10% and mortality from 29% to 10%. Following an episode of SBP patients should be considered for NORFLOXACIN 400 mg OD as prophylaxis. QUINOLONES have been used but increase risk of *Clostridium difficile*. ▶Section 6.11.
- **Fluid/salt balance:** restrict dietary Na <90 mmol/day (5.2 g). Lowers diuretic requirement and increases resolution of ascites and shorter hospital stay.
- **Diuretics:** start SPIRONOLACTONE 100 mg OD. There is a 3–5 day lag before natriuresis (urine Na > K) then add a loop diuretic, e.g. FUROSEMIDE 40–160 mg/d. Use Spironolactone and Furosemide in a ratio 50mg to 20mg, respectively.

Spironolactone should not exceed 400 mg. Review diuretics and take advice if Na < 125 mmol/L or serum creatinine rising > 0% from baseline.

- **Steroids:** have been advocated for severe alcohol hepatitis but evidence is contentious. They increase risk of serious infections. Exclude/treat infection first. Use under expert guidance. Pentoxifylline has also been recommended but evidence again is not clear.
- **Therapeutic paracentesis:** recommended with large ascites. If renal function normal then administer **1 unit (100 ml) HAS 20%** following every 3 L drained or for every 2 L if there is impaired renal function. Failure to volume expand risks circulatory dysfunction + renal failure. Albumin better than artificial plasma expanders. Ascites recurs in 90% of patients if diuretics not begun and in 20% despite diuretics. **Do NOT leave drain *in situ* overnight or more than 6 h.** ▶ Section 20.6.
- **Hyponatraemia:** ratio of Na >126 mmol/L, no need for H_2O restriction and continue diuretics if renal function stable. If Na <125 mmol/L consider stopping diuretics, especially if Na <121 mmol/L if creatinine rising (>150 µmol/L), volume expansion maintaining renal function is crucial. The maximum recommended weight loss during diuretic therapy should be 0.5 kg/day in patients without oedema and 1 kg/day in patients with oedema. ▶ Section 5.10.
- **Prevent AKI:** increase in serum creatinine ≥26 µmol/L within 48 h, or ≥50% rise in serum creatinine over the last 7 days, or urine output <0.5 ml/kg/h for more than 6 h based on dry weight, or clinically dehydrated then suspend all diuretics and nephrotoxic drugs. Fluid resuscitate with 5% HAS or 0.9% NS (250 ml boluses with regular reassessment: 1–2 L will correct most losses). Monitor daily weights and aim for MAP >80 mmHg to achieve urine output >0.5 ml/kg/h based on dry weight. At 6 h, if target not achieved or EWS worsening then consider escalation to higher level of care. ▶ Section 10.4.
- **GI bleed:** fluid resuscitate according to BP, pulse and venous pressure (aim for MAP >65 mmHg), suspected variceal bleed TERLIPRESSIN IV (caution if IHD or PVD; perform ECG in >65 y). If PT prolonged give IV VITAMIN K 10 mg stat. If PT >20 s (or INR >2.0) – give FFP (2–4 units). If platelets <50 give IV platelets. Transfuse blood if Hb <7.0 g/L or massive bleeding (aim for Hb >8 g/L). Early endoscopy after resuscitation (ideally within 12 h). ▶ Section 6.4.
- **Encephalopathy:** LACTULOSE 30 ml QDS or phosphate enema (aiming for 2 soft stools/day). CT if SDH in differential. ▶ Section 7.11.
- **Antibiotics:** sepsis start TAZOCIN 4.5 g 8 h IV or CEFTAZIDIME 1–2 g 8 h IV. Alternatives include CIPROFLOXACIN 500 mg 12 h PO/400 mg 12 h IV. Resolution is seen in 90%. Prophylaxis should also be considered.
- **Liver transplant:** those who survive an episode of SBP should be considered for liver transplantation.
- **Transjugular intrahepatic portosystemic shunt** (TIPS) for refractory ascites. 25% risk encephalopathy. Can cause heart failure.
- **VTE prophylaxis:** prescribe prophylactic LMWH (patients with liver disease are at a high risk of thromboembolism even with a prolonged PT; withhold if patient is actively bleeding or platelets <50).

References: European Association for the Study of the Liver (2010) EASL Clinical practice guidelines. *J Hepatol*, 533:97. Wiest *et al.* (2012) Spontaneous bacterial peritonitis: recent guidelines and beyond. *Gut*, 61:297.

7.10 Hepatorenal syndrome

- **About:** AKI in patient with acute liver failure and cirrhosis – presents with oliguria. Exclude other causes of AKI first especially prerenal.
- **Aetiology:** systemic vasodilation and renal hypoperfusion and afferent renal vasoconstriction. Exclude prerenal failure as a cause by a trial of volume expansion.

- **Causes:** 40% of patients with cirrhosis and ascites develop AKI. Causes are shock, diarrhoea, diuretics, sepsis, ATN, prerenal disease, drugs, paracentesis, obstruction or parenchymal renal disease. Exclude SBP as a cause.
- **Risk factors:** low MAP (<80 mmHg), dilutional hyponatraemia, urinary Na <5 mmol/L.
- **Differentials: prerenal failure, ATN**, nephrotoxic drugs, parenchymal renal disease (proteinuria/haematuria, abnormal renal USS), obstructive nephropathy, glomerulonephritis.
- **Classification: Type 1:** rapid AKI with oliguria. Creatinine quickly >350 µmol/L. Precipitated by spontaneous bacterial peritonitis (25% of patients), bleed or infection. Characterised by diuretic-resistant ascites, encephalopathy. Most die within 10 weeks. May respond to TERLIPRESSIN (see below). **Type 2:** moderate and stable reduction in the GFR, median survival of 3–6 months. Slower. Creatinine rarely >180 µmol/L.
- **Criteria for diagnosis of hepatorenal syndrome in cirrhosis:** (1) cirrhosis with ascites + serum creatinine >133 µmol/L (1.5 mg/dL). (2) No sustained improvement of serum creatinine (to <133 µmol/L) despite 2 d of diuretic withdrawal and volume expansion with albumin (1 g/kg of body weight per day up to a maximum of 100 g/d). (3) Absence of shock. No current or recent nephrotoxic drugs, e.g. NSAIDs, etc. No parenchymal disease (no proteinuria >500 mg/d or microhaematuria (>50 RBC/high powered field)) and normal renal USS.
- **Clinical:** fatigue, malaise, progressive uraemia with oliguria without significant proteinuria. Chronic liver disease, ascites, jaundice, encephalopathy. Abdominal pain/ascites, e.g. <u>SBP</u>, ▶ Section 7.9.
- **Investigations:** FBC, U&E, creatinine >130 µmol/L, ↓creatinine clearance <40 ml/min. Check LFTs, PT. Urine culture and urinalysis: urine volume <500 ml/day. ↓Proteinuria <500 mg/d. Urine Na <10 mmol/d. Urine osmolarity > plasma osmolarity. Urine RBC count <50 cells/High powered field. **Abdominal USS:** no renal parenchymal disease or obstruction to explain AKI, cirrhosis, ascites. **General sepsis screen** and diagnostic paracentesis to look for SBP, CXR, urinalysis, blood cultures.
- **Management:** specialist supportive care and nephrology review. Exclude other causes of AKI such as shock, ongoing infection or recent treatment with nephrotoxic drugs. Treat hypovolaemia with fluid challenge. Failure to respond suggests hepatorenal. Withdraw diuretics and other nephrotoxic drugs. Look for SBP and treat usually with CEFOTAXIME. **In alcoholic hepatitis:** PENTOXIFYLLINE 400 mg PO TDS may be used. VASOPRESSIN and NORADRENALINE may be used but get specialist help. TERLIPRESSIN 0.5–2.0 mg IV 6 h especially in Type 1 in addition to Day 1: 1 g HAS/kg; Day 2–16: 20–40 g HAS/day. Diuretics are usually avoided. Continue until serum creatinine falls below 130 µmol/l. Where creatinine is rising despite treatment, 60 g HAS/day may be clinically indicated. As ever take expert guidance. OCTREOTIDE 100–200 mcg SC 8 h may be used instead of Terlipressin. Liver transplantation is usually indicated in Types 1 and 2 and is the main definitive therapy. Transjugular intrahepatic porto-systemic shunting may be considered. Also see <u>AKI</u>, ▶Section 10.4.

References: European Association for the Study of the Liver (2010) EASL clinical practice guidelines. *J Hepatol*, 533:97. Ginès & Schrier (2009) Renal failure in cirrhosis. *N Engl J Med*, 361:1279.

7.11 Hepatic encephalopathy

- **About:** potentially reversible neuropsychiatric disorder in those with liver failure. Exclude unrelated neurologic and/or metabolic abnormalities.
- **Aetiology:** associated with arterial NH_4 levels and other protein breakdown products crossing blood–brain barrier.

- **Identify likely precipitants: sepsis:** chest, urine, biliary, spontaneous bacterial peritonitis. **Metabolic:** fluid overload or electrolyte, e.g. low Na, low K, diuretic overuse. Transjugular intrahepatic porto-systemic shunt, renal failure. **Drugs:** sedatives, NSAIDs, CNS suppressants. **GI bleeding:** which may be variceal or non-variceal. Ischaemic liver injury: ↓BP, sepsis. **Acute portal vein thrombosis:** needs USS. Development of hepatocellular carcinoma, continued alcohol intake.
- **Clinical:** reversal of day/night sleeping, psychomotor dysfunction, impaired memory. Sensory abnormalities, poor concentration, disorientation, tremor, shuffling gait. Melena, haematemesis. Fetor hepaticus, flapping tremor, asterixis.

Grades of encephalopathy
- Stage I: anxiety, mild confusion, reversed sleep/wake cycles, apathy, asterixis.
- Stage II: + moderate confusion, disorientation, rigidity.
- Stage III: + severe confusion, somnolence, incontinent, Babinski's sign.
- Stage IV: + coma, decerebrate posturing.

Investigations
- **FBC, U&E and LFT:** ↑WCC, AST/ALT, PT, alpha-fetoprotein.
- **Abdominal USS:** cholangitis, hepatocellular cancer, ascites, liver size.
- **Blood ammonia level:** ↑. Other causes of ↑ammonia are GI bleeding, renal failure, hypovolaemia, urea cycle disorder, TPN, urosepsis, valproic acid.
- **CT head:** rules out acute bleeding.
- **Lumbar puncture:** if encephalitis suspected (check coag and plt first).
- **Diagnostic ascitic tap:** for spontaneous bacterial peritonitis.
- **EEG:** symmetrical slowing with characteristic (but nonspecific) triphasic waves.
- **Others:** exclude hypoxia, hypercarbia, uraemia, hypoglycaemia.
- **Ascitic tap always:** exclude spontaneous bacterial peritonitis.

Management
- **Supportive:** manage dietary input including adequate protein (1.5 g/kg/day) and calories (30 kcal/kg/day). Watch for re-feeding issues. Assessment by a dietitian with experience in liver disease is useful. Grade III or more encephalopathy consider intubation to protect airways and other supportive treatment often needed.
- **Drugs:** avoid NS, opiates, NSAIDs, benzodiazepines. Check all other drugs for safety.
- **Precipitants:** look for and treat any cause, e.g. antibiotics for infection, paracetamol overdose, dehydration, manage bleeding, volume replace cautiously, avoid alcohol, diagnostic paracentesis for SBP and review all drugs.
- **LACTULOSE 20–50 ml BD** to give 3 loose stools per day. PHOSPHATE ENEMA BD may be needed. Lactulose is metabolised by bacteria in the colon to acetic and lactic acid, which reduces colonic pH, decreases survival of urease-producing bacteria in the gut, and aids conversion of ammonia (NH_3) to ammonium (NH_4), which is less readily absorbed by the gut.
- **Antibiotics:** CEFTRIAXONE 1–2 g/day. Consider RIFAXIMIN 600 mg BD for 6 months, maintained remission from hepatic encephalopathy compared with placebo and significantly reduced hospitalization (91% of the patients were using concomitant lactulose). METRONIDAZOLE 250 mg BD is also useful. Avoid neomycin.
- **ORNITHINE ASPARTASE:** effective in treating hepatic encephalopathy in a number of European trials.

References: Bass *et al*. (2010) Rifaximin treatment in hepatic encephalopathy. *N Engl J Med*, 362:1071. Ginès & Schrier (2009) Renal failure in cirrhosis. *N Engl J Med*, 361:1279.

7.12 Chronic liver disease

- **About:** chronic liver disease (CLD) contrasts with ALF as management of declining liver function. Complications such as SBP, varices, acute decompensation need management. The aim is to preserve function long enough for transplant if possible.

Assess mortality risk in cirrhosis: use Child–Pugh score	
Encephalopathy	None = +1, controlled/minimal = +2, advanced = +3.
Ascites	None = +1, mild = +2, moderate/severe = +3.
Bilirubin	(μmol/L): <34 = +1, 34–51 = +2, >51 = +3; in PSC/PBC the score levels are set higher: 68 = +1, and 170 = +2.
Albumin	(g/L): >35 = +1, 28–35 = +2, <28 = +3.
Prothrombin time (INR)	<4 s (INR 1.7) = +1, 4–6 s (INR 1.7–2.2) = +2, >6 s (INR >2.2) = +3.
Add Scores	5–6 – Class A has 100% 1 y survival, 7–9 – Class B 81%, 10–15 – Class C 45%.

Initial investigation for CLD of unknown aetiology

- FBC, LFTs, clotting screen, immunoglobulins – increased IgG in autoimmune, IgA in alcohol, IgM in PBC.
- Anti-mitochondrial (PBC), anti-smooth muscle, ANA in autoimmune hepatitis and renal failure in the presence of cryoglobulins (seen in viral disease specifically).
- Hepatitis viral/bacterial serology, alpha-1-antitrypsin, alpha-fetoprotein.
- Ferritin, copper, caeruloplasmin and urinary copper ± penicillamine challenge test (in patients <40 with unexplained CLD or seronegative hepatitis).
- Urinalysis and 24 h urine for creatinine clearance and protein, ECG, CXR, ultrasound and doppler studies of abdomen, CT, MRI/MRCP studies may be needed.

Complications/associations of CLD

- Ascites in liver disease and spontaneous bacterial peritonitis (▶Section 7.9).
- Hepatic encephalopathy (▶Section 7.11).
- Coagulopathy: upper GI bleed and varices (▶Section 6.4).
- Renal impairment or hepatorenal syndrome (▶Section 7.10).

7.13 Liver abscess

- **Three types:** local bacteria, amoebic (*Entamoeba histolytica*), echinococcus (*E. granulosus*).
- **Clinical:** fever, abdominal pain, hepatomegaly, jaundice. Right pleural effusion, pleural rub. Occasionally abscesses are well tolerated and may present as PUO. Anaphylaxis (*E. granulosus*).
- **Investigations:** FBC: ↓Hb, ↑neutrophil, ↑CRP, ↑ALP, ↑B12. Serology can be useful – see below. CXR: ↑right hemidiaphragm. Abdominal USS and CT diagnostic for liver abscess.
- **Differential:** liver cyst, hepatoma, metastases.
- **Management:** antibiotics are the first line in therapy and then some require open or radiologically guided percutaneous drainage depending on the response (see below).

Causes

- **Pyogenic:** from appendicitis, cholecystitis, diverticulitis. Older patients. Multiple lesions, possible bowel malignancy. Diagnosis: USS, raised LFTs. Management: IV antibiotics and drainage. Foul smelling pus. Treat COAMOXICLAV 1.2 g

8 h or TAZOCIN 4.5 g 8 h IV. Alternatives are CEFOTAXIME. Consider adding METRONIDAZOLE if causative organism unclear.

- **Amoebic:** see Amoebiasis, ▶ Section 9.48.
- **Hydatid disease:** tapeworm infection. *E. granulosus* cysts in liver, lungs and bones usually asymptomatic and patients are well unless secondarily infected. Hydatid cyst rupture can lead to anaphylaxis. Hydatid serology 90% positive. Mortality is related to anaphylaxis and sudden death reported. Management: surgery remains the primary treatment and the only hope for complete cure. The puncture, aspiration, injection, and reaspiration (PAIR) technique is suggested with open surgery as a further option along with appropriate agents such as ALBENDAZOLE and MEBENDAZOLE combination. Risk of anaphylaxis is, however, significant.

7.14 ▶ Gallstone disease and local complications

- **About:** commoner in women. Gallstones are seen in 10% of the population. Gallstones mostly silent.
- **Risks:** seen mainly in females, middle age and beyond, obesity, those on Octreotide. Liver disease, e.g. cirrhosis, rapid weight loss and fasting. Rare in black people other than sickle cell disease with haemolysis.
- **Aetiology:** lithogenic bile, ↑ insoluble cholesterol and insufficient bile acids. Obstruction of the gallbladder neck or cystic duct by a gallstone. Inflammation is more likely chemical rather than infective as bile is usually sterile.
- **Bacterial infection:** may be seen with: *E. coli*, *Klebsiella*, *Strep. faecalis*, and anaerobic organisms.

Pathophysiology and clinical presentations of gallstones	
Biliary colic	Gallstone stuck at cystic duct. Waves of RUQ or epigastric pain, N&V. Lasts 20 min then may return.
Acute cholecystitis	Inflamed gallbladder. Blocked cystic duct. May be bacterial infection and infected bile. Severe RUQ pain, fever. Murphy's sign is positive pressure on RUQ catches patient on inspiration.
Emphysematous cholecystitis	Gas-producing bacteria in gallbladder. Blocked cystic duct. Classically male diabetics. Similar to cholecystitis. Toxic. Gas seen on AXR/CT.
Acalculous cholecystitis	Seen in critical care. Trauma or burns, those on TPN, etc. High mortality (see below).
Chronic cholecystitis	Ongoing inflamed gallbladder. Colic. May be asymptomatic. Develops 'porcelain gallbladder'.
Gallbladder perforation	Gallbladder perforates due to erosion and ischaemia. Stones pass into peritoneal cavity. Peritonitis. Fever, RUQ mass. High mortality.
Acute cholangitis	Fever, jaundice, rigors, sepsis (▶ Section 7.15).
Gallstone acute pancreatitis	With stones in common bile duct (▶ Section 7.16).

Investigation: FBC and U&E: ↑WCC, ↑CRP, ↑creatinine, ↑urea. LFT: ↑bilirubin, ↑ALP, ↑↑GGT (especially if common bile duct blocked), ↑mild ALT and AST. **Abdominal USS:** gallstones, enlarged hydropic gallbladder with a thickened wall in the region of maximum tenderness. Gallstones in gallbladder and/or cystic duct or common bile duct. USS is more sensitive than CT for acute gallstone disease. USS can pick up stones as small as 2 mm. Identifies thickened wall gallbladder and gallbladder distension

(>4 cm short axis) and pericholecystic fluid. Operator can also look for a positive Murphy's sign. Stones in common bile duct suggested if duct diameter >5–7 mm. **ERCP with cholangiogram** may be needed for ductal stones.

- **Complications:** biliary sepsis and cholangitis, empyema (pus) of the gallbladder. Perforation and peritonitis.
- **Management:** ABC and O$_2$ as per BTS guidelines + IV access + NBM. NG tube if vomiting. **Fluids:** 1 L crystalloids (NS or Hartmann's) over 2–4 h and assess volume needs and replace.
- **Pain relief:** IM NSAIDs or MORPHINE 5–10 mg IV. Anti-emetics: CYCLIZINE 50 mg slow IV or ONDANSETRON 8 mg PO/IV BD.
- **Antibiotics:** TAZOCIN 4.5 g 8 h IV for 7–10 d. Penicillin allergy CEFUROXIME 1.5 g 8 h IV + METRONIDAZOLE 500 mg 8 h IV.
- **Surgical Management:** A laparoscopic cholecystectomy should be carried out urgently or within 5 days of onset of symptoms otherwise the patient is prone to further episodes. It has shorter stay, less pain and mortality than open surgery. Those unfit for surgery may have temporary drainage. Commonest complication is bile leak which can be managed by ERCP and stenting. In those with **biliary colic alone which settles within 6 h and no cholecystitis can go home with adequate pain control and have surgical review later**. Ask to return if worsens especially fever or worsening pain or severe vomiting. Murphy's negative.
- **Acalculous cholecystitis** can occur with no stones seen but a typical acute cholecystitis picture. Prognosis is worse. Seen with diabetes, fasting, TPN, sepsis, trauma, burns, opiates, IHD. Treat with antibiotics and supportive management. Gangrene and perforation are more common. Urgent cholecystectomy may be indicated. Other methods to treat chronic stones are oral bile acids (ursodeoxycholic acid) or extracorporeal shock wave lithotripsy (ESWL).

7.15 Acute cholangitis

- **Aetiology:** bacterial infection of the biliary tree usually due to stones or impaired drainage within the common bile duct.
- **Causes:** gallstones predominantly, strictures, sclerosing cholangitis, chronic pancreatitis, HIV-related cholangiopathy. **Rare:** clonorchis, ascarisis.
- **Clinical:** Charcot's triad of non-colicky RUQ pain to right shoulder, jaundice and fever. Biliary obstruction – dark urine and pale stool.
- **Investigation:** FBC, U&E, LFT: ↑WCC, ↑bilirubin, ↑ALP, ↑GGT, ↑ALT. Blood cultures positive in half. **Abdominal USS:** enlarged hydropic gallbladder with a thickened wall and stones. Stones in common bile duct suggested if duct diameter >5–7 mm. Abdominal CT: can be useful to see obstruction and measure common bile duct. Can also exclude pancreatic carcinoma/other pathologies. **Magnetic resonance cholangiopancreatography (MRCP):** can visualise biliary tree anatomy and stones. Not possible if patient has pacemaker, etc. **ERCP:** may also be done as investigations to assess for stones in common bile duct and exclude tumour.

Management

- **Supportive:** IV fluids, crystalloids and basic ABC + O$_2$ as per BTS guidelines. NBM, NG if vomiting. Get an abdominal USS as soon as possible.
- **Antibiotics:** TAZOCIN 4.5 g 8 h IV for 7–10 d. Alternative consider CEFUROXIME 1.5 g 8 h IV + METRONIDAZOLE 500 mg 8 h IV.
- **ERCP +/– sphincterotomy:** can allow biliary drainage and passage of a stone +/– spontaneously or pulled out with a basket device. If there is a malignant lesion or stricture a stent can be placed. Consider laparoscopic cholecystectomy at 6–12 weeks for gallbladder stones.
- **Complications:** sepsis, ARDS, multiorgan failure.

7.16 ▶ Acute pancreatitis

- **About:** significant morbidity and mortality. Under surgeons/gastroenterology.
- **Diagnosis:** needs 2/3 of typical abdominal pain, ↑amylase, ↑lipase and imaging (CECT/MRI).

Causes	
Gallstones (45%)	A gallstone in ampulla of Vater can allow bile reflux into pancreatic duct activating enzymes.
Alcohol (45%)	Chronic alcohol for several years or occasional binge.
Hypertriglyceridaemia	Look at fundi for lipaemia retinalis.
Primary hyperparathyroidism	Check Ca and PTH.
Cancer	Pancreatic cancer, biliary cancer.
Miscellaneous	Trauma, snake-bite, HIV, CMV, EBV, post ERCP, sphincter of Oddi dysfunction.
Drugs	Steroids, thiazides, azathioprine, sulphonamide.
Congenital	Pancreas divisum, familial non-X-linked dominant.

- **Aetiology:** Activation of trypsin, lipase and amylase and autodigestion leads to an inflamed oedematous/haemorrhagic pancreas. On-going tissue damage can activate complement with a progressive systemic inflammatory response syndrome. Revised Atlanta classification 2012: two phases of the disease: early and late. Severity is classified as mild, moderate or severe. Two types of acute pancreatitis (interstitial oedematous pancreatitis and necrotising pancreatitis).

Clinical

- ↑HR, ↓BP, shock from sepsis, haemorrhagic pancreatitis. Severe epigastric pain to back eased with sitting up and forwards. Peritonitis with guarding, signs of causes, e.g. gallstones, alcoholism. Shocked, sepsis – generalised, pneumonia, ↓Hb. Bruising in flanks – Grey–Turner's sign. Peri-umbilical bruising – Cullen's sign (haemorrhagic pancreatitis). Coagulopathy from DIC. Cyanosed, dyspnoea from ARDS. Oliguria from AKI and/or hypovolaemia.

Diagnostic criteria for acute pancreatitis

- Requires two of the following three features: (1) abdominal pain consistent with acute pancreatitis (acute onset of a persistent, severe, epigastric pain often radiating to the back), (2) ↑serum lipase activity (or amylase activity) >3× upper limit of normal (ULN), (3) characteristic findings on contrast-enhanced CT or MRI or USS.
- If clinical picture suggests acute pancreatitis, the serum amylase/lipase activity is <3× ULN (e.g. delayed presentation); imaging is needed to confirm the diagnosis otherwise the clinical picture + ↑serum pancreatic enzyme activities suffices and a CT is not usually required for diagnosis acutely.

Investigations

- **FBC:** ↓Hb with haem pancreatitis; ↑MCV with alcohol. **U&E:** AKI, ↓Ca, ↑triglycerides (familial hypertriglyceridaemia). **CRP:** ↑>200 within first 4 days suggests acute severe attack – risk of complications, e.g. infection, pseudocyst, abscess formation.
- **Pancreatic lipase**↑ (>3× ULN): more sensitive and specific than amylase. Elevated longer than amylase after disease presentation. **Amylase**↑(>3× ULN is diagnostic): usually >1000 IU/ml (levels up to 10 000 may be seen). Mild elevations

>200 IU/ml not unique to pancreatitis but may also be seen in abdominal pain due to perforation of a viscus, small bowel obstruction, leaking AAA, ectopic pregnancy. A level of >1000 is more diagnostic, *but there is not a close correlation between amylase level and clinical severity*. Very rarely a normal amylase suggests little remaining amylase-producing pancreatic tissue left. Amylase may be normal if alcohol-induced or hypertriglyceridemia. False positive serum amylase with macroamylasaemia – the level is constant. **Urinary trypsinogen-2↑** is now considered as a new test in development and **IL-6 and IL-8** may predict severity.

- **Arterial blood gases:** ↓pH, ↓HCO_3, ↓pO_2 in severe cases, ↑↑lactate.
- **Imaging: erect CXR/AXR:** exclude perforation, small bowel obstruction. Left pleural effusion may be seen. Look for calcification and sentinel loop. Bowel gas is seen in small bowel in centre of abdomen. **Contrast-enhanced CT/MRI abdomen:** reserved for patients in whom the diagnosis is unclear or who fail to improve clinically within the first 48–72 h after hospital admission or to evaluate complications. Best done at or after 3 days to support diagnosis and determine full extent of pancreatic necrosis and the presence of any fluid. CT may show fat-stranding surrounding the inflamed pancreas. Fluid may be aspirated to detect infection. Necrotic pancreas is identified by failure to opacify when CT with contrast is carried out. Gas bubbles may suggest infection. In a patient older than 40 years, a pancreatic tumour should always be considered as a cause.
- **USS abdomen:** should be performed in all. Detect pancreatic mass, gallstones, pseudocyst, liver disease.
- **ERCP:** may be diagnostically important when aetiology unclear and may show a cause, e.g. ampullary tumour, stricture, gallstones, pancreas divisum and may allow sphincterotomy. In those at high risk of pancreatitis post ERCP advise guidewire cannulation, pancreatic duct stents, rectal NSAIDs.

Severity scoring

- <u>**Balthazar CT Severity Index:**</u> **calculated on the basis of CT findings:** (A) normal pancreas +0, (B) focal or diffuse enlargement of the pancreas, contour irregularities, heterogeneous attenuation, no peripancreatic inflammation +1, (C) grade B plus peripancreatic inflammation +2, (D) grade C plus a single fluid collection +3, (E) grade C plus multiple fluid collections or gas +4. Percentage necrosis present on CT score: none +0, <33% +2, 33–50% +4, >50% +6. **Severe = score >6.**
- **Modified Glasgow Score: P**aO_2 <60 mmHg; **A**ge >55 years; **N**eutrophils (WCC) >15 × 10^9/L; **C**alcium <2 mmol/L; **R**aised urea >16 mmol/L; **E**nzyme LDH >600 units/L; **A**lbumin <32 g/L; **S**ugar (glucose) >10 mmol/L. Note spells out PANCREAS. A score >3 suggests severe and ITU/HDU care should be considered (Ann R Coll Surg Engl (2000); **82:** 16–17).

Local and systemic complications

- **Acute kidney injury:** Multiple factors. Optimise fluid status, treat infection, stop nephrotoxins. <u>AKI</u>, ▶Section 10.4.
- **Pancreatic pseudocyst and fluid collections:** can form around the pancreatic mass and may need laparoscopic drainage.
- **Necrotising pancreatitis:** more than 50% of gland necrosed on imaging. Can lead to infection and abscess formation. Needs antibiotics and occasionally surgery. May get walled off necrosis. Can erode into retroperitoneal vessels, e.g. splenic artery with acute haemorrhage.
- **Pancreatic abscess:** CT shows a ring-enhancing fluid collection with gas. Surgical or percutaneous drainage. IV antibiotics.
- **Others:** exocrine damage with malabsorption (low faecal elastase), endocrine – secondary diabetes.

- **Systemic:** recurrent acute pancreatitis, ARDS, AKI, DIC, multiorgan failure, generalised or local sepsis.
- **Chronic pancreatitis:** repeated episodes of pancreatic injury often alcohol related and frequent admissions. Alcohol cessation is the key in those who drink. Symptoms mimic acute pancreatitis. Develops exocrine and later endocrine dysfunction with steatorrhoea and weight loss. **Diagnosis with CT/USS/ERCP.** Exclude gallstones. **Differential** is autoimmune pancreatitis, inherited causes that start in early adult life and pancreatic cancer. Treatment is alcohol avoidance, nutritional support, manage exocrine and endocrine needs. Acutely these patients may be seen for mainly pain relief and managing acute flares. Pancreatic duct stenting if local stenosis.
- **Portal vein/splenic thrombosis:** localised inflammation. Develop portal hypertension with splenomegaly and variceal bleeds.

Management

- **ABC** and O_2 as per BTS guidance. Give early aggressive hydration (250–500 ml/h depending on cardiac/renal status) with 0.9% NS or Hartmann's solution to give urine output >30 ml/h. Baseline volume loss is 4–6 L but assess case by case. Consider CVP monitoring, monitor urine output, and clinical assessments of hydration, oxygenation, etc. There may be significant '3rd space' losses, which will need to be accounted for. ITU/HDU admission with any signs of organ failure. Look for and correct any significant hypocalcaemia. Severe cases need CT at 3–7 d and assess severity with CT severity score.
- **Nutrition:** In mild/mod disease normal oral feeding can be considered if no significant gastroparesis and there are normal bowel sounds and no signs of ileus. Early feeding by naso/gastric/jejunal (NG/NJ) tube is advised if there is ongoing vomiting. Enteral feeding is preferred to TPN. However, those with severe disease may be initially NBM. Calcium and magnesium should be checked and replaced if needed and adequate hydration given.
- **Analgesia:** TRAMADOL IV is preferred. MORPHINE 1–5 mg IV every 4 h is widely used. PETHIDINE 25–50 mg IV/SC/IM historically advocated as concerns that MORPHINE increased sphincter of Oddi tone or caused spasm. Combine with antiemetic ONDANSETRON 2–4 mg IV every 4–6 h when required.
- **Diabetes: variable rate insulin infusion** initially if hyperglycaemic or known diabetes convert to regular regimen.
- **Alcohol withdrawal:** consider CHLORDIAZEPOXIDE or LORAZEPAM 1–2 mg PO/IV/IM 8 hourly and PABRINEX IV paired vials TDS for 1–2 days.
- **Antibiotics:** are given if evidence of specific infections. Advice now against prophylaxis. Fever often due to inflammatory nature of the disease. If infected necrosis suspected then either IV CEFUROXIME or TAZOCIN, or MEROPENEM if penicillin allergic. (choice of carbapenems, quinolones, metronidazole).
- **Nutrition:** can feed normally if mild, no N&V, and abdominal pain resolved. In moderate to severe disease try to continue enteral nutrition which may be by NG/NJ tube. Try to avoid parenteral nutrition unless the enteral route is not available, not tolerated, or insufficient for caloric requirements.
- **ERCP +/– sphincterotomy** should be considered, usually within 24 h where there is a cholangitis or jaundice and a common duct stone, which requires removal. A sphincterotomy may be performed and/or stone removed. ERCP is not needed in most patients with gallstone pancreatitis without evidence of biliary obstruction.

Manage gallstones with either cholecystectomy, ERCP or, ursodeoxycholic acid can be considered.

- **MRCP or endoscopic ultrasound** (EUS) rather than diagnostic ERCP should be used to screen for choledocholithiasis if highly suspected.
- **CT-guided FNA:** consider infected necrosis in those with pancreatic or extrapancreatic necrosis who deteriorate or fail to improve after 7–10 days; consider either CT-guided FNA for Gram stain and culture to guide antibiotic prescribing, or empiric use of antibiotics without CT FNA.
- **Respiratory support:** patient with severe upper abdominal pain can experience basal atelectasis and hypoventilation and develop respiratory failure and may need a mixture of analgesia with a trial of high FiO$_2$ with humidification, chest physiotherapy to help expectorate secretions, CPAP or even invasive ventilation on ITU.
- **SURGERY** may be required where there is a **severe necrotising pancreatitis** or if there is an **abscess or pseudocyst.** Usually delayed about 4 weeks. A pancreatic necrosectomy involves removing dead pancreatic tissue, which may be done by laparoscopy. Minimally invasive methods are preferred to open necrosectomy. Consider cholecystectomy prior to discharge if gallstone pancreatitis. Asymptomatic pseudocysts may be observed and often resolve but some may need to be managed endoscopically.
- **Behavioural:** offer advice and help with good nutrition and in cessation of alcohol and smoking.

References: Tenner *et al*. (2013) Management of acute pancreatitis. *Am J Gastroenterol*, 108:1400. UK Working Party on Acute Pancreatitis (2005) UK guidelines for the management of acute pancreatitis. *Gut*, 54(Suppl III):iii1. Banks *et al*. (2013) Classification of acute pancreatitis. *Gut*, 62:102.

08 Haematological emergencies

8.1 Anaemia

- **About:** Hb depends on sex and age. Look at Hb, MCV and MCH. Anaemia may be acute or chronic but is better tolerated in young. Anaemia Hb <130 g/L in men, 120 g/L in women, 110 g/L pregnant women.
- **Pathophysiology:** we require bone marrow, B12, folate, iron, erythropoietin to produce RBCs with Hb. Haem: Fe^{2+} + protoporphyrin IX. Globins are haem-containing oxygen binding proteins. B12 and folate and bone marrow needed to make white cells and platelets.
- **Aetiology of anaemia:** deficiency of B12/folate causes megaloblasts in bone marrow and increased MCV. Deficiency of iron causes microcytosis with insufficient Hb (low MCV and MCH concentration). Lack of both causes a dimorphic anaemia with a mixture of small and large RBCs. Reduced bone marrow function: congenital, chemotherapy, infiltration, drugs, parvovirus B19, CKD. Excess blood loss/destruction of red cells, acute or chronic bleeding, chronic or acute haemolysis.

Causes/notes on anaemia	
Acute haemorrhage	Acute blood loss and haemodilution later with a lower Hb. Acutely Hb normal. Usually obvious – external wound or GI with melena/urinary/pelvic fracture/retroperitoneal. See also Haemorrhagic shock, ▶ Section 2.22; Bleeding disorders, ▶ Section 8.8.
Iron deficiency	Menstrual blood loss, GI blood loss. ↓Hb, ↓MCV, ↓MCH concentration, ↓ferritin (unreliable if CRP elevated), ↓serum iron, ↑TIBC, ↑soluble transferrin receptor. Iron/TIBC <19%. Upper and lower GI endoscopy, coeliac screen (duodenal biopsy, IgA TTG, anti-endomysial antibody). Capsule endoscopy. CT abdomen. Bone marrow – lack of iron and erythroid hyperplasia. Look for and treat cause and replace if needed.
B12 deficiency	Megaloblastic marrow. ↓Hb, ↑MCV >110. ↓B12 <50 ng/L and folate low too. ↑Bilirubin, ↑LDH. ↓WCC, ↓platelets. Neuropathy, SACD, optic atrophy. Usually pernicious anaemia, malabsorption, gastric surgery. Check intrinsic factor/parietal antibody. Treat with IM or Oral B12 2 mg/d.
Folate deficiency	Dietary or malabsorption, drugs. Megaloblastic marrow. ↑MCV >100. Red cell folate (better than tissue level) low. Folic acid 5 mg od.
Anaemia chronic disease	CKD, malignancy, connective tissue disease, RA, hypothyroid (macrocytic). Usually small or normal sized red cells.
Haemoglobinopathy	Congenital abnormal Hb reduces red cell half life with chronic anaemia, e.g. thalassaemia (very low MCV), sickle cell, etc. Sickle cell, ▶ Section 8.5.
Pregnancy	Dilutional anaemia is normal. Folate recommended pre-pregnancy for CNS development.
Haemolytic anaemia	Shortened RBC survival. Low Hb, low haptoglobin, elevated bilirubin, high LDH. Can be due to RBC structural issues (Spherocytosis/Elliptocytosis), abnormal Hb (sickle/thalassaemia), faulty RBC metabolism (phenylketonuria/G6PD), immune (warm IgG/cold IgM), physical, e.g. metal valves, malaria, microangiopathic haemolytic anaemia, PNH.

Sideroblastic anaemia	Rare. Dysfunctional haem synthesis. Marrow – ringed sideroblasts. Alcohol excess, lead, isoniazid. Treat cause. May benefit from vitamin B6.
Aplastic anaemia	Congenital, acquired, bone marrow infiltration, radiation, cytotoxic drugs, HIV, TB, PNH, drugs. Low RCC/WCC/platelets. Aplastic bone marrow. May be pancytopenia or more selective. Low/no reticulocytes. Identify cause and support. May need bone marrow transplant so caution with blood products. Urgent haem review. If neutropenic, see Neutropenic sepsis, ▶ Section 16.5.
Pancytopenia	Aplastic anaemia, B12/folate loss, TB, sepsis, leukaemia, myeloma, malignancy, PNH, SLE, drugs.

Clinical signs of abnormal FBC

- ↓Hb pale sclerae, hand creases. Fatigue, headache, breathlessness. Symptoms depend on rapidity of onset, cardiorespiratory status, age.
- ↓WCC if affected: fever, sore throat, sepsis.
- ↓Platelets: petechiae, menorrhagia, epistaxis, haematuria.
- Broad assessment of any coexisting illness which can be very varied. Look for fever, large spleen/liver/lymph glands. Look at congenital, racial (thalassaemia/sickle), contacts, travel.
- **Examine drug chart and recent drugs:** phenytoin, cytotoxics, alcohol, quinine.
- **Investigation: FBC:** ↓Hb, WCC, platelets. **Haematinics:** B12, red cell folate, ferritin/serum iron/TIBC, reticulocytes. **U&E:** AKI/CKD and CRP. TSH and T4. Bilirubin (red cell breakdown). CXR: infection, malignancy, TB. **Blood film:** schistocytes, fragmented, deformed, irregular, or helmet-shaped RBCs suggests DIC. **Reticulocytes:** usually increased except in aplastic anaemia. **Bone marrow:** hypocellular with aplasia, ringed sideroblasts, megaloblastic. Lack of iron. **Infiltration** – cancer, infection. **Intravascular haemolysis:** ↑LDH, reticulocytes, bilirubin, low haptoglobin, Coomb's test negative. AKI (HUS/TTP or uraemic platelet dysfunction). **Upper GI endoscopy** with D2 biopsies for coeliac, **lower GI endoscopy, capsule endoscopy and CT abdomen for iron deficiency anaemia**.
- **Management: establish cause. Treat and replace. Supportive measures – blood components.** Caution with giving Hb in pernicious anaemia with circulatory overload, if future need for bone marrow transplant, check if need irradiated blood (▶Section 8.17). Take haematology advice if unsure. Bone marrow transplant recipients and patients with cellular immunodeficiency should be considered for CMV negative blood. Focused management on determining cause and replacing components or treating disorder.

8.2 Severe thrombocytopenia

- **About:** thrombocytopenia is platelet count <150 × 10⁹/L. Severe bleeding if count <20–50 × 10⁹/L, worsened by antiplatelets.
- **Pathophysiology:** platelets survive 7–10 days. 35% of all platelets are found in the spleen. Reaction to vessel wall injury is rapid adhesion of platelets to the subendothelium and formation of a haemostatic plug, composed primarily of platelets. This is further stabilised by a fibrin mesh generated in secondary haemostasis. Significant quantitative or qualitative platelet dysfunction results in mucocutaneous bleeding. Platelet count <20 × 10⁹/L can be associated with severe bleeding.
- **Aetiology:** platelets formed from developing megakaryocytes in the bone marrow. Low platelets can be due to a fall in production or increased consumption or sequestration. Platelet dysfunction with antiplatelets, drugs and diseases, e.g. uraemia.

Causes of low platelets

- **Sampling error:** platelet clumping can spuriously lower platelet count. Repeat if any doubt. It is evident on a peripheral smear by the presence of platelet clumps.
- **Acute idiopathic thrombocytopenic purpura (ITP):** all ages. Immune-mediated destruction of platelets/megakaryocytes due to the platelet GP IIb/IIIa complex. May be postviral or drug-induced. Rarely SLE or HIV. Treat with steroids (PREDNISOLONE 1 mg/kg) or other immunosuppression and IVIg and splenectomy if severe and persisting. Avoid platelets if possible. ITP in pregnancy can lead to fetal thrombocytopenia with neonatal intracranial haemorrhage. Other newer agents include Danazol, Eltrombopag, Rituximab, Romiplostim.
- **Chronic ITP:** adults with on-going thrombocytopenia. Insidious onset. Smear shows giant platelets.
- **Heparin-induced thrombocytopenic purpura (HIT/T):** on UFH or LMWH and develops thrombocytopenia and thrombosis. Stop all heparins. Confirmed by *in vitro* testing to detect **heparin-dependent platelet antibodies.** ▶ Section 8.3.
- **HUS/TTP:** Neurological involvement, renal failure and diarrhoea. ▶ Sections 8.6 and 8.7.
- **Pregnancy-related thrombocytopenia:** usually mild thrombocytopenia in an otherwise healthy pregnancy. May resemble a mild ITP. Infant does not develop thrombocytopenia.
- **Pre-eclampsia/eclampsia syndrome:** causes increased platelet turnover, even when the platelet count is normal. Controlling BP and delivering the fetus leads to restoration of the platelet count. ▶ Section 15.5.
- **HELLP syndrome:** sometimes thrombocytopenia is associated with haemolysis and ↑liver enzymes and low platelet (HELLP) syndrome. Treat BP and deliver fetus.
- **Post-transfusion purpura:** typically occurs 10 days following a transfusion.
- **Disseminated intravascular coagulation:** pathological thrombin generation. There is consumption of platelets with thrombosis and bleeding. Seen in those with other overwhelming pathology. ▶ Section 8.4.
- **Drug-induced thrombocytopenia:** drugs such as gold, ibuprofen, quinine, quinidine, methotrexate, amiodarone, valproate, cimetidine, captopril, carbamazepine, sulfonamides, glibenclamide, tamoxifen, ranitidine, phenytoin, vancomycin, piperacillin, cocaine.
- **Bone marrow failure:** malignancy, infiltration, myelodysplasia, marrow failure.
- **Severe fever with thrombocytopenia syndrome:** infectious disease with a 12% case-fatality rate in China due to a novel bunyavirus.
- **Dengue fever, HIV:** endemic area or in risk groups. HIV test, CD4 count, viral load. ▶ Sections 9.8 and 9.33.
- **SLE:** check ANA dsDNA. Look for classical signs and laboratory results.
- **Hypersplenism:** thrombocytopenia rarely below 40×10^9/L.
- **Platelet dysfunction:** platelet numbers normal. Aspirin, Clopidogrel, Prasugrel, Ticagrelor, uraemia, etc. all prolong bleeding time.

- **Clinical:** spontaneous petechiae, purpura, bleeding. Mouth may show evidence of bleeding. Check drug chart. Look for splenomegaly and lymph nodes, which may suggest a cause. Menorrhagia, epistaxis, haematuria.
- **Investigation: FBC:** ↓Hb, ↓platelets. If bleeding and platelets $>40 \times 10^9$/L look for exacerbating cause. **U&E:** ↑creatinine, check B12, folate, ferritin. **Blood film:** schistocytes, fragmented, deformed, irregular, or helmet-shaped RBCs suggests DIC. **Intravascular haemolysis:** ↑LDH, ↑reticulocytes, ↑bilirubin, ↓haptoglobin, Coomb's test negative. (HUS/TTP or uraemic platelet dysfunction). **Coagulation:** normal PT, APTT, D-dimer and fibrinogen levels. Increased bleeding time. Renal biopsy if HUS may be indicated to see degree and nature of kidney damage. ADAMTS13 levels of limited use.
- **Management:** treat cause: look for underlying sepsis, drugs, other causes, and treat. **Bleeding:** direct pressure. If bleeding and ↓count $<50 \times 10^9$/L then consider IV

platelet transfusion and treat cause. Use local physical methods/surgery to stem bleeding. VITAMIN K 5–10 mg IV or orally: if liver disease or VITAMIN K deficiency possible. Avoid NSAIDs, ASPIRIN, and CLOPIDOGREL, warfarin, heparins and DOACs. Augment good mouth care with TRANEXAMIC ACID mouthwashes added if there is bleeding from the oral mucosa. Consider TRANEXAMIC ACID 1 g PO 8 h. Do not give if there is on-going haematuria and/or DIC. Uraemia: consider omitting antiplatelets. Manage uraemia. Pre-eclampsia/eclampsia/HELLP: **BP control and fetal delivery.**

When to transfuse platelets

- **General advice:** The use of platelet transfusion to keep the count above 10×10^9/L reduces the risk of haemorrhage as effectively as a higher threshold. May replace to higher levels if patient has taken antiplatelets or has platelet dysfunction or need for surgery or bleeding. Take haematological advice. Must determine cause before transfusion and exclude TTP by examining blood film. Platelets not usually indicated for TTP/HUS/HIT syndromes. In acute ITP only used for real risk of or actual bleeding. The decision to transfuse should be supported by the need to prevent or treat bleeding. There may be a role for desmopressin in patients taking aspirin or uraemia.
- **Platelets ($\times 10^9$/L) and advice when to transfuse platelets: 0–10:** prophylactic transfusion. **10–20:** bleeding, fever, infection, platelet dysfunction, coagulopathy. **20–50:** prior to minor procedures or in actively anticoagulated patients or in the presence of active bleeding. **50–100:** sufficient for most invasive procedures, including gastroscopy and biopsy, insertion of indwelling lines, transbronchial biopsy, liver biopsy, laparotomy, or similar procedures. **50–75:** prior to general surgery/childbirth. **50–100:** prior to ophthalmic surgery or neurosurgery.

Reference: Lin & Foltz (2005) Proposed guidelines for platelet transfusion. *Br Columbia Med J*, 47:245.

8.3 Heparin-induced thrombocytopenia

- **About:** heparin-induced thrombocytopenia (HIT) + thrombosis (HITT). Heparin induces formation of antibodies with thrombosis and a fall in platelets. Consider HIT in any patient with ↓platelets on heparin started within past 5–10 days.
- **Types: Type I HIT** is a relatively common, non-immune, clinically innocuous and benign reaction. **Type II HIT** is a rare, immune-mediated, potentially serious form.
- **Aetiology:** formation of platelet-rich thrombosis 5–10 days after starting heparin therapy. Target antigen is a complex between heparin and platelet factor 4 (PF4). More common with UFH, rarer with LMWH. IgG activates platelets via their FcIIa receptors.
- **Clinical:** arterial thrombosis: limb, stroke, MI, PE, renal artery, mesenteric arteries. Skin necrosis at injection sites. Adrenal failure due to vein thrombosis and haemorrhagic necrosis. DVT and HIT can cause venous limb gangrene. Seen day 10 post-UFH.
- **The 4Ts pre-test probability score:** This can assist in determining if HIT is present. Generally, scores of less than 3 suggest the absence of HIT. Higher scores send ELISA for heparin/PF4 antibodies. Not included here for brevity but scoring can be found on www.mdcalc.com.
- **Investigations: FBC:** ↓platelets <150×10^9/L or ↓ by 30–50% after starting heparin therapy (the platelet count may still be normal). **U&E:** look for AKI. **Blood film:** fragmented RBCs. **Specific test: ELISA for heparin/PF4 antibodies.**
- **Management: stop all heparins** (UFH/LMWH/heparin line flushes) in suspected HIT. Urgent haematology advice should be sought. Replace with agents such as the thrombin inhibitor ARGATROBAN. DANAPAROID SODIUM may be used in those with a history of HIT. Also warfarin but needs additional anticoagulation in interim whilst loading as it is a prothrombotic state (protein C levels fall).

8.4 Disseminated intravascular coagulation

- **About:** seen in 1% of inpatients. Uncontrolled microvascular clotting consumes platelets and clotting factors. Coagulopathy leads to massive haemorrhage, organ failure. Dreadful prognosis. Some say DIC = 'death is coming'.
- **Aetiology:** endothelial disruption and other initiators lead to a procoagulant state. Formation of microvascular thrombi consumes clotting factors, fibrinogen and platelets. Microthrombi can cause organ dysfunction. Bleeding due to coagulopathy. In malignancy, DIC can be a more chronic process over weeks and months.
- **Clinical:** severe spontaneous bleeding and bruising in an unwell patient. Haemorrhagic shock due to bleeding from lines, GI tract, genitourinary tract, epistaxis. Spontaneous intracerebral haemorrhage, post-operative wound bleed. Bleeding may be hidden, e.g. retroperitoneal, psoas. See also Haemorrhagic shock, ▶Section 2.22.
- **Causes:** trauma and tissue damage, sepsis and septicaemic shock (Gram-negative). Malignancy, acute promyelocytic leukaemia/M3, massive transfusions. Obstetric emergencies (placental abruption, amniotic fluid embolism, eclampsia). Pancreatitis, vascular abnormalities, snake bites, recreational drugs. ABO transfusion incompatibility, transplant rejection, severe liver failure.
- **Differential:** ALF, HUS/TTP, HITT.
- **Investigations:** (*markers of severity) **FBC, blood film:** anaemia, ↓platelets, fragmented red cells. **U&E:** AKI, ↑LDH and evidence of haemolysis. **Coagulation screen:** ↑PT* (>6 s) and ↑APTT, ↑TT, ↓fibrinogen* (<1 g/L), ↓platelets* (50 × 10⁹/L). ↑↑FDPs* due to fibrinolysis (high).
- **Differential:** TTP, HUS, severe hypertension, pregnancy: pre-eclampsia, HELLP syndrome. Microangiopathic haemolytic anaemia.
- **Management: supportive care:** admit ITU. ABC, O₂. Care with central lines, coagulopathy. Find and treat the underlying cause. Involve haematology. **Clotting factors:** give VITAMIN K slow IV 10 mg stat. Replace clotting factors FFP, cryoprecipitate, platelets and red cell concentrates based on bleeding risk more than laboratory results. If there is a prolonged PT and APTT then consider FFP if ↑risk of bleed or procedure or active bleeding. If fibrinogen low (<1 g/L) despite FFP replacement, consider fibrinogen concentrate or cryoprecipitate. **Platelets:** platelet half-life is short and platelets only given for acute bleeding when less than 50 × 10⁹/L, or the need for a procedure and less than 50 × 10⁹/L. If not bleeding and platelets low, consider transfusing when bleed risk high, e.g. platelets 10–20 × 10⁹/L. Take advice if unsure. **Treatment targets:** platelets >50 × 10⁹/L, fibrinogen >1 g/L, Hb >80 g/L, PT and APTT <1.5× normal. IV HEPARIN: may rarely be used to reduce the clotting. Indications include arterial or venous thromboembolism, severe purpura fulminans with acral ischaemia or vascular skin infarction. It should possibly not be stopped if patient already on it. Avoid IV TRANEXAMIC ACID except where there is severe bleeding and a hyperfibrinolytic state. One can augment mouth care with oral TRANEXAMIC ACID solution as a mouthwash which can help reduce oozing from friable oral mucosa.

Reference: British Committee for Standards in Haematology (2009) Guidelines for the diagnosis and management of DIC. *Br J Haematol*, 145:24.

8.5 Sickle cell crisis

- **About:** chronic haemolytic anaemia. Abnormal Hb first described by Linus Pauling in 1946. Commoner in black patients but may also affect other groups. Homozygous inheritance of HbSS or HbSC. Most painful crises are managed at home.

- **Aetiology:** HbSS contains 2 defective β-globin chains due to a Valine to Glutamate substitution on the β6 position. Structural change and HbS polymerisation and sickling at low O_2 tensions. HbAS: symptoms with extreme hypoxia (sickle cell trait).
- **Acute crises seen with HbSS:** (sickle cell anaemia) HbSS who only have HbS. HbSC: HbS and HbC from either parent. HbS–βO: sickle cell + β-thalassaemia.
- **Clinical:** crises triggered by infections and other illness or hypoxia. Usually severe chest/bone/back/limb/abdominal pain and anaemia. Anaemia from shortened RBC half-life needs transfusion but cost is iron overload.

Complications
- Haemolytic anaemia, aplastic crises, lung fibrosis, stroke, hepatosplenomegaly.
- *Salmonella* osteomyelitis, sickling crisis, avascular necrosis of the hips, HiB infection.
- Renal failure, renal concentrating defects, renal papillary necrosis.
- Priapism – sequestration of red cells in corpus cavernosum.
- Acute chest syndrome due to pneumococcal pneumonia, lung infarction or fat embolism, bleeding in anterior chamber of eye (hyphaema).
- Osteoporosis: vertebral collapse, avascular necrosis of femoral head or dactylitis or swollen joints, skin ulcers, pigment gallstones, splenic infarction – autosplenectomy.
- Stroke – seen mainly in children (see below).

Investigations
- **FBC:** ↓Hb 60–90 g/L, ↑retics. **Blood film:** sickled RBC, target cells, polychromasia.
- **U&E, LFT, LDH, CRP. CXR, ABG,** ECG, troponin and D-dimer if SOB/chest pain.
- **Exclude infection:** blood/urine cultures and CXR. USS abdomen.
- **Sickle solubility test:** positive in disease and trait.
- **Hb electrophoresis** 80–95% HbSS and no HbA.
- **Cross-match** if symptoms severe and transfusion needed. Close matching of blood is needed to reduce antibody formation.

Acute general management (consult with haematology early)
- **Supportive:** most painful crises are self-managed in the community with NSAIDs/paracetamol. Admission for uncontrolled pain or suspicion of complications. ABC, O_2 as per BTS guidelines. Eat and drink freely as able. If not able to take oral fluids then IV fluids to maintain good hydration.
- **Analgesia:** pain is often the dominating symptom and reason for admission. Offer analgesia within 30 min of presentation if needed. Avoid pethidine. Mild pains try PARACETAMOL 1 g 8 h and IBUPROFEN 400–600 mg 8 h or DICLOFENAC 50 mg TDS PO. If severe pains then in addition to NSAID give IV MORPHINE repeated until pain free, usually with an antiemetic e.g. CYCLIZINE 50 mg PO/IM/IV. Consider continuous infusion pump or patient controlled anaesthesia. Add a laxative e.g. SENNA 15 mg PO and/or LACTULOSE 10–20 ml. HYDROXYZINE 25 mg 12 h may be given for itch. HALOPERIDOL 1–3 mg PO/IM for anxiety.
- **Exchange blood transfusion:** Basically venesect and transfuse (e.g. 6 units in and 6 units out). Emergency indications are acute ischaemic stroke, multiple organ failure, acute chest syndrome, hepatic sequestration. Outcome for acute chest syndrome improved. Replacement of sickle cells by normal cells can help prevent further vaso-occlusion, although pre-existing vaso-occlusion may not be reversed. The goal for acute stroke and acute chest syndrome is a HbS under 30% (for patients with SCD-SS) while keeping the Hb less than 10.
- **LMWH:** VTE prophylaxis may reduce the length of stay of patients with an acute painful sickle cell episode.
- **HYDROXYCARBAMIDE (HYDROXYUREA):** raises HbF, reduces crisis by 50% so consider in all with severe disease.
- **FOLATE** – ensure supplementation given.

- **PROPHYLAXIS:** hyposplenism consider PENICILLIN 500 mg OD PO prophylaxis and pneumococcal/Hib vaccination.
- **Allogeneic bone marrow transplantation.** Curative with success in 90–95%. Usually from matched siblings. Requires myeloablative therapy. Outcome excellent.
- **Pregnancy:** screen pregnant patients. Acute care is the same. Transfuse to reduce proportion of HbS and so sickling crises. Liaise with obstetric team.

Specific syndromes

- **Acute chest syndrome:** chest pain, cough, fever, CXR infiltrates (may appear late), hypoxia. Precipitated by excess opiates/PE/fat embolism/microvascular infarction/ infection or fluid overload. Give O_2 as per BTS guidance. Bronchodilators for wheeze. Consider CPAP with escalation to ITU admission and ventilation if unable to keep PO_2 >8 kPa despite an FiO_2 of 0.6. May need a CTPA and anticoagulation if PE suspected. Take haematology advice and ITU help early. Antibiotics and antivirals if H1N1 suspected. May be prevented using incentive spirometry. Consider blood/ exchange transfusion. Need antibiotic coverage which also covers atypical, e.g. CO-AMOXICLAV and CLARITHROMYCIN. Penicillin-allergic – CEFTRIAXONE 1–2 g 12 h and CLARITHROMYCIN. May develop pulmonary arterial hypertension. Screen with transthoracic echo. PAH associated with increased mortality. Treat with hydroxyurea, chronic transfusions, oxygen. Consider prostacyclin and bosentan, and sildenafil.
- **(Splenic) sequestration crisis:** painful rapidly enlarging liver/spleen due to occluded organ venous outflow. In children the spleen is involved. Severe anaemia, ↓BP and fatal. In adults the liver more affected with severe RUQ pain and liver enlargement. Treat with good IV hydration, O_2, analgesia and blood transfusion. Exchange transfusion may be warranted. Treat infection. Rare in adults except with haemoglobin SC disease or SB + thalassaemia.
- **Aplastic crisis:** temporary red cell aplasia due to infection by parvovirus B19. Low Hb and ↓reticulocyte count. Supportive management.
- **Priapism:** penile venous outflow obstructed with a sustained painful erection. Can result in impotence. Treatment is ice, IV hydration, analgesia, transfusion if needed and urology referral. Injected α-blocker. May settle with conservative therapy.
- **Renal:** tubular necrosis and haematuria and potential urinary obstruction. Damage to collecting ducts can lead to impaired concentrating ability and dehydration. Nephritic syndrome and chronic kidney disease can develop.
- **Sickle cell stroke:** children/young adults. Transfuse to reduce the sickle fraction to <30%. Screen children with transcranial doppler. If high velocity flow should receive a preventative transfusion regimen. This has a 90% absolute risk reduction of first stroke.
- **Avascular necrosis of the femoral and humeral heads.** Adults. Plain films show advanced changes. MRI gold standard diagnostic tool. Needs analgesia and steroid joint injections, and some may need joint replacement.

References: Howard *et al.* (2015) Guideline on the management of acute chest syndrome in sickle cell disease. *Br J Haematol*, 169:492. NICE (2012) CG143: Sickle cell acute painful episode: Management of an acute painful sickle cell episode in hospital.

8.6 Haemolytic uraemic syndrome

- **About:** children with diarrhoeal illness and AKI (D+). May also be seen in adults without a diarrhoeal illness (D–). There is intravascular haemolysis and a microangiopathic haemolytic anaemia and AKI. Unlike DIC the coagulation tests are normal in HUS/TTP. Avoid antibiotics with *E. coli* 0157:H7 as it may precipitate HUS.
- **Aetiology: children:** AKI due to verocytotoxin-producing *E. coli*, e.g. *E. coli* strain 0157:H7.60. **Adults:** drugs that damage endothelial cells. Familial (congenital) HUS – deficiency of factor H, a plasma protein synthesised by the liver, which regulates the complement pathway.

- **Pathophysiology:** ADAMTS13 is a protease which breaks down clumps of vWF factor and deficiency can stimulate thrombosis and cause TTP/HUS without diarrhoea (D–). Toxin causes endothelial cell damage and renal microvascular thrombosis. Platelet aggregation causes consumptive thrombocytopenia. Microangiopathic haemolytic anaemia as RBCs circulate through partially occluded microcirculation.

Classification of haemolytic uraemic syndrome

- **Typical (D+) HUS involves diarrhoea**. Mainly children. Single episode. Normal ADAMTS13 levels. *E. coli* strain 0157:H7. Verocytotoxin (shiga toxin 1/2). New strain *E. coli* O104:H4 with high rate of complications. Toxins damage endothelium. Infective cause as 95% of cases of HUS in children and infants.
- **Atypical (D–) aHUS no diarrhoea:** many, unknown aetiology. *Strep pneumoniae* accounts for 40% of aHUS all ages. Recurrent episodes. Low ADAMTS13 levels. Inherited defect in complement levels. Drugs – mitomycin C, ticlopidine, ciclosporin, tacrolimus, quinine, chemotherapy. Congenital, malignancies – prostate, gastric, pancreatic, scleroderma, SLE/APLS. Often severe, with respiratory, neurology, coma; the mortality rate is 12%. Genetic – several genes detected.

Clinical

- **Diarrhoea +ve HUS:** haematuria, proteinuria, oliguria, gastroenteritis, bloody diarrhoea usually in children.
- **Diarrhoea –ve HUS atypical HUS:** AKI, illness (HIV, *Strep.*), genetics, drugs.
- **Both:** Red/brown urine, petechial rash (low platelets), malaise, hypertension, uraemia. Jaundice, easy bruising and pallor from anaemia.

Investigations

- **FBC:** ↓Hb <8 g/dL, ↓platelets. **U&E:** ↑creatinine. **LFTs:** ↑bilirubin (haemolysis).
- **Blood film:** schistocytes, fragmented, deformed, irregular, or helmet-shaped RBCs.
- **Intravascular haemolysis:** ↑LDH, ↑reticulocytes, ↓haptoglobin.
- **Coagulation:** normal PT, APTT, D-dimer, fibrinogen. **Coomb's test** negative.
- **Stool samples:** will be cultured for *E. coli* 0157:H7 and *E. coli* O104:H4.
- **Kidney biopsy** may be indicated to see degree and nature of kidney damage.
- **ADAMTS13** levels normal in diarrhoea +ve disease. Low in aHUS.
- **Others:** ANA, dsDNA, HIV test.

Management of HUS (urgent renal/haem consult)

- **Diarrhoea +ve:** children. Avoid antibiotics, antimotility agents, NSAIDs with *E. coli* 0157:H7 as can precipitate HUS and worsen severity. Avoid platelet transfusions. Transfer to renal unit or ITU. Dialysis in 50%. 85% can go on to make a full recovery. Manage hypertension, Input/Output, anaemia, K. Daily plasma exchange (plasmapheresis + FFP replacement) is treatment of choice. Other agents: unresponsive cases have been treated with VINCRISTINE or CICLOSPORIN A. No role for steroids. Children often recover completely. Irreversible renal damage and death in more severe cases. AKI, ▶ Section 10.4.
- **Atypical (no diarrhoea) aHUS:** prognosis worse. Therapy is directed mainly towards underlying cause. Initial mortality 10–15% and 70% go on to End stage renal failure. Consider plasmapheresis. Consider ECULIZUMAB (Soliris) which binds terminal complement C5. NICE and the FDA approved use but very expensive. Improves platelet count, reduces thrombotic episodes and maintains or improves kidney function. Main side effects are headache and leukopenia. Congenital disease may need liver transplant.
- **Avoid plasmapheresis** with HUS post *Strep. pneumoniae*.

References: Kavanagh & Goodship (2011) Atypical hemolytic uremic syndrome, genetic basis, and clinical manifestations. *ASH Education Book*, 15. NICE (2015) HST1: Eculizumab for treating atypical haemolytic uraemic syndrome.

8.7 Thrombotic thrombocytopenic purpura

- **About:** activation and consumption of platelets, vessel occlusion, microangiopathic anaemia. Neurological events. Plasmapheresis improves outcome.
- **Aetiology:** inhibition or congenital/acquired lack of ADAMTS13 increases platelet adhesion to endothelium by vWF. Causes thrombosis, platelet consumption.
- **Causes:** low ADAMTS13, acquired due to antibodies to ADAMTS13. Ticlopidine, clopidogrel, ciclosporin, OCP, pregnancy, SLE, HIV, hepatitis.
- **Pathophysiology:** platelet activation causes cerebral renal/gut microvascular thrombosis. Platelet aggregation and a consumptive thrombocytopenia. RBCs damaged passing through partially occluded microcirculation.
- **Differential:** DIC (coagulopathy), drugs, e.g. quinine, simvastatin, interferon, and calcineurin inhibitors, malignant hypertension, viral infections, CMV, autoimmune disease (lupus nephritis, acute scleroderma), vasculitis, HUS (diarrhoea positive/negative), malignancy, catastrophic APLS.
- **Clinical:** anaemia, fever. Thrombosis: phlebitis with superficial vein thrombosis. Thrombotic stroke, delirium, coma, cardiac/gut/renal ischaemia/infarction. Bleeding, e.g. mucosal, petechiae, purpura and bruising may be seen.

Investigation

- **FBC:** ↓Hb <8 g/dL, ↓platelets. **Clotting:** normal PT, APTT, D-dimer, fibrinogen.
- **Blood film:** microangiopathic haemolytic anaemia (MAHA) with schistocytes. Fragmented, deformed, irregular, or helmet-shaped RBCs.
- **Intravascular haemolysis:** ↑LDH, ↑reticulocytes, ↑bilirubin, ↓haptoglobin.
- **U&E:** ↑creatinine ↑K. **Kidney biopsy** may be indicated.
- **ADAMTS13 levels** low but wide variation of normal.
- **Renal CT/MRI** may show areas of infarction.
- **Serology:** HIV (+CD4 count), HAV, HBV, HCV. CT brain (if neurological signs).
- **CT chest/abdomen/pelvis** to check for underlying malignancy (if indicated).
- **Pregnancy test** where appropriate.

Management (urgent haem consult and transfer to tertiary centre)

- **Medical emergency**. High risk of preventable, early deaths in TTP. Needs plasma exchange as soon as possible, preferably within 4–8 h. May need immediate transfer to specialist haematology centre that offers PLEX.
- **High volume total plasmapheresis (PLEX)** reduces 3 month mortality from 90% to almost 15%. Removes circulating antibody and ↑ADAMTS13. Replace total plasma volume daily (some replace 1.5 × plasma volume). Low BP seen in those on ACE inhibitors. After PLEX consider steroids; either IV METHYLPREDNISOLONE 1 g/day for 3 days or oral PREDNISOLONE 1 mg/kg/day with an oral PPI.
- **HIV positive**, then consider starting HAART.
- If CNS/Cardiac involvement, start RITUXIMAB.
- **Platelets** avoided generally as can cause thrombosis. Take specialist advice if active bleeding and low platelets. Watch daily bloods for response. Relapses may require steroids, RITUXIMAB or other immunosuppressive agents and splenectomy. Red cells given as needed for anaemia. Give FOLATE 5 mg OD. Low dose ASPIRIN 75 mg OD started once platelets >50 × 10⁹/L. Long term avoid quinine and oestrogen-containing medications which can cause relapse.

Reference: Scully *et al.* (2012) Guidelines on the diagnosis and management of TTP and other thrombotic microangiopathies. *Br J Haematol*, 158:323.

8.8 Bleeding disorders and reversal of anticoagulation

- **About:** the body tries to maintain a constant balance of clot formation and breakdown. We produce prothrombotic as well as antithrombotic factors. Effective haemostasis requires vessel endothelial integrity, platelets, clotting factors as part of the coagulation cascade, vWF and fibrinogen.
- **Coagulation cascade:** two systems which function together to ultimately produce nets of fibrin. Extrinsic is initiated by tissue factor, a molecule found on smooth muscle, fibroblasts. Exposure-activated Factor VIIa forms Factors IXa and Xa. Alternative contact pathway involves formation of XIIa by high molecular weight kininogens and calcium. This activates XI to XIa, which forms Xa and then IX to IXa. This forms VIIIa which activates X to Xa which is the common focal point. Factor Xa converts prothrombin to thrombin and thrombin cleaves fibrinogen to fibrin which forms on the surface of platelets.
- **Platelets:** damage to vascular endothelium causes localised vasoconstriction and platelet activation. Platelet adhesion to damaged endothelium requires vWF.
- **Presentation:** bleeding may be obvious or occult with evidence of shock. It may be more chronic with progressive anaemia. Inherited conditions. There may be a long standing history of excess bleeding, e.g. with challenges such as dental extraction, circumcision and other surgery, menstruation, etc. Current bleeding – bruising, petechiae. GI – melena, PR bleeding, retroperitoneal. Renal – haematuria, Mucosal – epistaxis or from gums, bleeding into joints or intracerebral haemorrhage.
- **Investigations:** FBC: MCV may show anaemia, thrombocytopenia and low ferritin. PT (tissue factor and VII to VIIa) and APTT (XIIa/XIa, IXa), ↑D-dimers in DIC, ↑APTT with haemophilia A/B. ↑PT in vitamin K deficiency/warfarin and liver disease. Individual factors can be assayed as needed.

Clinical actions

- **Platelet disorders** – qualitative and quantitative defects. Thrombocytopenia is covered elsewhere. Antiplatelet agents, e.g. aspirin, clopidogrel. NSAIDs. Impaired function – uraemia, liver disease, acquired von Willebrand disease, cancer. New drugs – Prasugrel, Ticagrelor.
- **Drug-induced bleeding:** warfarin, heparin and DOACs covered below.
- **Consumptive coagulopathy:** inappropriate activation of coagulation system with ↓platelets, ↓fibrinogen (see DIC, ▶ Section 8.4).
- **von Willebrand disease:** seen in 1–2% population on testing but fewer clinically ever have problems. vWF binds platelets and endothelium and it also carries Factor VIII. Different forms mean that vWF can be reduced or simply faulty. Mucosal bleeding is main issue. Nose bleeds, menorrhagia. Can treat with TRANEXAMIC ACID 25 mg/kg TDS or DESMOPRESSIN. Severe bleeding Factor VIII and vWF concentrates may be given. Most are autosomal dominant, potentially mild to moderately severe. Test: ↓vWF antigen, ↓ristocetin cofactor activity, and in some ↓Factor XIII.
- **Haemophilia A/B:** haem A is commonest form. Lack of Factor VIII or IX, respectively. Clinically identical. Half of haem A have *de novo* mutations with unaffected parents. Affects males – X-linked recessive. Can be mild/moderate/severe. Treat with recombinant factors. Suffer from bleeding into joints, or related to minor traumas or post-surgery.

Bleeding while anticoagulated

- A careful balance must be struck if anticoagulation is important. The risk of death from active haemorrhage usually outweighs risk of lack of anticoagulation acutely and achieving haemostasis should be the priority in the first 24 h.
- Take advice with metal valves and stents. Simple actions such as pressure and surgical ligation and even radiological embolisation can assist in controlling bleeding. 'Bleeding comes first'. Risk of further PE can be reduced with IVC filter without a need to anticoagulate.

8.9 Bleeding on warfarin

Clinical	Escalation actions – omit warfarin dose, oral vitamin K, IV vitamin K, FFP, PCC
Life, limb or sight-threatening (intra-ocular not sub-conjunctival) haemorrhage on warfarin	High risk patients: age >70; hypertension; diabetes; renal failure; previous MI, stroke or GI bleed. ABC, stop warfarin, get IV access and resuscitate depending on bleeding source. Check INR, FBC, LFTs and give 5–10 mg vitamin K IV over 2–3 min. If INR 2–6 give OCTAPLEX 25 units/kg. If INR >6 or intracerebral bleed on warfarin give OCTAPLEX 50 units/kg stat by slow IV infusion. Maximum dose of 3000 units. If Octaplex not available give FFP 15 ml/kg (approximately 1 L in an adult). Repeat FBC and coagulation screen immediately after infusion and at regular intervals until stable.
Major, non-life-threatening haemorrhage on warfarin	Stop warfarin. Take bloods. Give vitamin K 2–5 mg IV. Consider FFP 15 ml/kg followed by repeat tests as above. Discuss with Haem need for PCC.
Less severe haemorrhage on warfarin	Withhold warfarin for 1 or more days and re-start at reduced dose when INR <5.0. Consider vitamin K 1–2 mg IV/PO.
INR >8.0 no bleeding	Stop warfarin and give VITAMIN K 1–5 mg PO or 0.5 mg IV. A 10 mg oral dose or 2 mg IV dose can be given if no further oral anticoagulation is required. If further anticoagulation required, re-start warfarin at reduced dose when INR <5.0.
INR 5.0–8.0 no bleeding	Consider 1 mg PO vitamin K. Repeat INR next day. Withhold warfarin for 1–2 days and review. Re-start at reduced dose when INR <5.0. Discuss with Haem if metal valve.

8.10 Bleeding on heparin

Bleeding on unfractionated heparin (UFH)

- As heparin has a half-life of <2 h, it is usually sufficient to stop the infusion. If bleeding is severe, reverse anticoagulation with PROTAMINE 1 mg per 80–100 units of heparin when given within 15 min of heparin.
- Give protamine at a rate not exceeding 5 mg/min, not more than 50 mg at one time. Halve protamine dose if heparin infusion has been stopped for 1 h, quarter dose if stopped for 2 h. Repeat treatment is rarely necessary. Discuss with haematology.

Bleeding on low molecular weight heparin (LMWH)

- Peak effect of LMWH is at 3–4 hours post dose and falls to a low level after 12 h. If bleeding is severe during the 12 h after a dose of SC LMWH, reverse anticoagulation with IV protamine sulphate as follows. Take blood for anti-Xa assay, coagulation screen and FBC.
- 1 mg PROTAMINE per 100 units heparin. Give 25–50 mg protamine IV infusion at 5 mg/min. Give remainder of the calculated protamine dose slow IV infusion over 8–16 h. The total dose will depend on the time since the injection and the nature of the bleed. Repeat treatment is rarely necessary. Discuss with haematology.

8.11 Bleeding on direct oral anticoagulants

- **About:** new anticoagulants tend to have a higher incidence of GI bleed than traditional therapy, but this varies based on indication of therapy and needs further evaluation to clarify risk [*Gastroenterology*, 2013;145:105].
- **General:** evaluate any signs or symptoms of blood loss. If there is active pathological bleeding stop the drug and any additional anti-thrombotics. Consider local pressure, surgical haemostasis, Group and cross-match. Volume replacement, or blood products. Consider TRANEXAMIC ACID 1 g bolus over 10 min, followed by 1 g slow IV 8 h. Red cell transfusion: aim for Hb >7 g/dL. Platelet transfusion: aim for platelets $>50 \times 10^9$ or if CNS bleed aim for $>100 \times 10^9$. Life-threatening, haematologist may advise prothrombin complex concentrate (PCC: Octaplex/ Beriplex) 25–50 IU/kg bolus dose (maximum dose 3000 IU) but data on clinical efficacy is not available. Always discuss with haematology as changing guidance.
- **Dabigatran:** check APTT to estimate exposure. Dabigatran is dialysable. Half can be cleared from plasma over 4 h. Check FBC/U&E. The $t_{1/2}$ is 12–17 h and increases with renal impairment. Antidote is PRAXBIND/IDARUCIZUMAB IV infusion as one split dose of 5 g (two vials of 2.5 g each).
- **Rivaroxaban:** as above. Check FBC/U&Es. If INR (neoplastin) and/or Xa ↑ then effects remain. Consider using IV PCC as above on advice of a haematologist. Not dialysable. Maintain BP and urine output to aid excretion. A new antidote Andexanet-alfa is being trialled.
- **Apixaban:** as above. Coagulation screen (determine time of last dose). Check FBC and U&Es. If Xa ↑ then effects remain. Consider using IV PCC as above on advice of a haematologist. Maintain BP and urine output to aid excretion. Andexanet-alfa may also have a role but is currently undergoing trials.

8.12 Bleeding on/after thrombolysis

- **About:** Alteplase is used for stroke, PE and cardiac thrombolysis and some other indications. Always monitor for bleeding.
- **Intracranial:** suspect bleed if fall in GCS, headache, new seizure, ↑NIHSS, acute hypertension, N&V, pupillary changes. STOP ALTEPLASE or other agent and CT SCAN. If bleed seen resuscitate and give CRYOPRECIPITATE 10 units or 2–4 units FFP with a target fibrinogen level of 1 g/L. TRANEXAMIC ACID may also be considered. Neurosurgical consult as indicated.
- **Extracranial:** suspect if there is a fall in BP, rise in HR, shock, epistaxis, melena, haematuria, haematemesis, abdominal pain and bruising or pain in flanks or thighs. Appropriate referral, e.g. ENT for persisting epistaxis, gastroenterology for melena, haematemesis, etc. *Immediately stop infusion of ALTEPLASE or other agent.* Use direct pressure if possible to control bleeding from arterial or venous puncture sites. Check fibrinogen, PT, APTT, FBC and cross-match and transfusion as needed. Low fibrinogen can be replaced by CRYOPRECIPITATE 10 units or 2–4 units FFP with a target fibrinogen level of 1 g/L. TRANEXAMIC ACID may also be considered.

8.13 Blood transfusion and blood products

- Risk of death is 3 in 1 million transfusions. Infection transmission is rare. Most deaths now tend to occur from transfusion-associated circulatory overload (TACO). Red cell needs are falling but platelets and plasma rises. Helped by using TRANEXAMIC acid in major traumatic haemorrhage and studies show a restrictive policy with respect to red cell transfusion in critical care and surgical patient is safe.
- There is increasing recognition of the lack of a precise trigger point but that this should reflect the patient's clinical needs and quality of life and symptomatology.

Important issues are to ensure that transfusion is necessary, the right blood, right patient, right time and right place and the right amount. Use only if benefits outweigh risks. Ensure informed consent of risks of blood and alternatives considered. Indications must always be recorded. Transfusion must never happen if there is any uncertainty about identity. Monitoring is vital. Never give Rh –ve or Kell –ve girls or fertile females Rh +ve or Kell +ve blood as they develop IgG anti-D antibodies which may cause haemolytic anaemia of the newborn.

- Whole blood is rarely used and instead individual products are used so 'blood' transfusion is a misnomer. It's a 'blood product' transfusion. Determine which product best fits the clinical need. Blood stocks come from unpaid altruistic donors and are tested for HBsAg, anti-HIV1/HIV2, anti-HCV, anti HTLV-1 and 2, syphilis antibodies. CMV may be tested to deliver stocks of CMV negative blood. May also be tested for serology to malaria, West Nile Virus and *Trypanosoma cruzi*. Those at risk of CJD are excluded from donor pool. Blood products are red cells, platelets, FFP and cryoprecipitate. Plasma comes only come from males to reduce TRALI and derivatives include albumin, IVIg, coagulation factors. ABO compatibility is desirable for FFP and cryoprecipitate but not for plasma. No need to worry about rhesus or irradiation.

8.14 Which blood/plasma product?

- **Red cell concentrates**. For bleeding/anaemia. Find and treat underlying cause. Red cells are needed for oxygen delivering capacity but due to low levels of DPG this can take several days to optimize. It is thought that transfusion in non-haemorrhagic anaemia may not be needed until Hb <70–80 g/L. Severe sepsis, traumatic brain injury or brain ischaemia, consider if <90 g/L. Consider for chronic anaemia (sickle cell, marrow disease, etc.) if Hb <70–80 g/L, though the exact threshold for transfusion depends on symptoms and context. In the setting of acute bleeding the Hb may be an unreliable indicator of need for transfusion. <30% loss (1500 ml adult) then replace with crystalloid, 30–40% crystalloid + red cell concentrates, >40% (2000 ml) rapid replacement with red cells. Blood with plasma and as many leucocytes removed as possible (reduces risk of vCJD) and an additive solution added. Stored at 4°C. Laboratory need to ensure ABO and rhesus compatibility. A bag of packed cells lasts 35 days and is kept refrigerated at 4°C. Volume is between 220 and 320 ml and should raise Hb by 10 g/L. Risks of infection, TACO, transfusion reactions, etc.

- **Platelets:** platelet function is reduced by drugs such as aspirin, ticlopidine, clopidogrel, abciximab, tirofiban, prasugrel, and ticagrelor, and systemic disease, e.g. renal failure. Platelet count can be a poor estimate of platelet functional activity. Each bag contains 300×10^9/L platelets in 300 ml and raises count by $20–30 \times 10^9$/L. **Indications:** any cause of severe thrombocytopenia with risk of bleeding. Avoid in HITT and TTP. Usually avoided in ITP. Use when platelet count $<10 \times 10^9$/L or when $<20 \times 10^9$/L and risks such as sepsis or bleeding. Pre-procedure (LP, biopsy/central line) then a level of 50×10^9/L should be aimed for. 80×10^9/L before spinal epidural and over 100×10^9/L prior to brain or eye surgery. Massive surgery then maintains levels $>75–100 \times 10^9$/L. Use in ITP if haemorrhage or need for surgery to get levels $>80 \times 10^9$/L. Rhesus compatibility and ABO compatibility: ABO compatible platelets are more effective. Side effects: include all those seen with a blood transfusion. One therapeutic dose for adults.

- **Fresh frozen plasma (15 ml/kg typical dose).** For acquired coagulation deficiencies. Stored at –25°C. Plasma derivative. Contains stable components of the coagulation, fibrinolytic and complement systems, proteins that maintain oncotic pressure and modulate immunity and others. **Indications:** used for single/multiple clotting factor deficiencies, acute DIC with bleeding, TTP with plasma exchange, or for inherited coagulation deficiencies undergoing major surgery, major haemorrhage in a ratio of 0.5–1 unit FFP per unit of red cells aiming for a PT and APTT ratio of <1.5 and a fibrinogen level of >1.5 g/L. Dose: **FFP 15 ml/kg body weight equivalent to four units for an adult).** For warfarin reversal (use only if PCC unavailable). **SE:** Reactions can include all those seen with a blood transfusion.

- **Cryoprecipitate.** Used for DIC and low fibrinogen and bleeding, is a plasma derivative from FFP and contains 100 IU of Factor VIII (missing with haemophilia A) and 250 mg of fibrinogen, vWF, Factor XIII and fibronectin. Used originally for haemophilia. Used with FFP unless isolated deficiency of fibrinogen. **Indications:** DIC with bleeding and a fibrinogen level <1.5 g/L, advanced liver disease, to correct bleeding or as prophylaxis before surgery, when the fibrinogen level <1.5g/L, bleeding associated with thrombolytic therapy causing low fibrinogen, renal failure or liver failure associated with abnormal bleeding where DDAVP is contraindicated or ineffective. Inherited hypofibrinogenaemia, where fibrinogen concentrate is not available. **SE:** Reactions can include all those seen with a blood transfusion. Dose: two pooled units, equivalent to ten donor units, for an adult (contains 3 g of fibrinogen).

- **Low levels of Ig:** IVIg for treatment of ITP and GBS.

- **Severe low albumin:** human albumin solution (HAS) is a plasma derivative. No cross-matching needed. Isotonic forms 50–500 ml of 4.5–5% used in burns, pancreatitis, trauma or plasma exchange. Concentrated amount of 20% 50–100 ml in nephrotic syndrome, liver cirrhosis, removal of ascites.

- **Warfarin reversal: prothrombin complex concentrates (PCC):** use for immediate reversal of warfarin (or equivalent) induced bleeding. It is a combination of blood clotting Factors II, VII, IX and X, as well as protein C and S. It is used to reverse the effect of warfarin rapidly reducing INR to 1.0. See *Section 22.3* for the Drug formulary.

Reference: Norfolk (ed.) and the UK Blood Services (2013) Indication codes for transfusion. In: *Handbook of Transfusion Medicine* 5e.

8.15 Cross-matching

- Blood transfusion has significant risks as well as benefits. The report *Serious Hazards of Transfusion* (SHOT) continues to highlight potentially fatal mistakes in the administration of blood. Follow your hospital policy on pre-transfusion sample collection, which should detail who can collect samples. Do not use addressograph labels to label blood samples for cross-matching.

- **Vital steps:** identify patient in whom a cross-match sample is indicated. Prepare kit and bring to bedside – do not pre-label bottle yet. Identify patient by asking name and DOB and check with wristband; take blood at bedside and label and date and sign the sample. Only cross-match and bleed one patient at a time to minimise the risk of error. Label the sample immediately at the bedside after taking the blood, before leaving the patient.

- **Never prelabel sample tubes.** Labelling of request: last name, first name(s) in full, DOB (not age or year of birth), NHS number or address or other unique patient identifier, reason for the request. Labelling of sample tubes: patient last and first name in full, NHS number or other unique patient identification number, DOB (not age or year of birth), date and time of collection, signature or initials of the collector. As the sample collector you must sign the request form and the sample label to verify patient identification. Check identity by asking the patient to state and spell his or her name, and check the wrist band and check that the request form and sample match the patient and wrist band. If not possible, e.g. coma or confused then check identity with spouse or carer at the bedside and then check wristband. Transfusion monitoring: pulse, BP, temp and RR every 15 min and most transfusions can be given over 90–120 min. Observation continued for additional 60 min.

References: British Committee for Standards in Haematology (1999) The administration of blood and blood components and the management of transfused patients. *Transfusion Med*, 9:227. Norfolk (ed.) and the UK Blood Services (2013) *Handbook of Transfusion Medicine* 5e.

8.16 Acute transfusion reactions

- **Febrile non-haemolytic** (temp >38°C, can be seen with blood, FFP, platelets): febrile non-haemolytic reactions are usually clinically mild. If unsure, slow blood and observe patient over minutes. If worsening or any haemodynamic compromise, then stop transfusion and start crystalloid and take senior advice. Minor symptoms are not uncommon. Check the name and the bag and ensure no identification errors. Seen in 1% of transfusions. Check correct patient/transfusion. Restart about 30 min of observations. Slow transfusion, paracetamol, continue if settles. Due to pyrogens and leucocyte antibodies.
- **Allergic transfusion reactions** (with blood, FFP, platelets): can range from urticaria to anaphylaxis. Urticarial: check correct patient/transfusion. Consider CHLORPHENAMINE 10 mg IV/IM. Continue if settles. Mucosal swelling: consider checking IgA levels. Anaphylaxis: stop transfusion, treat as for anaphylaxis with 1 L NS IV and HYDROCORTISONE 200 mg IV. Consider ADRENALINE 0.5 ml of 1 in 1000 IM. May occur with IgA deficiency being exposed to IgA. Consider checking IgA levels. Check mast cell tryptase immediately and at 3 and 24 h. Get a CXR if dyspnoea. Anaphylaxis, ▶ Section 2.18.
- **ABO incompatibility (with blood, rarely with platelets and FFP):** even 30 ml of Type A to group O can be fatal. Keep the implicated blood unit. Transfused red cell antigen meeting recipient's anti-A and/or -B antibodies rapidly leads to complement-mediated haemolysis to DIC, AKI and haemoglobinuria/aemia. Acutely unwell, tachycardic and ↓BP and progressively worse. Fever, chills, pain, flushed face, vomiting, diarrhoea all due to complement fragments. If transfusion reaction, stop blood. Take full bloods from patient and repeat cross-match. Direct antiglobin test, LDH, haptoglobin. Coagulation screen. Start IV NS. Give ADRENALINE IM if anaphylaxis. Consider FUROSEMIDE IV to initiate diuresis. Discuss with ITU. Discuss with haematologist. Keep opened unit and any unused units and return to lab for checking. If ↓BP, oliguria and anuria may cause AKI and need FUROSEMIDE IV. ABO incompatibility has 10% mortality. Extravascular lysis is milder with fever and chills and is usually delayed with anaemia and jaundice and usually due to anti-D. Check all bloods and coagulation screen. Commonest cause is mislabelling pre-transfusion samples and failures in identity checking. There is only a 30% risk of ABO incompatibility reactions so errors may go undetected.
- **Bacterial contamination:** commoner with platelets as stored at 20–24°C. Fever usually >39°C, ↓BP, rigors, septic shock, oliguria, DIC. Usually immediate and often lethal. Stop transfusion. Take blood cultures. Consider antibiotic.
- **Viral contamination:** HBV, HTLV, HIV, HCV. Testing is done for these. Use CMV-negative donors for those receiving bone marrow transplants or solid organ transplants on immunosuppression.
- **Other infections:** include syphilis and malaria and toxoplasmosis. Syphilis is screened for.
- **Transfusion-associated circulatory overload (TACO):** usually elderly medical; TACO any age but more in age >70. Leads to breathlessness and cardiogenic pulmonary oedema within 6 h, CXR changes. Treat as cardiogenic pulmonary oedema. It is one of the more common causes of transfusion-related death. Patients should be monitored and reassessed between transfusions. JVP ↑, BP ↑, O₂ sats ↓. Worsens with fluid challenge. Improves with diuretics. Abnormal echo.

- **Transfusion-related lung injury (TRALI):** haematology and surgical patients. Plasma antibodies react to host white cell antigens and pulmonary endothelium. Comes on acutely usually <2–6 h with breathlessness, rigors, non-cardiogenic pulmonary oedema, cough, CXR changes. Due to donor antibodies to white cells. Treat as ARDS. Seen with plasma or platelets. JVP ↓, BP ↓. CXR bihilar shadowing. ↓. O_2 sats. ↓WCC. Improves with fluid challenge. Worsens with diuretics.
- **Transfusion-associated graft versus host disease** (TA-GvHD): immunocompromised host. TA-GvHD occurs when donor lymphocytes from transfused blood engraft in the recipient and cause disease and destroy recipient's bone marrow. Occurs 10–14 days post-transfusion with clinical features of fever, skin rash, hepatitis, diarrhoea and pancytopenia. It is fatal in more than 90% of cases. Prevent by giving irradiated blood to groups at risk. See table below.
- **Post-transfusion purpura:** later fall in platelets after 10–14 days. Recipient develops antibodies to human platelet antigen 1a. Treat with IVIg or plasma exchange.

Reference: Serious Hazards of Transfusion website: www.shotuk.org.

8.17 Indications for irradiated blood

These patients require irradiated blood products in adults to prevent TA-GvHD

- Transfusions from a 1st or 2nd degree relative, patients receiving a granulocyte transfusion.
- Patients receiving HLA – selected components even if immunocompetent.
- Purine analogues (e.g. fludarabine, cladrabine, deoxycoformicin, bendamustine, clofarabine).
- Hodgkin's lymphoma, at any stage of the disease (for life).
- Patients receiving allogeneic haemopoietic stem cell (HSC) grafts, from the start of conditioning therapy and while the patient remains on GvHD prophylaxis (usually 6 months post-transplant). If chronic GvHD is present or the patient is taking immunosuppressants, continue irradiated blood components indefinitely.
- Allogeneic HSC donors being transfused 7 days prior to or during the harvest of their HSC.
- Patients who will have autologous HSC graft: any transfusion 7 days prior to/during the bone marrow/stem cell harvest.
- Transfusion from start of conditioning chemo-radiotherapy until 3 months post-transplant (6 months if total body irradiation was used).
- Those receiving anti-thymocyte globulin (ATG) and/or alemtuzumab (anti-CD52).
- Patients with known or suspected T-cell immunodeficiency, such as DiGeorge syndrome irradiation.
- There is also no indication for routine irradiation of cellular blood components for adults who are HIV antibody positive or who have AIDS.

8.18 Immunocompromised patients

Introduction

- Those with HIV or acquired/congenital immune deficiency.
- Those on steroid therapy – depends on dose and duration.
- Those on drugs for organ rejection post-transplant.
- Immunosuppression for RA, SLE and autoimmune disease.
- Use of Ciclosporin, Tacrolimus, Azathioprine, Mycophenolate, Steroids.
- Myeloma, lymphoma, hypersplenism, asplenia.
- Diabetes, hypophosphataemia (on TPN).
- Infections – influenza, rubella, measles, AIDS. Malnourished, malignancy.

Problems
- Meningitis.
- Severe overwhelming sepsis with fewer typical signs and symptoms.
- Pneumonias, meningoencephalitis, PCP pneumonias.
- Mucocutaneous and systemic fungal infections. Severe gastroenteritis, diarrhoea.
- Vulnerable to viral infections – isolate and need prophylactic and treatment antivirals.
- Avoid live vaccines. Culture, LP, treat with lower threshold.
- Stop immunosuppressive agents if significant infection detected.
- Increased malignancy risk – skin, renal, cervical.
- Take expert infectious diseases or transplant team help early.

Plasmapheresis/plasma exchange (PLEX)

- **About:** plasmapheresis means removal of plasma 'take away', which either involves some form of filtering by centrifugation or membrane separation that can remove products from plasma at a rate greater than the body can make and distribute the toxic immunoglobulins. With centrifuge devices, citrate is the anticoagulant of choice and this can cause hypocalcaemia. Plasmapheresis is used when a substance in the plasma, such as immunoglobulin, is acutely toxic and can be efficiently removed. It may be combined with other treatments such as Rituximab which destroys both normal and malignant B cells that have CD20 on their surfaces. These make immunoglobulins.
- **Indications:** GBS, myasthenia gravis, CIDP, hyperviscosity in monoclonal gammopathies, TTP, Goodpasture syndrome (anti-GBM disease), atypical HUS (autoantibody to factor H), neuromyelitis optica.
- **Method:** patients require central line placement. Dose 40–50 ml/kg of plasma is removed and the plasma replaced with albumin or saline. Up to 3–6 exchanges on a daily or alternate day regimen.
- **Side effects:** include a flu-like illness, haemodynamic instability with arrhythmias and ↓BP, and autonomic dysfunction. There may be problems from the access with thrombophlebitis, bleeding, line infections and PTX.

09 Infectious disease emergencies

9.1 Pyrexia of unknown origin

- **About:** Modern definition: PUO in hospital >38.3°C on several occasions, caused by a process not present or incubating on admission, where initial cultures are negative and diagnosis unknown after 3 days of investigation. Specialist PUO scenarios – HIV-positive and neutropenic PUO. Most are infection, malignancy or inflammatory/ autoimmune diseases.
- **Causes and strategy:** full and comprehensive history and repeated examination.
- **Common:** tuberculosis, endocarditis, gallbladder disease and HIV infection.
- **Rare:** tropical unless clear travel history or exotic diseases. Always consider: exposure to an infection, travel to a high-risk area, environmental exposure, contact with an infected individual, occupation and leisure activity history, e.g. canoeing (leptospirosis), animal exposure, sexual contacts, IV drug use/needles, blood transfusion, vaccinations. HIV test should be done in all.

Clinical clues: check frequently and observe fever

- **Lymphadenopathy and hepatosplenomegaly** give foci for tissue diagnosis.
- **Top to toe examination including orifices:** mouth, throat, perineum, axillae, skin.
- **Check for tenderness:** skin, spinal tenderness, bone pain, murmurs, rashes.
- **Abscesses:** skin, subphrenic, pelvic, brain, look for pain, risks, recent surgery, abdominal pain.
- **Tuberculosis:** weight loss, cough, confusion, immigrant.
- **Perinephric abscess:** complicated UTI, renal TB.
- **Endocarditis:** look for signs. Get TTE/TOE. blood cultures, HACEK group.
- **Cholangitis:** LFTs may be minimally deranged, USS, look for stones.
- **Drugs can cause a fever.** Consider stopping any likely ones.
- **PAN/RA/SLE:** check autoantibodies, check U&E, urine, juvenile idiopathic arthritis.
- **Others:** sarcoidosis, Crohn's disease, ulcerative colitis.
- **Rare:** familial Mediterranean fever, thyrotoxicosis.
- **Kikuchi's disease:** histiocytic necrotizing lymphadenitis, young women, rare, benign condition, cervical lymphadenopathy and fever.
- **Malignancy:** lymphomas, leukaemia, solid tumours, e.g. renal cell, hepatocellular.
- **Brucellosis:** travel to affected areas, exposure to animals, or work in food preparation and ingestion of unpasteurised dairy or raw meats.
- **Dental abscesses:** check the mouth and dentition and tap the teeth for pain and discharge and get dental review.
- **Bioterrorism:** anthrax, plague, smallpox (was eradicated, fever, aches, vomiting, centrifugal pustular rash use vaccination, Cidofovir/ST-246), tularaemia.

Investigations

- **FBC and DWCC:** neutrophilia suggests bacterial infection. Lymphocytosis: ? viral infection. Lymphopenia: HIV infection. Neutropenia: viral infection. Eosinophilia: ? parasitic infection, ↓platelets, ? malaria (parasites on film indicative).
- **ESR/CRP:** elevated confirms disease but poor specificity for aetiology.
- **Serology:** HIV1 and HIV2, HBV, HCV, monospot, CMV/EBV.
- **Blood cultures:** preferably having been off antibiotics for several days. Aerobic and anaerobic bottle using strict asepsis. Contaminants can seriously jeopardise diagnosis and care.
- **LFTS:** hepatitis, cholangitis, alcoholic liver disease. Can suggest liver biopsy.

- **Imaging:** CXR in all. Consider USS abdomen and pelvis or CT chest/abdomen/pelvis for pus collection, malignancy.
- **Biopsy:** nodes or liver biopsy or bone marrow can help with diagnosis.
- **Labelled white cell scanning:** can help isolate any white cell collection.
- **Echocardiogram:** transthoracic and TOE if endocarditis suspected.
- **Lumbar puncture:** if any suggestion of CNS infection – headache, delirium.
- **Tuberculosis suspected:** culture urine, sputum, stool, CSF and morning gastric aspirates.
- **Therapeutic trials** can be considered as a test if a diagnosis is strongly suspected, e.g. tuberculosis, brucellosis.
- **Autoimmune screen:** ANA, dsDNA, ANCA, RF, anti-CCP.
- **Syphilis:** TPHA/FTA/FTI. **Leptospirosis:** IgM, blood cultures. **Lyme disease** serology.

Management
- Resuscitate: ABC. Severe sepsis, ▶ Section 2.21; Hypovolaemia, ▶ Section 2.20. If possible try to avoid starting antimicrobials without at first getting CSF and multiple blood cultures off and discussing with infectious diseases or microbiology.
- Logically work through common diagnoses first. Consider second opinion as these can be challenging and arrange rheumatology review.

9.2 ▶ Assessment of the febrile traveller

- **About:** 1 in 12 travellers acquire an infection needing medical attention. Differential is all the home grown local infective and perhaps non-infective causes plus exotic ones. In any infective presentation a travel history should be always be obtained. Anyone with fever and flu-like illness who has travelled to an endemic area has falciparum malaria until proven otherwise.
- **Main killers:** meningococcaemia, cerebral malaria and viral haemorrhagic fevers. They are uncommon but rapidly fatal. If malaria considered determine what prophylaxis taken, areas visited and likely dates of infection.
- **Clinical:** business, leisure. Where stayed, town vs. countryside, medications taken, night nets, unprotected sex with new person(s). Game parks, farms, caves, health facilities, exotic foods, activities involving fresh or salt-water exposure. Any bites, e.g. bats, dogs.
- **Symptoms:** malaise, photophobia, rash, dysuria, cough, phlegm, rash, eschar on legs/inguinal/axilla (typhus), rose spots on torso (typhoid) hepatosplenomegaly, lymphadenopathy or jaundice.

Consider usual causes first
Always consider the usual familiar causes – influenza, UTI, chest infection, meningitis, endocarditis, TB or a lymphoma, Lyme disease.

Clues to infective causes where unclear
- ↑**Lymphocytes:** viral infection, TB, pertussis, brucellosis, syphilis.
- ↓**Lymphocytes:** HIV, *Legionella*, steroids.
- ↑**Neutrophils:** bacterial infection.
- ↓**Neutrophils:** sepsis, viral, brucella, typhoid (WCC normal), kala-azar, TB.
- ↑**Eosinophils:** parasites, drugs, polyarteritis nodosa.

Sources of infection endemic locations
- **Anywhere:** HIV, bacterial sepsis, UTI, meningitis, HSV encephalitis, influenza, leptospirosis, rabies.
- **Africa:** malaria, dengue fever, rickettsial disease, enteric fever, viral haemorrhagic fevers, Ebola, amoebic liver abscess, Katayama syndrome.
- **African safari:** rickettsial disease, African trypanosomiasis.

- **West Africa (Nigeria, Niger, Mali, Senegal, etc.):** viral haemorrhagic fever.
- **Horn of Africa:** visceral leishmaniasis.
- **Southeast Asia:** malaria, dengue fever, enteric fever, chikungunya disease, rickettsial disease.
- **Africa, Asia, Caribbean, South America:** malaria, typhoid 'enteric' fever, viral hepatitis, dengue fever, poliomyelitis.
- **Southwestern USA** (desert areas): coccidioidomycosis.
- **Sexual contact:** HIV, gonorrhoea, syphilis, Chlamydophila, chancroid, hepatitis B.
- **Blood borne:** hepatitis B/C, HIV.
- **IV drug users:** *Staph. aureus*, hepatitis B/C, HIV, anthrax, botulism.
- **Mosquito bite:** malaria, dengue fever, chikungunya disease, tularaemia, filiariasis, Zika virus, yellow fever, West Nile virus, Japanese encephalitis.
- **Tsetse fly:** African trypanosomiasis.
- **Animals:** brucellosis, rabies, Q fever, plague, tularaemia.
- **Dog, fox, skunk, bat contact (bite):** rabies.
- **Bats:** rabies, histoplasmosis, Marburg haemorrhagic fever, Nipah virus encephalitis, Hendra virus disease.
- **Faeco–oral:** hepatitis A and E, enteric fever, gastroenteritis.
- **Fresh water:** leptospirosis, schistosomiasis (Katayama fever).
- **Tick bites:** often painless. Rickettsia, Lyme disease, Rocky Mountain spotted fever, ehrlichosis.
- **Hotels and air conditioning and shower heads:** *Legionella*.

Incubation periods: time between acquiring pathogen and disease symptoms/signs
- **<21 days malaria**, typhoid fever, dengue, rickettsia, leptospirosis. May occur whilst on holiday.
- **>21 days malaria**, TB, viral hepatitis, Katayama fever usually on getting home.
- Work out all the dates and relevant activities and exposure. Count days.

Clinical signs
- **Eschar:** 'patch of black necrotic tissue'. Tick bites. Typhus/Rickettsial infection, anthrax, *Pasteurella multocida*.
- **Buboes:** bubonic plague, gonorrhoea, tuberculosis, chancroid or syphilis.
- **Cold sores:** *Herpes simplex* encephalitis, pneumococcal pneumonia.
- **Sore throat:** teenager, adult <30, infectious mononucleosis (EBV or CMV), epiglottitis, tonsillitis, quinsy, Lemierre's syndrome.
- **Fever without tachycardia** (ignore if on beta-blockers): typhoid fever, legionnaire's disease, malaria, dengue, yellow fever, VHF, chlamydial pneumonia.

Other considerations
- **Preventative measures:** vaccines against hepatitis A/B, and yellow fever usually rules out these infections. *Anti-malarial chemoprophylaxis does not exclude malaria.* Protective clothing, use of netting, avoiding being outdoors in peak times for feeding, etc.
- **Historical clues:** travel itinerary: the risk of acquiring a travel-related infection depends on the precise geographic location and the length of stay at each destination. Modern hotel or with locals or family. Infections can be acquired en route, so layovers and intermediate stops should be recorded. Mode of transport should be recorded.
- **Sexual history:** with whom, male/female, frequency, protected, prostitution, condom use, what type of sex. Risk of infection. Other STIs.

Management of pyrexia in a traveller (infective, inflammatory, malignancy)
- **Cerebral/falciparum malaria:** if in endemic malarial area then assume falciparum malaria until you have a total of three negative smears which should be obtained

8–12 h apart over the course of 2 days. Discuss with infectious diseases specialist. If any signs of complications then consider starting treatment immediately (see *Section 10.3* below).

- **Bloods:** get FBC, blood film, U&E, LFT, HIV test, acute viral serology, blood cultures and CXR and CT head if any neurology. Lumbar puncture if CNS symptoms (check coagulation first). Serology and liver USS if liver abscess suspected. If bacterial meningitis or HSV encephalitis are a possibility, then treat appropriately.
- **Echocardiogram, cultures, CRP** if any cardiac signs. TFTs as thyrotoxic crisis could resemble infection. Repeat history and examination to make sure all information extracted. Take expert advice. Work through differential.
- **Others:** is there another cause – medications, malignancy, vasculitis, rheumatological, factitious?

9.3   Falciparum malaria

- **About:** incubation period (IP) usually <4 weeks but cases seen up to 6 months.
- **High risk groups:** children, pregnant, HIV/immunocompromised, travellers. **Protective:** sickle cell trait, G6PD deficiency.
- **Expert advice** local team or London 0845 155 5000, Liverpool 0151 706 2000.
- **Assume malaria until proven otherwise if patient has been in endemic area.** Fatal disease may present like 'flu' and moribund before post take ward round. Asking about travel is the golden question with urgent serial thick and thin films which can be falsely negative. Rapid stick tests. Treat quickly on clinical acumen as it can kill within hours. Appropriate prophylaxis with full adherence does not exclude fatal falciparum malaria. Take expert advice.
- **Endemic areas:** Africa, Asia, Papua New Guinea, South America, Western Pacific. Milder disease in older children and adults from endemic areas.
- **Aetiology:** a bite from an infected female *Anopheles* mosquito injects sporozoites which infect hepatocytes. Hepatocytes release merozoites which infect erythrocytes. Bite to RBC infection takes 7–30 days. Infected RBCs release more merozoites which infect more RBCs and cause pyrexia. Lethality due to cytoadherence of infected red cells to the walls which block post-capillary venules. Mechanism is formation of *P. falciparum* erythrocyte membrane protein (PfEMP)-1. Rosetting is another finding where infected cells adhere to uninfected RBCs.
- **Clinical:** flu-like malaise, fever >39°C (may be absent), headache, vomiting, malaise, myalgia. Coma, fits, hemiparesis, blindness, brisk reflexes, extensor plantars, decorticate or decerebrate posturing, diarrhoea, rigors, backache, drenching fevers, hepatosplenomegaly. AKI needing dialysis in 10%, intravascular haemolysis, jaundice, haemoglobinuria. Malaria does not cause lymphadenopathy or rash (consider other or additional diseases, e.g. HIV, malignancy).
- **Complications:** ↓GCS, seizures, oliguria <20 ml/h, ARDS/pulmonary oedema. Spontaneous bleeding/DIC, shock (algid malaria BP <90/60 mmHg). Haemoglobinuria (without G6PD deficiency).
- **Markers of severity:** Hb <8 g/dL, glucose <2.2 mmol/L, HCO3 <15 mmol/L, pH <7.3, lactate >5 mmol/L, parasites >2%. Creatinine >265 µmol/L, ↑bilirubin and jaundice.
- **Differential:** malaria must first be excluded in any pyrexial illness from, or in, an endemic area. Typhoid, hepatitis, dengue, avian influenza, SARS, HIV. Meningitis/encephalitis and viral haemorrhagic fevers.

Investigations

- **FBC and U&E:** ↓Hb, haemolysis, ↑reticulocytes, ↑urea and ↑creatinine, ↑LDH.
- **Thick and thin peripheral blood films:** (EDTA sample) to identify parasite infection. Thick films identify parasite. Thin films show the number of red cells infected and type. Need serial 3× thick/thin negative slides over 48–72 h to fully

exclude malaria. Consider stopping antimalarial prophylaxis, as these may reduce parasitaemia and so reduce test sensitivity. Examination should identify the degree of parasitaemia.

- **Antigen tests:** some rapid tests are available but treatment may give false negatives. Chronic infection: ↑IgM and marked splenomegaly and ↓Hb.
- **Coagulation screen:** DIC seen: CXR: non-cardiogenic pulmonary oedema, exclude pneumonia and other causes of fever.

Complications

- **Coma** (cerebral malaria): manage ABCs, exclude other causes (e.g. hypoglycaemia, bacterial meningitis). Avoid steroids, heparin and adrenaline; intubate and ventilate if necessary.
- **Hyperpyrexia:** tepid sponging, fanning, cooling blanket and antipyretics.
- **Convulsions:** ABC; treat promptly. IV/PR DIAZEPAM if on-going.
- **Hypoglycaemia:** monitor glucose and treat hypoglycaemia. Consider IV 10% Dextrose infusion.
- **Severe anaemia:** (Hb <5 g/100 ml, ↓PCV <15%) transfuse with screened fresh whole blood.
- **Acute pulmonary oedema:** over-enthusiastic rehydration should be avoided so as to prevent pulmonary oedema. Prop patient up at an angle of 45°, give oxygen, give a diuretic, stop IV fluids, intubate and add PEEP/CPAP in life-threatening hypoxaemia.
- **Acute kidney injury:** exclude pre-renal causes, check fluid balance and urinary sodium; if severe AKI consider haemofiltration or haemodialysis, or if unavailable, peritoneal dialysis. The benefits of diuretics/dopamine in acute renal failure are not proven (▶Section 10.4).
- **Spontaneous bleeding and coagulopathy:** transfuse with screened fresh whole blood (cryoprecipitate, FFP and platelets if available); give VITAMIN K injection.
- **Metabolic acidosis:** exclude or treat hypoglycaemia, hypovolaemia and septicaemia. If severe, add haemofiltration or haemodialysis.
- **Shock:** suspect septicaemia, take blood for cultures; give parenteral antimicrobials, correct haemodynamic disturbances.
- **Hyperparasitaemia:** treat as below.

Management (take expert individualised advice)

- Oral/IV rehydration may be needed with fever, polyuria, poor intake. Give O₂ to achieve 94% saturation. Treat hypoglycaemia with IV glucose. Admit complicated malaria to the ITU. Use parenteral therapy or oral/NG QUININE until pharmacy can provide an IV preparation. Do not delay antimalarial if patient has signs of complicated falciparum malaria. If the diagnosis unclear stop antimalarial to improve test accuracy. If unsure take expert help.
- **Pregnancy** (take expert advice – these patients are at higher risk of complications). Falciparum malaria in pregnancy may be more severe than suggested by the peripheral blood film due to marked placental sequestration. Most dangerous in 3rd trimester. Use Quinine and Clindamycin (as per *BNF*). Avoid Doxycycline in pregnancy or breastfeeding. Fetus usually unaffected. Quinine is safe and effective in all stages of pregnancy and is used in standard doses. IV ARTESUNATE may be used in severe cases under expert guidance.

Antimalarial treatment (follow expert guidance)

- Record what anti-malarial prophylaxis. May influence treatment.
- **Non-falciparum malaria in adults:** CHLOROQUINE 600 mg PO stat then 300 mg at 6, 24 and 48 h. If vivax/ovale then PRIMAQUINE 30 mg (15 mg if ovale) base/day for hypnozoites for 14 days, but check for G6PD deficiency first as can cause haemolysis.

- **Uncomplicated falciparum malaria:** choice of (1) QUININE 600 mg PO 8 h + (DOXYCYCLINE 200 mg OD OR CLINDAMYCIN 450 mg 8 h) all for 7 days. QUININE is treatment of choice; if pregnant avoid Doxycycline and use CLINDAMYCIN. (2) MALARONE 4 'standard' tablets daily for 3 days. (3) RIAMET (artemether and lumefantrine) 8 tablets 12 h for 3 days.
- **Complicated falciparum malaria** (seriously ill or unable to take tablets, or if >2% of red blood cell are parasitized): Loading dose QUININE 20 mg/kg in G5 over 4 h. Followed by QUININE 10 mg/kg every 8 h for first 48 h (or until patient can swallow). Reduce dosing frequency to 12 h if IV QUININE continues >48 h. Once able to take oral therapy then QUININE SULPHATE 600 mg TDS for 5–7 days. Must be accompanied by a second drug: DOXYCYCLINE 100 mg BD PO for 7 days (or CLINDAMYCIN 450 mg TDS for pregnant women) from when the patient can swallow. Note there are QUININE-resistant areas of SE Asia and ARTESUNATE may need to be considered. QUININE IV/PO is safe in pregnancy for treatment of falciparum malaria.
- **ARTESUNATE:** drug of choice (34% ↓mortality) used on named patient basis under specialist advice. Rapid effect on parasite clearance. Most effective with parasitaemias >10%. If not available, then QUININE. ARTESUNATE 2.4 mg/kg as an IV injection at 0, 12, 24 h, then daily thereafter. A 7-day course of DOXYCYCLINE should also be given as above.

9.4 Traveller's diarrhoea

- **About:** half of travellers in developing countries. Poor sanitation, use only boiled or bottled water, unpeeled fruit, avoid ice cubes, salads. Most bacterial spread faeco-oral. More common with acid suppression, e.g. PPI. Malaria can cause diarrhoea.
- **Cause:** E. coli (ETEC/EAEC below), Salmonella, Campylobacter, Shigella, enteric fever, Cholera, Giardia, Cryptosporidium, rotavirus, malaria.
- **Clinical:** loose watery diarrhoea, colic and dehydration. Severe: bloody diarrhoea, fever, abdominal pain and severely dehydrated.
- **Investigate:** U&E <LFTS, stools for ova, cysts, parasites and culture.
- **Management:** limit spread, hand washing. Most self-limit with oral rehydration therapies. Some need medical care and IV hydration. Severe give CIPROFLOXACIN. If amoebiasis suspected (bloody diarrhoea) then add METRONIDAZOLE for 10 days. Caution with antimotility agents. Some later develop lactose intolerance. Need lactose hydrogen breath test. Hypovolaemia, ▶Section 2.20.

9.5 Tick typhus

- **About:** tick bite. Rickettsia. Obligate intracellular, Gram –ve bacteria. African tick typhus commonest seen in UK. S/E Africa. Walking with uncovered legs.
- **Clinical:** IP <10 days, high fever, headache, myalgia, maculopapular rash, eschar at site of tick bite, lymphadenitis and reactive arthritis.
- **Complications:** pneumonitis, meningo-encephalitis. Occasionally DIC or AKI with fatality rates up to nearly 20%.
- **Diagnosis** exclude malaria. Confirmation diagnosis retrospectively on paired initial and convalescent-phase serum sample.
- **Management:** DOXYCYCLINE 100 mg BD PO/IV for least 7 days very effective.

9.6 Rocky Mountain Spotted fever

- **About:** tick bite is source of rickettsia. *Rickettsia rickettsia*. Central and Southern US states (far from the Rockies).
- **Aetiology:** Gram –ve intracellular coccobacillus which invades endothelial cells causing vascular injury.

- **Clinical:** fever, headache, myalgia, maculopapular rash, no eschars. Reduced GCS, gangrene, focal neurology, organ failure, fatality 5%.
- **Diagnosis:** low Hb, raised WCC, raised LFT, AKI. Send serology.
- **Management:** treat on clinical suspicions in patient who was in endemic area. DOXYCYCLINE 100 mg BD PO/IV for least 7 days very effective.

9.7   Schistosomiasis (Katayama fever)

- **Source:** endemic in parts of Africa. From fresh water lakes/rivers allows cercariae from snails to penetrate intact skin. *Schistosoma mansoni, S. haematobium* and *S. japonicum.* Also called bilharzia.
- **Clinical:** (1) Swimmer's itch following skin penetration with papular rash. (2) Katayama fever 4–10 weeks (longer than other traveller-acquired febrile illnesses, e.g. dengue, leptospirosis). Systemic schistosomal infection, fever, lethargy, myalgia, arthralgia, cough, headache. Urticarial rash, diarrhoea +/– blood, hepatosplenomegaly and wheeze. (3) Chronic infection liver, GI tract and bladder.
- **Diagnosis:** stool – eggs can be seen. peripheral eosinophilia. Ova seen in urine.
- **Management:** PRAZIQUANTEL will kill mature but not immature schistosomes so repeat. Treat at the time of diagnosis of Katayama fever and 3 months later. A short course of steroids may help alleviate acute symptoms.

9.8   Dengue

- **Source:** flavivirus with 4 serotypes endemic in Asia, S America, Caribbean; transmitted by day-biting mosquito *Aedes aegypti*. Incubation period 7 days (3–14 days; mean 7 d) of mosquito bite. No effective vaccine.
- **Aetiology:** primary infection is usually benign. Secondary infection with a different serotype or multiple infections with different serotypes may lead to severe disease with dengue haemorrhagic fever (DHF) or dengue shock syndrome (DSS).
- **Clinical: initial infection:** mild febrile, headache, retro-orbital pain, myalgia, arthralgia (back pain) and erythrodermic rash which may become petechial. **2nd exposure** (local or staying >2 weeks): initial fever often abrupt spiking at 40°C for 5–7 days then signs of DHF with petechiae, melena, drop in Hb +/– DSS with capillary leak, postural ↓BP, narrow pulse pressure, ascites, effusion, SBP <90 mmHg. Secondary infection rare in travellers. Critical phase of DSS/DHF lasts 24–48 h.
- **Investigations:** FBC: ↓WCC, ↓platelets <100 × 10^9/L and 20% ↑PCV due to plasma leak, low protein. ↑LFTs. DIC. PCR or positive IgM-capture ELISA. Needs daily FBC and haematocrit and platelet count.
- **Management:** supportive. Access to ITU to monitor organ failure. Transfuse if required. IV crystalloids and colloids given rapidly in severe disease. Avoid aspirin as antipyretic. Mortality 1–2%. Steroids/antivirals have no evidence base. See Hypovolaemia, ▶Section 2.20; Sepsis, ▶Section 2.21; DIC, ▶Section 8.4.

9.9   Viral haemorrhagic fever

- **RNA viruses:** arenaviruses, filoviruses, bunya viruses and flaviviruses. Urgent isolation and senior advice if contact with Ebola or from affected area. Do not do bloods without discussing with infectious disease specialist.
- **Source:** Africa, S America and Asia. Very rare with a handful of cases per decade in the UK. Delayed diagnosis leads to further cases. Zoonosis. Usually from monkeys. As viruses depend on a host they are usually restricted to the geographical area inhabited by those animals. Humans are not the natural host for these viruses, which normally live in wild animals.

- **Types:** Lassa fever: visitors to Nigeria, Liberia, Sierra Leone. Crimean–Congo haemorrhagic fever, Marburg and Ebola. Contact with dead. Sick animals.
- **Pathogenesis:** haemorrhage, severe capillary leak and shock.
- **Clinical:** Incubation <3 weeks. Some cause mild illnesses, others cause severe, life-threatening disease. Fever, fatigue, dizziness, muscle aches, loss of strength, and exhaustion. Petechiae, bruising, haemorrhage, mucosal bleeding, PR bleeding. Hypovolaemic shock, coma, delirium, and seizures. AKI.
- **Investigations:** (take advice if safe to do bloods as high risk) send serology, **FBC:** fall in Hb and ↑haematocrit, **U&E:** AKI, coagulation screen, sickle test, ABG, ↑LFT. Blood films for malaria.
- **Management:** isolate. Personal protective gear. Exclude/treat for malaria if suspected. Contact local infectious disease specialist and follow local policy. Immediately isolate patient, protective clothing, waste disposal. Largely supportive. *Person-to-person spread possible so strict precautions must be taken.* IV RIBAVIRIN has been effective in treating some individuals with Lassa fever or HRS. Convalescent-phase plasma has been used in some patients with Argentine haemorrhagic fever. Transfer to specialist unit. See <u>Hypovolaemia, ▶ Section 2.20; Sepsis, ▶ Section 2.21; DIC, ▶ Section 8.4.</u>

9.10 Chikungunya

- **Source:** alphavirus transmitted by day-biting *Aedes* mosquitos. Seen in Africa and SE Asia.
- **Clinical:** flu-like, malaise, headache, rash, severe joint pain.
- **Rare sequelae:** encephalitis, GBS, seizures.
- **Management:** check serology. Supportive care.

9.11 Plague/tularaemia

- **Source:** *Yersinia pestis*. sub-Saharan Africa. Gram –ve coccobacillus. Reservoir in rodents. Passed by bites containing blood-stained vomit from fleas who bit infected rodent. Untreated mortality >70%. Potential bioterrorism. Tularaemia can present similarly. Same treatment.
- **Clinical:** bubonic plague – swellings (buboes) in groin, axilla, neck lymph nodes, septicaemia, pneumonia (haemoptysis), meningitis.
- **Investigations:** diagnosis by blood culture or from aspirate from bubo.
- **Management:** isolate, protection. GENTAMICIN 5 mg/kg/day IV, CIPROFLOXACIN 400 mg IV BD, DOXYCYCLINE 100 mg IV BD.

9.12 Brucellosis

- **About:** *Brucella abortus, B. melitensis, B. suis, B. canis*. Gram –ve intracellular infection.
- **Source:** animal contact (goats, sheep, cattle, camels, pigs, dogs), unpasteurised milk, cheeses. S Europe, India. Incubation period 2–4 weeks.
- **Clinical:** undulant fever. Enlarged nodes, liver, spleen, foul swelling sweat, arthritis, osteomyelitis, meningoencephalitis. Scrotal pain.
- **Investigations:** WCC and CRP may not be ↑. Diagnosis serology. Culture is prolonged – blood, CSF, lymph nodes.
- **Management:** DOXYCYCLINE 200 mg OD ×6 weeks. Rifampicin. Combined with streptomycin for 2 weeks.

9.13 Pseudomonas infection

- **Source:** *Pseudomonas aeruginosa*, Gram −ve, rod-shaped bacterium.
- **Clinical:** hospital-acquired pneumonia, UTI, soft tissue and wounds, chronic lung disease, cystic fibrosis.
- **Investigations:** WCC and CRP may or may not be ↑. Culture.
- **Management:** CIPROFLOXACIN PO or TAZOCIN, MEROPENEM, GENTAMICIN IV. Often combined.

9.14 Q fever

- **Source:** *Coxiella burnetii*. From animals. Transmission via dust, aerolised media, spores, and unpasteurised milk.
- **Clinical:** IP 2–4 weeks, fever, headaches, myalgia, pneumonia, hepatitis, rarely endocarditis.
- **Investigations:** diagnosis by serology titres.
- **Management:** DOXYCYCLINE ×14 days. <u>Endocarditis, ▶Section 3.22; Pneumonia, ▶Section 4.14.</u>

9.15 Anthrax

- **Source:** *Bacillus anthracis*. Gram +ve rods. Found naturally in soil as spores. May be used in bioterrorism. Releases a three protein exotoxin with components called oedema factor and lethal factor causing oedema and tissue necrosis.
- **Clinical: cutaneous:** handling infected material – blisters, itching and a black eschar (anthrax – greek for coal). Lymphadenopathy. **Pulmonary:** inhalation of spores – breathlessness, haemoptysis, chest pain, cough, sweats, haemorrhagic mediastinitis. **Gastrointestinal:** eating raw infected meat – fever, chills, neck lymphadenopathy, bloody diarrhoea. **Injection:** a few cases of a heroin batch contaminated with spores – fever, skin abscess.
- **Investigations:** FBC, U&E, CRP: blood/sputum/CSF/skin swab for *B. anthracis* before antibiotics. Serology for *B. anthracis*. **CXR/chest CT:** enlarged mediastinum, nodes and pleural effusion often bloody.
- **Management:** no person to person spread except rarely with cutaneous form, however, until risks and source established full protection should be used and local guidance and isolate. **Those at-risk without symptoms: anthrax vaccination can be considered.** CIPROFLOXACIN and/or DOXYCYCLINE can be given to exposed individuals before symptoms. **Cutaneous disease:** DOXYCYCLINE PO for 7–14 days as outpatient. **Systemic/inhalational anthrax:** ABC, ITU, antibiotics (CIPROFLOXACIN IV and/or DOXYCYCLINE IV) and antitoxin. RAXIBACUMAB a monoclonal antibody, may be useful against an anthrax bacterial antigen. Another is OBILTOXAXIMAB. Prognosis is very poor for those with pulmonary/mediastinal, gastrointestinal or meningeal anthrax. Death is toxin-mediated and results in haemorrhagic/septicaemic shock. <u>Sepsis, ▶Section 2.21.</u>

9.16 Leptospirosis

- **Source:** *Leptospira interrogans*. Worldwide including UK. Direct (water sports, canoeing, swimming) exposure to infected urine of rats, dogs, cattle and other domestic and wild animals. IP <10 days.
- **Clinical:** biphasic. Initial flu-like 'septicaemic' symptoms for 7 days, followed by immune period (IgM +ve) of 2–3 weeks with fever, myalgia (sore back and legs), jaundice, hepatorenal syndrome and haemorrhage. Conjunctival suffusion is suggestive.

- **Can develop:** aseptic meningitis, AKI, liver failure, myocarditis, pancreatitis, purpura, ecchymosis, pulmonary and gastrointestinal haemorrhage. Most are self-limiting but occasionally severe and even fatal. Jaundice, hepatomegaly and bleeding, respiratory failure, ARDS, DIC.
- **Differential in tropics:** malaria, dengue, typhoid, scrub typhus, hantavirus.
- **Investigations:** FBC: ↑↑neutrophils, ↓platelets, ↓Hb if haemorrhage. ↑↑CK. ↑LFTs. **Coagulation screen:** normal, usually slightly ↑PT and bleeding is due to capillary fragility. U&E: AKI, ↑bilirubin, ↑ALT. **Urinalysis:** may show proteinuria and haematuria. Urine is not a suitable sample for the isolation of leptospira seen in 2nd week. **Serology:** cultures slow. Diagnosis needs serology with IgM titre >1 in 320 and convalescent serology >10 days for IgM ELISA and microscopic agglutination test (MAT). CSF and aerobic blood cultures: (taken within the first 5 days of onset, before antibiotics) can be referred to the UK Leptospira Reference Unit. Keep blood cultures at room temperature prior to sending.
- **Management:** mainly symptomatic and supportive. AKI managed with dialysis if needed. Blood transfusion as needed. DOXYCYCLINE or AMOXICILLIN PO for mild disease or BENZYLPENICILLIN or CEFTRIAXONE IV if more severe. Evidence for antibiotic effectiveness is unproven. Note penicillins can cause Jarisch–Herxheimer reaction with fever, low BP, myalgia, ↑HR. Those with jaundice can become very unwell despite therapy and may need liver support. Severe disease is probably immunologically mediated.

9.17 Listeriosis

- **Source:** *Listeria monocytogenes*. Gram +ve. Found in environment. Contaminates food: salads, soft cheese, undercooked meat, chicken, patés. At risk: more severe infection in elderly, pregnant, immunocompromised.
- **Clinical:** N&V, backache and diarrhoea. **Complications:** meningism, progressive coma, stroke-like episode, adult brainstem encephalitis (CSF may be normal), meningitis, stillbirth or premature labour, neonatal listeriosis causes sepsis or meningitis.
- **Investigations:** ↑WCC. ↑CRP, ↑ESR. MRI sign of encephalitis. CSF culture, ↑WCC and normal glucose.
- **Management:** AMPICILLIN IV (confirmed listerial meningitis 21 days). Take specialist advice if penicillin-allergic. Add DEXAMETHASONE 0.15 mg/kg 6 h for meningitis. Bacterial meningitis, ▶ Section 11.11.

9.18 Botulism

- **About:** potent neurotoxin causes a descending paralysis.
- **Source:** large anaerobic Gram +ve spore-forming bacillus *Clostridium botulinum* is found in soil. Releases neurotoxin which blocks presynaptic Ach release causing paralysis at motor nerve endings. Most powerful neurotoxin known to date.
- **Clinical:** food-borne, intestinal, wound infection. Progressive blurred vision, bulbar and facial weakness, dysphagia, unable to speak. Progressive descending symmetrical paralysis, respiratory failure. Death in 10%. Diarrhoea, vomiting, dry mouth, constipation.
- **Differential:** Guillain–Barré syndrome and myasthenia.
- **Investigations:** FBC, U&E, ABG: hypoxia and hypercarbia, FVC measurements TDS. NCS show defect is at neuromuscular junction.
- **Management:** ABC, ITU, severe cases (FVC <1 L) may need to be intubated/ventilated to avoid respiratory failure. Chest/passive physiotherapy. Antibiotics and debridement if wound-based infection (IV PENICILLIN G or CLINDAMYCIN). NG/PEG feeding if no swallow. PPI or Ranitidine to prevent stress ulcer. Urinary

catheterisation if needed, DVT prophylaxis. Wound infection: debridement and antitoxin and antibiotics EQUINE BOTULINUM ANTI-TOXIN: neutralises toxin. Halts but does not reverse neurology. Recovery takes months.

9.19 Clostridial infection

- **Source:** *Clostridium perfringens* forms gas. Large Gram +ve anaerobic spore-forming rods. Five types (A–E) differentiated by surface antigens. A is commonest cause of human disease. Alpha-toxin causes gas gangrene (lecithinase, haemolysis and necrosis). Found in soil, dust, faeces.
- **Pathogenicity:** gas gangrene – pain, massive tissue necrosis due to release of toxins, e.g. phospholipase C, lecithinase. Destroys polymorph. Local fermentation produces gas in the tissue. Potentially and rapidly fatal.
- **Clinical:** food poisoning onset 12–24 h post-ingestion with diarrhoea. Anaerobic cellulitis or infection of ischaemic limb.
- **Investigations:** Gram +ve spore-forming bacilli which grows on anaerobic culture.
- **Management:** debridement, hyperbaric O_2 chamber, BENZYLPENICILLIN IV + CLINDAMYCIN IV. Also see <u>Necrotising fasciitis</u>, ▶Section 18.6.

9.20 Acute bacterial sepsis

- **About:** don't forget about common infections. Renal/urine, chest, cardiac, GI, cholecystitis, bone and joint.
- **Investigations:** screen if temperature, ↑ or ↓WCC, malaise, confusion. FBC, U&E, LFT. ↑CRP. Screen urine, aerobic and anaerobic blood cultures, CXR, lumbar puncture, ascitic aspirate, echocardiogram, joint aspirate, serology where useful. CT head, USS abdomen/pelvis.
- **Management:** if unwell send samples and give broad spectrum antibiotics within 1 h. See <u>Sepsis</u>, ▶Section 2.21.

9.21 Measles

- **Note:** prevent with vaccine (MMR). Severe in the immunocompromised patient (take urgent advice). Paramyxovirus. Notifiable.
- **Source:** IP 12 days. In those unvaccinated non-immune. Respiratory droplets. Severe infection in older children/adults. Lifelong immunity. Infectious for 1–2 weeks.
- **Clinical:** prodrome of URTI, Koplik spots in buccal mucosa, macular papular rash. Lymphadenopathy, diarrhoea, otitis media, bacterial pneumonia. Viral encephalitis, seizures acutely. Malnourished/immunocompromised get pneumonitis, encephalitis. Secondary bacterial pneumonia or severe diarrhoea or cancrum oris. Can be lethal particularly in developing countries.
- **Diagnosis:** serology or PCR. **Complications:** Viral, later bacterial pneumonia, encephalitis; very late: subacute sclerosing panencephalitis.
- **Management:** IVIg may help immunocompromised if given early. Vitamin A can help. Antibiotics for bacterial superinfections.

9.22 Chickenpox/varicella zoster virus (Shingles)

- **About:** More severe in adults, immunosuppressed, pregnant. Varicella pneumonia has a 10% mortality. Lives in dorsal root ganglion and can reactivate. Increased risk with pregnant, smokers, immunosuppressed.
- **Clinical:** crops of vesicles to pustules, crust and dry on face, scalp and trunk. Feverish. IP from contact to symptoms 2–3 weeks. Hypoxia, breathlessness and

respiratory failure. Can recur in later life as shingles with a dermatomal spread of vesicles with redness, pain and inflammation.

- **Investigations:** ABG: hypoxia, serology if immunity unclear. Long-term calcification on CXR. Viral DNA on PCR or electron microscopy.
- **Management:** stop any immunosuppression. Take expert guidance. HDU/ITU care for respiratory support in severe varicella pneumonia. Broad-spectrum antibiotics for secondary bacterial infection (Staph. aureus, pneumococcus, haemophilus). High dose ACICLOVIR. Vaccination in those over 50 seems to dramatically lower the risk of post herpetic neuralgia.
- **Adolescents/adults:** childhood uncomplicated infection needs only supportive care. Age >16 presenting <3 days of onset needs to be treated. Shingles/adult chicken pox: oral ACICLOVIR. May need treatment for neuropathic pain. Severe complicated infection: IV ACICLOVIR.
- **Pregnant women:** need Zoster immune globulin (ZIG). They need ACICLOVIR if they develop signs. Take advice.

9.23 Mumps infection

- **About:** Paramyxovirus.
- **Clinical:** IP is 2 weeks. Parotitis, orchitis (sterility is uncommon), meningitis, pancreatitis, encephalitis is rare.
- **Investigations:** CSF: lymphocytic. (Salivary) Amylase may be high due to parotitis and confuse pancreatitis diagnosis. Serology/PCR for confirmation.
- **Management:** Isolate if admitted. Supportive management.

9.24 Herpes simplex 1 and 2

- **About:** usually benign but watch for HSV encephalitis.
- **Clinical:** severe mucocutaneous lesions – mouth, genital, anorectal, vaginal, oesophagus, systemic. HSV2 more genital. Often reactivation rather than new infection. Visceral involvement can be fatal, e.g. encephalitis.
- **Investigations:** LP for CSF. Stop immunosuppression. Expert consult. HSV DNA PCR on lesions.
- **Management:** oral ACICLOVIR for 1 week. Severe complicated infection: IV ACICLOVIR, also consider VALACICLOVIR and FAMCICLOVIR. Look for and treat any bacterial superinfection. Viral encephalitis (▶ Section 11.9).

9.25 Infectious mononucleosis

- **About:** seen with EBV, CMV, HHV6 and HIV and toxoplasmosis.
- **Clinical:** syndromic presentation with severe sore throat and fever and malaise. Teenagers or young adults. Pharyngeal oedema/respiratory obstruction, rash with Ampicillin, post-viral fatigue. Hepatitis 80%, jaundice, myelitis, encephalitis. GBS, ↓platelets, splenomegaly, nephritis, myopericarditis, splenic rupture.
- **Investigations:** positive monospot with EBV. Viral Serology for usual causes. Atypical lymphocytes (activated CD8 +ve T lymphocytes) may be seen. USS abdomen if splenomegaly.
- **Management:** largely supportive. Avoid sports and trauma with splenomegaly. Manage complications as they arise. Steroids may be given for encephalitis, thrombocytopenia and other complications. Avoid amoxicillin/ampicillin.

9.26 Cytomegalovirus

- **About:** Close contact human to human, saliva. Screen blood to ensure CMV non immune not exposed if immunocompromised.
- **Clinical:** immunocompetent: get hepatitis and infectious mononucleosis, rarely GBS. Immunocompromised: (solid organ and stem cell transplant) get a CMV pneumonitis usually 1–4 months post transplant. Mortality of 50%. AIDS patients CD4 < 50: retinitis, CMV colitis and polyradiculopathy. Pregnancy: primary infections can affect fetus. With rash, hepatosplenomegaly and CNS complications.
- **Investigations:** swab, microscopy, serology (high +ve in most population) and biopsy. PCR samples. Biopsy: Owl eye inclusion bodies and giant cells.
- **Management:** CMV infection is VALGANCICLOVIR (solid organ transplant patients) otherwise IV GANCICLOVIR. Needs expert help, particularly if pregnancy or immunosuppressed. Others FOSACANET, CIDOFOVIR. Consider HAART if AIDS.

9.27 Influenza

- **About:** caused by influenza A and B. Orthomyxoviruses. Most extensive and severe outbreaks are due to influenza A.
- **Virology:** surface haemagglutinin (H) and neuraminidase (N) antigens. Haemagglutinin binds erythrocytes and initiates infection. Neuraminidase cleaves haemagglutinin and releases virus from cells.
- **Variants:** avian influenza: influenza A infection (H5N1) caused a more severe pneumonia. Seen mainly in SE Asia. Treat as for influenza with neuraminidase inhibitors. Swine influenza: Mexico 2009. Influenza A infection (H1N1).
- **Clinical:** comes on within days of contact. Fever, headache, severe myalgia and malaise. Cough, sputum and respiratory tract symptoms. Diarrhoea. Secondary infection is common. *Staph. aureus* pneumonia.
- **Complications:** secondary bacterial pneumonia, myositis, GBS, myocarditis, transverse myelitis, encephalitis, pericarditis.
- **Investigations:** PCR of nose swab. CXR cavitating secondary pneumonia.
- **Management:** supportive, hydration, analgesia, isolation, hand washing. Pandemic flu: needs special isolation and barrier nursing with staff wearing appropriate masks, goggles, gloves and protective gear. Patient wears a surgical mask. Neuraminidase inhibitors: OSELTAMIVIR PO or inhaled ZANAMIVIR inhibit neuraminidase and work against influenza A and B, but must be given within 48 h to reduce duration of illness. Sepsis, ▶Section 2.21; Pneumonia, ▶Section 4.14.

9.28 Severe acute respiratory syndrome

- **About:** isolate suspected SARS immediately. SARS is a coronavirus respiratory illness (SARS-CoV). Since 2004, no known cases of SARS anywhere in the world. Prior to 2004, patients had had close contact with infected person.
- **Clinical:** sore throat, rhinorrhoea, chills, rigors, myalgia, headache, D&V.
- **Investigations:** ↑WCC, ↑CRP, ↑ALT, ↑CK, ↑LDH. Get FBC, WCC, CXR. Blood cultures, test for viral respiratory pathogens, influenza A and B and respiratory syncytial virus. Legionella and pneumococcal urinary antigen testing if CXR/CT evidence of pneumonia (adults only).
- **Management:** supportive. Isolate, analgesia, oxygen. See advice for MERS below regarding PPE. Take local expert advice. Sepsis, ▶Section 2.21; Pneumonia, ▶Section 4.14.

9.29 Middle Eastern respiratory syndrome

- **About:** isolate immediately. Coronavirus new to humans. Travel from Saudi Arabia and environs should raise suspicion.
- **Clinical:** severe acute respiratory illness, fever, cough, and shortness of breath. Case fatality 52%.
- **Management:** supportive. Isolate, analgesia, O_2. Deadlier than SARS. Ensure respiratory isolation. Ask patient to wear a surgical mask. Wear personal protective equipment (PPE) – this should be a correctly fitted FFP3 respirator, gown, gloves and eye protection. If not available, wear a surgical mask, plastic apron and gloves. Take local expert advice. Sepsis, ▶ Section 2.21.

9.30 Zika virus infection

- **About:** outbreak in Brazil 2015 led to reports of birth defects (microcephaly) and poor pregnancy outcomes.
- **Clinical:** fever, rash, joint pain, and conjunctivitis (red eyes). Usually mild with symptoms lasting from several days to a week. GBS documented. Severe disease uncommon.
- **Investigations:** pregnant women with Zika symptoms should be tested.
- **Management:** avoid mosquito bites. Found in semen. Avoid unprotected sex with infected person. Mosquitoes that spread Zika virus also spread dengue and chikungunya viruses.

9.31 Needlestick injury

- **About:** concern is potential infection with HBV, HIV, HCV. Needle used to take blood or give IM/IV/SC injection pierces the skin of another. Infected fluids in eyes or ingested or on contact with mucocutaneous surfaces. Hepatitis C risk 3%, HIV risk 0.3%. All NHS staff should be immunised against hepatitis B.
- **Aetiology:** passage of blood-borne viruses. HBV risk in HBV patient much higher but clinical staff should have been immunised. If there is a reasonable risk that the patient is HIV positive, then treat as a medical emergency and seek urgent help – see below.
- **Management:** encourage wound to bleed freely and then wash with soap and water. Don't scrub such that further tissue damage occurs. Cover with waterproof dressing. If oral or eye contamination, then wash and irrigate thoroughly with IV NS via giving set or tap water. Mouth contamination should rinse but don't swallow. Report incident promptly to line manager and complete incident form when appropriate. In working hours contact occupational health, out of hours go to local emergency department (A&E). Do not try to manage this on the ward yourself or with your team.
- **Inform the patient and explore any particular risks** for HIV/HBV/HCV, e.g. IV drug use, sexual history. Patient may allow a clotted sample for HBV/HCV/HIV. Patient should be aware that results will be divulged to the injured person. The consent should be recorded in their notes. All NHS clinical staff should be immunised against hepatitis B. Hepatitis B immunoglobulin may be given if required following expert assessment with emergency department or occupational health who may liaise with microbiology. The risk of hepatitis C is 3% and there is no post-exposure prophylaxis (PEP) but follow up should be carried out. For HIV the risk is 0.3% and depends on depth of wound, visible blood on device, needle from artery or vein and terminal HIV disease. Risk of HIV transmission = risk that source is HIV positive × risk of exposure. As part of risk assessment record size and volume of the inoculum, i.e. whether the needle was hollow, etc. Depth of injury. Visible blood on the device that caused the

injury. Injury with a needle that had been placed in an artery or vein. If HIV possible, AZT reduces infection 5-fold. PEP is given which involves three antiretrovirals for 1 month and is started immediately. PEP should be taken following local expert risk assessment and guidance and policies; an exact protocol is not included here because local practice should be followed.

Reference: Kuhar *et al.* (2013) Updated US Public Health Service Guidelines for the management of occupational exposures to HIV and recommendations for post-exposure prophylaxis. *Infection Control and Hospital Epidemiology*, 34:875.

9.32 Tuberculosis (*Mycobacterium tuberculosis*)

- **About:** *Mycobacterium tuberculosis* is the most common form in humans. *M. bovis* seen in developing countries from infected milk products (non-pasteurized). Pulmonary cavitation is synonymous with infectivity but may be absent in those with AIDS. Isolate patient.
- **Risks:** increasing due to HIV/AIDS, homelessness, alcohol dependency. Immigrants from Sub-Saharan Africa, Bangladesh, India, Pakistan. Drug and multidrug resistant (rifampicin) TB is a problem. Age, malignancy, alcohol, immunodeficiency, malnutrition. Use of immunosuppression, anti-TNF-alpha drugs.
- **Pathology:** classed as one of the granulomatous inflammatory conditions. Th1 reaction with epithelioid macrophages, Langhans giant cells, lymphocytes. Central caseous necrosis and production of interferon-gamma by T helper cells. The Ghon focus + local hilar lymphadenopathy is called a Ghon complex.
- **Clinical:** night sweats, fevers, weight loss, cervical or generalized lymphadenopathy, hepatosplenomegaly. Pyrexia of unknown origin, cervical lymph node (scrofula). **Gastro:** TB of terminal ileum with a RIF mass, peritonitis, ascites, psoas abscess. **Resp:** breathlessness, cough, sputum and consolidation and upper lobe scarring on CXR, pleural effusion. **Renal TB:** sterile pyuria with WCC in urine and normal cultures negative. **Skin:** lupus vulgaris and erythema induratum. **CNS TB:** TB meningitis – headache, cranial nerve palsies, etc. **Vertebral disease:** back pain – spinal infection, discitis, disc collapse, spinal cord compression. **Cardiac:** TB pericardial effusion and constrictive pericarditis. **Endocrine:** Addison's disease with adrenal TB.

Investigations

- **FBC:** ↓Hb, ↑WCC, ↑ESR, ↑CRP. ↑**LFTs:** ↑AST, ↑ALT. **CXR:** pleural effusion, hilar lymphadenopathy, consolidation, fibrosis, upper and middle lobe infection, millet seed-like opacities on chest film <5 mm with miliary TB. Cavitatory disease suggests infectivity, right mid zone collapse. Pneumothorax. Send **sputum smear:** direct staining and microscopy of a smear from recently expectorated sputum. If bacilli seen it is classed as 'smear positive' and is infectious. Inducing sputum is said to be as effective as broncho-alveolar lavage. Auramine O is an alternative to Ziehl–Neelsen especially as the dye fluoresces under UV light and so the bacilli are easier to see. **Sputum cultures** are the gold standard but take 3–6 weeks to grow and then identify species. **Sputum analysis:** DNA analysis using PCR identifying serotype and drug sensitivity. **Serology:** HIV test and CD4 count.
- **Tuberculin test:** uses purified protein derivative (PPD) to elicit a delayed-type hypersensitivity response which is mediated by T lymphocytes. The reaction is maximal at 2–3 days after inoculation. Positive tuberculin testing does not always suggest active disease, it suggests a prior immune response, previous infection or BCG. So only a grade 3/4 (10 mm induration) or a negative test are useful in those with history of BCG. It is important to elicit a weal to demonstrate that it is intradermal and not subcutaneous. Most with active TB will have a positive skin test (=10 mm). Must measure the induration, not erythema. Tuberculin skin tests are not contraindicated in BCG-vaccinated people and skin test reactivity should

be interpreted and treated as for unvaccinated people. False negatives occur in immunosuppressed, steroids, malnourished, HIV, severe TB (e.g. miliary disease), early primary disease – becomes positive 2–12 weeks post primary infection. **Lumbar puncture:** CSF – ↑lymphocyte, ↑protein low glucose but smears rarely positive in TB meningitis. Check CT to exclude any space occupying lesion. **Early morning urines** to culture for TB in suspected renal disease. **Renal imaging:** image with CT or intravenous urogram. **Bronchoscopy and lavage:** may be useful to get samples in difficult cases when there is an unproductive cough and high clinical suspicion. It may help to exclude other causes such as tumours with a potential for biopsy of abnormal tissue. **Microbiological culture** from sputum analysis, gastric aspirate (used in children), urine for renal TB, bone marrow biopsy, CSF, liver biopsy, bronchoalveolar lavage. **Interferon gamma release assays:** ↑level does not differentiate active and latent disease. Main use is alongside Mantoux testing to detect latent disease.

Management

- Needs to be a high level of suspicion in the high-risk groups identified and TB with widespread manifestations should always be considered. Those with smear-positive disease need to be isolated. It is a notifiable disease. Smear-negative patients are rarely infectious. Smear-positive patients can be considered not infectious after 2 weeks of treatment. Should be referred to specialist. Adequate tissue samples for diagnosis should be taken before treatment started. Patients should be treated with 4 drug regimen (RIPE) for 2 months and 2 drug regimen for 4 months. In those with a low chance of resistance then RIFAMPICIN, ISONIAZID and PYRAZINAMIDE only without ETHAMBUTOL may be used (RIP): RIPE 2 months and RI 4 months; RIP 2 months and RI 4 months – low chance of resistance. Exceptions: TB of CNS – treatment is for 12 months. Resistance to any of the drugs (isoniazid or rifampicin) means a 9 month course.

9.33   HIV/acquired immunodeficiency syndrome

- WHO guidelines now agree that all HIV-positive patients should receive antiretroviral therapy (ART) after diagnosis regardless of CD4 count. When to start depends on a person's unique needs and circumstances.
- Evidence is strongest with a CD4 count <350 cells/mm^3 (WHO Guideline HIV, September 2015).

Seroconversion illness/acute retroviral syndrome

- **About:** HIV testing should be considered as routine in all who are sexually active or who use IV drugs.
- **Source:** worldwide. Symptoms within 2–6 weeks of infection. HIV1 Europe/America/Asia, HIV2 Africa.
- **Risk groups:** men having sex with men. IV drug use and needle sharing. Casual unprotected sex with sex worker. Their sexual partners. Children of HIV-positive mothers.
- **Clinical** (seroconversion 2 weeks after contact): fever, rash, joint pains, malaise, lymphadenopathy, headache, myalgia, pharyngitis. Lasts for days to 3 weeks. Medical attention often sought as severe. Highly infectious period. Differential diagnosis of acute seroconversion: exclude malaria in endemic area, glandular fever, influenza, and dengue.
- **Investigations:** HIV1/HIV2 antibody not detected but there is HIV RNA or HIV p24 antigen in plasma. HIV test and repeat after 6 weeks and CD4 count and viral titres. CXR and ABG if suspected *Pneumocystis carinii* pneumonia (PCP).
- **Management:** patient highly infectious. Test also for syphilis and other sexually transmitted infections. Take expert advice as to need for post exposure prophylaxis.

Refer to GUM for contact tracing and treatment with ART. Over time the CD4 count falls. Those with a CD4 <200 cells/mm³ are at high risk for opportunistic infections. If the CD4 <50 then high risk of CMV and atypical mycobacterial infections, e.g. disseminated *Mycobacterium avium* intracellulare.

Acquired immunodeficiency syndrome (AIDS)

- It is later with the clinical occurrence of infections and malignancies in the setting of a low CD4 count that AIDS is defined. All those with symptomatic disease should be offered ART, usually as the count is <350 cells/mm³.
- Those who are pregnant, need treatment for hepatitis B infection or have HIV nephropathy are treated regardless of CD4 count. Aim is to reduce the plasma viral load (PVL) and improve CD4 count and avoid resistance. This requires 3 or more drugs which are potentially toxic.

Nervous system

- **Stroke:** ischaemic stroke. Exclude other causes. Easy to confuse subcortical lesions on CT with PML. Low threshold for MRI and CSF.
- **Cryptococcal meningitis:** CD4 <50. Headache, neck stiffness, fever, photophobia, cranial nerve palsies and papilloedema. Chronic meningitis. CT: may be normal or cryptococcomas, hydrocephalus. Serum cryptococcal neoformans antigen (CRAG) in serum and CSF (100% sensitivity for meningitis). CSF: ↑WCC, ↑protein but occasionally normal. Start ART: IV AMPHOTERICIN B and FLUCYTOSINE for 2 weeks followed by FLUCONAZOLE for 8–12 weeks.
- **Cerebral toxoplasmosis:** host is cat. Ingestion of eggs. Infection before and held under check by immunity. Reactivates when CD4 <50 cells/mm³. Progressive symptoms over days. Seizures, fever and reduced GCS, hemiballismus/chorea. CT/MR shows multiple ring enhancing lesions in cortex and basal ganglia. Capsule formation is poor due to reduced immune response so there is good antibiotic penetration. Positive IgG serology useful. Take advice. Good response to Pyrimethamine, sulfadiazine and folinic acid. Repeat CT after 2 weeks shows improvement; if not then consider brain biopsy.
- **Progressive multifocal leucoencephalopathy:** onset can be over weeks. Usually CD4 <100 cells/mm³. Can mimic white matter disease. Due to JC virus. One or more focal non-enhancing lesions of gradual onset. Fever, headache uncommon suggests toxoplasmosis. Can mimic stroke. CSF: PCR for JC virus. Optimise ART.
- **Tubercular meningitis:** cervical lymphadenopathy, headache, N&V, pyrexia, meningism. IIIrd and VIth nerve palsies. CSF: ↑opening pressure, ↑protein and ↓sugar and ↑lymphocytes, ↓CD4 <200 cells/mm³. Needs ART and 12+ months antitubercular therapy.
- **Primary cerebral lymphoma:** progressive symptoms over weeks. Headache and focal neurology. No fever. More likely if toxoplasma serology negative or failure to respond to treatment for toxoplasmosis. Multiple periventricular lesions on imaging. Irregular and weakly enhancing. CD4 <100 cells/mm³.
- **AIDS dementia complex:** progressive cognitive and functional decline. CSF normal. CT shows atrophy.
- **Transverse myelitis:** sensory level with motor weakness, autonomic loss.
- **Guillain–Barré syndrome:** ▶ Section 11.27.
- **Peripheral neuropathy:** typically, a sensory neuropathy.

Cardiopulmonary

- **Bacterial pneumonias:** Fever, breathless, productive cough. Will depend on degree of immunocompromise. 10 times commoner than in HIV negatives. Higher risks with IV drug abuse. Cover as well for PCP. Treat early. ▶ Section 4.15.

- **Pneumocystis pneumonia:** CD4 <200 cells/mm^3. High LDH. Breathless, dry cough, fever, for 2 weeks, desaturation. If the CD4 >200 cells/mm^3 or on prophylaxis and compliant then PCP much less likely. ▶ Section 4.15.
- **Tuberculosis:** test HIV in all those with evidence of TB. Assume infectious. Isolate and get sputum cultures and respiratory review once diagnosis confirmed. May be insidious and atypical and no cavitation and lower lobe involved. ▶ Section 4.15.
- **Cardiac:** may have a dilated cardiomyopathy and myocarditis. Needs Echo. Manage heart failure and arrhythmias.

Gastroenterology – requires endoscopy and biopsy of lesions

- **Oro-oesophageal candidiasis:** painful swallowing. Red, painful bleeding mucosa. Can be candida. Treat with FLUCONAZOLE 7–14 d. Differential if ulcerated is CMV or HSV infection and OGD and swabs taken.
- **CMV colitis, oesophagitis, hepatitis:** Owl's eye inclusion bodies. consider IV GANCICLOVIR. HSV then IV ACICLOVIR.
- **Chronic diarrhoea:** some have an unknown cause. Others due to cryptosporidiosis infection. Also vulnerable to *Salmonella, Shigella, Campylobacter*, giardiasis and some may be mixed pathogens. Leads to dehydration, weight loss due to malabsorption. Send stool cultures.
- **Others:** HIV enteropathy, gastrointestinal TB, sclerosing cholangitis.

Dermatology

- **Multi-dermatomal herpes zoster:** can be seen with CD4 >500 cells/mm^3. Treat with ACICLOVIR PO 5/day. Alternative is FAMCICLOVIR. Severe or ophthalmic involvement, switch to IV ACICLOVIR.
- **Herpes simplex:** oral, mucosal disease, hands, face. Crusted vesicles. Treat with ACICLOVIR PO 5/day. Alternative is FAMCICLOVIR.
- **Kaposi sarcoma:** purplish skin lesions. HHV6 infection. May be in skin or in lung and other organs.

Haematology

- Thrombocytopenia: ▶ Section 8.2.

Ophthalmic

- **CMV retinitis:** CD4 count <50 cells/mm^3 or as part of IRIS (see below). Ophthalmology consult. GANCICLOVIR may be given directly into the eye.
- **Varicella zoster:** can affect ophthalmic branch of V and so the cornea. It can also cause an acute retinal necrosis simultaneously. Look for vesicular tingling and then painful rash over V1 distribution or may be multi-dermatomal. IV ACICLOVIR is given.

Antiretroviral drugs

Combination therapy is key to avoid resistance. May also require prophylaxis, e.g. for pneumocystis. ART reduces viral load and improves survival. **BHIVA** recommends therapy-naïve patients start ART containing two nucleos(t)ide reverse transcriptase inhibitors (NRTIs) plus one of the following: a ritonavir-boosted protease inhibitor (PI/r), an NNRTI or an integrase inhibitor (INI). They recommend therapy-naïve patients start combination ART containing tenofovir (TDF) and emtricitabine (FTC) as the NRTI backbone combined with a third agent. This should be managed by experts in HIV medicine.

Different medications

- Nucleos(t)ide reverse transcriptase inhibitors (NRTIs): zidovudine, abacavir, lamivudine, didanosine, tenofovir.

- Protease inhibitors (PIs): e.g. ritonavir/saquinavir/indinavir.
- Non-nucleos(t)ide reverse transcriptase inhibitors (NNRTIs): active against HIV1, e.g. nevirapine/efavirenz.
- HIV cell fusion inhibitors, e.g. enfuvirtide.

Antiretroviral drugs side effects
- **Lactic acidosis:** with NRTI. ↑mortality. N&V, ↑lactate.
- **Pancreatitis:** see with ddI, d4T and ddC drugs.
- **Lipodystrophy syndrome:** (insulin resistance/dyslipidaemia/fat redistribution), d4T.
- **Rhabdomyolysis:** protease inhibitors + statin. PIs are cytochrome p450 inhibitors: ↑toxicity of drugs metabolised on this pathway. Check BNF or equivalent.
- **Toxic epidermal necrolysis/Stevens–Johnson syndrome:** Nevirapine.

Immune reconstitution inflammatory syndrome (IRIS)
- Seen with introduction of ART. Rapid ↓viral load and ↑CD4 count. More likely from a very low CD4 count.
- There is a rise in T cells and enhanced immune response to infections that had been subclinical. Certain infections involved are: *Mycobacterium avium* complex, CMV retinitis, worsening pulmonary TB, worsening cryptococcal meningitis.

CD4 count (per mm³) and opportunistic infections
- **CD4 any:** Kaposi sarcoma, pulmonary TB, HZV, bacterial pneumonia, lymphoma.
- **CD4 <250:** PCP, oesophageal candidiasis, PML, HSV.
- **CD4 <100:** cerebral toxoplasmosis, HIV encephalopathy, cryptococciosis, miliary TB.
- **CD4 <50:** CMV retinitis, atypical mycobacterial infection.

Reference: www.bhiva.org/documents/guidelines/treatment/2012/hiv1029_2.pdf.

9.34 Syphilis

- **About:** spirochete. *Treponema pallidum*. Sexual transmitted.
- **Clinical: primary:** painless oral, rectal or genital ulcer with painless nodes. **Secondary:** fever, malaise, rash. Maculopapular. Lymphadenopathy, Nephritis, hepatitis, uveitis. **Tertiary:** Skin, bone destructive lesions. **Quaternary:** Aortic aneurysm, Neurosyphilis, Dementia, tabes dorsalis, Argyll Robertson pupils.
- **Investigations:** Swab of ulcer dark ground microscopy. Serology: VDRL/TPPA/FTA. CSF testing when appropriate. Neurosyphilis WBC > 20 cells/μL or greater or a reactive CSF (VDRL) test result. HIV test.
- **Management:** Primary: DOXYCYCLINE 100 mg BD 10d, BENZATHINE PENICILLIN 2.4 g IM × 2. Late: DOXYCYCLINE 100 mg BD 28d, BENZATHINE PENICILLIN 2.4 g IM × 3. Neurosyphilis PROCAINE PENICILLIN 2 g IM OD plus PROBENICID 500 mg QDS 17 days or DOXYCYCLINE 200 mg bd 28 days. Screen for other sexually transmitted infections and contact screen.

9.35 Oropharyngeal bacterial infections

- **Glandular fever:** mentioned elsewhere – caused by CMV, EBV. Avoid Amoxil/Ampicillin as causes rash.
- **Common viral:** measles, mumps, rubella, coryza and many of the common viral illnesses may cause some throat pain and associated pharyngitis.
- **Acute pharyngitis:** avoid AMPICILLIN or AMOXIL. Mainly viral (adenovirus, rhinovirus, RSV). Management is supportive. Bacterial (*Strep. pyogenes* – Group A beta-haemolytic streptococci) more likely if fever and purulent tonsillar exudate and cervical lymphadenopathy without significant cough. Can confirm with rapid

antigen detection test (RADT) and throat culture. Local complications include peritonsillar abscess. Treat with oral PENICILLIN V for 10 d or CLARITHROMYCIN for 10 d. Complications: acute rheumatic fever, scarlet fever, post-streptococcal glomerulonephritis.

- **Acute epiglottitis:** see entry for Stridor, ▶Section 4.4.

9.36 Diphtheria

- **About:** *Corynebacterium diphtheria, C. ulcerans.* Fatality 5–10%.
- **Aetiology:** releases an exotoxin which blocks protein synthesis. Mild cases can go undiagnosed. Toxin acts as an RNA translational inhibitor. Local tissue necrosis. Toxaemia and paralysis due to demyelinating peripheral neuritis. Cardiac failure due to myocarditis.
- **Microbiology:** Gram +ve, aerobic, non-motile, rod-shaped bacteria. From direct physical contact or aerosolized from infected person.
- **Clinical:** produces a grey thick membrane in pharynx. Nasal, laryngeal and pharyngeal mucosa affected. Can lead to airway obstruction and stridor. Sore throat, fever, malaise. Heart failure, heart block and arrhythmias. Cranial nerve palsies, diplopia, dysarthria, dysphagia. Sensorimotor Polyneuropathy.
- **Investigations:** FBC, U&E, CRP, CXR. ECG: heart block and arrhythmias. NCS shows demyelination. Culture of swabs from larynx/pharynx. Echocardiogram to assess LV function.
- **Management:** ABCs, O_2. Bed rest and telemetry initially. Isolation and treatment of the index case. Prevention with diphtheria toxoid immunisation and is also given with suspected diphtheria infection. Give 2 weeks of BENZYLPENICILLIN IV or AMOXICILLIN IV or ERYTHROMYCIN IV if penicillin allergic. Horse serum derived ANTITOXIN is given for acute infection. Remove membrane by laryngoscopy or bronchoscopy to prevent airways obstruction. Also treat contacts. Seek expert help.

9.37 Lemierre's syndrome (*Fusobacterium necrophorum*)

- **About:** mortality 5%. Septic thrombosis of internal jugular vein (IJV).
- **Microbiology:** *Fusobacterium necrophorum* produces a lipopolysaccharide endotoxin (leukocidin) and haemolysin which increases virulence. Also *Streptococcus* sp., *Bacteroides* sp., *Peptostreptococcus* sp., and *Eikenella corrodens*.
- **Aetiology:** disseminated abscesses. Septic thrombophlebitis of the internal jugular vein. Associated infection of the oropharynx due to G-ve anaerobic bacillus. Main sources of infection are tonsil, pharynx, and chest.
- **Clinical:** sore throat, painful swelling of the neck, fever, rigors. Haemoptysis and dyspnoea if lungs involved. Pus on tonsils. Thrombophlebitis of the IJV. Palsies of cranial nerves IX to XII. Septic emboli – joints, liver, spleen, osteomyelitis, meningitis.
- **Investigation:** FBC: ↑WCC, ↑CRP, ↑ESR. Blood cultures. CXR: cavitatory abscesses from septic emboli, pleural effusions. CT thorax: may find septic pulmonary emboli and internal jugular venous thrombosis and lung cavitation from abscesses. Pleural fluid/empyema. Doppler USS of neck veins shows occluded IJV.
- **Differential:** infectious endocarditis. Wegener's as lung lesions and ENT issues (check cANCA).
- **Management:** HDU/ITU level care. O_2. Supportive. Antibiotics: take microbiological advice. High dose IV antibiotics, e.g. TAZOCIN IV + METRONIDAZOLE IV. Often sensitive to penicillin, clindamycin, chloramphenicol. Some beta-lactamase activity may be seen. Anticoagulation with IV heparin/LMWH: controversial and may speed recovery, though there may be worries about bleeding from septic emboli. Some

reserve it only for evidence of clot progression towards cavernous sinuses, others for SVC thrombophlebitis. In those with uncontrolled sepsis and repeated septic emboli despite appropriate medical therapy, surgical ligation or excision of the IJV should be performed, although this treatment is rarely needed today.

Reference: Golpe *et al.* (1999) Lemierre's syndrome. *Postgrad Med J*, 75:141.

 Meticillin sensitive/resistant *Staph. aureus*

- **About:** *Staph. aureus* with acquired resistance to meticillin, flucloxacillin and oxacillin by acquiring the mec-A gene.
- **Clinical:** line infections, bone and soft tissue infections, pneumonias and septicaemia. MRSA is associated with a higher mortality than MSSA. Needs good asepsis, hand washing and eradication policies.
- **Investigations:** blood culture, skin swabs, nasal and groin often screened. Lines.
- **Management:** Any *Staph. aureus* bacteraemia "always" gets at least 2 weeks of IV antibiotics and needs microbiological advice. *Staph. aureus* in the urine should also initiate concerns and blood cultures should be done. Look for cardiac or bone infections. Metastatic infections seen in those inadequately treated, to bone, spine and joint and heart. MRSA septicaemia should receive VANCOMYCIN or TEICOPLANIN. DOXYCYCLINE may be used for soft tissue infections.

 Bacterial resistance: VRE, ESBL, CRE/CRO

- **Vancomycin resistant enterococcus (VRE):** enterococci common commensals. VRE may be difficult to treat because of the limited range of effective antibiotics. May cause UTI, wounds and vascular catheter site infections. Many simply colonised and non-pathogenic. Limit spread. Single room isolation especially if diarrhoea and handwashing measures. Decolonisation generally unsuccessful and therefore not recommended. VRE are of limited virulence (unlike MRSA) and mostly colonise rather than infect. If detected in faeces needs no treatment. VRE rarely causes infection in the healthy. Take local microbiological advice. Uncomplicated cystitis due to VRE can usually be treated with NITROFURANTOIN.
- **Extended-spectrum beta-lactamases (ESBL):** bacteria that produce ESBLs are resistant to many penicillin and cephalosporin antibiotics. Usually *E. coli* and *Klebsiella* sp. *E. coli* produce CTX-M enzymes and may cause UTIs, more serious infections and septicaemia. Difficult to treat. In most fit and healthy individuals ESBL not a problem and they are well. Immunocompromised and elderly at greater risk. Management is based on isolation and limiting spread by hand washing and other means.
- **Carbapenem-resistant enterobacteriaceae/organisms (CRE/CRO):** CRE are Enterobacteriaceae such as *E. coli*, *Klebsiella* resistant to carbapenems e.g. meropenem. CRO are *Pseudomonas*, *Acinetobacter* with similar resistance. These organisms are endemic and often imported in those who have exposure to overseas healthcare. Infections with CRE/CRO have increased morbidity, mortality, prolonged hospital stay and expense. They are normal gut commensals. Can cause infection in the critically ill. Anyone who has been an inpatient in a hospital abroad should be isolated and screened within 24 h of admission, usually by a rectal swab or stool sample, or from a wound, or urine if catheter, or sputum if productive. Most patients are colonised but have no symptoms. Needs two negative swabs to be clear. All positives must remain isolated. Aim is preventing spread. Hand hygiene using soap and water is the only effective way of removing this organism from the hands. Visitors should wear disposable aprons and gloves.

9.40 Gastroenteritis and similar infections

- **About:** usually a self-limiting bowel infection. Rarely can result in severe fluid/electrolyte loss. More severe in elderly, pregnant, immunocompromised, co-morbidities who may need admission.
- **Causes:** viral: norovirus, rotavirus, adenovirus, etc. Bacterial: non-typhoidal *Salmonella*, *Campylobacter*, *Shigella* (blood dysentery stools), cholera (*Vibrio cholera*, rice water stool).
- **Inflammatory diarrhoea:** abdominal pain, fever, small volume bloody stool. Involves distal small bowel and colon with invasion and mucosal cell death. Similar to ulcerative colitis. An example causative infection is with *Shigella*.
- **Secretory diarrhoea:** nausea, vomiting, high volume water stool with early dehydration and ↓BP, less fever, less bloody stools. E.g. cholera.
- **Clinical:** colicky abdominal pain, diarrhoea and dehydration are main symptoms, with ↓BP. Oliguria, syncope. Can be bloody diarrhoea.
- **Investigations:** FBC, U&E, LFT, CRP, stools for microscopy and culture. Prevention is key: avoid contact for 24–48 h after symptoms have stopped. Side room or home if can manage and hydrated. Hand washing with soap and water. Wear glove and aprons where advised.
- **Management:** isolation and good hand washing and infection control. Oral rehydration therapy for mild cases. More severe need IV fluids. Most resolve without antibiotics. Severe cases consider antibiotics as below. Antibiotics: treat if >6 type unformed stools per day, fever, blood or significant co-morbidities; beware that antibiotics should be restricted to most severe cases and most will resolve naturally. CIPROFLOXACIN PO is the antibiotic of choice in most infections. However, antibiotics best avoided if you suspect *E. coli* 0157 as increases risk of HUS. METRONIDAZOLE for giardiasis and amoebiasis. For *Campylobacter* CLARITHROMYCIN.

9.41 *E. coli* infections

- **Enteropathogenic** (EPEC) mild to severe disease with bloody diarrhoea.
- **Enterotoxigenic** (ETEC) causes marked diarrhoea and vomiting.
- **Enteroinvasive** (EIEC) damages colonic cells with watery (bloody) diarrhoea but no toxin, usually mild and self-limiting.
- **Enterohaemorrhagic** (EHEC) with verocytoxin (VTEC) such as 0157:H7 and others. Usually from poorly cooked food: milk and meat. The enterotoxins can affect kidneys, heart and brain and cause HUS. Made worse by antibiotics. Clinical: watery or bloody diarrhoea, dehydration, AKI.
- **Management:** self-limiting so usually supportive and oral or IV rehydration as needed. Avoid antibiotics, especially if 0157:H7 suspected.

9.42 *Staphylococcal* food poisoning

- **Source:** cheese, meats. Poor hygiene and storage.
- **Clinical:** sickness within 3–6 h. Mostly severe vomiting > diarrhoea. Toxins may act as superantigens. Severe dehydration can occur.
- **Management:** needs oral/IV rehydration and anti-emetics.

9.43 Shigella dysenteriae

- **About:** *Sh. flexneri, Sh. boydii, Sh. sonnei.* 10 bacteria sufficient. Gram –ve. Invade colonic mucosa. Release Shiga toxin. Contaminated food, flies, men having sex with men. Institutions.
- **Clinical:** inflammatory diarrhoea, colic, abdominal pain. Bloody purulent stools. Fever and dehydration. Later Reiter's syndrome (red eye, arthritis, urethritis).
- **Investigations:** send stool for culture.
- **Differential:** acute severe colitis. **Complications:** rectal prolapse, megacolon, Reiter's syndrome, HUS.
- **Management:** supportive. Consider CIPROFLOXACIN 500 mg BD 5d or CO-TRIMOXAZOLE.

9.44 Enteric fever (typhoid/paratyphoid)

- **About:** *Salmonella typhi* causes typhoid fever (TF) and *Salmonella paratyphi* causes paratyphoid fever. Can be life-threatening unless treated promptly.
- **Aetiology:** infects terminal ileum mucosal associated lymphoid tissue. Spreads via thoracic duct to lymph nodes and reticuloendothelial system.
- **Clinical:** 2–3 weeks of progressive symptoms. Dry cough. IP 5–21 days. Fever, headache, ↓HR (TF). Constipation or diarrhoea. Rose spots (easily missed), meningism, encephalopathy. Apathy, hypo- and hyperactive delirium is frequent (TF), hepatosplenomegaly (TF). Worsening over 2–3 week period leading to intestinal haemorrhage, bowel perforation, and death.
- **Investigations:** blood and stool cultures positive in first 2 weeks (stools positive in chronic carriers). FBC: fall in WCC and platelets. U&E: AKI, ↑LFTs. Serology is possible.
- **Management:** CEFTRIAXONE IV for 14 days for severe cases or where resistance suspected (acquired in Asia). Supportive care is required. Surgery for any bowel perforation. Fever may take 3–5 days to resolve. Non-typhoidal *Salmonella* CIPROFLOXACIN PO 5 d or CEFTRIAXONE

Reference: Fiddian–Green (2009) Treatment of enteric fever. *BMJ*, 338:b1159.

9.45 Bacillus cereus

- **Source:** seen classically from fresh rice. Heat stable exotoxin.
- **Clinical:** severe vomiting. If toxin-producing organisms ingested may be more of a watery diarrhoea presentation. Self-limiting <1 day.
- **Management:** needs oral rehydration. IV if severe and dehydrated.

9.46 Cholera

- **About:** faeco-oral or vomitus. Water-borne as survives in fresh and salt water.
- **Aetiology:** *Vibrio cholera* serotype 01. Toxin activates acetylate cyclase in intestinal mucosa. Active secretion of water and chloride.
- **Clinical:** acute secretory diarrhoea. Volume loss ++ and hypovolaemic shock.
- **Investigations:** U&E: ↑urea, creatinine. AKI. Diagnosis: dark field microscopy.
- **Management:** needs salt and water replacement. Oral rehydration but usually needs IV replacement. Use IV Ringer–lactate. Can lose 10 L/day, which needs to be replaced. Give DOXYCYCLINE 300 mg single dose or CIPROFLOXACIN.

9.47 Giardiasis

- **About:** *Giardia intestinalis* from contaminated water.
- **Clinical:** acute watery secretory diarrhoea, malabsorption, weakness.

- **Investigations:** send stool ova, cysts, parasites – motile trophozoites in stool.
- **Management:** prevent – boil water for 1 min. METRONIDAZOLE 400 mg 8 h for 5 days. Rehydration and electrolyte correction.

9.48 Amoebiasis

- **About:** *Entamoeba histolytica* cyst ingestion. Contaminated water, salads, ice cubes. Seen worldwide.
- **Clinical:** (1) Acute colitis with bloody diarrhoea, even perforation. Lasts days to weeks. (2) Liver abscess: 2–5 months post ingestion, RUQ pain, weight loss, enlarged liver, +ve serology. USS/CT liver. Aspirate if needed – non-foul smelling 'anchovy sauce'. Left lobe abscesses are higher risk to rupturing into critical sites (e.g. the pericardium), which justifies more intervention.
- **Investigations:** cysts are commonly seen in faeces but not diagnostic. USS liver, Check serology +ve in 90%.
- **Management:** prevent – boil suspect water for 1 min. METRONIDAZOLE PO for 7–10 days then DILOXANIDE FUROATE PO to clear organism from bowel.

9.49 Neurocysticercosis

- **About:** tapeworm (*Taenia solium*) infection ingested from infected food or water. Seen where pigs kept in close contact with human faeces. 2nd commonest infective cause of epilepsy worldwide (1st is TB). Dying cysts in muscle, eye, brain elicit inflammatory reaction.
- **Clinical:** epilepsy, cerebellar and brainstem signs, dementia, obstructive hydrocephalus. Headaches, backache if in spine. Eyes – blindness. Fundoscopy.
- **Investigations:** bloods: leucocytosis, eosinophilia, and ↑ESR. Plain X-rays of muscles show calcified cysts. Brain CT calcified lesions. MR lesions in different stages: vesicular, colloidal and nodular–granular stage. May show obstructive hydrocephalus. CSF: ↑protein, oligoclonal bands, eosinophilia.
- **Management:** may develop hydrocephalus needing external ventricular drainage. Initiate PHENYTOIN 150–300 mg OD or VALPROATE 300 mg BD for seizures. Needs PRAZIQUANTEL or ALBENDAZOLE combined with STEROIDS to dampen inflammatory response (but screen for TB first).

9.50 Tetanus

- **About:** *Clostridium tetani* infection in the west seen in older non-immunised adults. Preventable. Clean wounds and tetanus booster if need. Severely contaminated wounds give human tetanus immunoglobulin (HTIG).
- **Aetiology:** obligate anaerobe Gram +ve bacillus with drumstick spore, produces tetanospasmin which leaves the motor neurons without inhibition causing severe spasms and lethality.
- **Prevent:** childhood DTaP vaccine series. Adults tetanus booster every 10 years.
- **Clinical:** symptoms seen weeks after contaminated wounds or injection drug use. Hypertonic muscles with rigidity, spasms, clonus, risus sardonicus, ophisthotonus. Trismus 'lockjaw' (cephalic tetanus).
- **Investigations:** FBC, U&E, LFT, check FVC, ABG, ECG. Poor prognosis: short IP, rapid onset, acquired from burns, wound, umbilical stump, septic abortion, delayed treatment, head or neck lesion.
- **Management:** ABC. Admit to ITU. Neuromuscular blockade. Tracheostomy. Give HTIG 500 units IM. IV METRONIDAZOLE may improve outcome. Skin care,

physiotherapy, sedation. Manage any seizures/spasm with DIAZEPAM 5–10 mg or LORAZEPAM 1–2 mg IV. Baclofen, muscle relaxants, magnesium. Monitor for autonomic complications – labetalol. Survival usually results in a full recovery over 6 weeks.

9.51 Lyme disease

- **About:** *Borrelia burgdorferi* transmitted by Ixodes ticks. Early treatment can prevent infection.
- **Clinical:** can cause initial skin rash (bull's eye target erythema migrans) and headache and arthralgia. Later: heart (heart block), neuropathy, neuritis, Lyme arthritis and cranial neuropathy (bilateral VII), meningitis.
- **Diagnosis:** IgG/IgM serology +ve later so treat clinically (false +ves are seen). CSF not needed.
- **Treatment:** look for and remove all ticks. Removal <24 h usually prevents transmission. Check all over and scalp. DOXYCYCLINE within 72 h of a tick bite is more than 80% effective in preventing Lyme disease. Suspected infection DOXYCYCLINE or AMOXICILLIN or CEFUROXIME for 2 weeks. Persisting fatigue. Late CNS disease: CEFTRIAXONE 2 g/d IV for 1 month. Overall prognosis good.

235

10 Renal and urological emergencies

10.1 Pathophysiology

- 2 Kidneys lie retroperitoneally at level of T12–L3 vertebrae. Left kidney somewhat more superior than the right. On average 11 cm in length, 6 cm wide and 3 cm thick. Composed of inner cortex, outer medulla, calyces, pelvis and ureter.
- Supplied by renal arteries from aorta. 20% of cardiac output so 1 L blood (600 ml plasma) per minute. 20% is filtered into Bowman's space. GFR 120 ml/min. Drain into renal veins. GFR depends on BP, renal perfusion, afferent and efferent arteriole tone.

10.2 Haematuria

Taking referral/answering bleep
- When did it start? Quantity? Clots? Is patient passing urine or in retention? Is patient pyrexial, pain – cystitis/pyelonephritis? Recent catheterisation? Prostate disease?
- Pregnant? Known bladder malignancy? On any anticoagulants? 30% of patients with painless haematuria have a malignancy.

Definitions and causes
- **Microscopic haematuria:** non-visible haematuria. Two or more red cells per high power field in MSU unrelated to exercise, menses or trauma.
- **Macroscopic haematuria:** visible haematuria.
- **Haematuria:** bleeding from glomerulus to urethra. Can be divided into glomerular and non-glomerular. **Glomerular haematuria:** usually with proteinuria, hypertension and renal dysfunction. Commonest is IgA Nephropathy, Type IV collagen nephropathy, Alport's disease. **Non-glomerular haematuria:** stones, tumour, papillary necrosis.
- **Investigations:** FBC, U&E, CRP, urinalysis. Cystoscopy, intravenous urogram, renal USS. β-hCG. PSA and formal microscopy, culture and sensitivities. False positive dipstick for blood may be seen with menstruation or trauma (exercise or recent sex or local lesions – ulcers, warts). Haematuria, red cell casts, proteinuria – consider glomerulonephritis. CRP/echocardiogram/blood cultures if endocarditis considered (rare). Renal biopsy: to diagnose renal glomerular disease.
- **Red flags:** painless macroscopic haematuria, symptomatic microscopic haematuria in absence of UTI. Age >50, abdominal mass on examination, smokers.

Referral guidance for haematuria
- **Urology referral:** unexplained macroscopic (visible) haematuria at any age, microscopic haematuria (all ages) with hesitancy, dysuria, frequency or urgency and absence of UTI, persisting asymptomatic microscopic haematuria age 40 or older.
- **Nephrology referral:** microscopic haematuria and ↓eGFR, haematuria and HTN >140/90 mmHg, proteinuria (ACR >30 mg/mmol or PCR >50 mg/mmol), macroscopic haematuria and intercurrent infection, usually chest, family history of renal disease or haematuria.

On arrival
- **Indications for admission:** look for UTI and coagulopathy. Admit if clot retention, cardiovascular instability, uncontrolled pain, sepsis, acute renal failure, coagulopathy, severe co-morbidity, heavy haematuria or social restrictions. Those not needing admission should drink plenty of clear fluids and return for further medical attention if the following occur: clot retention or worsening haematuria

despite adequate fluid intake, uncontrolled pain or fever, or inability to cope at home. Repeat observations and review medications and consider stopping anticoagulants depending on their need. ↓BP or ↑HR may suggest sepsis or haemorrhage.

- **Follow-up by a urological team** ideally within the 2 week cancer referral target. Consider bladder and prostate cancer in those males over 40. In those under 40, cystoscopy may not be mandatory if another cause found.
- **Significant macroscopic (visible) bleeding** can cause clot retention resulting in outflow obstruction and often a three-way catheter irrigation system should be used. In bleeding of this severity, reverse all anticoagulation and get urological advice. Ensure check Hb and replace blood. **Will need urgent cystoscopy** if persists and imaging of whole renal tract.
- **Microscopic haematuria** (not visible but positive dipstick) and protein consider as UTI. Lack of protein in dipstick could suggest tumour or stones.
- **Microscopic haematuria and proteinuria** consider nephrology and a more medical cause, e.g. glomerulonephritis.

Causes of haematuria	
Urinary tract infection (cystitis and pyelonephritis)	Commonest cause. Pain, dysuria, blood, protein, leucocytes in urine. Positive cultures. Confusion, suprapubic discomfort. Usually ↑WCC and CRP. May present as delirium or 'off legs' in the elderly.
Traumatic bladder catheterisation	Often seen post-catheter or any form of instrumentation. Exacerbated by any antithrombotics. Bleed should settle, but if it persists investigate.
Bladder cancer	Common in older population and needs cystoscopy for diagnosis, biopsy and staging and treatment.
Renal cell cancer	Look for a renal mass, fever, USS or CT abdomen. Bladder cancer: persisting haematuria. Cystoscopy.
Prostate cancer	↑PSA, bony metastases, prostatism, hard craggy prostate on PR. Urology referral.
Prostatitis	Pain and UTI-like symptoms.
Renal stones	Pain loin to groin. Passing grit in the urine. ▶Section 10.8.
Thrombocytopenia	Check FBC and causes. ▶Section 8.2.
Antithrombotics and anticoagulants	Warfarin, dabigatran and other DOAC, aspirin, clopidogrel and heparin can worsen bleeding and are not uncommon causes. Need risk assessed on temporary stopping or reduction of dose. ▶Section 8.8.
Infective endocarditis	Murmur, fever, ↑CRP, stigmata of endocarditis, needs echo.
Acute glomerulonephritis	Haematuria and proteinuria. May be RBC casts and dysmorphic RBCs. Check anti-GBM, ANCA, ASO titres and usual renal work up.
Nephropathies causing microscopic haematuria	IgA nephropathy: commonest glomerulonephritis worldwide. Familial incidence. Younger patients than other causes. Proteinuria. Micro/macroscopic haematuria during respiratory infection, proteinuria and reduced eGFR. Follow up needed. Some progress to end stage renal failure.
Type IV collagen nephropathy	Causes a familial microscopic haematuria.
Alport syndrome	Seen in 1 in 50 000. Microscopic haematuria in children. Sensorineural deafness. Eye disease. Mutation COL4A5. Needs BP control, RAS blockade, renal replacement.

Thin basement membrane nephropathy	Family history of renal disease.
Tuberculosis	Weight loss, overseas, CXR, sterile pyuria classically.
Sickle cell	Usually known sickle cell anaemia.
Schistosomiasis	Overseas exposure due to *Schistosoma haematobium*. Also called bilharzia. Chronic bladder inflammation. Risk factor for bladder cancer.
False positive dipstick	Myoglobinuria, e.g. rhabdomyolysis.

 Reduced urinary output (anuria/oliguria)

- **Taking referral/answering bleep/attending:** (attend quickly if low BP, hypoxic, ↑temp, ↑HR, ↑EWS).
- **Resuscitate if needed:** ABC. Oxygen, check BP, HR, temperature. If low BP then get IV access, check bloods and manage as for shock. Cardiac monitor if AKI and hyperkalaemia. Ensure accurate fluid balance chart. Omit antihypertensive on drug chart. Correct any volume loss. If biochemical evidence of AKI then suspend nephrotoxic medications and ensure all drugs have been assessed for correct dose in AKI. In most cases simply increasing oral or IV fluids is sufficient. A cautious fluid challenge of 250–500 ml over 30 min and then repeated should cause some response.
- **Measure urine output:** determine exact urine output and assess patient's hydration status. Quantify input oral and IV and losses in the past few days. Weight changes are useful: 1 kg = 1 L.
- **Reduced urine output:** oliguria: <500 ml/day urine output (which is about 20 ml/h). Oliguria is usually pre-renal but may be renal. If pre-renal and patient is dry then give fluids, e.g. 500 ml IV NS over 1 h and review. If the patient has poor intake and is not in heart failure then further fluids needed to improve urine output. Oliguria might suggest hypoperfusion and sepsis or other causes of shock. Attend quickly if low BP, ↑temp, ↑HR, ↑EWS (could be subacute obstruction so consider bladder scan and catheter). If low BP assess as for ↓BP. If renal cause suspected ask about new drugs or IV contrast for an X-ray or angiogram that could precipitate or cause AKI. Is there rhabdomyolysis or severe infection? Check bloods and lactate and possible venous blood gases if AKI. Seek help.
- **No urine:** anuric think obstruction first. Has patient any suprapubic pain or is catheter blocked or is it acute retention? Reasonable to ask staff to flush or change the catheter if one is in place. Bladder scan will tell you if bladder full or empty and then catheterise. If obstruction still considered, then a renal USS is usually diagnostic. The question is at what level: is it urethra, prostate, bladder, ureters, renal? Those with post-renal causes need to be discussed with urology for surgical or radiologically placed drainage before definitive management.
- **Differential: recording error** – fluid balance underestimates urine output. **Pre-renal failure** – oliguria and recent ↓BP. Cardiogenic, haemorrhagic shock, sepsis, obstructive shock. Excessive antihypertensives. **Renal** – ischaemic, nephrotoxic drugs, nephritis. **Post-renal** – obstruction at renal pelvis, ureters, bladder, urethra. Stones, tumour, prostate.

 Acute kidney injury

- **About:** AKI has replaced the term 'acute renal failure' to emphasis potential reversibility. AKI is a sudden rapid reduction in GFR and there may be oliguria and anuria. Mortality varies from 10 to 80% depending on population studied. About half have sepsis or hypovolaemia and others have obstruction, nephrotoxic drugs and parenchymal renal diseases. Increased length of stay, mortality and expense. Prevalence of AKI is about 5% in hospital patients. A minority need a nephrologist. Most managed by generalists. Only 1% need dialysis.

- **Aetiology:** reduced renal function: impaired control of water and electrolytes. Impaired excretion of drugs and other metabolites. Impaired acid–base control – need to excrete acid load. Impaired BP control, impaired EPO synthesis, impaired vitamin D hydroxylation.
- **Note:** if you suspect vasculitis, e.g. systemically unwell, rash, fever, ↑CRP, pulmonary haemorrhage, send ANCA/anti-GBM and seek nephrology help immediately.

RIFLE and AKIN classification for AKI in adults

Stage	Creatinine (µmol/L)	Urinary output
1: Risk	Creatinine >120, increased by >26 within 48 h or > × 1.5–1.99 baseline value <7 days	<0.5 ml/kg/h for >6 consecutive hours
2: Injury	Creatinine × 2 (creatinine >240) or × 2.0–2.99 baseline value <7 days	<0.5 ml/kg/h for >12 consecutive hours
3: Failure	Creatinine increased ×3 or >354 mmol/L or dialysis needed	<0.3 ml/kg/h for >24 consecutive hours or anuria for 12 h
Loss	Complete loss of function needing RRT >4 weeks	

Risk factors for AKI and poor outcome: age >75, CKD (eGFR <60 ml/min/1.73 m^2) cardiac failure, liver disease, DM. Peripheral vascular disease, nephrotoxic medication, hypovolaemia, sepsis.

Causes and investigations	Notes
Pre-renal failure (60%) Low urine Na <20 mmol/L. High osmolality. Avid retention of Na and water.	Shock, hypovolaemia, haemorrhage, severe sepsis, heart failure, cirrhosis and liver failure, renal artery stenosis. Clinical: ↓BP, shocked, ↑HR. Acute setting. Burns, gastrointestinal losses, sepsis. **Uraemia:** drowsiness, poor appetite, itch, encephalopathy, pericardial rub. Late: seizures and coma.
Renal failure (25%) Normal urine Na >40 mmol/L. Intrinsic renal disease: proteinuria and haematuria and red cell casts. Normal or low urine osmolality.	• **Acute tubular necrosis (45%):** acute fall in GFR: tubule cell damage and cell death. Ischaemia or toxin driven. Ischaemia usually due to prolonged pre-renal failure. There can be recovery over 1–3 weeks with diuresis. May also be due to nephrotoxic drugs or DIC or myoglobinuria, radiocontrast. • **Glomerulonephritis (GN):** neoplasia, autoimmune, drugs, genetic abnormalities and infections. • **Rapidly progressive GN:** vascular/vasculitis (4%) – Wegener's granulomatosis, HUS, TTP, hypertension, scleroderma, renal artery stenosis. • **Acute interstitial nephritis:** hereditary, systemic, toxic and drug-induced. • **Acute on chronic renal failure** (13%): mostly due to ATN and pre-renal disease. • **Haemolytic uraemic syndrome:** microangiopathic anaemia, ↓Hb, ↑LDH, ↑bilirubin. Myeloma kidney: ↑ESR, monoclonal band. • **Malignant hypertension:** control BP.
Post-renal USS: evidence of obstruction with dilated system.	Urinary tract obstruction (10%): stones, tumour, papillary necrosis, surgical ligation of ureters, extrinsic compression, retroperitoneal fibrosis. Catheterise if distended bladder. Admit to urology for relief of obstruction.

| Chronic | Renal USS usually small kidneys but may show normal/large kidneys if amyloid or diabetes or polycystic kidney disease. Normocytic normochromic anaemia, low calcium, ↑phosphate. Old tests: ↑creatinine. No signs or symptoms of acute illness. Progressive uraemic symptoms. Usually diabetes, HTN, APKD. Chronic fatigue. Multiple co-morbidities. Polyuria and nocturia and low urine osmolality if concentrating defect. |

Clinical assessment and initial management

- **ABCs:** O_2, IV access, bloods, urine, cultures, ECG (particularly for high K). Don't rush to catheterise unless oliguria/anuria.
- **Assess hydration:** measure temp, BP and pulse, JVP and capillary refill (should be <3 sec) and GCS. A postural drop even lying to sitting may suggest hypovolaemia. Consider 250–500 ml IV fluids if 'dry' over 30 min. Reassess symptoms and signs.
- **Symptoms:** determine if new or longstanding malaise, lethargy, delirium, N&V, generalised anorexia. **Chest:** breathless and haemoptysis – pulmonary oedema, consolidation, alveolar haemorrhage with vasculitis (Wegener's granulomatosis or Goodpasture's syndrome). **Cardiac:** pericardial rub due to uraemic pericarditis. A pericardial effusion may be seen on echo or CXR. Occasionally this may progress to tamponade. **Skin:** palpable purpura, neuropathy might suggest vasculitis. Skin pigmentation, pallor and itch are common with evident scratch marks. Impaired platelet function and bruising is seen.
- **Urine output:** oliguria helps define AKI but is non-specific. Anuria suggests post-renal obstruction. Polyuria: CKD with impaired renal concentrating ability or high Ca or an osmotic load (glucose), or diabetes insipidus which may worsen hypovolaemia. A low volume concentrated urine with low Na suggests prerenal causes.
- **Drug chart:** always examine the drug chart – current and recent. Evaluate each drug with BNF looking for **nephrotoxins, e.g.** aminoglycosides (Gentamicin, etc.), Vancomycin, Cisplatin, Lithium, NSAIDs, ACEI, ARBs, Ciclosporin, radiocontrast, paracetamol OD. **Intrinsic nephrotoxins** are myoglobin, haemoglobin.

Syndromic renal presentations to recognise

- **Nephrotic syndrome:** proteinuria (frothy urine) exceeding 3.5 g/24 h, hyperlipidaemia, lipiduria, oedema (puffy eyes in morning to generalised oedema/anasarca), hypoalbuminaemia <25 g/L, hypercoagulability. **Causes:** primary GN, minimal change disease (children), focal segmental glomerulosclerosis (most common cause in adults), membranous GN. Others: diabetic nephropathy, sarcoidosis, autoimmune: SLE, Sjögren's, infection: syphilis, hepatitis B, HIV, amyloidosis, multiple myeloma, vasculitis, cancer, drugs: gold, penicillamine, captopril, NSAIDs.
- **Nephritic syndrome:** haematuria/red cell casts, HTN, oliguria, uraemia, proteinuria (<3 g/24 h). **Causes:** post-infectious GN, primary, IgA nephropathy (Berger's disease), RPGN, proliferative GN, secondary GN, Henoch–Schönlein purpura, vasculitis.
- **Investigations:** urine dipstick, urine microscopy, CXR, U&E, LFTs, CRP, ESR, Ca, immunoglobulins, PPE, BJP, complement (C3, C4) autoantibodies (ANA, ANCA, anti-dsDNA, anti-GBM), renal ultrasound, renal biopsy.

Investigations

- **FBC and film:** ↓Hb not typical with AKI. ↑WCC, platelets? Haemolysis? Microangiopathic anaemia – check blood films.
- **Urinalysis** shows blood, protein and red cell casts on microscopy. Positive protein values of 3+ and 4+ on reagent strip testing of the urine suggest intrinsic glomerular disease and this is reinforced if there are a high number of red cells. Increased white cells (>5 per high power field) are non-specific but are found more commonly with acute interstitial nephritis, renal or UTI and GN. If proteinuria do an urgent spot urine protein : creatinine ratio.

- **U&E:** ↑urea, ↑creatinine, ↑potassium. ↑**Lactate:** in tissue hypoxia/sepsis.
- **Calcium/phosphate:** ↓Ca – CKD, ↑Ca – malignancy, myeloma, primary hyperparathyroidism. ↑phosphate.
- **LFTs:** ↓albumin with nephrotic syndrome. ↑Blood glucose: with diabetes.
- **ABG:** ↓pH and ↓HCO₃ associated with AKI.
- **Coagulation tests:** can be abnormal if DIC associated with sepsis.
- **Blood cultures:** if sepsis is suspected.
- **Creatine kinase:** rise suggests rhabdomyolysis or acute MI.
- **CXR:** pulmonary oedema or alveolar haemorrhage. Cavitating lesions suggesting a pulmonary/renal syndrome.
- **ECG:** look for cardiac disease (LVH, STEMI/non-STEMI) or high K.
- **CT renal tracts:** exclude structural lesion or retroperitoneal fibrosis.
- **Renal USS:** perform within 24 h if obstruction suspected. Assess renal size and exclude obstruction.
- **Renal biopsy:** shows a crescentic type picture in RPGN. Biopsy if suspected GN/RPGN/tubulointerstitial nephritis or vasculitis. ↑ESR – myeloma or infection. ↑CRP if infection/vasculitis/autoimmune disorder.
- **PPE and urine Bence–Jones:** always do both when looking for multiple myeloma.
- **Autoantibodies:** ANCA (MPO and PR3), anti-GBM, ANA, dsDNA.
- **Complement:** C3 and C4 and cryoglobulins. **HIV test:** where risk factors exist.
- **Magnetic resonance angiography** (MRA): if suspicion of renal artery stenosis.
- **Body weight:** measured daily gives a good idea of fluid balance.

Prevention

- Avoiding ↓BP and dehydration and reducing and stopping potentially nephrotoxic drugs. Some causes are predictable and preventable. If at risk of contrast-induced AKI (CI-AKI) give pre-procedure volume expansion with IV NS or isotonic sodium bicarbonate. No compelling evidence for the routine use of *N*-ACETYLCYSTEINE to prevent CI-AKI. Manage rhabdomyolysis with IV volume expansion with 0.9% SALINE IV and sodium bicarbonate.
- AKI following the administration of radiological contrast tends to occur within 72 h and often resolves after around 5 days.

Management

Escalate early, use critical care outreach and/or nephrology if ↑EWS or need advice.

- **Medical management:** ABCs, resuscitate, IV access, O₂. If non-obstructive liaise closely with renal physicians. The cause may be volume depletion or intravascular loss or nephrotoxic drugs or a mixed picture.
- **Manage vascular filling status:** determine using clinical signs and other results if under, normal or overfilled. Cautiously correct fluid balance, stop or adjust doses of all renally excreted or nephrotoxic drugs. In mild cases renal function will improve over several days with cautious fluid management. In those with impaired cardiac function small challenges with 250 ml IV NS over 10 min and then reassessment of urine output and fluid balance and pulse and postural BP is reasonable. More fluid may be given. In selected severe cases a CVP line may help guide fluid replacement. Once fluid balance is normal, then watch for an improvement in urine output suggesting pre-renal cause. If a hydrated patient is oliguric and non-obstructed then a diuretic stimulus with FUROSEMIDE 100–120 mg may be given slowly IV over 10–20 min. A failure to respond suggests that things have progressed beyond simple pre-renal failure and we may be dealing with ATN. In those with ongoing oliguria and rising urea and creatinine consider renal referral.
- **Fluid balance and nutrition:** Fluid replacement = output + 500 ml per day usually with NS. Normal enteral nutrition should be maintained as much as possible.
- **Inotropes:** there is no evidence for DOPAMINE in improving outcome in AKI. Use of inotropes should be led by specialists.

- **Protect veins.** In case that haemodialysis will be needed at a later stage the non-dominant arm upper limb vasculature should be preserved as a contingency for future permanent access.
- **Exclude post-renal cause with USS:** if obstruction is possible (oliguria/anuria), then get a renal USS <24 h to exclude an obstructive cause and if so liaise with urology. A bladder catheter relieves prostatic or urethral obstruction. If a per-urethral catheter cannot be placed due to an enlarged prostate or urethral stricture then a suprapubic catheter is needed (ask urology). Imaging evidence of a dilated ureter and hydronephrosis will require **percutaneous nephrostomy**. A urinary catheter is a source of infection. If no obstruction and good output then assess need particularly in mild AKI. **Avoid GENTAMICIN cover, as nephrotoxic.** Remove catheter as soon as it is not adding value. Once post-renal causes are treated there may be a marked diuresis which needs to be anticipated and compensated for in the fluid management plan. Frequent monitoring of fluid balance and U&E is required.
- **Stop nephrotoxic drugs:** stop/avoid drugs such as ACE inhibitors, NSAIDs, AT2 blockers and reduce the dose of other drugs that are renally cleared. See BNF.
- **Specialist management:** escalate where creatinine >×3 baseline, or >354 µmol/L to critical care/nephrology or complications as below or where advice needed. Look for **autoimmune disease or GN** (if RPGN/Wegener's or Goodpasture's is suspected then quick card test for cANCA and anti-GBM), **myeloma kidney, HUS, TTP,** suspected poisoning. Further investigations such as renal biopsy are for the nephrologists to deal with. There may well be a return of function in the short term over the first few weeks, but in some patients cortical scarring means a progressive course into chronic renal failure and a need for lifelong renal replacement therapy (RRT).

Complications

- **Hyperkalaemia:** refractory high K related to AKI needs dialysis so urgently contact the renal team. Needs 10 ml 10% CALIUM GLUCONATE over 5 min. INSULIN 10 units in 50 ml 50% GLUCOSE over 10 min. SALBUTAMOL 5–10 mg nebulised, calcium resonium. See *Section 5.3* on hyperkalaemia for further guidance. Consider IV NaHCO₃ 1.26% in AKI if HCO₃ <22 mmol/L and not in fluid overload as 500 ml over 1 h. Can cause sodium overload. These actions work for 4 hrs. May need dialysis. ▶Section 5.3.
- **Metabolic acidosis:** as medical treatment for management of hyperkalaemia. A pH <7.15 requires critical care referral. May need dialysis.
- **Pulmonary oedema:** sit up and give oxygen as per BTS guidance. If haemodynamically stable try **FUROSEMIDE 80 mg IV** and then an infusion at 10 mg/h. Also consider if not ↓BP, 2 × **GTN spray (800 mcg)** and prepare **GTN infusion at 1–10 mg/h** (infusion of 50 mg in 50 ml). May need dialysis if cannot get rid of fluid.

Renal replacement

- **Renal replacement management:** it may be that conservative measures are insufficient and urgent RRT is indicated. Usual indications are listed below. The patient will need either ITU for haemofiltration or renal unit transfer. Haemofiltration is most commonly used acutely as volume shifts are less and can be provided in an ITU set-up and can remove endotoxins in those who are septic. Be sure to talk to your intensivists and renal physicians early before this situation arises if at all possible.
- **Indications for discussing urgent renal replacement in AKI:** urea >35 mmol/L, high K >6 mmol/L pulmonary oedema, severe acidosis (pH <7.2), HCO₃ <15, encephalopathy, bleeding due to uraemia and pericarditis. Ethylene glycol poisoning.

References: www.renal.org/clinical/guidelinessection/AcuteKidneyInjury.aspx. KDIGO Group (2012) Clinical practice guideline for acute kidney injury. *Kidney Int Suppl*, 2:1.

10.5 Chronic kidney disease

- **About:** irreversible decline in kidney function over years. Asymptomatic until advanced. Glomerular filtration rate (GFR) is the best estimate of kidney function and is based on serum creatinine level, age, sex, and race. Most will die from heart disease. eGFR/creatinine need to be stable to diagnose CKD.

Classification
- **Normal:** normal GFR is approximately 100 ml/min/1.73 m^2.
- **Stage 1:** function is normal. Proteinuria or haematuria or known renal pathology eGFR >90 ml/min. Managed in primary care. Annual assessment.
- **Stage 2:** mild, GFR 60–89 ml/min/1.73 m^2 with proteinuria or haematuria or known renal pathology. Managed in primary care. Annual assessment.
- **Stage 3:** eGFR 45–59 ml/min and **Stage 3B:** eGFR 30–44 ml/min: 6–12 month reviews.
- **Stage 4:** eGFR 15–29 ml/min/1.73 m^2.
- **Stage 5:** end-stage renal failure/disease, eGFR <15 ml/min.

Causes
- Type 1/2 diabetes and hypertension, glomerulonephritis, interstitial nephritis, polycystic kidney disease, obstructive nephropathy, vesicoureteral reflux, recurrent kidney infection.

Clinical
- Symptoms with stages 4/5. ↓Hb (low EPO and platelet dysfunction bleeding). Fatigue, nausea, vomiting, fluid retention, hiccups, pericardial rub, cachexia.
- Look for sepsis, heart failure, hypovolaemia, examination for bladder enlargement. CKD causes HTN and HTN causes CKD, encephalopathy. Avoid non-dominant forearm veins with Venflons as may need AV fistula.

Investigations
- **FBC:** if low Hb, exclude non-renal cause. Check haematinics.
- **U&E:** measure creatinine. Watch for hyperkalaemia. **CRP** – inflammation/infection.
- **Bone:** low Ca and ↑phosphate, ↑Ca, consider myeloma. Oral phosphate binders will often be necessary.
- **Urinary protein is always renal:** albumin/creatinine or protein/creatinine ratio (ACR or PCR). Microalbuminuria predicts End stage disease with diabetes.
- **USS renal tracts:** exclude obstruction, APKD, asymmetrical, e.g. renal artery stenosis, small kidneys with CKD.
- **CT/MRA:** structural lesions, renal artery stenosis.
- **Renal biopsy:** when benefits outweigh risks, e.g. IgA nephropathy or focal glomerulosclerosis.
- **Serology:** ANCA/GBM when appropriate.

Management
- Look for acute or chronic reversible causes and manage as AKI.
- **Anaemia:** develops with Stage 3B or 4 diseases. Check haematinics. Target 110–120 g/L. Consider iron ± erythropoiesis stimulating agents.
- **Blood pressure:** aim for 130/80 mmHg for patients with proteinuria: urinary ACR >30 or PCR >50.
- **Urinary protein:** ACR >30 or PCR >50 suggests worsening renal function. Start ACEI/ARB if HTN: target BP 130/80 mmHg. ACR >70 or PCR >100 needs strict BP control and specialist referral/discussion.

- **Cardiovascular risk:** advice on smoking, exercise and lifestyle. Consider cholesterol lowering therapy if macrovascular disease, or 10 year risk of events >20%.
- **Immunisation:** influenza and pneumococcal, hepatitis B if RRT contemplated.
- **Medication review:** stop nephrotoxic drugs (particularly NSAIDs) and ensure doses of others are appropriate to renal function.

Reference: SIGN (2008) 103: Diagnosis and management of chronic kidney disease: a national clinical guideline.

Urinary tract infection

- **About:** UTI usually symptomatic bacterial infection of the urinary tract. Kidney (acute pyelonephritis) – young females. Bladder (acute cystitis) – young females. Prostate (prostatitis) – older males, due to urinary infection, in younger often an STI.
- **Note:** asymptomatic bacteriuria (ABU) does not itself require treating in uncomplicated patients. UTI denotes symptomatic disease. However, ABU during pregnancy is associated with complications such as preterm birth and perinatal mortality for the fetus and with pyelonephritis for the mother. Treatment of ABU in pregnant women decreases the risk of pyelonephritis by 75%. Uncomplicated UTI refers to acute cystitis or pyelonephritis in non-pregnant outpatient women with a normal anatomy and no instrumentation of the urinary tract.
- **Risks:** catheterisation or instrumentation of urinary tract, pregnancy. Post-coital: void afterwards because organisms milked into bladder. Diabetes mellitus (women only), incontinence, lack of circumcision in men. Structural abnormalities, neurogenic bladder, dehydration.
- **Microbiology:** *E. coli* 85%. *Staph. saprophyticus* 10%. Others include *Klebsiella, Proteus, Citrobacter, Pseudomonas aeruginosa*. G+ve enterococci and *Staph. aureus* and even yeasts.
- **Clinical:** general malaise, fever, N&V, most often female. <u>Pyelonephritis</u>: classically unilateral loin pain, rarely bilateral, fever, rigors. <u>Cystitis</u>: suprapubic discomfort, frequency, dysuria. <u>Prostatitis</u>: dysuria, perineal pain, frequency. <u>Elderly</u>: delirium, falls, instability, agitation.
- **Investigations:** FBC, U&E, CRP: ↑WCC, ↑CRP. U&E typically normal unless underlying renal issues. **Urine dipstick:** protein and blood support infection but may have other causes. **Nitrites:** not all bacteria convert nitrate to nitrite, and a sufficient concentration must be present to be detectable. Positive test strongly supports infection. **Leukocyte esterase:** enzyme found in polymorphs in the urine. Either is a positive test when the clinical picture is suggestive. A negative dipstick test is not good enough to exclude bacteriuria in pregnant women – send a sample for culture. **Urine microscopy:** WCC can be a helpful marker before culture results available at 24 h. A lower diagnostic threshold is used in women than men. **Urine culture:** gold standard but contamination from poor sampling can complicate matters. USS renal can be considered in recurrent UTI to exclude anatomical issue.

Diagnostic criteria for UTI

Level of proof to call it a UTI	Patient group
≥10^2 CFU/ml + 2 samples WCC ≥10/mm³	Symptomatic women
≥10^2 CFU/ml	Symptomatic young females
≥10^3 CFU/ml	Symptomatic male or catheterised patient
≥10^5 CFU/ml on two occasions	Asymptomatic individuals

- **Complications:** bacteraemia and urosepsis. SIRS. Delirium. Falls. AKI. **Diabetic:** obstructive uropathy associated with acute papillary necrosis causing AKI if bilateral. Staghorn calculi if chronic infection develops, renal/perinephric abscess formation. Emphysematous pyelonephritis where gas-forming bacteria proliferate.
- **Management:** ABC, O_2 etc. if septic. Ensure adequate hydration, analgesia and nutrition and IV fluids. Look for and treat any causes. Start antibiotics once urine has been sent for culture unless sterile sampling difficult where it can be prudent and pragmatic to treat empirically rather than wait for a contaminated sample that can never be obtained.

Infection	Management
Cystitis/lower UTI (simple cystitis without fever or loin pain)	Take advice if urosepsis or there has been a multi-resistant pattern in antibiotic sensitivity seen in previous isolates. NITROFURANTOIN PO (avoid if eGFR <60 ml/min, G6PD deficiency, porphyria). Duration of treatment: 3 days in non-pregnant women/uncomplicated UTI, 7 days in men.
Cystitis/lower UTI: as above but also PREGNANT	Approximately 2–10% of pregnancies are accompanied by ABU and of these 40% develop infection. Most due to *E. coli*. Screening at 12–16 weeks. Send a sample for culture and sensitivities. AMOXICILLIN and Cephalosporins for 1 week are safe and effective. Avoid trimethoprim in pregnancy.
Acute pyelonephritis	CO-AMOXICLAV IV. Switch to CO-AMOXICLAV PO when apyrexial >48 h. If pyrexial after 48 h, consider renal USS to exclude renal abscess. Review with results of culture. Treat for 2 weeks. ERTAPENEM IV or GENTAMICIN IV. Take advice if pregnant.
Indwelling urinary catheters	Antibiotic treatment is not required unless patient is systemically unwell. Treatment should follow antibiotic sensitivity test result with changing/removal of the catheter. For empirical management discuss with consultant microbiologist.
Catheter change	Urinary catheter insertion or change of antibiotics are no longer routinely recommended. unless previous catheter-related bacteraemia when GENTAMICIN 120 mg IV stat is given if renal function normal.

10.7 Renal obstruction (obstructive uropathy)

- **Cause of post-renal AKI:** complete obstruction causes anuria, partial causes oliguria. Early treatment (usually surgical/radiological) can restore renal function. Can occur at any level from renal calyces to the distal urethra. Admit under urology.
- **Aetiology:** normal sites of narrowing are junctions between renal pelvis and ureter, ureter and bladder, bladder and urethra (bladder neck) and urethral meatus. Acquired causes and congenital cases seen in children. Depends on degree of obstruction, whether obstruction is slow and progressive. Depends if it affects both or a single kidney. Is there underlying renal disease?
- **Causes:** congenital narrowing usual at sites mentioned above; posterior urethral valves. Phimosis and meatal stenosis. Infection with oedema and scarring. Tumour – cervix, uterus, colorectal, bladder, prostate. Debris: blood clots, sloughed papillae, benign prostatic hypertrophy. Pregnant uterus pressure, retroperitoneal fibrosis. Malignancy extrinsic compression – cervical, ovarian, bowel. Abdominal aortic aneurysm. Trauma at any level. Neurological – diabetic neuropathy, spinal cord disease. Accidental ligation at abdominal surgery.
- **Clinical:** acute obstruction: pain due to build up of hydrostatic pressure in kidney. Bilateral acute obstruction: anuria and AKI. Partial obstruction: polyuria and nocturia as concentrating ability impaired. Chronic picture: hypertension and polycythaemia.

Look for phimosis or meatal stricture, full bladder, flank pain or abdominal masses. PR examination for prostate enlargement and rectal tumour. Gynaecological exam: uterine or cervical or ovarian disease.

Investigations

- **Bloods:** FBC: ↑WCC, ↑U&E – ? AKI, ↑CRP. Check Ca.
- **Urinalysis:** protein, leucocytes, glucose.
- **Imaging: bladder scan:** urine in bladder, post-voiding volume. **USS renal tracts:** useful to see obstruction and a dilated system with hydronephrosis or hydroureter.
- **Non-contrast CT** is modality of choice for stones. **IVU:** can delineate level of stenosis.
- **Voiding cystourethrography**. Antegrade/retrograde urography for renal pelvis and ureter.

Management

- **Supportive:** ABC, manage hydration, electrolytes and acid–base balance. May be AKI. Watch K. Treat any infection.
- **Imaging, usually USS or non-contrast CT**, should be done quickly and urological referral if signs of obstruction. Urgent relief of obstruction to restore function and reduce risk of urosepsis. May be simple urethral catheterisation or drainage by nephrostomy/ureterostomy or suprapubic catheter as is appropriate.
- **Individualised treatment of particular cause**. There is often a post-obstruction diuresis (even 1 L/h) following treatment requiring appropriate fluid replacement to avoid pre-renal problems.

10.8 ▶ Nephrolithiasis

- **About:** calculi in kidney and/or ureters. Care in those with single kidney or CKD. Renal stones seen in 10% of adults at some time. Admit under urology. Most are men aged 20–50 and recurrence is common.
- **Stones:** reduced urine output leads to supersaturation and stone formation. Calcium oxalate and calcium phosphate in 80% (radio-opaque). Urate stones in 10% (radio-lucent). Cystine in 1% (radio-opaque). Struvite (magnesium ammonium phosphate) in 5% (radio-opaque).
- **Causes:** distal RTA, gout, T2DM, primary hyperparathyroidism, idiopathic hypercalcaemia, cystinuria, polycystic kidneys, dietary or internal hyperoxaluria. Hyperuricosuria. Stone formation exacerbated by hot climates with resultant oliguria.
- **Clinical:** excruciating back or abdominal or flank pain: 'loin to groin/labia'. Patient writhing around in agony, unlike peritonitis who lie still. The pain can last minutes or hours and there can be intervals of no pain. N&V, frequency, dysuria, oliguria, and haematuria. Chronic distension may be painless. Fever suggests infection. ↓BP may suggest sepsis or alternative diagnosis, e.g. AAA. Check testes to exclude torsion. Check hernia orifices. Renal angle ? pyelonephritis.

Investigation

- **FBC:** ↑WCC, ↑CRP with infection. **β-hCG:** always if pregnancy possible.
- **Urinalysis:** nitrites suggest UTI. Red cells compatible with stone disease but not always seen. Culture if WCC/nitrites. Alkaline urine pH >7.6 seen with struvite stones. pH <5 suggests uric acid.
- **AXR (kidneys–ureter–bladder):** sensitivity for stones 45–60%.
- **U&E** calcium and urate and PTH if ↑calcium: ensure no stone-forming causes and renal function.
- **Non-contrast helical CT urogram:** sensitivity and specificity >95%. Detects radio-opaque and radio-lucent stones. No need for intravenous contrast medium.

Impaction is usually at ureter/bladder junction or ureter/pelvis or pelvic brim. CT excludes differential which includes AAA.

- **Intravenous urography (IVU):** shows level of ureteric obstruction and defines pelvi-caliceal anatomy. It can miss some radio-lucent ureteric or renal stones (10–20% of stones). It is about 70–90% accurate.
- **USS renal tracts:** use in pregnancy, in children, and in febrile people. A low 50% diagnostic accuracy for stone detection, but main use is to diagnose hydronephrosis in people with complicated renal colic.
- **Differentials:** appendicitis (pain is right-sided), diverticulitis (pain is left-sided). Ectopic pregnancy, pyelonephritis, salpingitis in women, ruptured AAA.
- **Complications:** urinary tract obstruction and upper UTI. Pyelonephritis, pyonephrosis, urosepsis can ensue. AKI.
- **Cautions:** special care must be taken with those with renal stones and pre-existing renal disease, single kidney, kidney transplant, bilateral renal obstruction, pregnancy. Stone >5 mm or larger where impaction likely. Any signs of infection. Unusual for stones to present age >60 so look for alternative diagnoses.

Management

- **Conservative:** collect and sieve all urine to catch stones. Send for biochemical analysis. Encourage oral fluids and maintain hydration and urine flow. Most stones 5 mm or less in diameter pass in 90% of cases. Stones >8 mm impact in 95%. Management is conservative. Pain control and in uncomplicated cases care may be at home. Advise the discharged person to seek urgent medical assistance if fevers or rigors, pain worsens or abrupt recurrence of severe pain.
- **Caution:** admit under urology those with signs of infection, single or transplanted kidney, pre-existing renal impairment, bilateral obstructing stones are suspected, significant analgesic need, dehydration and unable to maintain oral intake, pregnancy, patient preference, diagnosis uncertain in older patient or ectopic pregnancy in younger female. Choices for analgesia include DICLOFENAC PR or IM (max 150 mg per day). DIAMORPHINE or MORPHINE. Antiemetic: consider IV CYCLIZINE or IV/IM METOCLOPRAMIDE (avoid in those <20 years). Reduce the dose by 25–50% in moderate or severe renal impairment.
- **Medical expulsive therapy:** α1-adrenergic blockers are indicated for those with adequate renal function reserve with a newly diagnosed distal ureteric stone (less than 10 mm), whose symptoms are controlled, and who have no clinical evidence of sepsis. TAMSULOSIN 0.4 mg od is the drug of choice and has been shown to reduce time to expulsion and need for intervention and increases the probability that larger 5–10 mm distal ureteric stones will pass (*Ann Emerg Med*, 2016;67:86). NIFEDIPINE XL 30 mg daily can also increase stone expulsion rate from 35% to 79% when combined with a steroid. PREDNISOLONE 10 mg BD in a 5 day burst can be added to both. This may help reduce the intense inflammatory reaction.
- **Surgical removal:** consider if stone does not pass with basket extraction, surgical removal or lithotripsy.
- **ESWL** (extracorporeal shock-wave lithotripsy): focused sound waves fracture stone. Non-invasive and can be done as outpatient.
- **Percutaneous nephrolithotomy:** used for larger stones and staghorn calculi. A nephroscope is inserted into renal pelvis and collecting system and stone broken up and extracted.
- **Ureteroscopy** can be done with a laser to break up the stone. Ureteric injury low in experienced hands.
- **Open surgery:** done with large stones, multiple stones, etc.
- **Discharge:** if pain settles and there is no stone or the stone is 5 mm or less on X-ray kidney–ureter–bladder, the patient may be discharged with an NSAID orally, e.g. DICLOFENAC 50 mg tds. An urgent IVU should be requested and referral to urology.

If the pain does not settle admit. Higher risk patients are those with a solitary or transplanted kidney, pre-existing renal impairment or where bilateral obstructing stones are suspected.
- **Prevention:** high fluid intake, urine volume 2 L per day, coffee, tea, beer, wine, orange juice reduce stone formation. Avoid sugar sweetened drinks.

10.9 Ischaemic priapism

- **About:** unwanted/painful erection >4 h unrelated to sexual interest/stimulation. 95% ischaemic with sluggish or non-existent blood flow.
- **Aetiology:** vascular disease affecting normal penile erectile function. Sludging and obstruction to blood flow.
- **Causes:** sickle cell disease, leukaemia, neoplasia, drugs, e.g. cocaine, etc. and drugs injected to cause erection. Erection may be seen with spinal cord transection.
- **Clinical:** penis may be swollen, rigid and painful.
- **Investigations:** FBC, sickle test, blood film, U&E. Penile doppler – no flow and penile blood gas – hypoxia.
- **Management:** cooling, rest, ice packs over penis, pain relief, discuss with urology. Irrigation with NS aspirate 20–50 ml usual dark hypoxic blood from corpus cavernosum with butterfly needle until bright red blood seen. Sympathomimetics: Intracavernosal phenylephrine 100–200 mcg every 5–10 min; maximum 1 mg in 1 h. Dilute to 100 mcg/ml and inject in 1–2 ml aliquots. Observe for palpitations, arrhythmias, headache.
- **UROLOGY:** surgical shunts used only after a trial of intracavernous injection of sympathomimetics has failed.

Reference: European Association of Urology (2015) Guidelines on priapism.

11 Neurological emergencies

11.1 Neuroscience and neuroanatomy

- **Physiology:** the brain is 1% of body weight but gets over 10% of cardiac output for its high metabolic demand. It is sensitive to embolism and ischaemia and any reduction in global cerebral perfusion for more than a few seconds causes collapse. The brain is irrigated by four arteries: two internal carotid arteries anteriorly (anterior circulation) and the two vertebrals posteriorly which then join to form the basilar (posterior circulation). Vertebrals arise from ipsilateral subclavians. The branches of these arteries meet again with the circle of Willis with posterior communicating artery connecting ICA to PCA and the anterior communicating between R and L anterior cerebral arteries.

- **Pathophysiology:** the brain is contained within a bony box and so as pressure increases the largest exit is the foramen magnum. The skull contains, by volume, 80% brain, 10% blood, 10% CSF. Within the skull there are further compartments due to the falx and tentorium. These limit the scope of expansion such that any increase in intracranial volume will cause a gradual and ultimately exponential rise in ICP which leads to brainstem compression and death. ↑ICP will also reduce cerebral perfusion pressure, which is mean systemic arterial pressure (MAP) minus ICP. Normal 'opening' pressure is 10–25 cm CSF. Always measure opening pressure at LP. Rising ICP can result in focal signs and herniation syndromes.

Motor

- **About:** cell bodies for the corticospinal/nuclear tracts lie in layer V of the primary motor cortex (PMC) in the precentral gyrus. Voluntary precise motor movements are decided within centres within the frontal lobe and relayed to the PMC. There are only two cells between brain and muscle, the upper (UMN) and lower motor neurons (LMN).

- **Upper motor neuron:** myelinated motor axons exit the PMC and pass inferiorly as the corona radiata via the posterior limb of the internal capsule to form the cerebral peduncle in front of the midbrain. Corticonuclear fibres synapse with local cranial nerve motor nuclei to the eyes (III, IV, VI), face (X, VII), tongue (XII) and pharynx and larynx (IX, X). Corticospinal tracts pass to the spinal cord to innervate respiratory, trunk, arms and leg muscles. Within the brainstem the motor fibres lie ventrally. At the level of the medulla (pyramid) the motor fibres cross right to left and left to right, accounting for the contralaterality of the motor system. At the level of the foramen magnum the fibres pass laterally to form the lateral corticospinal tracts in the spinal cord. The axon descends until it reaches its corresponding nerve root level where it synapses with the anterior horn cell. Structural lesions cause a C/L UMN weakness. Structural lesions within the brainstem cause an ipsilateral cranial nerve palsy and C/L UMN weakness.

- **Lower motor neuron:** the UMN axon synapses with the corresponding LMN cell body called the anterior horn cell. This axon passes out in the spinal canal and fuses with the posterior nerve root and forms a nerve root that passes out via the spinal foramina. Motor to arms joins the brachial plexus and to legs the sacral plexus. Here the peripheral nerves form and pass to their respective muscles. Structural lesions will simply cause an ipsilateral LMN weakness and sensory loss.

- **Neuromuscular junction:** the action potential reaches the terminal bouton and releases Ach. If sufficient Ach is released there is then summation of the stimulus and the generation of an action potential that leads to muscular contraction. Ach is broken down by local cholinesterases. Weakness (myasthenia) can be caused by a lack of Ach – denervation or even excess Ach, e.g. organophosphates, or damage to the post-synaptic nicotinic acetyl choline receptor – such that an action potential cannot form.

Types of weakness

- **UMN:** ↑tone (spasticity), hyperreflexia, clonus, extensor plantar, upper limb flexors > extensors. Lower limb extensors > flexors.
- **LMN:** ↓tone, absent or reflexes, muscle wasting, absent plantar response.
- **Muscle end plate:** fatigability, no wasting, reflexes normal/↓, plantar normal or reduced.
- **Myopathy:** proximal weakness, ↓tone, ↓reflexes, ↓plantar response, mild wasting.

Brainstem

Contains cranial nerve nuclei and descending motor and ascending sensory tracts, the reticular formation required for sleep and wakefulness. The important clinical anatomical facts are below. The brainstem has three levels. Neuroanatomy books show the images inverted compared with CT/MRI imaging.

- **Midbrain:** almost V shaped on cross-sectional imaging. Corticospinal/nuclear fibres form the front of the V. At the back on either side are the nuclei for the IIIrd nerve and below the IVth nerve. The IIIrd nerve exits ventrally and lies close to the Pcomm artery. The aqueduct lies at the back of the midbrain.
- **Pons:** almost bulbous appearance on imaging. Motor fibres anteriorly. Packed with fibres passing via pons to cerebellum. Contains the V, VI, VII and VIII cranial nerves. The VII and VI lie close together. Any LMN facial weakness with an ipsilateral VI suggests an ipsilateral pontine lesion affecting both nuclei. Behind the pons lies the IVth ventricle. In front of the pons lies the basilar artery.
- **Medulla:** more of the spinal cord butterfly-like shape. Motor fibres lie anteriorly forming the pyramids and decussate. The posterolateral aspect is vulnerable to infarction due to posterior inferior cerebellar artery occlusion resulting in Horner's syndrome due to damage to sympathetic tract, damage to nucleus ambiguus (IX, X, XI) involved in swallowing and to the vestibular nuclei and inferior cerebellar peduncle and spinal trigeminal nucleus.

Cranial nerves

(I) **Olfactory:** smell. Damaged by frontal meningiomas. Most often loss of smell is due to ENT issues. (II) **Optic nerve:** see below. (III) **Oculomotor** (midbrain): levator palpebrae superioris, superior, inferior and medial rectus, inferior oblique. Parasympathetic to constrict pupils for accommodation and light (Edinger–Westphal nucleus to ciliary ganglion). (IV) **Trochlear** (midbrain): superior oblique. Unable to look down and in. (V) **Trigeminal** (pons): muscles of mastication, sensory to face (ophthalmic/maxillary/mandibular divisions), dura mater, intracranial blood vessels, teeth. (VI) **Abducent** (pons): lateral rectus. (VII) **Facial** (pons): facial expression and eye closure, stapedius. Sensory external auditory meatus and taste from anterior 2/3rds of tongue. Salivary and lacrimal glands. (VIII) **Vestibulocochlear** (pons): balance (vestibular apparatus) and hearing (cochlea). (IX) **Glossopharyngeal** (medulla): sensory from pharynx, middle ear, carotid sinus and body, posterior 1/3rd tongue. Salivary glands.

Stylopharyngeus (X) **Vagus** (medulla): sensory from pharynx, larynx, oesophagus, aortic bodies and arch. Parasympathetic to chest and abdominal organs. (XI) **Spinal accessory** (medulla): sternomastoid and trapezius. (XII) **Hypoglossal** (medulla): motor to tongue.

Cerebellum

Primary role is coordinating motor function with other parts of the brain. Lies behind the IVth ventricle. Receives sensory and motor input from the motor and premotor cortex and returns feedback to these same centres. Hemispheres deal with ipsilateral movement. Hemispheric damage causes ipsilateral cerebellar signs. Midline damage causes a truncal ataxia. Signs are past pointing, dysarthric speech, nystagmus and dysdiadochokinesia. Acute cerebellar dysfunction is a feature of acute and chronic alcohol and drug toxicities e.g. anticonvulsants and stroke disease. Structural damage lateralises, toxic issues are generalised.

Autonomic

Composed of **sympathetic** and **parasympathetic** systems both using two neurons. Sympathetic fight and flight responses increase heart rate, are inotropic, dilate pupils, bronchodilate and increase muscle blood flow and decrease cutaneous, reduce lacrimation and intestinal motility and salivation and increase sweating. They stimulate the internal urinary sphincter to prevent voiding. Parasympathetic antagonises these with bradycardia, increased lacrimal and salivary secretions and pupil constriction and bronchoconstriction and detrusor stimulation and urination and defecation. There are pre- and post-ganglionic neurons which synapse in an autonomic ganglion. The sympathetic ganglion lies in the sympathetic chain lateral to the spinal cord. Parasympathetic ganglion lies close to the target organ. Sympathetic preganglionic fibres release Ach and postganglionic fibres release noradrenaline to adrenergic receptors, except for Ach at sweat glands. Parasympathetic releases Ach at pre- and post-ganglionic neurons. Initial synapse for both is a nicotinic Ach receptor. The parasympathetic final synaptic target for Ach is a muscarinic Ach receptor. Impaired autonomic function seen long term with diabetes and amyloid, but acutely with GBS and drug toxicities. These may cause severe autonomic instability. Monitoring and support is key and the use of appropriate drugs. For example, Atropine is an anticholinergic that blocks muscarinic Ach receptors and so blocks parasympathetic activity, therefore raising heart rate, dilating pupils, drying secretions and causing urinary retention. Most pharmacological interventions in illness seek to support the circulation mimicking fight/flight responses with agents producing sympathetic activity and blocking parasympathetic. Sympathetic excess and its effects due to drugs or disease need to be managed with alpha and beta adrenergic blockers and other drugs that lower BP and heart rate.

Vision

- **Optic nerve lesion:** Mild will cause altered colour perception, reduced acuity and even loss of vision. There may be nothing to find clinically. Later optic atrophy. Classically with MS.
- **Optic chiasm:** A central lesion usually a pituitary macroadenoma +/– haemorrhage or some other tumour type can compress chiasm often causing an asymmetrical bitemporal hemianopia. Sudden acute onset with pituitary apoplexy.

- **Cortical Vision:** Left parietal, temporal and occipital cortex all contain parts of the visual pathways for vision from the right side of the midline. Damage causes a right partial or complete homonymous hemianopia. An isolated temporal lesion will cause a superior quadrantanopia and parietal an inferior quadrantanopia.

Sensory pathways (ascends to contralateral parietal lobe)

- **Cortical level sensory:** Left parietal cortex receives the sensory input from the right – touch, vibration and all sensation other than smell.
- **Anatomy of ascending sensory function** (3 cells and 3 synapses): sensation is a much more subtle and subjective sign. Different modalities are carried in different tracts and this can help to localize a lesion and so different modalities are tested. All perceived sensation terminates eventually in the contralateral post central gyrus of the parietal lobe.
- **Posterior column/medial lemniscus pathway:** vibration and proprioception enter via the dorsal root and pass into the ipsilateral posterior columns (lower body sensation in the medial gracile fasciculus and upper body in the lateral cuneate fasciculus). This ascends to form the medial lemniscus tract within the brainstem which then crosses at the medulla to synapse in the contralateral thalamus higher up and then passes via the internal capsule up to terminate in the primary sensory cortex on the post central gyrus of the parietal lobe.
- **Spinothalamic:** pain and temperature enter via the dorsal root and pass to opposite side close to the central canal. They then pass up the cord to synapse in the ipsilateral thalamus and pass as axons via the internal capsule on the post central gyrus of the parietal lobe.

 Clinical assessment

Determine pathology using duration and onset

- **Sudden and immediate:** dramatic. Usually vascular or electrical. Vascular (embolic stroke is sudden, thrombotic stroke tends to stutter in onset, haemorrhage can be sudden but usually slow and progressive), seizure, SAH, functional, migraine (usually over minutes).
- **Minutes to hours:** migrainous aura, seizure, thrombotic stroke rarely, an expanding haemorrhagic stroke, SDH, EDH.
- **Hours to days:** demyelination, inflammation, infections, e.g. viral encephalitis, meningitis.
- **Months:** Creutzfeldt–Jakob disease, aggressive tumours, e.g. glioblastomas or metastases, MND/ALS.
- **Years:** low grade gliomas, progressive stroke disease, neurodegenerative diseases, e.g. Parkinson's, Alzheimer's, Huntington's. Primary progressive MS, secondary progressive MS. MND (ALS).
- **Recurrent:** migraine, epilepsy, demyelination, stroke, relapsing–remitting MS.

Determine pathology using positive vs. negative neurology

- **Positive:** tingling, flashing lights, allodynia, jerks and movements. Migrainous aura spreads over minutes (cortical spreading depression) or a focal seizure spreads over seconds usually due to an irritative focus.
- **Negative:** weakness, hemianopia, loss of sensation, incoordination, deafness. Suggests destructive pathology – inflammatory, vascular, demyelination, tumour, etc.

11.3 Patterns of weakness

Differentials for new weakness in adults

- **Functional "block":** diagnosis of exclusion – can mimic any neurological disorder or none. Absence of hard signs helps and normal tests. Expert review needed. Can occur and resolve quickly or slowly. Pattern of weakness/sensory loss can mimic true pathology. Paraplegia, stroke-like, seizure-like. Give-way weakness. Lots of extreme effort. A lifted leg can be held up against gravity but not lifted. Uneconomic gaits and postures. Contrast between exam findings and therapy findings. Positive Hoover's sign. Normal imaging. Give lots of positive support: "you have a block". Be supportive and sympathetic and especially reassuring. True malingerers are the exception. Poorly understood manifestation of non-structural illness.

Cortical/subcortical level/brainstem weakness, increased tone, hyperreflexia, upgoing plantar

- **Acute stroke:** comes on over seconds. Contralateral weakness, visual and sensory loss. ▶ Section 11.19.
- **Post seizure:** Todd's paralysis with weakness persisting post seizure for up to 24 hr ▶ Section 11.16.
- **Tumour:** progressive contralateral weakness, seizures. ▶ Section 16.4.
- **Cerebral abscess:** progressive contralateral weakness, seizures. ▶ Section 11.13.
- **Demyelination:** subacute progressive contralateral weakness. Consider MS or ADEM. ▶ Section 11.34.
- **Subdural haematoma: contralateral weakness.** Elderly head trauma, anticoagulants, ▶ Section 11.25.
- **Epidural haematoma:** head trauma, lucid then fall in GCS and contralateral weakness. ▶ Section 11.26.
- **Motor neurone disease (MND):** Mixed UMN/LMN and no sensory or eye signs, ▶ Section 11.36.
- **Parenchymal infection:** PML, HSV, neurocysticercosis, TB.
- **Parasagittal meningioma:** bilateral leg weakness as presses on both frontal motor cortices medially.

Spinal cord (myelopathy) weakness, increased tone, hyperreflexia, upgoing plantar

- **Notes:** Cord lesions – above lesion normal neurology, LMN at level of lesion and UMN below. Transection C1–4 quadriparesis, respiratory failure, C5–T1 arm and leg weakness, sensory level, below T1 paraparesis, sensory level. Lesions may be subtotal and asymmetrical. Cord damage may be complete. However, often it is incomplete and this can lead to several syndromes:
- **Central cord syndrome:** significant traumatic cervical hyperextension can cause ischaemic central cord damage. Weakness and loss of sensation in both arms, intact motor and sensation in leg. Will need neurorehabilitation and usually seen on Trauma ward.
- **Hemisection of cord:** loss of ipsilateral posterior columns (vibration and proprioception) and corticospinal (UMN weakness) and C/L spinothalamic (pain and temperature). Also called Brown–Séquard syndrome. Any aetiology causing unilateral cord damage and dysfunction.
- **Subacute combined degeneration** – B12 deficiency with UMN weakness and dorsal column loss. May be peripheral neuropathy and loss of ankle jerks.
- **Transverse Myelitis:** UMN weakness and sensory level. Depends on level. Lhermitte's signs. Clumsy hand. Asymmetry. May be urinary retention. Autonomic dysfunction. Commonly due to multiple sclerosis and may find other signs of lesions. MS, ▶ Section 11.34. Other causes are neuromyelitis optica (myelitis and optic neuritis and Ab to Aquaporin 4. ▶ Section 11.34), viral, e.g. HIV, CMV, HSV, post mycoplasma, vasculitis and even paraneoplastic. The CSF and MRI show inflammatory changes. Steroids, IVIg and PLEX for inflammatory causes.
- **Cervical spondylotic myelopathy:** canal stenosis can cause progressive damage to cord. Affects lower limbs first. Can have numb and clumsy hands and progressive upper limb neurology. Nerve roots may be compressed with pain and weakness. Usually C5/6 or C4/5 or C6/7. Neck and pain down roots into shoulders and arms. C6/7 compresses C7 weak triceps and dermatomal sensory loss. C5/C6 lesion C6 affects biceps. Diagnosis with MRI. May settle conservatively. Surgical decompression for progressive neurological disability.

Differentials for new weakness in adults

- **Syringomyelia:** cape-like dissociated sensory loss and loss of pain and temperature. Syrinx seen on MRI often with Chiari malformation.
- **Physical injury to cord:** an acute cord lesion due to trauma or some space occupying lesion will cause UMN weakness below the level, sensory level, affect sphincters. Early on motor may be flaccid then replaced by a spastic paraparesis, affects arms if above T1. Pain is an important feature in conscious patients. Also retention. Priapism seen. Needs immobilisation of neck and back and appropriate care in transfers. Needs imaging and trauma management. ABC, labile BP may be autonomic sympathetic damage so cautious with anaesthesia. Care of local trauma/orthopaedics team.
- **Vascular:** anterior cord infarction or haemorrhage 'spinal stroke', e.g. related to aortic aneurysm surgery or embolism/thrombosis, cavernomas and AVM or coagulopathies. Anterior cord syndrome: spastic bilateral weakness and spinothalamic loss. Preserved posterior columns (seen with anterior spinal artery infarction). Central cord syndrome: cervical level hyperextension can cause ischaemic central cord damage. Weakness and loss of sensation in both arms, intact motor and sensation in leg.
- **Malignant cord compression:** there is little space for lesions lying in the canal to expand without compressing neural structures. Spinal metastases can impinge the vascular supply to the cord as well as cause direct pressure. Most are epidural and secondaries. Most commonly thoracic then lumbar then cervical. Image whole cord. ▶ Section 16.8.
- **Metabolic:** B12 deficiency – posterior column and UMN corticospinal loss. Megaloblastic anaemia. High LDH, Low B12 Check levels and replace.
- **Infections:** syphilis (tertiary): tabes dorsalis – dorsal column loss. Pain variable, can be severe. Immunosuppressed, HIV.
- **Spinal cord abscess** with pain and swelling. Can be at any level including below L1. Pott's disease of spine with kyphosis due to TB.P CXR, plain films MRI
- **Spinal cord AVM or haemorrhage.** Tortuous vessels on surface of cord. May not be seen on MRI needs angiogram. It can bleed. Other causes of bleed Hereditary haemorrhagic telangiectasia, cavernoma, coagulopathy.
- **Epidural haematoma/abscess** can cause sudden acute cord injury (on anticoagulants or bleed from AV malformation, post lumbar puncture/epidural). Epidural abscess, e.g. spinal tuberculosis or other infection. Reverse anticoagulants. Urgent neurosurgical consult.

Anterior horn cell to cauda equina weakness, reduced tone and reflexes

- **Poliomyelitis:** causes an acute flaccid paralysis. Usually asymmetrical. May be limbs, bulbar or respiratory. Non-vaccinated from endemic areas.
- **Acute myelopathy or cauda equina lesion:** sudden or subacute onset of quadriplegia or paraplegia and loss of sphincter control and sensory level. Need to identify if this is a compressive lesion or medical cause, e.g. spinal stroke or transverse myelitis. Urgent MRI indicated and if non-compression then LP for CSF. Cord lesions often cause initial flaccid weakness but becomes hypertonic within 24–48 h. Pain may help identify level and suggests a more surgical compressive cause. ▶ Section 11.29.
- **Infections and abscess formation** – see above.
- **Motor neurone disease:** death of anterior horn cell with LMN, fasciculations and wasting. Also UMN, ▶ Section 11.36.
- **Disc prolapse:** soft central part of the disc, the nucleus pulposus, may rupture through the outer layers of the disc (annulus fibrosis). Most commonly posterolateral. If fragment of nucleus compresses nerve root patient experiences pain, e.g. sciatica. Also numbness and weakness in dermatome/myotome. Commonest discs to prolapse are the L4/5 on L5 root and the L5/S1 discs on S1 root. Causes pain (sciatica) with straight leg raise as nerve stretched. Others are possible including L3/4. There will be loss of

Differentials for new weakness in adults

corresponding reflex. A central disc protrusion can compress the central part of the canal. Effects depend on size and position of herniated disc and canal size. Central disc prolapses below L1 can cause the rare conus medullaris or cauda equina syndrome. Discs can also rarely herniate at cervical level with nerve root pain into arm and LMN signs in the region of the compressed root. A central cervical disc lesion may cause progressive spasticity and abnormal gait below as well as acute pain and needs urgent imaging.

- **Malignant cauda equina compression:** there will be pain, sphincters with reduced anal tone and incontinence and LMN leg weakness. Most are epidural and secondaries. Consider steroids and urgent imaging and referral to oncology and spinal team. ▶ Section 16.8.
- **Acute trauma injury to spine below L1 affecting cauda:** trauma team review. Severe pain and tenderness (if conscious) and LMN weak legs, atonic bladder, loss of vasomotor control, atonic bowel. Neurology may be asymmetrical and partial. Can last 2 weeks. Needs urgent imaging and surgical review.

Peripheral neuropathy (weakness, wasting, fasciculations, absent reflexes)

- **Ascending polyneuropathy (GBS/CIDP):** *ascending inflammatory demyelinating polyneuropathy:* ascending usually symmetrical weakness of both legs over days with areflexia; Motor, sensory and autonomic symptoms. Areflexia is a useful sign but reflexes may be present first 2 days. Needs IVIG. May follow illness. CIDP slower in onset and is steroid responsive. ▶ Section 11.27.
- **Polyneuropathy:** most commonly GBS with a progressive LMN weakness. No reflexes. Others are CIDP, HIV polyneuropathy GBS ▶ Section 11.27.
- **Symmetrical peripheral neuropathy:** can be motor, e.g. Charcot–Marie–Tooth and related conditions. ▶ Section 11.35. Multiple chronic causes, e.g. alcohol (peripheral symmetrical sensory), diabetes, lead toxicity, drugs, leprosy worldwide, paraneoplastic (lung cancer), etc.
- **Peripheral mononeuropathy:** median, ulnar, radial, common peroneal. Motor and sensory characteristics. Use NCS to confirm.
- **Multifocal motor neuropathy with conduction block:** middle aged, slowly progressive weakness, wrist drop, foot drop, asymmetrical. Minimal wasting, fasciculations. Diagnose with NCS/EMG anti GM1 ab. Responds to IVIg; can be confused with MND.
- **Critical illness polyneuropathy:** (CIP) weakness on the ITU. Can be face, arms, legs, respiratory muscles. Usually post ventilation. Similar critical illness myopathy may be seen. Needs NCS/EMG. CSF normal. Axonal. Intensive insulin therapy.
- **Diphtheria:** descending paralysis, unable to focus with vision, oropharyngeal weakness, limb weakness, quadriparesis. Sensorimotor. NCS show demyelination. Give diphtheria antitoxin as early as possible and supportive care.
- **Porphyria:** severe acute axonal polyradiculopathy or neuronopathy. Asymmetrical and proximal weakness and sensory loss. Motor of face, eyes, limbs, respiratory. Raised delta-aminolaevulinic acid. Can mimic GBS. Needs IV haem arginate (▶ Section 5.17).

Neuromuscular junction weakness, reduced tone and reflexes and fatiguability

- **Myasthenia gravis (MG):** progressive fatigable weakness: proximal limbs and neck flexion are weak, face (bilateral ptosis) and diplopia and difficulty swallowing. Consider myasthenia. Check antibodies against acetylcholine receptors. Ice cube/tensilon test. ▶ Section 11.28.
- **Lambert–Eaton syndrome** weakness and fatiguability. Exercise may improve strength then fatigues. Paraneoplastic in many. Get EMG. Treatment 3,4 diaminopyridine. PLEX and IVIG can be tried.
- **Botulism:** *Clostridium botulinum.* Progressive descending bulbar weakness and generalised flaccid paralysis. ▶ Section 9.18.

Differentials for new weakness in adults

- **Tick paralysis:** seen in Australia and North America. Weakness 2–5 days after tick exposure. Usually children. Female tick releases a neurotoxin in saliva. Might find large engorged tick on skin (often scalp); when tick removed symptoms improve and resolve – grasp the tick as close to the skin as possible and pull in a firm steady manner ensuring all parts removed. Tick toxin blocks Ach release. Progressive ascending weakness like GBS.

Muscle (usually wasting symmetrical proximal weakness) weakness, reduced reflexes and tone

- **Proximal myopathy:** proximal weakness – raising hands above head or standing is impaired. Look for rash, cushingoid features, osteomalacia, etc.
- **(Dermato/poly)myositis:** elderly. Insidious onset of weakness. Proximal upper limb muscles. Dysphagia, weak neck flexion. Skin lesions. Lung fibrosis, cardiac arrhythmias. Paraneoplastic in some. Raised CK/ESR helps. Positive ANA and EMG findings. Muscle biopsy. Needs Methylprednisolone.
- **Inclusion body myositis:** Age >50. Progressive quad weakness. Unable to do stairs. Forearm wasting. Wasting. Foot drop. Diabetes. ESR/CK are normal. Get EMG and biopsy. Poor response to steroids and IVIG.

Transient/episodic weakness

- **Myasthenia gravis** and similar conditions above.
- **Sleep paralysis:** transient inability to move or speak on waking. Linked to narcolepsy. May have daytime sleepiness, cataplexy, hypnagogic hallucinations, sleep paralysis.
- **TIA:** will correspond with a transient arterial occlusion – see stroke.
- **Electrolytes:** ↓↓K, ↓↓Ca, ↓↓Mg all cause generalised weakness until recover.
- **Periodic paralysis:** onset usually childhood, ↓↓K and ↑K levels, associated with thyroid disease. Seen more in Asians. Sudden episodic generalised weakness. Provoked by fasting or high carbohydrate meals or exercise. Measure electrolytes. Replace K if needed.
- **Post ictal "Todd's paralysis" weakness.**
- **Migraine with aura/ hemiplegic migraine:** associated migrainous syndrome.
- **Multiple sclerosis** and worsening in warm environment.

11.4 Coma

About: wakefulness is controlled by the reticular activating system (RAS) which is a fine network of nerves within the brainstem ascending as far as the thalamus and hypothalamus bilaterally. Compression, stroke, tumours and any other pathology can cause disruption with coma. Progressive rises in ICP result in brainstem ischaemia and dysfunction and finally respiration ceases. It is important to understand the different forms of cerebral oedema which are detailed below. The RAS is closely associated with the cranial nerve nuclei for eye movement as well as the medial longitudinal fasciculus, so associated eye signs are commonly seen and help with localisation. Pupillary response is important as the IIIrd nerve lies close to the tentorium and can be subject to external pressure from above from a local aneurysm (post communicating artery). The pupillomotor constrictor fibres lie on the surface of the nerve so the ability of the eye to respond to light is impaired if the nerve is compressed resulting in a sluggish pupil response to light. With isolated pontine lesions there may be pinpoint pupils which are responsive but difficult to determine. This is an important eye sign in a comatose patient. Another important sign in the comatose patient is to look for meningism. Assuming no cervical injury then use passive neck flexion so that chin is almost touching chest. If there is any flexion of the knees then consider meningeal irritation and the need for CT/LP to exclude meningitis or SAH as a cause of coma. Structural lesions causing coma must be within the brainstem or involve both cerebral hemispheres and must be large enough to cause compression/ischaemia and impaired function of brainstem and diencephalon.

Glasgow Coma Scale

- Developed in the 1970s when the only brain imaging was a plain skull X-ray, as a clinical way to identify worsening neurological function that would necessitate neurosurgical intervention. **Advice:** communicate what patients can do rather than just the absolute score.
- Describe score as X out of 15 to ensure no misunderstanding. Changes may be more important than actual values. Difficult to deal with aphasic patients who get a reduced score of 1 out of 5 for best verbal.
- An aphasic alert patient has only a baseline score of 11. Possibly ignore speech and mark best eye and best motor out of 10. Coma is generally defined as a GCS of 3–8. Consciousness depends upon the brainstem reticular activating system and its cortical projections being intact and functioning.

Eye opening E4	Best verbal V5	Best motor M6
E1: Nothing	V1: Nothing	M1: Nothing
E2: Eye opens to pain (supraorbital, sternal pressure/rub)	V2: Incomprehensible sounds (moans)	M2: Arm extends to pain (decerebrate response), adduction, internal rotation of shoulder, pronation of forearm
E3: Eye opens to speech (wake patient if asleep)	V3: Inappropriate words (random words no conversation)	M3: Arm flexes to pain (decorticate response)
E4: Eye opens spontaneously	V4: Confused (disorientation and confusion)	M4: Arm withdraws from pain (retracts arm when pinched; flexion ok)
	V5: Normal (coherently and appropriate – month, age)	M5: Hand localises to pain (e.g. gets above chin when supra-orbital pressure applied)
		M6: Obeys commands (patient follows simple commands)

On arrival to a comatose patient: always consider treating **hypoglycaemia and opiate excess** if unexplained coma

- **ABC: high flow O_2.** Examine if breathing. If not then institute BLS/ALS. If GCS <9 place patient in recovery position. If airway unsafe, breathing difficult, then place in recovery position and oro/nasopharyngeal airway. Get ITU review or if rapidly worsening, apnoeic then arrest team. Suction secretions. If there is poor respiratory effort then BVM ventilation manually whilst preparing for intubation. Check core temperature.
- **What is the GCS?** Why are they in hospital? Any trauma? Medications – hypoglycaemics? Opiates/Codeine? Anticoagulants? What is the temperature, pulse, BP, O_2 sats, respiratory rate? Look all over for a petechial rash, meningism, seizure-like episodes or known epilepsy. If reduced GCS, place patient in the recovery position. Get anaesthetic review. Look at drug chart. A single dose of codeine or oramorph can be enough to reduce GCS.
- **Perform top to toe assessment** if new patient to look for any signs of trauma or any other signs, e.g. petechiae from meningococcaemia, Kernig's signs. If any concerns of spinal injury then immobilise.
- **Check observations:** temp/HR/BP/O_2 sats, RR and ensure not hypothermic (exposure, hypothyroid) and if so treat. Quickly check bedside capillary blood glucose. If any doubts treat for hypoglycaemia (20–50 ml of 50% GLUCOSE into large vein and flush). If alcoholism or any suggestion of dietary issues give PABRINEX IV paired vials TDS for 1–2 days.
- **Opiate toxicity:** consider NALOXONE 100–400 mcg IV repeated as needed. Beware opiate patches: search for and remove any opiate, fentanyl, buprenorphine patches. Repeat GCS and get notes and determine potential causes. Take senior advice.

On arrival to a comatose patient: always consider treating **hypoglycaemia and opiate excess** if unexplained coma

- **CT head** will quickly exclude structural problem: SAH, subdural, extradural, intracerebral or cerebellar bleed, tumour, oedema, herniation syndromes, hydrocephalus and make it a medical coma rather than surgical.
- **Recent travel in malarial area.** Send films. Look for haemolysis. Recent flu-like illness before deterioration. Investigate and treat quickly if falciparum malaria considered.
- **Encephalitis/meningitis:** if CT shows no surgical cause then needs LP with opening CSF pressures to be performed – check no coagulopathy first.
- **Post-seizure or non-convulsive status:** consider LORAZEPAM 2–4 mg IV and PHENYTOIN 20 mg/kg if ongoing seizure activity.
- **Stroke:** usually obvious on scan, e.g. large bleed with coning or malignant MCA with oedema and midline shift. Bilateral thalamic and top of the basilar artery infarcts can give coma disproportionate to CT findings. MRI can help when stable.
- **Toxicology screen:** thick/thin films, ketones, ABG, blood cultures.
- **TCA overdose:** can cause coma and fixed dilated pupils, upgoing plantars.
- **Consider the coma cocktail** of management below.

Clinical clues

- **Signs of trauma and injury:** Battle's sign, panda eyes, skull lacerations or haematomas. If so consider immobilising the spine and appropriate imaging to exclude spinal and brain injury and any other trauma-associated injuries.
- **Asymmetry:** an asymmetrical motor response to pain may suggest a lateralising structural lesion rather than toxic metabolic cause unless the lower brainstem is affected when symmetry returns.
- **Post-ictal:** headache, incontinent, known epilepsy, alcohol (DTs), bitten (usually the side) tongue may suggest seizure and post-ictal drowsiness.
- **Dilated pupil** (cocaine, IIIrd nerve) and may suggest pressure on ipsilateral IIIrd nerve. Pupil constricting fibres lie superficially and liable to pressure. Suspect coning if sluggish to constrict or fixed and dilated. As progresses both pupils may become fixed and dilated. Rarely in a non-comatose patient Ipratropium nebuliser with mask close to eye causes dilation. TCA overdose can cause coma and fixed dilated pupils, up going plantars.
- **Constricted pupil** and usually reactive but very hard to detect (consider opiates and a test dose of Naloxone, Horner's syndrome). Rarely an isolated pontine bleed or infarct will cause pinpoint pontine pupils which are just about reactive. Toxic conditions often also cause small symmetrical reactive pupils.
- **Bilateral fixed dilated:** massive brainstem injury. Exclude hypothermia and drug toxicity/adrenergic syndrome.
- **Dysconjugate gaze suggests brainstem pathology.** If the head can be safely turned (no spinal injury) then usually the eye moves relative to the orbit fixated at same position. If the eyes are static within the orbit this is abnormal loss of 'doll's eye movement'.
- **Look for meningism:** comatose patient always use passive neck flexion (unless there is a history of head trauma and possible neck injury) so that chin is almost touching chest. If there is any flexion of the knees then consider meningeal irritation and needs CT/LP to exclude meningitis or SAH.
- **Averted gaze with the eyes looking fixedly to one side** suggests a contralateral irritative lesion, e.g. a tumour causing seizure.
- **Coma is unlikely to be stroke** if patient moves all limbs symmetrically, pupils and eye movements normal, CT is normal, coma is deep, e.g. GCS 3–6, gaze is not averted to one side, there are other signs such as fever. Look for toxic metabolic causes and consider LP. Patients often too ill and unstable to MRI acutely.

- **Jaundiced:** hepatic encephalopathy, falciparum malaria, and malignancy. Check skin for petechiae – meningococcal meningitis, DIC. Pyrexia, cold sores: HSV encephalitis.
- **Back:** turn patient and check back including along spinal cord and orifices. Abdominal, chest and cardiac exam are needed.
- **Investigations:** FBC, U&E CRP: WCC, glucose, TSH/FT4 (myxoedema coma), infection. ABG: hypoxia, hypercarbia, acidosis. For metabolic acidosis calculate anion gap. Urine: blood, protein, WCC, toxicology if overdose suspected (check blood paracetamol/salicylates). LP: if no contraindications and suspected meningitis or encephalitis. MRI scan and EEG: done later. Difficult to monitor sick restless patient in MRI scanner. Treat for seizures acutely if suspected. IV anticonvulsant: (**PHENYTOIN 20 mg/kg over 1 h**) if persisting seizures (always consider non-convulsive status). CT head: often the most discriminating test in unexplained coma and needs to be done immediately post arrival in the emergency department. Get a neurosurgical consult if abnormal head CT and surgically amenable finding +/– mannitol or steroids – see doses below.
- **Coma and normal CT:** treat medical, infective, toxicology, metabolic causes. Consider LP, EEG, toxicology, etc. Rare 'stroke and normal CT' causes of coma would be basilar artery thrombosis of artery of Percheron infarct. Look for a bright basilar artery.

Differentials for coma

- **Obvious or occult head injury:** was there head trauma which has been missed by emergency department? Look for injury. Blood in ear canal. Trauma review should highlight issues. Get CT head. Look for haemorrhage, oedema. Exclude cervical spine injury? Do not accept trauma patients with 'medical' problems medically unless a full trauma survey has been done. CT may look normal if there is diffuse neuronal injury with perhaps signs of cerebral oedema.
- **SAH:** thunderclap headache, persisting headache, N&V, low GCS. May be localising signs. Blood in subarachnoid space on CT and aneurysm/AVM may be seen. Site of blood helps locate aneurysmal site. Unilateral dilated pupil (IIIrd nerve) due to ↑ICP or PCOMM/superior cerebellar aneurysm. Urgent neurosurgical consult. CT negative suspected SAH is unlikely to cause coma or lateralising neurology. Look for hydrocephalus. ▶Section 11.23.
- **Haemorrhagic stroke:** large haemorrhage with ↑ICP (cerebellar bleeds and possibly supratentorial superficial cortical bleeds benefit from surgery). Look for and manage secondary hydrocephalus with external ventricular drainage. ▶Section 11.22.
- **Subdural haematoma:** may be astonishingly little to find even with marked changes if gradual onset; even a minor TIA episode. Stop anticoagulants. CT is diagnostic. Neurosurgical referral. ▶Section 11.25.
- **Ischaemic stroke:** large infarct with oedema (consider hemicraniectomy). Assess for thrombolysis. Strokes generally do not cause coma unless ↑ICP and pressure on brainstem, e.g. malignant MCA syndrome or large cerebral, subthalamic, cerebellar haemorrhage. The very rare exception is unilateral or bilateral thalamic strokes or top of the basilar artery stroke (if suspected get MRI) and extensive brainstem strokes.
- **Non-convulsive SE:** may be few or no outward sign of on-going seizures except perhaps eye flickering. Needs EEG. Treat with anticonvulsants, e.g. PHENYTOIN 20 mg/kg IV. ▶Section 11.16.
- **Post cardiac arrest:** often undergo urgent PCI and consider therapeutic hypothermia (cooled to 32–34°C for 12–24 h if rhythm was VF). Supportive management after PCI. May be significant hypoxic brain damage. ▶Section 1.11.

- **Severe renal failure:** uraemia can reduce GCS. Can reduce clearance of opiates. Bloods show AKI. ▶ Section 10.4.
- **Drug overdose:** alcohol, ethylene glycol (specific antidote), benzodiazepines (flumazenil in selected cases), tricyclic antidepressants with coma and fixed dilated pupils, upgoing plantars. This list is not comprehensive.
- **Opiates/codeine:** causes miosis, respiratory depression. Opiate medications, transdermal patches NALOXONE 100–400 mcg IV stat and repeated as $t_{1/2}$ short if required.
- **CNS infections:** meningitis: purpura, fever, neck stiffness. Meningism. CT/LP. Give CEFTRIAXONE 1–2 g 12 h IV. ▶ Section 11.11.
- **Encephalitis:** seizure, focal signs, fever, neck stiffness, delirium. Assume HSV and give IV ACICLOVIR. Needs CT/LP. ▶ Section 11.9.
- **Cerebral malaria:** travel in endemic area <6 months. Get blood films to lab. Urgent expert advice. QUININE IV. ▶ Section 9.3.
- **Post-ictal/Non Convulsive status:** supportive ABCs if fitting has stopped. May need anticonvulsant if SE. Should gradually awaken within 2 h – if not then start to look for causes. ▶ Sections 11.16 and 11.17.
- **Raised ICP:** space occupying lesion, e.g. abscess, tumour, haematoma will be seen on CT.
- **Cerebral oedema:** post-hypoxic brain damage or proximal MCA stroke, tumour, vasogenic oedema, diabetic ketoacidosis, high altitude, Reye's syndrome, hypoxic injury, carbon monoxide, SIADH.
- **Liver failure:** jaundice, abnormal LFTs, signs of liver failure; recent paracetamol overdose – N-acetyl cysteine. ▶ Section 7.11.
- **Encephalopathy:** drug-induced, metabolic, liver failure. Sodium valproate can cause coma and associated with ↑blood ammonia.
- **Endocrine:** hypothyroid: hypothyroid appearance, thyroidectomy scar, ↓HR, give thyroxine +/– steroids. ▶ Section 5.7.
- **Hypoglycaemia:** check blood glucose, give 20–50 ml 50% GLUCOSE or GLUCAGON 1 mg IM. Look for cause.
- **Hyperglycaemia:** DKA/HHS with dehydration, ketones in urine/breath, ↑Na, cerebral oedema. ▶ Section 5.18.
- **Addisonian crisis:** ↓BP, pigmentation, ↑K, ↓Na. ▶ Section 5.1.
- **Pituitary apoplexy:** CT may show bleeding, visual loss ▶ Section 5.9.

Coma management: the 'coma cocktail'

Consider where cause of coma is uncertain

- **ABCDE high flow oxygen** intubation and ventilation if hypoxic and GCS <9. Recovery position, NP airway.
- **GLUCOSE 20–50 ml of 50% IV** or equivalent if hypoglycaemia possible. Check blood sugar. Send lab glucose.
- **NALOXONE 400 mcg – 1.2 mg IV** repeated as needed. Lower dose in chronic opiate users or end of life.
- **PABRINEX IV paired vials TDS for 1–2 days** for any suspected malnutrition/alcoholism.
- **CEFTRIAXONE 2 g IV stat +/– BENZYLPENICILLIN 2.4 g IV stat + STEROIDS** for bacterial meningitis.
- **IV ACICLOVIR 10 mg/kg** for any suspicion of HSV encephalitis.
- **DEXAMETHASONE 8 mg IV** stat for tumour-related cerebral oedema then 3.3 mg 6-hourly.
- **MANNITOL 200 ml of 20% (20 g/100 ml) IV** infusion should be given for ↑ICP/incipient coning to bridge towards a definitive procedure, e.g. surgery or shunting hydrocephalus.
- **FLUMAZENIL 0.2–0.5 mg slow IV** if benzodiazepine overdose. May need infusion. Caution if risk of seizures.

Management (G5 = 5% Glucose, NS = 0.9% Saline)

* **Supportive:** ABC, oxygen, physiological monitoring. Ideally HDU or ITU bed. Correct positioning, skin care, recovery position. Nasopharyngeal airway. May need intubation and ventilation if airway and breathing unsafe or GCS <9. Discuss with ITU and critical care outreach team. Escalate for consultant to consultant referral if appropriate on a case-by-case basis. Consider coma cocktail above.
* **Initial:** all patients need rapid blood glucose determination and 50 ml of 20–50% GLUCOSE IV where indicated and PABRINEX IV paired vials TDS for 1–2 days if deficiency suspected.
* **NALOXONE 100–400 mcg IV** (lower dose in chronic users) if opiate abuse/use suspected. Up to **NALOXONE 2 mg** may be needed.
* **CNS infection:** consider empirical treatment for meningitis + encephalitis if suspicions (get LP if not contraindicated). Give ACICLOVIR if encephalitis or CEFTRIAXONE + DEXAMETHASONE if bacterial meningitis confirmed on LP.
* **FLUMAZENIL 0.2–0.5 mg slow IV** if benzodiazepine excess and compromised and no history of epilepsy. An infusion may be needed.
* **Differential is wide:** if unclear despite history and examination and initial bloods then a CT brain will help to separate potential surgical/physical causes from medical causes. A normal CT brain has its own diagnostic differential (see below).
* **Urinary catheters:** only if essential. Patients can be padded and simple suprapubic pressure can result in reflex bladder emptying. Only if retention or close does output need monitoring.
* **Seizures:** if continuing then **LORAZEPAM 2–4 mg IV** and **PHENYTOIN 20 mg/kg IV** loading dose. ▶Section 11.16.
* **Hydration:** can be difficult to assess. Fluid replacement 25–30 ml/kg per day in all comatose patients, initially to match normal losses. If coma persists then manage feeding and nutritional issues.
* **Medications:** these will often be stopped. If they are vital then try other routes, e.g. PR for ASPIRIN. A NG tube can be placed for vital medications. Some important medications to continue – steroids (may need to be increased) or immunosuppression, anti-Parkinsonian medications, anti-anginals, antibiotic prophylaxis, warfarin or other anticoagulants where appropriate, rate-controlling medications, e.g. DIGOXIN (give IV or NG) or beta-blockers, HAART therapies, anticonvulsants.
* **Exposure:** avoid possible hypothermia with blankets or 'space blankets' and warmers as needed.
* **Stress ulcers:** stress ulceration – consider PPI/H2 blocker in selected patients.
* **Resuscitation status:** determine ceiling of care, particularly in patients with poor prognosis.
* **Management of ↑ICP:** see below.

Coma with a normal/near normal (initial) CT head

* Head injury, hypoglycaemia, sepsis, low Na, myxoedema.
* Post-cardiac arrest, hypoxic brain damage.
* Drug toxicity – TCA overdose, anticonvulsants, benzodiazepines, TCA, opiates/codeine/sedation.
* Post seizure, non-convulsive status (EEG).
* Top of the basilar artery occlusion (bright basilar), bilateral thalamic ischaemic stroke.
* Encephalopathy, encephalitis, meningoencephalitis, cerebral malaria.
* Hypoactive delirium, malingering/psychiatric.

11.5 Acute headache

- **Physiology:** the brain is insensitive to pain. However, meningeal arteries, proximal portions of the cerebral arteries, dura at the base of the brain, venous sinuses and cranial nerves 5, 7, 9, and 10, and cervical nerves 1, 2, and 3 can generate pain.
- **About:** on referral if thunderclap (peak less than 5 min) and/or worst ever at onset then SAH is the immediate concern. What is the GCS and observations? How is the patient? Symptoms/signs other than headache? Has there been a head injury? Meningism, fever, rash or malaise? Meningitis/encephalitis. Medications causing headache: nitrates, dipyridamole, beta-blockers, sildenafil, calcium channel blockers, ACEI, alcohol, analgesia headaches with opiates, triptans, NSAIDs.
- **Discussion:** most will be benign (only 7% of suspected SAH are SAH) but all need to be taken seriously. The human and medicolegal cost of missing SAH is high. Keep a low threshold to CT/LP. Note red flag signs and symptoms below of serious pathology. Caution as nearly half of secondary headaches (SAH, tumours, ↑ICP, etc.) respond to triptans.
- **Note:** When to worry: the old adage is 'worry about the "first, worst or cursed"'. The first, in someone who doesn't have headaches; the worst, in someone who does; or headaches "cursed" with some other significant symptoms like weakness or confusion or meningism. **Further reading:** Forbes, R. Acute Headache. *Ulster Med J* (2014); 83(1): 3–9.

Immediate assessment

- ABC, assess GCS and look for focal neurology. A reduced GCS or thunderclap headache or possible head injury or on anticoagulants requires immediate CT brain. Thunderclap encompasses headaches which proceed from nil to maximal within 4–5 min and not just those that feel like hit round the head with baseball bat. Cluster headache seen more often in middle-aged males – responds to high flow O_2. Ask about recent LP or epidural with low-pressure headache. Horner's syndrome (small pupil, partial ptosis are the main signs) – think carotid dissection or lateral medullary infarct, or lung tumour and cerebral metastases. Eye symptoms – for red eye with injected conjunctiva consider acute angle closure glaucoma especially in an older patient.
- **Investigations: ESR/CRP/temporal artery ultrasound or biopsy:** if temporal arteritis considered (age >50 y). **CT head:** will exclude bleeding and tumour. If CT negative and recent SAH suspected then LP may be needed; however, modern scanners very sensitive. LP risks other disabling headaches. If concerns of SAH (wait 12 h post max headache), meningitis or encephalitis and no contraindications. Measure opening pressure. **CT angiogram or MR angiogram:** if carotid/vertebral dissection or aneurysm or RCVS suspected.

Red flags related to headache

- Sudden onset severe (max <4 min): exclude SAH. Needs CT/LP.
- ↑Headache with cough or bending: MRI for posterior fossa lesion.
- ↑Headache in morning with nausea/vomiting (exclude SOL).
- ↑Severity over time: consider SOL/mass.
- ↑When standing: low ICP, CSF leak, colloid cyst of IIIrd ventricle.
- Headache + neurological symptoms/signs need investigation.
- Headache + visual loss age >50 y: check ESR/CRP, ?GCA.
- Headache + immunosuppressed, HIV, TB, meningitis, lymphoma.
- Headache + cancer: exclude cerebral metastases.

11.6 Primary headaches

- **About:** primary headaches are so called as there is no identifiable structural pathology and the outcome is good. The paradox is that their headaches are often more severe and debilitating than those with an underlying pathology with a few exceptions, e.g. SAH. The diagnosis is clinical and often no tests needed, but in some, where there may be diagnostic uncertainty or changing symptoms or red flags or onset later in life, then imaging is indicated to exclude structural pathology.

Causes

- **Migraine (no aura):** aura absent but severe often pulsating, often recurring unilateral headache may last 4–72 h. Shorter with effective treatment, longer than 72 h in others. Desire to be alone, quiet, lie down and sleep. Severe attack looks ill, nauseated, grey pallor. Feels very miserable. Headache often worse than those with aura. Manage as migraine with aura.
- **Migraine with aura:** recurrent episodic headache with systemic symptoms. Comes on gradually, and there may be preceding aura such as tingling, weakness, and altered speech, word finding difficulties, flashing lights, scotomas or fortification spectra. Positive family history. Headache then comes on and lasts 4–72 h by definition but some are shorter and some longer. Patients feel awful; look grey, usual response for severe attacks is to want to lie down and sleep. First line: ASPIRIN 900 mg or IBUPROFEN 600 mg PO if not vomiting or else DICLOFENAC 100 mg PR + METOCLOPRAMIDE. Second line: triptans, e.g. SUMATRIPTAN 50 mg PO or 6 mg SC (C/I with IHD/TIA, stroke). If severe vomiting, consider IV NS.
- **Cluster headaches** (commonest of the trigeminal autonomic cephalgias). Occur in repeated attacks. Severe. Unilateral. Retro-orbital stabbing. Tearing, miosis, ptosis. Restless patient pacing floor. Give 100% O_2 and SUMATRIPTAN 6 mg SC as the first choice treatment for the relief of acute attacks of cluster headache. Prevent with PREDNISOLONE or VERAPAMIL. Commoner in men.
- **Paroxysmal hemicranias:** severe, unilateral orbital, supraorbital, and/or temporal pain, always same side, lasting 2–45 min up to 5–10 times/day. With either conjunctival injection, lacrimation, nasal congestion, runny nose, ptosis, eyelid oedema. Dramatic effect of INDOMETHACIN 150 mg daily.
- **Short-lasting unilateral neuralgiform headache attacks with conjunctival injection and tearing (SUNCT) syndrome:** rare, males > females in middle age. Moderate headache lasts 1 minute. Ipsilateral conjunctival injection, lacrimation. Nasal stuffiness/rhinorrhoea and increased intraocular pressure on the symptomatic side and swelling of the eyelids. Usually frontal and periocular. Intractable to medications.
- **Medication overuse headache:** must be excluded in all patients with chronic daily headache (headache >15 days per month for more than 3 m) and those using opioid-containing medications or overusing triptans are at most risk. Resembles migraine or tension type headache. Chronic analgesic ingestion especially codeine. Gradual withdrawal. Prevent with AMITRIPTYLINE or GABAPENTIN.
- **Tension headache:** usually a chronic band-like headache but many variants. Rarely truly thunderclap. Often long history of similar episodes. No associated symptoms or signs beyond headache. Give NSAID or paracetamol.
- **Coital/post-coital headache:** diagnosis once SAH excluded. May be experienced with orgasm. There is a real possibility that this could be SAH but it would be less likely if it has occurred several times before without incident. In future take NSAIDs prior to sex. Exclude SAH in all cases with LP/CT. Benign form is orgasmic cephalgia once SAH safely excluded.
- **Exploding head syndrome:** not a true headache but can be misunderstood with poor history. Auditory hallucination that occurs whilst falling asleep – sound

like a gun going off in one's head. May be unable to speak or move. Benign condition – avoid extensive investigations or treatment.

11.7 Secondary headaches

- **About:** identifiable structural pathology needs to be identified and managed. Primary and secondary headaches can co-exist.
- **Subarachnoid haemorrhage:** 'red flags – worst ever headache, neck stiffness, meningism, vomited, onset with exercise'. Rupture of an aneurysm or AVM is usually catastrophic and presents with thunderclap headache and often collapse and coma. ▶ Section 11.23.
- **Acute stroke:** both ischaemic and acute haemorrhagic stroke can cause sudden headache but more common with haemorrhage. CT scan will be diagnostic. Particularly worrying is patient on anticoagulation or with any focal neurology. In those with ischaemic stroke it is often on the affected side and is a vascular headache which represents shunted blood through collaterals due to a major arterial obstruction, e.g. MCA occlusion. Needs urgent CT head. ▶ Section 11.19.
- **Cerebral venous thrombosis:** consider this within the differential of thunderclap presentation. CT head may be normal, show clot or venous infarction +/– haemorrhage. Suspect if LP shows high red cells, high opening pressure and increased lymphocytes. Diagnose formally with CT venography or MR venography, whichever available. Anticoagulate. ▶ Section 11.21.
- **Space occupying lesion:** gradually increasing size or oedema or bleed into a focal lesion, e.g. tumour or abscess.
- **Acute infection:** bacterial meningitis: look for petechiae if meningococcaemia, neck stiffness, Kernig's sign, meningism. Acute delirium in elderly, pyrexia. Treat empirically if any suspicion. Many with fever of recent onset and headache will have a systemic illness headache. This is poorly understood. Usually self-limiting with good outcome, when the underlying infection resolves. Some, however, end up with a non-specific persistent headache for months.
- **Viral meningitis:** similar presentation to bacterial meningitis so investigate and treat as for bacterial meningitis until diagnosis excluded. ▶ Section 11.12.
- **Encephalitis:** fever, obtunded, seizures, focal neurology, cold sores. Needs LP and antivirals: IV ACICLOVIR if diagnosis considered. ▶ Section 11.9.
- **Pituitary apoplexy:** severe headache and IIIrd nerve palsy and visual loss as severe pressure around optic nerve from haematoma. CT/MRI may show infarction/bleeding. May have known pituitary tumour. Needs neurosurgical decompression if vision affected. Needs IV HYDROCORTISONE because acute hypopituitarism is possible. Neurosurgical consult. ▶ Section 5.9.
- **Cervical (internal carotid or vertebral) arterial dissection:** neck, retro-orbital pain or occipital pain. Associated focal neurological signs. Horner's syndrome with ipsilateral carotid dissection. Brainstem signs with vertebral dissection and may also have a Horner's from PICA thrombosis and lateral medullary syndrome. ▶ Section 11.21.
- **Colloid cysts:** headache, syncope. CT evidence of IIIrd ventricle cyst. May see acute hydrocephalus.
- **Reversible cerebral vasoconstriction syndrome** (RCVS): single or repeated severe, often bilateral thunderclap headaches. Seizures and focal neurological deficits, ischaemic stroke and non-aneurysmal SAH, LP – ↑blood and protein. MRA/CTA/DSA: "beads on a string" appearance of cerebral arteries which resolves at 3 months. Verapamil/Nimodipine may be given. Multiple suggested causes – idiopathic, pregnancy, vasoactive drugs, hypertensive crisis, etc. ▶ Section 11.21.

- **Temporal (giant cell) arteritis:** subacute headache in older patient. Check ESR or CRP. Temporal artery tenderness or polymyalgia symptoms or transient or persistent visual loss. Needs TAB. ▶ Section 13.4.
- **Acute angle closure glaucoma:** consider in a patient with headache associated with a red eye, halos or unilateral visual symptoms. Urgent ophthalmology referral. ▶ Section 13.1.
- **Carbon monoxide poisoning:** CO produced when gas, oil, coal or wood do not burn fully. Cold weather. More than one person affected in shared accommodation. Check ABG and COHb levels. SaO_2 falsely normal. ▶ Section 14.10.
- **Spontaneous intracranial hypotension:** marked low pressure headache on standing. Can come on suddenly. Relieved by remaining supine. Post LP or spontaneous leak. Give fluids and simple caffeinated drinks. May need epidural blood patches (usually done by anaesthetist). Typical meningeal enhancement on MRI and cerebellar tonsillar descent and bilateral SDH. CSF opening pressure <10 cmH_2O.

11.8 Acute delirium/confusion

Taking referral/answering bleep: What is patient doing and how long for? How were they yesterday? Is it new? Age, why is patient in hospital? Check set of observations. AMTS.

On arrival: See notes, review observations and medication. Confusion in new admissions with poor cognitive reserve is common and may suggest some serious issues and poorer prognosis. Is this confusion on a background of milder confusion or normality? Is this confusion, psychosis or dysphasia? Is this delirium or dementia, or dementia with delirium?

The confusion assessment method (CAM)

(A) **Acute onset and fluctuating course:** is there evidence of an acute change in mental status from baseline? Does abnormal behaviour come and go? Fluctuate during the day? Increase/decrease in severity?

(B) **Inattention:** does the patient have difficulty focusing attention? Are they easily distracted? Do they have difficulty keeping track of what is said?

(C) **Disorganised thinking:** is the patient's thinking disorganised, incoherent? Does the patient have rambling speech/irrelevant conversation? Unpredictable switching of subjects? Unclear or illogical flow of ideas?

(D) **Altered level of consciousness:** alert, vigilant, lethargic, stuporous, comatose? Confusion assessment method: delirium = A + B + either or both C and D (Inouye *et al.*).

General assessment

A comprehensive clinical assessment from head to toe needed as well as drug history and try to get as much corroborating history as possible. Work through common causes, e.g. infection (chest/urine), metabolic (low Na), malignancy (high Ca), drugs, e.g. codeine. Establish baseline. Use and record answers to the mental test score (AMTS) or some standard questions in terms of cognition, recall, orientation to time and place, speech, comprehension and attention span. The abbreviated MTS can be done or the more complex mini mental state examination. Any recording of cognition is useful.

Abbreviated mental test score

- What is your age? (1 point)
- What is the time to the nearest hour? (1 point)
- Memory test, e.g. an address which should be told and then tested at end (1 point)
- What is the year? (1 point)
- What is the name of the hospital or number of the residence where the patient is situated? (1 point)
- Can the patient recognise two people (the doctor, nurse, home help, etc.)? (1 point)
- What is your DOB? (day and month sufficient) (1 point)
- In what year did World War 1 begin? (1 point)
- Name the present monarch/dictator/prime minister/president (1 point)
- Count backwards from 20 down to 1 (1 point)

Causes of confusion/delirium

- **General sepsis:** examine chest and CXR, sats for pneumonia. Check urine for UTI, check lactate/WCC. U&E for sepsis. Intra-abdominal sepsis, skin sepsis. Assess temp, WCC, CRP. CXR. Check urine, stool and treat empirically.
- **Drugs: always examine drug chart and GP drugs:** illicit and prescribed drugs: cocaine, heroin, amphetamine; codeine, opiates (may be a patch), tramadol, morphine, ʟ-dopa, alcohol, large dose steroids, anticholinergics.
- **Hypoglycaemia:** check capillary blood glucose. On hypoglycaemic diabetic meds.
- **Occult head injury:** was there head trauma which has been missed by emergency department? Is a CT needed? Look for bumps and abrasions and cuts. Blood in ear canal.
- **CNS infections:** obtunded, neck stiffness, rash. Meningitis (a very common cause in elderly), encephalitis. Consider CT to exclude SOL/abscess and urgent LP and treatment. ▶ Section 11.11.
- **Delirium tremens:** agitated delirium with acute alcohol withdrawal. PABRINEX IV paired vials TDS for 1–2 days.
- **Wernicke's encephalopathy:** eye signs, delirium, ataxia, B1 deficiency. Often alcoholics, also hyperemesis, malnutrition. Give PABRINEX.
- **Acute stroke:** dysphasia often misinterpreted as confusion. Delirium vs. dysphasia. The dysphasic patient cannot follow simple tasks – close eyes, touch nose, touch left ear. Even the most confused patient can. Is there right sided weakness, hemianopia? ▶ Section 11.19.
- **Acute pain:** elderly person and acute urinary retention, or fractured neck of femur, or acute abdomen, or MI. Agitated. Incoherent.
- **Cardiac:** ACS/silent MI seen in elderly, diabetes. Pericarditis, fast AF and ↓BP.
- **Hypoxia and hypercarbia:** check ABG, CXR, COPD, carbon monoxide poisoning. Look for CO_2 retention.
- **Drug withdrawal:** alcohol, benzodiazepines, opiates, antidepressants.
- **Acute psychosis:** schizophrenia or other mental health disorder. Hyperactive, agitated, delusions, psychotic.
- **Metabolic:** low or high Na, liver failure, renal failure, myxoedema madness, apathetic thyrotoxicosis, high Ca, Addison's disease, pituitary failure, SIADH, porphyria.
- **Vitamin:** suspect if malnourished, alcoholic, hyperemesis, give THIAMINE. B12 deficiency with pernicious anaemia and other causes. Pellagra.
- **Malaria:** travel or endemic area send thick/thin films. Treat if real possibility. Also consider other tropical disease if recent travel. HIV conversion.
- **Autoimmune/limbic encephalitis:** autoimmune which may or may not be paraneoplastic. NMDA receptor antibody encephalitis, voltage-gated potassium channel-complex antibody-associated limbic encephalitis (VGKC-LE). MRI FLAIR

shows medial temporal signal changes. Cancers – lung, breast, testis, lymphoma, teratoma, thymoma. Treatment: remove tumour and/or immune modulation with varying success.

- **Hashimoto's encephalopathy:** females usually. Psychosis, seizures. Tremor, myoclonus. Stroke-like episodes but normal MRI. Elevated CSF protein. Positive thyroid antibodies. Responds to steroids.
- **Structural brain pathology:** abscess, stroke, SAH, encephalitis, meningitis, tumour, hydrocephalus, spongiform encephalopathy; CT scan helpful. Consider LP.
- **Seizure/NCSE:** EEG, CT/MRI/ LP. Treat and see if resolves. ▶ Sections 11.16 and 17.
- **Malignancy:** high Ca, liver metastases, brain metastases, paraneoplastic.
- **Inflammatory disease:** any acute inflammatory illness or flare up. Neurosarcoidosis, Behçet's disease, etc.
- **Encephalitis:** infectious – usually HSV infection, also HIV, Murray Valley and Japanese encephalitis can be seen in epidemics. Take expert advice. Send CSF and viral and PCR. ▶ Section 11.9.
- **Creutzfeldt–Jakob:** can quickly deteriorate over weeks. Myoclonus is a helpful clue. CSF elevated protein 14-3-3. Sporadic – rapid, older, myoclonus. Variant – younger, slower, ataxia.

Reversible and non-reversible dementias

- **Progressive dementias:** Alzheimer's, vascular, Lewy body, frontotemporal, alcoholic, Huntington's disease, CJD, Pick's disease, Parkinson's disease, HIV, SSPE, PML.
- **Reversible 'pseudodementias':** B12/folate/thiamine/thyroxine deficiency, SDH, normal pressure hydrocephalus (NPH), operable tumour (e.g. meningioma), depression.

Investigations

- **Blood:** glucose, FBC, ESR, U&E. Calcium, B12 and folate. TFTs. Urinalysis. **ABG:** hypoxia, hypercarbia, CO-Hb level.
- **CXR:** tumour, infection, hypoxia. **ECG:** silent MI. **ABG:** hypoxia, hypercarbia.
- **CT head:** can be difficult but looking for major pathology, e.g. SDH, haemorrhage, tumour, oedema, etc.
- **Lumbar puncture:** meningitis/encephalitis/SAH. CSF removed in NPH done to see if improvement in walking but controversial.
- **EEG:** focal seizure or non-convulsive status or encephalopathy.
- **Infections:** HIV test, malaria thin and thick films, LP.
- **Rare:** thyroid antibodies, NMDA receptor antibody, VGKC-LE.
- **Measure ammonia:** high with hepatic encephalopathy, drugs such as valproate and some chemotherapy can cause an ammonia encephalopathy.
- **MRI:** can help if encephalitis or inflammation or stroke or malignancy or other structural lesions are suspected.

Management

- **Supportive:** manage anxiety, keep lights on, calm, friendly reassurance, and involve familiar people or family members. Work through potential causes as listed above. May need mild sedation or even full sedation and airway management for a CT brain.
- **Sedation:** appropriate when patient at risk of harm and not used just for convenience. Go slow. LORAZEPAM 1–4 mg PO/IM/IV can be tried or HALOPERIDOL 0.5–2 mg PO/IV/IM/SC (low doses 0.5–2 mg in elderly) are useful but avoid if at risk of seizure. Get help if risk of over-sedation and airway management. Very low threshold for a CT head is needed. Avoid haloperidol in Lewy body dementia.
- **Antibiotics/Aciclovir:** treat if suspicion for bacterial meningitis and HSV encephalitis (treat both). Get LP if possible.

- **Give** PABRINEX IV paired vials TDS for 1–2 days prior to IV GLUCOSE. Look and treat hypoglycaemia quickly.
- **Stop opiates**. Remove any transdermal opiate pain patch and give NALOXONE 100–400 mcg IV.
- **Give** PHENYTOIN 20 mg/kg IV or LORAZEPAM 1 mg IM if non-convulsive status on EEG.

Reference: Inouye *et al.* (1990) Clarifying confusion: the confusion assessment method. A new method for detection of delirium. *Ann Intern Med*, 113:941.

11.9 Viral encephalitis

- **About:** high mortality. Most commonly due to *Herpes simplex 1* (HSV-1).
- **Aetiology:** acute inflammation of brain parenchyma +/– spinal cord in adults.
- **General:** headache, fever, pyrexia, ↓GCS, hemiparesis, altered speech, psychosis/delirium, brainstem signs.
- **Travel:** enquire about recent exposure to ticks or travel to areas with endemic viral encephalitides.

Causes of encephalitis

- **Herpes simplex virus 1:** 'general' + cold sores, high fever. Favours temporal lobes, frontal and limbic system. Can show haemorrhagic necrosis. Rarely HSV encephalitis (HSE) may later be complicated by an autoimmune encephalitis. Increased risk of HSV if deficient in toll-like receptor 3. Younger. IV ACICLOVIR dramatically reduces mortality and morbidity.
- **Herpes simplex virus 2** is more likely to cause a relapsing meningitis or meningoencephalitis in adults.
- **Varicella zoster virus:** 'general' + widespread vesicular rash. All ages.
- **West Nile virus (WNV):** arbovirus mosquito. Erythematous rash. Age >50. 10% fatality. Epidemic in the USA. Often a brainstem encephalitis with coma.
- **Japanese encephalitis:** arbovirus. 'General' + movement disorder. Epidemics.
- **Enterovirus:** Coxsackie/Echo virus. Seen in summer/autumn. General symptoms.
- **Others:** measles, mumps, rubella, rabies, EBV, HIV JC virus.
- **Immunocompromised:** toxoplasmosis, CMV, TB, cryptococcus, primary CNS lymphoma, PML.
- **Non-infectious:** post viral autoimmune.

Investigations

- **Bloods:** FBC: ↑WCC, ↑CRP. U&E: may see hyponatraemia.
- **Imaging:** urgent CT: to exclude abscess and to show asymmetric lesions in the temporal lobes with HSV. May be necrosis and haemorrhage. MRI: DWI is most sensitive. T2 changes in mesial temporal lobe/inferofrontal and insular cortex with oedema/necrosis with HSV (similar with autoimmune and HHV6). Thalamic changes with WNV.
- **Lumbar puncture:** if no C/I. CSF: ↑lymphocytes and protein. Polymorphs may be seen with WNV and CMV. Measure opening pressures. PCR for HSV and WNV virus if suspected. Bloody CSF can result in a falsely negative PCR.
- **EEG:** periodic high voltage sharp waves and slow wave complexes at 2–3 s intervals in temporal leads.
- **Stereotactic brain biopsy:** rarely needed. HSV shows neuronal inclusion bodies called Cowdry Type A, found in the neuronal nucleus.
- **Poor prognostic indicators for HSV:** age >30. Coma, Bilateral EEG abnormalities. ↑CNS viral load, treatment delayed (4 days), abnormal CT.
- **Differential:** autoimmune encephalitis (limbic with antibodies to VGKC, Hashimoto's with thyroid disease, antibodies to NMDA receptors), ADEM.

Management

- **ABC**, O_2 as per BTS guidelines. Arrange imaging, **LP** and **CSF** to confirm diagnosis. Monitor renal function. ITU involvement if low GCS. Specialist advice. Any suspicion of the diagnosis give ACICLOVIR 10 mg/kg 8 h IV × 14–21 days. Untreated HSV is a tragedy with disability and death. Treatment reduces mortality from 54% to 28%. Check CSF is free of HSV before ending treatment by later repeating LP and PCR. Suspected CMV infection: GANCICLOVIR. Ensure hydration and NG feeding as required. Often initially managed in HDU setting. Of those who survive there is a high risk of on-going neurological deficits. There is no evidence base for steroids.
- HSE survivors may deteriorate and should be investigated for recurrent HSV infection or for antibodies to NMDA-receptor and other synaptic proteins which can be a late complication. MRI may help. CSF and serum NMDA receptor antibodies checked. Immunotherapy may be indicated.

11.10 Rabies

- **About:** causes a fatal encephalitis. Found worldwide. Lyssavirus of rhabdovirus family. Disease may be delayed 1–3 months after contact.
- **Aetiology:** from dog or other animal bite. Saliva from dog, bat, fox, skunk or other animal comes into contact with a person's mouth, eyes, nose, or a fresh wound. Infectious phase 1–3 months. Less if wound is head and neck.
- **Clinical:** acute syndrome post bite. Fever, hydrophobia due to laryngospasm, agitation or coma, tremor, muscle spasms. Paralytic with ascending flaccid quadriparesis similar to GBS or polio with associated encephalitis.
- **Investigations:** saliva, CSF <100/mm³ lymphocytes. Protein mildly elevated. MRI – brain stem T2 changes. Immunology may be negative so use PCR for virus. Negri bodies in cytoplasm of brain biopsy of dog if available.
- **Management:** no effective treatment. ITU care. Supportive. Post-exposure prophylaxis (PEP) with rabies Ig and vaccination can be tried. The experimental Milwaukee protocol may be tried.

11.11 Acute bacterial meningitis

- **About:** bacterial infection in the subarachnoid space. Notifiable disease. Delayed treatment increases mortality and morbidity. Difficulty is those with an atypical and subacute presentation. Treat on clinical suspicion alone. Consider meningitis or meningococcal sepsis if ANY of the following are present: headache, fever, altered consciousness, neck stiffness, rash, seizures, shock.
- **NB.** Empirical therapy does not cover *Listeria* species. Suspect in older, diabetic or immunocompromised patients.
- **Aetiology:** pneumococcus/meningococcus/HiB all capsulated. They colonise nasopharynx and secrete IgA protease.
- **Pathology:** purulent exudate in the subarachnoid space. Loss of cerebral autoregulation. Localised thrombophlebitis and vasogenic oedema. Arterial/venous thrombosis and infarction. ↑Protein levels.

Infectious agents causing meningitis

- **Streptococcus pneumonia:** main adult cause. Related to pneumococcal pneumonia, sinusitis, otitis media. Commoner in alcoholics. Diabetes, post-splenectomy, complement deficiency, basal skull fractures and CSF rhinorrhoea. Can cause CVT, hemiplegia, hydrocephalus, ventriculitis with 20–40% mortality. Prevent with pneumococcal vaccination. Increasing penicillin resistance.

Give BENZYLPENICILLIN if sensitive. CEFTRIAXONE or CEFOTAXIME IV. VANCOMYCIN IV may be added. 2 week course.

- **Neisseria meningitidis:** Gram –ve diplococcus. Serotype B commonest (75%). Others A and C (reducing due to vaccination) commonest in developing world and W135. Affects children and adolescents. Petechial (non-blanching) rashes or purpura are vital to early diagnosis. Complement deficiencies, e.g. properdin, increase risk. Septicaemia – Waterhouse–Friderichsen syndrome with adrenal haemorrhage causing shock. DIC. Haemorrhagic rash. Diagnose with blood/CSF Gram stain and culture and PCR. BENZYLPENICILLIN if sensitive. CEFTRIAXONE or CEFOTAXIME IV.
- **Haemophilus influenzae:** small Gram –ve. Children. Capsulated type B strains. Reduced due to HiB vaccination. Related to ENT infection in some. Develop deafness, CVST, SIADH, subdural collections. CEFTRIAXONE or CEFOTAXIME IV. Give steroids.
- **Other Gram negatives:** seen in debilitated, diabetics and cirrhotics often with head injuries and post-craniotomy. CEFTRIAXONE or CEFOTAXIME IV. 3 week course.
- **Group B streptococci:** traditionally a neonatal infection. Now being seen in all ages including elderly. BENZYLPENICILLIN or AMPICILLIN.
- **Listeria monocytogenes:** elderly, pregnant and immunocompromised. Food-borne – soft cheese, patés, coleslaw and undercooked meats. Needs IV AMPICILLIN or GENTAMICIN. *Listeria* resistant to cephalosporin and so not covered by empirical treatment. May cause brainstem signs. Listeriosis, ▶ Section 9.17.
- **Staphylococcus aureus:** post neurosurgery, penetrating trauma, shunt-associated meningitis post invasive procedure with coagulase negative *Staph*.
- **Viral meningitis:** HSV, VZV, EBV, CMV, mumps, HIV. Others are echo/enterovirus and coxsackie. Usually benign. Suspected HSV meningitis consider ACICLOVIR if severe. Any neurology beyond headache and meningism consider encephalitis.
- **Cryptococcal (fungal):** seen in immunosuppression, HIV/AIDS (▶ Section 9.33), steroids, lymphoma. AMPHOTERICIN B IV.
- **Tuberculosis:** insidious, cranial nerve palsies. Raised lymphocytes and protein, low glucose. Give steroids. TB, ▶ Section 9.32.

Clinical

- Look for meningism. Neck stiffness (unable chin to chest), meningeal irritation, resists passive neck flexion; Kernig's sign: patient supine with thigh flexed back to abdomen and knee flexed. Pain elicited on straightening the knee; Brudzinski's sign: supine and flexing neck causes flexion of hips and knees.
- Signs may be muted in the young and elderly or immunocompromised. Chest infection, craniotomy, rhinorrhoea, petechiae (non-blanching), hands and feet and conjunctiva. Atypical presentation with delirium, stroke-like episodes, falls. Unexplained fever, N&V, photophobia, seizures, with progression, VI nerve palsy, papilloedema.
- Reduced level of consciousness, decerebrate posturing, falling heart rate, ↑BP.
- **Complications:** seizures, stroke from arterial/venous thrombosis, low Na. ↑ICP, hydrocephalus, cerebral abscess/empyema, and cerebral herniation.
- **Differentials: viral meningitis** due to enterovirus, mumps or HSV. Lymphocytes in CSF <300/mm³. Normal glucose and mild elevated protein. **TB meningitis:** lymphocytes 100–500/mm³ and ↑protein and low glucose. **Fungal meningitis:** e.g. cryptococcus on India ink stain.

Investigations

- **FBC, U&E, ↑CRP, blood cultures** immediately and antibiotics commenced.
- **CT scan and LP:** imaging not needed if fully conscious, no lateralising signs, no seizures and no HIV infection. In a fully conscious patient, a CT scan delays treatment and delays the LP. An early LP directs appropriate antibiotic treatment. It can aid diagnosis of aseptic meningitis, which avoids unnecessary antibiotics. Most cases

of headache and fever of recent onset will have a systemic illness headache. If LP delayed then antibiotics should be given. LP can be delayed if severe sepsis, rapidly evolving rash or severe cardiorespiratory compromise or coagulopathy. Blood cultures should be sent.

- **CSF:** check glucose (with concurrent blood glucose), protein, microscopy and culture, lactate, meningococcal and pneumococcal PCR, enteroviral, herpes simplex and varicella zoster PCR. Consider investigations for TB meningitis. Look for ↑WCC (neutrophils) >5–2000/mm³ (*note the huge range*). Normal CSF has 0–5 cells/mm³. ↑protein, ↓glucose and ↑CSF pressure. PCR for bacterial DNA. Latex agglutination to pneumococcus, meningococcus, influenzae, *E. coli* and Group B streptococci. Very high protein and low glucose are bad prognostic predictors. ↑CSF lactate >3.5 mmol/L suggests bacterial meningitis. ↑WCC and negative Gram stain may be due to previous antibiotic treatment or viral meningitis. Mumps virus can lower CSF glucose. **CSF:** Indian ink stain or Gram stain for cryptococcus. Cryptococcal antigen in CSF or blood.
- **Skin biopsy** of petechial skin lesions can reveal organisms.
- **Differential:** viral meningitis, HSV encephalitis, Rocky Mountain spotted fever in USA. SAH, acute disseminated encephalomyelitis, cerebral abscess, cerebral malaria. HIV/AIDS.

Management (antibiotics + steroids)

- **Supportive:** ABCs, O_2 as per BTS guidance. Discuss with microbiology to optimise antibiotics and expedite samples. Following require urgent senior review +/– critical care input: rapidly progressive rash, poor peripheral perfusion, capillary refill time >4 s, oliguria or SBP <90 mmHg, respiratory rate <8 or >30 /min, pulse rate <40 or >140 /min, acidosis (pH <7.3) or base excess worse than –5, WBC <4 × 10⁹/L, lactate >4 mmol/L, GCS <12 or a drop of 2 points, poor response to initial fluid resuscitation.
- **Antibiotics:** treat on suspicion. CSF: penetration of antibiotics depends on meningeal inflammation. Try to get blood cultures, LP and CSF before antibiotics. CEFTRIAXONE or CEFOTAXIME IV immediately as empirical therapy. Duration 7 days meningococcus, 14 days pneumococcal. CSF/blood cultures will guide therapy as will patient's age. This therapy does not cover *Listeria* so if considered (age >55, pregnant, immunocompromised) then add AMPICILLIN or AMOXICILLIN for 21 days and some may add GENTAMICIN 5 mg/kg/d for 10 days. If meningitis post-head injury/neurosurgery/brain abscess: MEROPENEM IV. If you suspect penicillin-resistant pneumococcus, then add VANCOMYCIN. Suspect pseudomonas then add VANCOMYCIN + CEFTRIAXONE.
- **Steroids:** adults with suspected pneumococcal or *H. influenzae* bacterial meningitis give DEXAMETHASONE 10 mg stat IV and then 0.15 mg/kg every 6 h for 2–4 days. Improves overall outcome with *H. influenzae*, tuberculous, and pneumococcal meningitis.
- **Antifungals:** cryptococcal meningitis needs LIPOSOMAL AMPHOTERICIN B 3 mg/kg IV/day and FLUCYTOSINE and then FLUCONAZOLE 400 mg OD. Discuss with infectious diseases experts.
- **Antivirals:** consider ACICLOVIR 10 mg/kg 8 h IV if HSV meningoencephalitis is within the differential. Have a low threshold for treatment whilst awaiting CSF PCR.
- **Notifiable disease.** Inform local public health. Consider prophylaxis for close adult contacts. Take local advice. RIFAMPICIN 600 mg BD for 2 days has been used. Take microbiological advice if unsure. Staff do not need prophylaxis unless they gave mouth to mouth resuscitation.

Reference: Cochrane Review (2016) Corticosteroids for acute bacterial meningitis. British Infection Society, Early Management of Suspected Meningitis and Meningococcal Sepsis in Immunocompetent Adults. 3rd Edition.

11.12 Acute viral (aseptic) meningitis

- **About:** meningeal inflammation but a more benign and self-limited illness than bacterial meningitis. There may be a microencephalitis.
- **Causes:** enteroviruses 80%, mumps, HSV-2, CMV, measles, influenza, HH6.
- **Clinical:** nausea, vomiting, irritability, delirium, headache, neck stiffness, photophobia, malaise. No focal neurology or seizures, etc.
- **Investigations:** FBC, WCC and CRP may show inflammatory response. HIV test advised. CT/MRI usually normal. Severe cases T1-weighted MRI may show diffuse enhancement of the meninges. LP and CSF: elevated lymphocytes. Virology: PCR to HSV, CMV, HIV. Toxoplasma serology if needed. Send blood, faeces, throat swabs for viral serology and cultures.
- **Differential:** partially treated bacterial meningitis so ask about prior antibiotic usage, other inflammatory and granulomatous or malignant conditions.
- **Management:** supportive usually recovery in 7–10 days with excellent prognosis. Manage headache and fever with analgesics and paracetamol. Ensure hydrated. Usually benign and self-limited and self-caring can be managed at home. Consider treating those with immunodeficiency. **HSV meningitis** treatment with ACICLOVIR should be only for those with evidence of associated encephalitis. Take advice if unsure. **CMV meningitis:** use Ganciclovir/Foscarnet in immunocompromised hosts.

11.13 Cerebral abscess

- **Types:** differentiate intracerebral and subdural pus collections. An abscess has pus in the parenchyma and the other pus in subdural space (empyema).
- **Risk factors:** alcoholism, immunosuppression, e.g. post-transplant, skull fracture, associated mastoiditis or localised infection. Dental abscess, bronchiectasis, TB, AIDS, bacterial endocarditis. All commoner in men.
- **Aetiology:** local spread, e.g. *Staph. aureus* from penetrating skull trauma. From sinus ENT infections. *Pseudomonas* from ears, anaerobes and streptococci from oral cavity. Systemic blood spread from lung abscess, bronchiectasis, congenital cyanotic heart disease (Fallot's), PFO, pulmonary AV fistula, endocarditis. Immunocompromised/HIV – toxoplasma and nocardia and fungal infections.
- **Pathology:** early cerebritis (local infection and infiltration) → late cerebritis (central necrosis) → collagen capsule formation with central necrosis takes 2 weeks. Steroids slow time course. The capsule can impede antibiotic penetration.
- **Clinical:** focal symptoms of space-occupying lesion. Headache, focal seizure. Delirium. ↑ICP – general malaise, drowsiness, progressive coma, hemianopia with temporal lobe abscess, movement disorder. Neurological signs, poor dentition. Evidence of neglect/alcoholism. Look for clubbing, murmurs, dental abscess, jaundice (look in ears). Patients can appear well if pus is well walled off.
- **Differential:** malignant glioma (also has ring enhancement but does not show DWI changes on MRI). Needle aspiration (may be only way to differentiate), metastatic tumour (look for primary), toxoplasmosis (HIV, positive serology, response to treatment), nocardia (brain biopsy, treat).
- **Investigations:** bloods: ↑ESR/CRP, ↑WCC may be normal. Blood cultures, HIV serology. Echocardiogram: endocarditis. CXR: bronchiectasis, exclude lung tumour. CT brain with contrast/MRI brain with gadolinium: shows ring-enhancing lesion with extensive surrounding oedema. Necrotic centre in early stages can show restricted diffusion on DWI. Look for hydrocephalus and signs of ↑ICP or signs of local sepsis, CT sinuses for sinusitis, mastoiditis. There may be a subdural collection. LP avoided if raised ICP and imminent herniation syndrome – take advice.

A brainstem abscess should raise concerns over *Listeria* but there is no capsule and antibiotics should be given.

- **Management:** take neurosurgical advice. Stereotactic biopsy and culture to confirm diagnosis and identify organism to direct antibiotic therapy. Drainage may be by needle aspiration or excision and drainage if superficial and non-eloquent area. Multiple small abscesses managed medically. A short course of steroids (Dexamethasone 16–24 mg/day) may have a role if significant oedema until definitive drainage. Antibiotics: empirical IV CEFTRIAXONE 2 g 12 h + IV METRONIDAZOLE 500 mg 8 h for 6–8 weeks and review. A capsule can prevent antibiotic penetration with low levels in the core. Take microbiology advice. Anticonvulsants may be needed for seizures. Occasionally abscess can rupture causing a ventriculitis with very poor prognosis. Neurorehabilitation.

11.14 Septic cavernous sinus thrombosis

- **About:** sinuses have no valves so retrograde infection from central face can spread. Cavernous sinuses lie on either side of pituitary fossa and include the internal carotid artery and III, IV and VI nerve on way to the orbit. Cavernous sinus thrombosis may at times be purely due to a procoagulant state.
- **Microbiology:** *Staph. aureus* 70%, others are streptococci, pneumococci, Gram negatives, spread usually from facial cellulitis or sinus infection of sphenoid and ethmoid sinuses.
- **Clinical:** fever, periorbital oedema, headache, photophobia, proptosis, ptosis, III/IV/VI nerve palsy, diplopia, papilloedema, retinal haemorrhage, visual loss. Spread can be rapid over 1–2 days with spread to deep veins and venous infarction and coma.
- **Investigations:** FBC, WCC, CRP, CT brain to exclude other diagnosis. MR/CT venography is definitive for diagnosis.
- **Differential: orbital cellulitis:** periorbital swelling, proptosis, chemosis, ophthalmoplegia, fever, decreased vision, and pain. Usually unilateral. CSF normal. **Preseptal cellulitis:** no proptosis or ophthalmoplegia. **Orbital apex syndrome:** infection in the posterior orbit causes visual loss and ophthalmoplegia out of proportion to proptosis and periorbital oedema which may be minimal. Also local malignancy and inflammatory diseases.
- **Management:** IV antibiotics with anti-staphylococcal cover. Surgery is rare other than to drain co-terminous sinus infections. Anticoagulation may be considered to prevent extension of venous thrombosis.

11.15 Idiopathic intracranial hypertension

- **About:** often seen in obese young females with a high opening pressure headache. Can result in visual loss. Not benign as sight may be permanently compromised.
- **Precipitants:** weight gain, tetracycline, steroids, amiodarone, Tamoxifen, Minocycline, Isotretinoin, all-trans-retinoic acid (ATRA) for APML, Ciclosporin.
- **Clinical:** classically but not always obese young females. Rapid weight gain. Chronic high pressure headache worse in morning, coughing, straining. Papilloedema and enlarged blind spot. Diplopia (VIth nerve). Pulsatile tinnitus.
- **Investigations:** FBC, U&E, ESR. CT at least initially to exclude SOL before LP. LP shows high opening pressures. Remove 20 ml helps headache/vision. CSF normal. Also consider CT/MR venography to exclude cerebral venous sinus thrombosis. Visual fields assessment.
- **Management:** stop any causative drugs, lose weight. Start ACETAZOLAMIDE. Monitor with neurology follow up. Optic nerve sheath fenestration or CSF shunting.

11.16   Seizures: status epilepticus

Treat if seizure is abnormally prolonged >5 min or repeats within 1 h. There may be long-term consequences if persists more than 30 min including neuronal death, neuronal injury, and alteration of neuronal networks, depending on the type and duration of seizures.

- **About:** epilepsy is a tendency to have seizures so need at least two to diagnose and start treatment, though one may do with a clear recurring structural cause. Few single seizures will last more than 5 min. Status epilepticus (SE) is a medical emergency. Mortality for SE is 17–26% (by older definition). 10–23% of patients who survive are left with new or disabling neurological deficits. Status applies to all seizure types but convulsive status epilepticus is most important. Half of those with convulsive SE have chronic epilepsy. Seizures are usually temporal or frontal lobe in origin. Stopping antiepileptic drugs is commonest cause and recommencing is the treatment. Convulsive SE causes severe metabolic and physiological damage as well as raised ICP. Damage may be permanent.

- **Causes and precipitants:** failure to take antiepileptic drugs, tiredness, alcohol, stress, fever, infection. Primary epilepsy, pre-eclampsia (pregnant >20 weeks, BP >140/90, proteinuria). Hypoglycaemia, encephalitis, meningitis, space occupying lesion. Brain tumour, brain abscess, haematoma, stroke – bleed or ischaemia. Cerebral vasculitis, severe low Na, severe low Ca, head trauma. Cocaine, opiates, overdose of tricyclics or phenothiazines. Idiopathic, pseudoseizures, cerebral malaria.

- **Advice:** things to check. Is there suspicion of a structural lesion needing CT brain and/or LP? Consider causes of coma and treating for such. Drugs that lower fit threshold: alcohol commonest, cocaine, TCAs, theophylline. Drug withdrawal, e.g. alcohol and sedatives. Exclude hypoglycaemia. Infection, particular HSE, chest and urine. Brain tumour/abscess.

- **Clinical:** usually generalised cry and then fall, rhythmic contraction of limbs, unresponsive. In SE the fit-like movement and unresponsiveness remains or recurs. A witnessed history of the fit is vital to making the diagnosis and all efforts must be made to get this information if diagnosis uncertain. Some will recall have a preceding aura: smells, tastes, especially with a temporal lobe focus. Tongue biting and urinary incontinence all suggest a generalised seizure as a differential. Most seizures are followed by a post-ictal phase of several hours for complete recovery which is useful in differentiating from other causes of collapse, which recover quickly, e.g. vasovagal and Stokes–Adams attacks. Nocturnal seizures – wake up with headache, wet bed, bruises, confused. A fertile fitting female with an abdominal mass may be pregnant with eclampsia.

Seizure classification

- **Generalised:** conceptualised as originating at some point within and rapidly engaging bilaterally distributed networks. There is typically a loss of consciousness. Divided into tonic–clonic ("grand mal" seizures, lose consciousness, muscles stiffen, then jerking movements), absence ("petit mal") where patient has lapses in awareness and may appear to be staring, atonic (characterized by an abrupt loss of muscle tone), tonic (stiffening), clonic (repeated jerking), and myoclonic (brief shock-like jerks of a muscle or muscles).

- **(Simple/complex) partial seizures:** clinical and EEG evidence shows focal origin at some point within networks limited to one hemisphere. Subdivided into simple (the patient was aware and maintained consciousness during the seizure) and complex (consciousness or awareness was impaired during the seizure). Seizures should be described accurately according to their semiologic features. These rarely need treatment acutely and need specialist review. Unclassified seizures are those that didn't fit into the other categories or those for which it is unclear where in the brain they began. Partial seizures evolving to a bilateral convulsive seizure (formally called secondary generalisation).

- **Semiological features:** these can often be associated to underlying contralateral cortical anatomical location. Dysphasia (L parietal/frontal), dysarthria, gelastic (laughing), dacrocystic (crying), vocal, verbal, sensory (somatosensory, visual (occipital), auditory (temporal), olfactory (usually bad smell temporal), gustatory (usually a bad taste temporal), epigastric, cephalic, autonomic (heart rate changes, sweating, piloerection), dyscognitive (bilateral) with loss of memory or awareness (was called complex partial), affective, illusionary. [*Epilepsia* 2001;42:1212.]

Differential of seizures

- **Non-epileptic attack disorder (NEAD):** not true seizures. Also known as 'pseudoseizures'. Often mistaken for epilepsy. Difficult to diagnose. Eyes usually closed, resist eye opening. Seizures come on gradually and last longer than 5 min. Can be incontinent. Lateral tongue bite uncommon. Increased respiratory rate. Diagnosis may need EEG monitoring and expert input. May be seen in those with epilepsy which makes management difficult.
- **Generalised convulsive movements:** syncope with jerking movements, severe rigors in obtunded patient, cardiorespiratory compromise with anoxic seizures, non-epileptic attack disorder.
- **Drop attacks:** cardiac disorders, cataplexy, metabolic disorders, vertebrobasilar ischaemia.
- **Transient motor attacks:** tics, TIA, spasms, movement disorders.
- **Confusion or fugue states:** transient global amnesia, hysteria, intermittent psychosis, encephalopathy.

Investigations (check glucose)

- **Bloods:** FBC, U&E (low or high Na), Ca and Mg. **LFTs:** alcohol withdrawal. **Glucose:** hypoglycaemia – unknown over diabetic excess insulin. Check anticonvulsant levels – SE may be due to lack of compliance. ↑CRP: infection, inflammation, vasculitis, malignancy. ECG and CXR should be done.
- **Pregnancy test:** urine/serum β-hCG in all fertile females (eclampsia).
- **Brain imaging:** low threshold to CT brain acutely in a first time seizure or where new neurology or trauma has occurred. MRI when stable if needed. Those with a clear seizure history who wake up quickly without deficit may not need imaging. In new patients MRI is the imaging modality of choice, but acutely CT is more available, quicker and allows monitoring. MRI can be done post discharge to look for structural lesions, developmental abnormalities, and also for medial temporal sclerosis, a cause of temporal lobe epilepsy due to paediatric febrile convulsions.
- **EEG:** may show spike and wave patterns suggesting high risk of recurrence. It may be done as outpatient. It is very useful acutely to help diagnose NEADs.
- **Lumbar puncture:** if encephalitis/meningitis or SAH or HIV suspected. Have a low threshold if there is no obvious acceptable explanation for the seizure. Check opening pressure, WCC count, protein, glucose, Gram stain, smear for acid-fast bacilli, cryptococcus, viral and bacterial cultures. PCR for herpesvirus.
- **Toxicology screen:** for cocaine or other drugs if suspected. Anticonvulsant levels should be taken for later assessment.
- **Prolactin level (PRL):** goes up with generalised and some focal seizures but not with pseudoseizures. Take within 30 min of post-ictal period. If elevated may be useful at a later date to determine baseline PRL level as mild hyperprolactinaemia is not uncommon in the general population for various reasons.

Status management

Watch the clock 0–10 min

- ABC and O$_2$ as per BTS guidelines. Monitor with 10 min temp, BP, pulse, capillary blood glucose, GCS and pupils. Note time of onset to know duration. Place in safe recovery position. Protect airway and head. Get IV access (send bloods: U&E, glucose, Ca, Mg, anticonvulsant level, toxicology if needed). Monitor closely. O$_2$ sats, HR, BP, respiratory rate, GCS.
- Manage in appropriate area with monitoring and staff. Do not insert anything in the mouth. Fits usually terminate in 2–5 min. Eyes often open, lateral tongue bite, may be incontinent. Often no need to give any medications and just get IV access, fluids and monitor. Consider nasopharyngeal airway. If at any time seizure has terminated then manage supportively and allow to wake up after post-ictal period.
- Continue to monitor for further seizures and look for precipitant.

0–30 min (with all these drugs be ready to manage respiratory depression)

- **Seizure persists >5 mins or further seizure:** LORAZEPAM 2–4 mg IV given at 2 mg/min repeated once after 10–20 min if needed or DIAZEPAM 5–10 mg IV or DIAZEPAM 10–20 mg PR if no IV access. Prehospital: MIDAZOLAM 10 mg buccal (unlicensed) given by oral syringe between gum and cheek divided between both sides of mouth may be used with good efficacy and safety.
- **Any suspicion of excess opiates** suspected: consider NALOXONE (0.2–2.0 mg slow IV).
- **Start fluids**, e.g. 1 L NS over 4–6 h.
- **Possible hypoglycaemia:** GLUCOSE (25 g) 30–50 ml of 50% solution.
- **Alcoholism or malnutrition:** PABRINEX IV paired vials TDS for 1–2 days if any suggestion of alcohol abuse or impaired nutrition.
- **Consider** PHENYTOIN: 20 mg/kg over 60 min IV in NS loading dose (max dose 2 g) with cardiac monitoring. If already on phenytoin then send level and consider maintenance dose only or consider another agents. DO NOT GIVE WITH G5. Phenytoin has zero order (saturation) kinetics, resulting in a large exponential rise in serum concentration as the dose increases. Watch levels (therapeutic range 10–20 mg/L or 40–80 µmol/L). If seizures persist with phenytoin try second line IV PHENOBARBITAL 10 mg/kg at a rate of not more than 100 mg/min; max. 1 g.

0–60 min: seizure fails to terminate or recurs

- Get anaesthetic help if airway unsafe or GCS <9 and not quickly improving. If fit continuing, then need to transfer to ITU. EEG monitoring. Consider monitoring intracranial pressure. Revision of antiepileptic drug therapy.
- **Refractory seizures after 30–40 min:** consider transfer to ITU for intubation and GA. Intensivists can consider loading dose of PROPOFOL and infusion or MIDAZOLAM or THIOPENTAL SODIUM titrated to effect (the dose regimen is beyond this text and the patient will be under ITU care); after 2–3 days infusion rate needs reduction as fat stores are saturated. Continued for 12–24 h after the last clinical or electrographic seizure, then dose tapered.
- **EEG monitoring:** necessary for refractory status. Consider the possibility of non-epileptic status. In refractory convulsive SE, the primary end-point is suppression of epileptic activity on the EEG, with a secondary end-point of burst-suppression pattern (that is, short intervals of up to 1 s between bursts of background rhythm).

Other considerations

- **Ask why.** Exclude meningoencephalitis. Consider IV ACICLOVIR 10 mg/kg 8 h and CEFTRIAXONE 1–2 g 12 h if possible but try to get an LP first after a CT has shown no contraindications, drug toxicity, metabolic causes, sepsis (check WCC, lactate), alcohol or other drug withdrawal. Look for head injury. **Have a low threshold to CT/MRI and LP.** Try to obtain collateral history and context so as to determine cause. Is there head injury, drugs, history of epilepsy and medications taken? If the patient is pregnant then always consider eclampsia.

- **Suspected vasculitis or vasogenic oedema (tumour):** should be evidence on imaging and in the right clinical context take expert advice and consider DEXAMETHASONE 10 mg IV. No role for steroids for acute ischaemic or haemorrhagic stroke or head injury.
- **Complications:** aspiration pneumonia, rhabdomyolysis, AKI, trauma, dislocated shoulder.
- **Recovery:** patients who present with generalised seizures are expected to awaken gradually. If the level of consciousness does not improve by 20 min after cessation of movements, or the mental status remains abnormal 30–60 min after the convulsions cease, non-convulsive status must be considered (do EEG) or some other explanation should be sought.
- **NEAD:** difficult diagnosis because many are incredibly convincing and a patient with enough drive can end up intubated and ventilated. EEG and neurology input should help. Some do also have genuine seizures and some have never had seizures but have convinced others including neurologists that they do and are on several agents and it can be near impossible to untangle.
- **Isoniazid related seizures:** take advice. May need large doses of PYRIDOXINE.
- **Post stroke epilepsy:** large cortical infarcts or haemorrhage. Increased risk if parahippocampal gyrus that surrounds the hippocampus is affected. Usually comes on several months after the stroke. Treat with Valproate or Levetiracetam.

Simple uncomplicated seizure

- **Discharge:** consider discharge if known epilepsy, full recovery to baseline, well, self-caring independent patient, seizure was short lasting and terminated without sedation. Prefer patient to be under supervision or a responsible adult to check-up on patient and on normal adequate anticonvulsant therapy.
- **Follow up:** arrange neurological follow-up with first fit clinic and in the meantime book an outpatient EEG and MRI. YOU MUST advise patient not drive AND DOCUMENT IT. Tell patient to inform DVLA. Usually licence withdrawn for 6–12 months but that is a DVLA decision. DVLA will write to the GP or neurologist for clinical information.

Starting anticonvulsants

Management of epilepsy is three-fold: avoiding precipitants – tiredness, alcohol, drugs. Compliance with antiepileptic drugs. Surgery in a small number to either resect the seizure focus or pathways that allow generalisation or deep brain stimulation. Refer first fit clinic.

- **For first seizure** the need for on-going antiepileptic drugs depends upon the presence of an on-going precipitant and the ability to avoid precipitants. In most cases medication is not commenced after a single seizure. There is a 45% risk of a further seizure in 2 years. Where there is an active on-going precipitant, e.g. a tumour or a structural abnormality, then it may be reasonable to start an anticonvulsant with the first seizure. Efficacy varies little between drugs and choice is more limited by side-effects and interactions and pregnancy, and now there is probably a trend to use the newer agents. All patients with first seizure should have a specialist neurology review. Pregnant patients, in fact fertile females who may become pregnant, require neurological consult before starting any agent which should be at the first fit clinic within weeks of diagnosis or discuss directly with neurology before discharge.

- Generally any of the following agents are used: PHENYTOIN 150–300 mg OD PO, VALPROATE 300 mg BD PO, LEVETIRACETAM 250 mg OD PO. Follow BNF advice.
- **General advice:** further refinement should be left to the neurologist. In the meantime advice regarding no driving, avoiding machinery or situations where unexpected loss of consciousness would cause significant harm, e.g. using hazardous machinery, cycling in traffic, climbing ladders, or swimming unaccompanied (this list is not comprehensive), then advice to curtail the activity should be given until more specialist assessment. Document driving advice in notes.
- **Sudden unexpected death in epilepsy** (SUDEP). Rare. May occur after a generalised tonic–clonic seizure (commoner in those with over 3 per year), those not on antiepileptic drugs or sub-therapeutic levels, early adulthood, and epilepsy of long duration and mental retardation. May be related to suffocation exacerbated by central apnoea. Related to nocturnal seizures and possibly poor control.
- **St John's wort:** avoid in those taking antiepileptic drugs as can affect drug levels of many of them.
- **Juvenile myoclonic epilepsy:** myoclonic jerks, tonic–clonic seizures, often after waking. First line are Valproate and Lamotrigine but Valproate avoided in fertile females due to fears of teratogenicity and side-effects. Needs life long drug therapy.
- **Catamential epilepsy:** associated with menstruation, usually worsens mid-cycle at ovulation. May be treated with Clobazam midcycle with usual antiepileptic drugs.
- **Pregnancy and epilepsy,** ▶ Section 15.11.
- **Antiepileptic hypersensitivity syndrome:** rare but potentially fatal syndrome. Seen with some antiepileptic drugs (Carbamazepine, Lamotrigine, Phenytoin and others (see BNF)). Starts within 8 weeks of commencement with fever, rash, and lymphadenopathy, liver dysfunction, haematological, renal, and pulmonary abnormalities, vasculitis, and multi-organ failure. STOP DRUG immediately and never restart. Take expert advice.

References: Arif *et al.* (2008) Treatment of status epilepticus. *Semin Neurol*, 28:342. NICE (2013) CG137: Epilepsy.

11.17 Non-convulsive status epilepticus

- **About:** patient is comatose or delirium due to ongoing seizures. Possibly under-diagnosed condition. Consider treatment with benzodiazepine. EEG is the gold standard test. Consider this diagnosis in all comatose patients.
- **Aetiology:** all age groups – infants to elderly. May follow benzodiazepine withdrawal. May follow a generalised seizure in a patient who fails to recover quickly. Less metabolic derangement. Risk of sustaining focal damage.
- **Different forms: simple partial:** without motor features. **Absence:** inappropriate treatment of idiopathic generalised epilepsy (e.g. carbamazepine). Responds to low dose lorazepam. **Complex partial:** EEG can be helpful but diagnosis is very much clinical in nature. Confusional state with variable clinical symptoms and absence of coma. Treat with benzodiazepines or oral clobazam.
- **Clinical** (suspicion of diagnosis then get an EEG): generalised tonic–clonic seizure and a long post-ictal period. Reduced GCS with mild subtle twitching or blinking or fluctuating mental status and behaviour. Reduced GCS with a history of a previous seizure. Elderly patients with hypoactive delirium or low GCS especially if on neuroleptic medications. Stroke patients who look clinically worse than expected.
- **Investigations:** FBC, U&E, LFT, Ca, ALP, CRP: as for SE. CT brain scan: may show underlying pathology, e.g. tumour, stroke, haemorrhage, abscess, encephalitis. EEG: diagnostic generalised spike and slow wave discharges.

- **Management:** minimal evidence of lasting neurologic deficits due to non-convulsive SE. There are various types as shown above with some differentials. Low dose LORAZEPAM 1–2 mg IM or equivalent. Assess for clinical or EEG improvement and respiratory depression, ↓BP, or other adverse effect. Consider PHENYTOIN 20 mg/kg IV over 1 h or other antiepileptic drug and assess clinical response. Investigations and management are much the same as <u>Status epilepticus</u> (▶Section 11.16).

Reference: NICE (2013) CG137: Epilepsy.

11.18 Neuroleptic malignant syndrome

- **About:** seen in 1 in 200 individuals taking antipsychotic drugs. Mortality 10%. Usually seen early within first month of treatment.
- **Causes:** neuroleptics, e.g. Haloperidol, Metoclopramide. Withdrawal of ʟ-dopa and Dopamine agonists. Restart medication.
- **Clinical:** often a psychiatric patient. ↑CK and fever >40°C. Drowsy, young, Parkinson's disease. Exhaustion, dehydration, low Na, catatonic. ↑HR, autonomic instability, severe muscle rigidity. Low BP, salivation, urinary incontinence.
- **Investigations:** FBC, U&E: ↑WCC, ↑CRP. AKI: ↑urea, ↑creatinine. ↑↑CK >1000 mmol/L with rhabdomyolysis. Check Ca, Mg, TFTs. Monitor for AKI, ARDS, DIC, aspiration.
- **Management:** ABC: high FiO$_2$ as per BTS guidelines. Consider ITU. Stop causative agent. Intensive care may be needed if GCS <8. Ensure cooling and adequate hydration. Consider DANTROLENE 1 mg/kg IV (up to 10 mg/kg). Consider BROMOCRIPTINE. Also consider levodopa, Pergolide, benzodiazepines.

11.19 Cerebrovascular disease

- **About:** the stroke physician's job is challenging – first reliably diagnose stroke and then identify the most likely underlying stroke aetiology and then develop a strategy to reduce risk of recurrence.
- **Physiology:** Brain is 1–2% body weight but gets 10% of flow. Normal blood flow is 50 ml/100 g/min. Reversible damage is possible at flows of 8–23 ml/100 g/min. Irreversible damage is seen at flows <8 ml/100 g/min. Grey matter has a higher metabolic demand than white matter.
- **Introduction:** third commonest cause of death. 80% are ischaemic and the remaining 15% haemorrhagic with 5% SAH. Similar pathologies can cause both – venous infarction famously can cause haemorrhage, dissections can lead to SAH, SAH can lead to delayed cerebral ischaemia, septic emboli from endocarditis can cause obstruction and bleeding. In the vast majority the cause is simple. In selected cases (beyond the scope of this book) one needs to think beyond the obvious.
- **Atypical or young stroke**, consider asking yourself the VIVID list: is this **vasculitis, infective, venous, and inflammatory or dissection**? If you never consider an unusual aetiology you will never diagnose it. However, avoid over-investigation and false positives. The management, for example, of PFOs and certain thrombophilias and other 'risk factors' is unclear and potentially hazardous therapies must be evidence-based. Association does not always mean causation.

11.20 Transient ischaemic attacks

- **Definition:** focal transient ischaemia of the brain or retina lasting <24 h (in reality often <20 min). TIAs are risk factors for large disabling strokes. Risk is greatest in the days following TIA. Patients should be seen urgently in a stroke prevention (TIA) clinic in order to confirm diagnosis, rapid screening and manage/reduce risks factors. An accurate diagnosis of TIA should only be, with few exceptions, made if all the symptoms can be ascribed to the transient occlusion of a single arterial vessel.

TIA differentials

- Have caution in diagnosing TIA where all the symptoms cannot be blamed on a single transient arterial occlusion. Stereotypical TIAs rarely recur more than 3–4 times and these are possibly migraine, seizure or functional. If unsure take expert advice. Repeated identical attacks are not cardioembolic. If the patient still has persisting neurology at point of referral then treat as stroke. This is important as persisting neurology can be haemorrhage and so anti-platelets would not be wise and these patients need urgent stroke referral and CT brain.
- **Migraine with aura:** usually the aura part is confused with TIA. May be positive flashing lights, fortification spectra, a moving scotoma with a bright margin, word-finding difficulties, stuttering expressive dysphasia-like episode (never receptive in my experience), tingling and paraesthesia. The headache usually comes on later. Common in young and females but may commence in later years. Migraine aura and no headache is acephalgic migraine. Stereotypical repeated episodes likely migraine.
- **Hypoglycaemia:** always exclude. Usually diabetics on hypoglycaemic agents. Acute alcohol. Quinine. Insulinoma.
- **Hypocalcaemia:** hypoparathyroid, renal failure, parathyroidectomy. Tingling. Twitching mouth.
- **Anxiety attack:** especially with hyperventilation, tingling, generalised weakness. Recent trauma, enquire sensitively.
- **Partial motor/sensory seizures:** sensory symptoms, tingling, slow progression over a minute moving over face and arm. Unwanted movements in face, hand or leg have been reported with TIA. Needs EEG and MRI to exclude irritative focus. Ask about other seizure-like activity (Seizures/epilepsy, ▶Section 11.16). Difficulty with speech associated with focal seizure 'speech arrest'.
- **Pre/syncope:** often easy as there is a global deficit. TIA does not cause presyncope or syncope, though a vasovagal may be associated with tingling and transient neurology.
- **Transient global amnesia:** a historical diagnosis and if the history is compatible then no further action needed. Not TIA. Aetiology unclear. Benign.
- **Optic neuritis:** a visual loss from optic neuritis. Sensory or motor symptoms. Usually coming on over hours rather than seconds.
- **Pressure neuropathy:** a radial, common peroneal nerve, median nerve, ulnar nerve. Usually in setting where nerve compressed.
- **Within the bounds of normal experience:** we all can experience tingling, paraesthesia, drop a cup, say the wrong word and many other symptoms which we would not regard as significant. Need to define significance and avoid overdiagnosis.
- **Others:** anything can be referred to a TIA clinic from dizziness caused by a PE, to SDH, to known brain metastases and anxiety states. A large SDH with midline shift can give recurrent transient focal neurology.

Clinical assessment

- **Clinical:** unilateral weakness of face/arm/leg. Variable hemisensory loss – face/arm/leg. Transient dysphasia, transient ataxia, transient hemianopia, or transient monocular blindness. Ask about headache – can suggest haemorrhage/stroke/

migraine/temporal arteritis. Look for AF, residual neurology, and temporal artery tenderness. Residual weakness, mild or subtle dysphasia, ataxia. Look for pronator drift. Difficulty heel/toe walking. Look for hemisensory loss. Listening for bruits is useful but the decision for carotid imaging depends on symptoms of ipsilateral carotid territory ischaemia.

- **Clinical TIA less likely with:** +ve phenomena, e.g. flashing lights, fortification spectra. Isolated vertigo without other brainstem symptoms. Bilateral symptoms. Syncope or presyncope or altered consciousness. Memory loss. Repeated stereotypical episodes for weeks/months would seem to be unusual for TIA – ?focal seizure. Unlikely to be cardioembolic if same neurological deficit each time. A complex progressive story.

ABCD₂ score (risk score)	
Age	>60 (+ 1). **BP:** SBP >140 and/or DBP >90 mmHg (+ 1).
Clinical	Unilateral weakness (+2), dysphasia/dysarthria, no weakness (+1), do not score both.
Duration	10–59 min (+1), >60 min (+2). **Diabetes** (+1).
	Repeated episodes in 1 week gives an automatic score of 4 (high risk). Those with repeated episode, a carotid bruit or AF are a high risk priority.
Risks	Score of 6–7 gives 2 day stroke risk of 8% and 7 day risk of 12%. Score of <4 gives 2 day risk of 1% and 7 day risk of 1% [*Lancet* 2007;369:283].

Note: New RCP guidance (2016) recommends that all TIA should be seen <24 h and that scoring systems such as ABCD₂ not needed. Telephone triage may help to select those with a convincing history as true TIAs are seen in less than half of all referrals. Patients with suspected TIA that happened over a week ago can be seen within 7 days.

Investigations

- **FBC, U&E, ESR** (giant cell arteritis) with headache or amaurosis fugax, age >50. Fasting blood glucose and lipids.
- **CXR:** especially in smokers (lung cancer + brain metastases).
- **ECG, echocardiogram** (age <50, abnormal ECG, murmur, recent MI).
- **Carotid doppler** scan in those with TIA and potential candidate for endarterectomy.
- **CT brain:** can help exclude TIA mimics or infarction/haemorrhage.
- **MRI with diffusion weighted imaging:** modality of choice (the more prolonged the episode the more likely to see changes).
- **Comments:** TIA can be a soft diagnosis – by definition there are no residual signs or symptoms and imaging may be entirely normal. With stroke and imaging the diagnosis is far more solid. The stroke physician must weigh up the history in the context of *a priori* risk and the likely probability of a TIA that could suggest imminent stroke. Avoid labelling unexplained 'odd spells' as TIA. Remember if you cannot ascribe all the symptoms to the transient blockage of a cerebral blood vessel then the diagnosis of TIA is unsafe and needs to be reviewed. Repeated stereotypical transient neurological episodes are migraine or focal seizures or consider another diagnosis. If very frequent a trial of an AED may be useful. Consider neurological opinion. Transient neurological symptoms immediately post syncope or seizure are unlikely to be TIA but due to the syncope or seizure. Take advice if unsure.

- **Management:** CLOPIDOGREL 300 mg loading then 75 mg OD immediately without CT scan (transient neurology is very rarely haemorrhagic). Start ATORVASTATIN 20–80 mg OD. DIPYRIDAMOLE MR 200 mg BD is used much less now but may be considered with aspirin if clopidogrel not tolerated. Can cause severe headache so start once daily and slowly increase.
- **Admission:** we rarely admit high risk TIA referrals unless very concerned (most are not TIAs, take advice if unsure) but see them immediately in TIA clinic same day with carotid doppler/CT or MRI, or next morning after commencing antiplatelet and statin. Some presenting after hours I do keep overnight if I am concerned and if that's the quickest and safest way to get earliest imaging and duplex for the patient next morning. Take expert advice if unsure.
- **Driving:** not to drive for 28 days (UK DVLA). There is usually no need to involve DVLA if complete resolution, but should inform motor insurance. The exception is if the patient drives a lorry, bus, coach or taxi when DVLA need to be involved and approval needed before can drive.
- **Carotid surgery:** if TIA confirmed with corresponding carotid stenosis >50% then consider carotid endarterectomy as soon as possible if good surgical candidate.
- **Atrial fibrillation:** consider rapid **warfarin** or **direct oral anticoagulant,** e.g. dabigatran/similar agent. Do not delay. We would commence DOAC in the clinic following conversation on risks and benefits.
- **Risks:** smoking cessation and hypertension management. Diet advice. Exercise.
- **Other tests:** depending on age and strength of diagnosis other tests such as echo/trans-oesophageal echo and thrombophilia screens may be undertaken.
- **Repeated TIAs.** Many are not TIA but migraine, focal seizures, anxiety, syncope and some remain unexplained. Repeated stereotypical episodes improve with anticonvulsants. May be useful to get MRI to exclude focal lesion and/or EEG. It would be unusual for AF or cardioembolism to cause identical TIAs.

11.21   Ischaemic stroke

- **About:** sudden onset of focal negative neurological symptoms and signs. Focal brain ischaemia and infarction. 80% of strokes are ischaemic. Try to predict vessel occluded as almost all ischaemic strokes have vessel-specific clinical syndromes.
- **Aetiology:** covered later in chapter.
- **Definitions:** WHO definition: neurological deficit of cerebrovascular cause that persists beyond 24 h or is interrupted by death within 24 h. It includes brain, retinal and spinal ischaemia. There is tissue damage but this may not be seen on initial early CT imaging. MRI will show immediate restricted diffusion.
- **Stroke onset is key to management choices:** strokes may be symptomless until an activity is attempted, e.g. movement, speech, etc., therefore onset is really from when patient last known to be well and fully functional with no deficit.

Differentials

- **Focal/generalised seizure:** motor or sensory. Todd's paresis. Usually as part of a generalised seizure which may not be witnessed or nocturnal. Weakness resolves. Patient obtunded. May be an epilepsy history. Nocturnal seizure: suspect if patient wakes up with sore head, incontinent, tongue bitten, feels unwell. Post-stroke seizures tend to be seen months after the stroke with a focus in the territory of the previous stroke.
- **Migraine with unilateral motor symptoms (MUMS):** younger patient with known history of stroke-like symptoms as part of migraine with aura. If this is first ever presentation then treat as stroke. Positive symptoms: flashing lights, scotomas, complete visual loss, speech disturbance/dysphasia, headache. Care needed as some strokes seem to be accompanied by migraine-like episodes. Consider thrombolysis

if first presentation and stroke is real possibility. If possible, rapid DWI can help. If recurrent stereotypical then migraine more likely.

- **Old stroke systemic illness** (I call these 'Ozzies'): CT shows old stroke, history of a stroke with a sudden worsening of symptomatology on same side and same weakness. Usually precipitated by fatigue, infection or metabolic cause. Once treated neurology resolves. May need MRI to be certain.
- **Functional:** younger patient, challenging life, often smokers and risk factors but atypical signs. Arms drift down, no pronation. Give way weakness. Excessive effort. Power stronger when limbs tested separately. Incongruent abilities with therapists. Bizarre gaits. Normal imaging. Need positive stroke team support with full expectation of recovery.
- **Bell's palsy/Ramsay Hunt syndrome:** facial weakness see Bell's palsy below (▶ Section 11.33).

Causes once stroke diagnosed

- **Large artery disease:** atherosclerosis within aortic arch and its branches, ICA especially at its bifurcation within carotid siphon and within large intracranial vessels. Same is seen in the vertebral artery and basilar artery. Disease is caused by progressive increase in plaque size and obstruction. Plaque rupture and thrombosis or even distal embolisation of thrombus and debris (artery to artery stroke). If stenosis comes on gradually over time there is a chance of development of collaterals making subsequent occlusion less severe, even symptomless. Atherosclerosis common within the aortic arch or its branches and can lead to obstruction or embolisation of thrombus. Arterial dissection of carotid or vertebral can cause local acute occlusion or thromboembolism into its area of perfusion.
- **Cardio-embolism (30%):** look for AF particularly when associated with valvular heart disease. Also endocarditis, MI and apical thrombus, atrial myxoma and paradoxical emboli across a patent foramen ovale (PFO)/atrial septal aneurysm. There is an increased incidence of PFO in young cryptogenic strokes, but association does not prove causality and evidence for closure is poor. Cardiac Echo (TTE and TOE) is indicated. 24 h tape may pick up paroxysmal AF. 7 day tape even better.
- **Small artery disease (40%):** there is localised stenosis and thrombosis usually of deep perforating arteries of the cerebral hemisphere and brainstem. The driver behind this is diabetes and hypertension. These are end arteries with little collateralisation. The result is lacunar infarction. These are small deep lesions usually less than 1.5 cm in diameter. Over time the cumulative effect of multiple lacunar infarcts is a subcortical vascular encephalopathy.
- **Venous thrombosis:** atypical, crosses arterial boundaries and may be bilateral parietal. Seizures, headache, stroke. Suspect infarct or haemorrhage in a prothrombotic state or local infection. Request an MR venography or CT venography.
- **Low flow:** low BP causing watershed infarction between ACA and MCA and MCA and PCA.
- **Alternative: rarely** consider are they microbleeds? May not show up on CT. Needs specific MRI sequences.

List of risk factors for ischaemic stroke

- Atherosclerosis – age, hypertension, DM, hyperlipidaemia, smoking.
- Arterial dissection – hypertension, trauma.
- Connective tissue disease, fibromuscular dysplasia. Vasculitis – temporal arteritis.
- Polyarteritis nodosa, Behçet's, arterial spasm – migraine, SAH.
- Embolic – AF, endocarditis, valve disease, atrial myxoma, PFO, LV dysfunction, mural thrombus.
- Thrombophilia – prothrombin, Factor V Leiden, protein C and S deficiency, malignancy. Oestrogens, antiphospholipid syndrome, hyperviscosity.

Clinical syndromes (ischaemic stroke)

Artery	Clinical – think "which is the culprit vessel?"
Middle cerebral artery	C/L hemiplegia face, arm >> leg. C/L hemisensory loss. C/L homonymous hemianopia. Aphasia if dominant side affected. Anosognosia/neglect if non-dominant.
Anterior cerebral artery	C/L hemiplegia leg >> face and arm. Gait disturbance. Urinary incontinence. Primitive reflexes. Abulia.
Posterior cerebral artery	C/L homonymous hemianopia with macular sparing. Memory loss, somnolescence, cognitive changes.
Vertebral and posterior inferior cerebellar artery	Lateral medullary syndrome, pontine and midbrain infarcts, Horner's syndrome, ipsilateral cerebellar signs, spinothalamic loss, dysphagia, hiccups, vertigo.
Lacunar strokes	**Medial and lateral lenticulostriate:** (from MCA/ACA) cause C/L lacunar syndromes involving internal capsule. Pure motor, pure sensory, dysarthria + clumsy hand, ataxic hemiplegia. **Pontine perforators:** pontine lacunar-type motor/ataxic syndromes. Cranial nerve syndromes. Also focal thalamic and cerebellar infarcts.
Basilar artery occlusion	Diplopia, hemianopia, vertigo, progressive coma, ophthalmoplegia.

Initial investigations

- **Bloods:** FBC, CRP, ESR, U&E, LFT, glucose, lipids.
- **ECG:** primarily to find AF or MI/LVH/cardiomyopathy.
- **CXR:** cardiomegaly, lung tumours with brain metastases mimicking stroke.
- **Non-contrast CT head** may initially be normal and may take 6–12 h for hypodensity to show. Earlier signs include subtle signs such as loss of grey/white matter, cortical differentiation, thrombus in MCA or basilar arteries, sulcal effacement, loss of insular ribbon. Cortical and subcortical atrophy and small vessel disease may be seen.
- **1–7 day tape:** done in most patients where paroxysmal AF suspected, e.g. cardioembolic strokes in different sides and both anterior and posterior circulations.

Additional tests in selected patients

- **Carotid doppler:** mild non-disabling anterior circulation stroke/TIA and fit and willing enough for a carotid endarterectomy if a symptomatic stenosis is found.
- **Echocardiogram:** age <50, significant murmur, ECG changes, cardiac symptoms.
- **CT angiogram:** can show up Circle of Willis demonstrating acute occlusion of a major branch, e.g. MCA. It can also show neck vessel stenosis of occlusion (carotid and vertebral). However, only done as initial work up in selected centres. It needs to be considered if there is a plan to refer for vascular intervention. May be done as option to look for AVM or dissection but most centres use MR angiography.
- **CT + contrast:** when a tumour is suspected. Looking for enhancement.
- **MRI:** DWI for infarction, gradient echo/T2* for haemorrhage. Selected patients where diagnosis uncertain, location of stroke needed.
- **MR/CT venography:** if cerebral venous/sinus thrombosis suspected.
- **MR angiography:** if carotid stenosis or intracranial stenosis or aneurysm or dissection or vascular anomaly considered.
- **Troponin:** ACS suspected. **BNP** if heart failure suspected.
- **Vasculitis screen:** ↑CRP. Younger, seizure, headache, multiple infarcts/bleed.

- **Sickle test:** if sickle cell anaemia suspected.
- **Thrombophilia** screen in those <45 with history of venous/arterial thrombosis or family history of VTE or venous thrombosis in unusual site, e.g. cerebral/portal/hepatic vein. Other than anti-cardiolipin there is a very poor correlation with arterial strokes and these thrombophilias. Most useful for venous infarcts.

Hyperacute management

- **Stroke unit:** regular neurological observations – temperature, pulse, BP, GCS, pupillary responses. Stroke unit admission reduces mortality.
- **Reperfusion therapies for ischaemic stroke:** intravenous thrombolysis (IVT) and mechanical thrombectomy: see guidance below if indicated.
- **General care:** IV hydration and swallowing assessment before eating, skin care, nutrition. Consider NG tube if unsafe swallow after 12 h.
- **VTE prevention:** for immobile patients, intermittent pneumatic calf compression for 30 days is preferred, as well as early mobilisation. UFH/LMWH should be avoided.
- **Medical:** if not for thrombolysis and non-haemorrhagic, start ASPIRIN 300 mg stat PO/PR for 2 weeks.
- **Hypertension** not treated acutely unless SBP persistently over 200 mmHg for ischaemic stroke and 180 mmHg for haemorrhage. Reductions in BP should be very gradual or can severely reduce cerebral perfusion.

Acute medical care

- **Antiplatelet:** ASPIRIN 300 mg PO/PR × 2 weeks. Add a PPI if history of dyspepsia. Then convert ASPIRIN 300 mg to CLOPIDOGREL 75 mg OD (1st line therapy). Use combined ASPIRIN 75 mg + DIPYRIDAMOLE 200 mg BD if unable to take clopidogrel.
- **Hypertension:** it is usual to delay treatment up to 1 week unless severe, i.e. BP >185/110 mmHg and if so then consider thiazide + ACEI/AT2 blocker or calcium channel blocker via NG or PO may be given. Lower BP slowly over hours and days.
- **Cholesterol:** ATORVASTATIN 20–80 mg start after 48 h if new, or continue if already on statin. Aim for total cholesterol <4.0 mmol/L or LDL < 2 mmol/L.
- **Anticoagulant:** DOAC or warfarin for those with AF or PAF with no C/I, after patient consent commence low dose Warfarin 3–4 mg/day around day 10. Aim for INR of 2–3 by day 14. Use CHA_2DS_2VaSc and HAS-BLED score (▶Section 3.16) to assess relative risks of anticoagulation. Those with a stroke or TIA with AF must be anticoagulated at 10–14 days unless contraindication.
- **Diabetes:** maintain blood glucose 5–15 mmol/L and avoid hypoglycaemia.
- **Oxygen:** give as per BTS guidelines.
- **Fluids/nutrition:** bedside swallow assessment ('SIP test') and if normal then allow normal intake but keep under review. Get speech and language therapy review if unsure. If nil orally start IV fluids, preferably IV NS at 100 ml/h initially. If swallow remains poor then start NG feeding if indicated after assessment at 24–48 h. Do not place NG immediately unless vital oral meds required, e.g. sinemet, etc. Take expert advice on PEG tube usage.
- **Carotid stenosis:** doppler or CTA to screen for symptomatic carotid stenosis in those who would be candidates for urgent carotid endarterectomy, i.e. **TIA and mild non-disabling strokes**.
- **Top of the basilar occlusion:** acute comatose, eye signs, extensor plantars. Bright basilar dot on CT. If suspected, then consider CTA to confirm thrombus. If no good other explanation and no other C/Is, then consider IVT <4.5 h and/or MT within 24 h of onset. Prognosis usually grim so worth attempting. Get consent. Specialist decision.
- **Artery of Percheron occlusion:** subtle coma/somnolescence and eye signs (full or partial IIIrd nerve) and normal CT. MRI may show bilateral thalamic infarction +/− midbrain. Might consider Alteplase off-licence but rapid diagnosis difficult within

time window, difficult with coma differentials. May need urgent DWI to confirm. Specialist decision.

- **Cerebral venous/sinus thrombosis:** infarction, oedema and haemorrhage seen. Does not respect arterial boundaries. May be bilateral about the midline. Bleeding due to RBC diapedesis and not vessel rupture. Anticoagulation can be given. Look for prothrombotic state, puerperium or local sepsis. Cerebral deep vein thrombosis worse prognosis. CT dense vein and cord sign. Delta sign if thrombus occupies the superior sagittal sinus. Needs CT venography or MR angiography/venography. Anticoagulate for at least 3 months. Investigate cause.

Acute stroke complications

- **Malignant MCA syndrome and hemicraniectomy:** analysis has shown that mortality is reduced from 70 to 30%; survival with good functional outcome is doubled from 20 to 40%. One-third survive with substantial disability. There is no age cut-off. **Consider** if: pre-stroke ranking <2, imaging evidence of >50% MCA infarction (involving deep and superficial MCA territory), >145 cm³ volume of infarction, within 48 h of stroke onset. Patients will usually have an NIHSS >15, particularly if dominant hemisphere infarct. Patients with dominant as well as non-dominant hemisphere infarcts are suitable for decompression. **The following may not be suitable:** older patients, significant co-morbidity that would hinder survival or rehabilitation, bilateral fixed dilated pupils, time >48 h after stroke onset, PCA/ACA involved. Referral tends to go via tertiary centre stroke physicians who arrange neurosurgical consult.
- **Haemorrhagic transformation:** withhold antiplatelets. Usually conservative management.
- **Pulmonary embolism/DVT:** confirm radiologically. Consider anticoagulation for at least 3 months.

Intravenous thrombolysis (IVT) and mechanical thrombectomy (MT) assessment (RCP Guidelines 2016)

NB: CTA usually needed pre-referral for MT to prove occlusion. In UK thrombectomy services outside large urban centres still being developed. Mechanical thrombectomy includes intra-arterial clot extraction using stent retriever and/or aspiration techniques.
In all patients with acute ischaemic stroke and an NIHSS >=4: consider IVT alone: presents <4.5 h of stroke onset. For those aged >80, at 3–4.5 h benefits less clear and so an individualised decision should be made. Details and screening below. No proximal large vessel occlusion then no MT referral.

In all patients with acute ischaemic stroke and an NIHSS >=6:

- Consider both IVT and MT if proven proximal intracranial large vessel occlusion and the procedure can begin (arterial puncture) <5 h after known onset.
- Consider MT alone: if proven proximal intracranial large vessel occlusion and the procedure can begin (arterial puncture) <5 h after known onset and there are contraindications to IVT, e.g. contraindication to anticoagulation.
- Consider late MT (with prior IVT unless contraindicated) beyond an onset-to-arterial puncture time of 5 h if: (1) the large artery occlusion is in the posterior circulation, and <24 h of onset, or (2) large vessel occlusion and imaging evidence of salvageable brain tissue and onset <12 h.

Clinical exclusion criteria to IV thrombolysis (IVT)

- GCS <9, rapidly resolving symptoms. NIH score <4 or >25 (caution >22). SBP >185 mmHg, DBP >110 mmHg despite treatment. Fixed head or eye deviation. Seizure at stroke onset and residual deficit is post-ictal weakness.
- Pathology other than stroke is more likely. Thunderclap headache suggestive of SAH (SAH with deficit should show blood on CT).

CT exclusion criteria for IV thrombolysis (IVT)

- CT hypodensity or sulcal effacement in >1/3 of MCA territory.
- CT shows bleeding, tumour, abscess, or developed stroke, AVM or aneurysm.

Lab results exclusion criteria (do not wait for these unless specific concerns)

- Blood glucose <3 mmol/L or >22 mmol/L. Platelet count <100 × 10^9/L.
- Hb <10 g/dL or haematocrit <25%. Abnormal INR >1.7 or APTT >36 sec.

Historical exclusion criteria to IV thrombolysis (IVT)

- **Heparin** within previous 48 h. Taking DOACs. Take advice if last dose >24 h.
- **Trauma:** recent puncture of non-compressible blood vessel, LP <7 days or traumatic CPR <10 days, surgery or visceral biopsy <4 weeks, major surgery <3 months, recent head injury, significant trauma (fracture or internal injuries) <3 months.
- **Bleeding:** history of recent bleeding (PR/PO/PU/gynae/epistaxis), any neoplasm with increased bleeding risk including intracranial neoplasm, endocarditis, pericarditis, arterial aneurysm, arteriovenous malformations: aortic aneurysm or ventricular aneurysm. Any known bleeding problem or blood disorder. Haemorrhagic retinopathy (untreated proliferative diabetic retinopathy).
- **Pregnancy:** pregnant (discuss) or childbirth <4 weeks ago, desire to breast-feed after treatment. Pregnancy is not a contraindication.
- **Stroke:** ischaemic stroke in past 3 months, haemorrhagic stroke any time in the past, arteriovenous malformation or aneurysm.
- **Gastrointestinal:** ulcerative GI disease <3 months, varices, active peptic ulcer disease, severe liver disease, coagulopathy or suspected varices.

Management pre and post IV thrombolysis (IVT)

- **Monitor BP every 15 min to ensure <185/110 mmHg.** If BP >185/110 mmHg and within pre-treatment thrombolysis window, then treat with LABETALOL 20–40 mg given IV push unless C/I, which may be repeated. Second line is GTN IV 1–10 mg/h. If, despite this, BP >185/110 mmHg then do not give ALTEPLASE especially if BP resistant and not confident that you can maintain BP <185/110 mmHg for the next 12–24 h.
- **ALTEPLASE:** give **0.9 mg/kg body weight** (maximum 90 mg) infused IV over 60 min. Give 10% of the total dose administered as an initial IV bolus.
- **Monitor closely before, during and after thrombolysis** for at least 24 h. Watch for potential side effects and complications. Should be prescribed by, and administration supervised by, a doctor once the approval has been obtained from the stroke/neurology consultant. In the first 24 h immediately after stroke thrombolysis try to avoid urinary catheter unless in retention. Avoid IM injection. Discuss with stroke team. Do not give any aspirin, NSAID, antiplatelet or anticoagulant. It is reasonable to give Paracetamol IV/oral/PR; safe for analgesia or pyrexia.
- **Admission to a Hyperacute Stroke unit:** is key for good outcome and reduces disability and mortality.

Complications of IV thrombolysis

- **Anaphylaxis/angioedema (0.7%):** manage as for anaphylaxis. Oral and tongue oedema may be seen and this can require expert airway management so involve anaesthetists early. Seen more so in those on ACEI and so should be monitored for during alteplase. Stop alteplase if detected and summon help. Give steroids. Bleeding into tongue is differential (CT will show it). If swelling is due to haematoma reverse anticoagulation.
- **Neurological deterioration** seen in 13%. May be due to bleeding, infarct extension, seizure, sepsis, malignant MCA. **Intracranial bleed:** suspect if fall in GCS,

headache, new seizure, ↑NIHSS, acute hypertension, N&V, pupillary changes STOP ALTEPLASE and SCAN.
- **Extracranial haemorrhage:** signs of bleeding or shock.

References: National clinical guideline for stroke, Fifth Edition. Royal College of Physicians, 2016.

11.22 Haemorrhagic stroke

- **About:** many different causes and patterns. Up to 15–20% of strokes are haemorrhagic. Intracerebral haemorrhage (ICH) is an important cause of stroke with a 30 day mortality rate of 20–30%. Leading causes include chronic hypertensive vasculopathy, amyloid angiopathy, and anticoagulant-related haemorrhage.
- **Types:** lobar cortical haemorrhages, deep subcortical bleeds. Putaminal, thalamic, brainstem bleeds. SAH.

Causes of haemorrhagic stroke	
Hypertension	Causes lobar and deep bleeds in the basal ganglia, thalamus, cerebellum, pons.
Arteriovenous malformations	Seizures, younger patients.
Cavernoma (cavernous angioma)	Seizures, bleeds in younger patients.
Cerebral amyloid angiopathy	Causes lobar haemorrhages in those over 70 usually without hypertension.
Warfarin/haemophilia/ thrombolysis/DIC	Warfarin or any coagulopathy.
Embolic stroke	Higher rate of haemorrhagic transformation seen with embolic strokes and any large stroke especially if hypertensive.
Cerebral venous thrombosis	Haemorrhagic and ischaemic stroke can be seen.
Endocarditis	Bleed from mycotic aneurysms from septic emboli bleed.
Sickle cell disease	Both ischaemic and haemorrhagic stroke. Seen in children.
Malignancy	Primary or metastatic cancer.
Vasculitis	Polyarteritis nodosa, SLE, Wegener's granulomatosis, Takayasu's, temporal arteritis.
Systemic	Sarcoid, Behçet's disease.
Trauma	History. Signs of head injury. Not stroke.

- **Haemorrhagic stroke mimics:** head trauma – look for soft tissue injury. Did patient fall and hit head and bled or did the bleed come first? Tumours, e.g. melanoma. Infarct with haemorrhagic transformation. Endocarditis with haemorrhage from septic emboli. Cortical vein thrombosis and secondary haemorrhage.
- **Pathology:** haematoma formation usually splits white fibre bundles. Secondary oedema exacerbates increased ICP and coma/coning. Progressive bleeding not uncommon, especially if anticoagulated. Older atrophied brain may allow more room for expansion. Some bleeds may be low pressure, e.g. cavernomas from venous side. Bleeding into ventricular system. Obstructive hydrocephalus.
- **Prognosis:** 15% of strokes are due to intracerebral haemorrhage. 5% are due to SAH. 30–50% death within 30 days.

Investigations

- **Bloods:** FBC: ↓platelets, ↑INR if warfarin/liver disease, CRP, ESR, glucose. U&E: (low Na with SAH). LFTs.
- **Non-contrast CT:** sensitive for blood and shows haematoma in brain substance +/− oedema, +/− extension into ventricles, +/− hydrocephalus and signs of ↑ICP. Presence of intraventricular blood is a poor prognostic indicator.
- **Contrast CT:** contrast may be given if tumour suspected or SAH to locate an aneurysm. A 'spot sign' in PICH suggests an area of active dynamic bleeding and marks a poorer prognosis. Contrast, however, is rarely given acutely outside teaching centres.
- **MRI:** T2* black blood sequences detect bleeding. Helpful acutely and later when the haematoma has resolved. Old bleeds show a slit-like appearance with signs of haemosiderin. Repeat interval scan at 6 weeks can help exclude an underlying vascular lesion, e.g. tumour, AVM, cavernoma, aneurysms.
- **MR venography:** consider if any suspicion of venous thrombosis with haemorrhage.
- **MRA/CTA:** allows imaging of aneurysms and dissections and vascular malformations. Also see vessel outline and signs of vasculitis or spasm.
- **Digital subtraction cerebral angiography:** reserved for selected cases in tertiary centres for those with SAH or AVM. 1% stroke risk associated with the procedure. Involves selective catheterisation of carotids and subclavian arteries.
- **Echocardiography:** CRP and work up if endocarditis suspected. Septic emboli can bleed.
- **Lumbar puncture** for red cells and xanthochromia if SAH suspected.

Management

- **Supportive:** ABC, IV fluids, ITU if GCS <9 and high EWS.
- **Admit to stroke unit.** monitor temperature, pulse, BP, GCS, pupillary responses. Swallow assessment, NG tube if needed. Multidisciplinary care and rehabilitation.
- **Coagulopathy:** if on warfarin give Vitamin K 5−10 mg IV stat and if INR elevated give 4-factor prothrombin complex concentrates (PCC), e.g. **Octaplex/Beriplex or FFP.** Warfarin must be stopped and reversed in the short term even with metal prosthetic cardiac valves. Give platelets if thrombocytopenic. Correct any coagulopathy. Patients with ICH in association with DOAC factor Xa inhibitor treatment should receive urgent treatment with 4-factor PCC. **Andexanet alfa** has been shown to reverse the effects of factor Xa inhibitors but is yet to be licensed. Patients with ICH on Dabigatran treatment should have the anticoagulant urgently reversed with Idarucizumab (Praxbind). **Antiplatelets:** if the patient has received antiplatelet therapy platelet transfusion should be avoided and can worsen outcome unless thrombocytopenic. **Protamine** should be considered if heparin has been administered within 4 h of the onset of bleeding.
- **Hypertension:** RCP (2016) recommends that those with primary ICH who present <6 h of onset with a SBP >150 mmHg should be treated urgently using a locally agreed protocol for SBP lowering to <140 mmHg for at least 7 days, unless: GCS <5, haematoma is very large and death is expected; a structural cause for the haematoma is identified; immediate surgery to evacuate the haematoma is planned.
- **Surgery:** refer to neurosurgeons, especially if cerebellar haematoma >3 cm diameter and/or developing hydrocephalus and falling GCS for **external ventricular drainage (EVD) and shunting,** or sub-occipital craniectomy for evacuation of the clot. Little evidence to suggest neurosurgical benefit in supratentorial bleeds, the exception being young patient with a superficial bleed close to the cortex and easily accessed. Deep hypertensive bleeds rarely benefit from surgery.

- **IV steroids** have no evidence base and may raise BP and glucose.
- **Mannitol** may be used to lower high ICP whilst en route for neurosurgery.
- **Stop statins:** controversial. Some evidence to stop them. A recent analysis suggests statins may be beneficial post bleed (*Int J Stroke* 2015;10:10). Follow local advice.
- **VTE prevention:** early mobility, intermittent pneumatic calf compression is the method of choice in all. LMWH/UFH should be avoided. In the event of PE then consider IVC filter insertion.
- **Manage diabetes:** (maintain blood glucose 5–15 mmol/L) avoiding hypoglycaemia.
- **Seizures:** anticonvulsants: e.g. IV Phenytoin, Levetiracetam, Valproate may be needed.
- **End of life care:** the decision may be for palliation, though some patients can make surprising recovery. Take experienced advice. May be reasonable to postpone DNACPR decisions for the first 24 h. See DNACPR, ▶Section 19.19.

References: National clinical guideline for stroke, Fifth Edition. Royal College of Physicians, 2016.

11.23 Subarachnoid haemorrhage

- **About:** a common challenge for the acute physician. Background knowledge helps manage the risks. Mortality rates are 30–45% for aneurysmal SAH. Approx. 20–50% of aneurysms rupture over a patient's life. Symptomatic aneurysms need clipping or coiling; asymptomatic aneurysms need an expert assessment of risks. 'Red flags – worst ever headache, neck stiffness, vomited, onset with exercise' – however, only 7% of those screened will have had SAH.
- **Main early risks** are rebleeding, vasospasm, arrhythmias, hydrocephalus, seizures. Traumatic SAH due to head injury is not covered here. Unruptured aneurysms found in 3% of population. Annual rupture rate is 0.5–1% per annum.
- **Note:** CT scan alone is sensitive enough to rule out SAH in patients presenting with lone acute severe headache, GCS = 15, no neurological features or neck pain, if performed <6 h of onset with a 3rd generation CT scanner with thin slices, reported by a radiologist experienced in reporting CT brain scans.
- **Pathophysiology:** spontaneous bleeding from aneurysm/AVM which lie in the subarachnoid space. Subarachnoid space surrounds the brain and spinal cord. Blood needs to reach below L1/2 to be detectable by LP. The pressures may cause bleeding into local brain parenchyma. Blood tends to track into sulci and ventricles and basal cisterns. Blood then pools around cisterns and circle of Willis and later can elicit vasospasm. *In vivo* conversion of Hb over 12 h to bilirubin detectable as xanthochromia. Seizures occur in 5–15% of patients. Cerebral vasospasm seen in 20–40% of patients and half die or suffer delayed cerebral ischaemia with infarction. The risk of developing hydrocephalus depends on volume of blood within the subarachnoid space and ventricles. Aneurysms can rebleed which can be catastrophic. Rebleeding is increased by measures that rapidly lower intracranial pressure. Aim to treat before this happens. 90% of aneurysms lie in the anterior circulation, usually on the anterior communicating artery (ACOMM 30%), and posterior communicating artery (PCOMM 25%), the MCA bifurcation (20%), the ICA bifurcation (8%), and other locations (7%); 10% of aneurysms arise from the posterior circulation usually at the basilar tip but also PICA/AICA and SCA. 10–15% of patients presenting with SAH have multiple aneurysms. Occasionally an aneurysm on the ICA in the cavernous sinus can rupture and be contained, causing a caroticocavernous fistula with pulsatile whooshing sound and an audible skull bruit. May follow thunderclap headache.

Causes of SAH

- **Aneurysmal SAH** (aSAH) **(80%):** aneurysms 5–7 mm diameter in the anterior circulation lowest risk of rupture, risk higher for those in posterior circulation. In contrast to sporadic aneurysms, familial aneurysms often larger (>10 mm) and multiple. Intracranial aneurysms develop with increasing age and usually arise at areas of vessel branching. Rupture rate increases with size. Small aneurysms are commoner, and so bleeds are seen more in smaller aneurysms. Related to smoking and excessive alcohol, connective tissue diseases. First degree relative with SAH. Smoking, binge drinking, illicit drugs. Increased incidence with adult polycystic kidney disease (10%). SLE. Marfan's and Ehlers–Danlos syndromes, pseudoxanthoma elasticum and sickle cell disease.

- **Arteriovenous malformations (10%):** these are vascular anomalies which consist of a plexiform network of abnormal arteries and veins linked by one or more fistulae. They lack the typical capillary bed interposed between the arteriole and venule and have arterioles with a thinner than normal muscularis. Annual rate of bleeding is about 2% amongst patients with no history of bleeding. Annual rate of repeat haemorrhage is 18%. Can present initially as bleeding or seizures.

- **Perimesencephalic:** SAH on CT and blood seen in the cisterns around the brainstem and suprasellar cistern. LP confirms SAH but angiography is normal. Tend to do well with rebleeding uncommon. Possibly venous tear or rupture with bleeding. Blood around brainstem.

- **Trauma:** SAH can be seen with head injury. Treat as per traumatic brain injury.

- **Vasculitis** (rare), bleeding from intracranial cervical arterial dissections (rare).

- **Cerebral amyloid angiopathy:** age >70, convexity SAH and cortical bleeding.

- **Reversible cerebral vasoconstriction syndrome:** thunderclap headache, focal deficits, and convexity SAH. Needs MR/CT/DS angiography.

- **Cerebral venous sinus thrombosis:** thunderclap headache and convexity SAH.

- **Dural arteriovenous fistula:** convexity SAH, diagnosed with DS angiography with bilateral external carotid injections.

- **Pituitary apoplexy,** posterior reversible encephalopathy syndrome (PRES) with convexity SAH.

- **Cortical or meningeal tumours:** convexity SAH.

- **Children:** Sickle cell, Moyamoya disease.

Clinical

- **Headache:** prior headaches may be experienced in 30–50% due to warning 'sentinel' bleeds or due to pressure from expansion of the aneurysm prior to rupture. Often described as 'worst ever headache' which comes on very acutely – 'hit around back of head'. The headache usually persists in some form. Some cases less acute. Definitions range from any with maximal headache onset <10 min. Headache may be occipital or cervical and bleeding from a cervical AVM may be missed on CT. Blood tracking down may cause some neck stiffness from meningeal irritation. Vomiting, syncope and seizure may accompany onset. Triptans and other anti-migraine therapies can improve the headache from SAH so be cautious. In an acute headache 1 in 10 are SAH but if there are additional signs then this becomes 1 in 4.

- **Timing:** comes on at rest or exertion, during sleep, coitus and straining. Enquire after associated collapse/syncope and then recovery, photophobia and neck stiffness, vomiting, diplopia. Beware the sore stiff neck with meningeal irritation.

- **Reduced GCS:** progressive bleeding leads to coma, coning and sudden death.

- **Localisation clues:** may be found but CT anyway. Some signs are useful. Headache and IIIrd nerve palsy suggest an ipsilateral PCOMM/superior cerebellar artery aneurysm. Leg weakness and extensor plantars suggest ACOMM aneurysm. Hemiparesis suggests MCA aneurysm. If there are signs and one suspects SAH there really should be blood on the CT. If there are lateralising sign and a normal CT within

6 h of headache, then SAH is very unlikely. Arterial or venous infarction both cause headache. Take urgent expert advice. Arrhythmias and myocardial dysfunction and even pulmonary oedema and cardiac arrest – aggressive resuscitation is warranted as outcome can be reasonable. 1 in 7 will have intraocular haemorrhages.

- **Differential of thunderclap headache:** primary thunderclap headache: when all tests are negative this is the presumed diagnosis. Cerebral venous thrombosis, benign orgasmic cephalgia. Migraine or cluster headache, reversible cerebral vasoconstriction syndrome. Primary parenchymal haemorrhage, tumour with bleed, carotid/vertebral dissection.

Grading of subarachnoid bleeds: World Federation of Neurosurgeons	Fisher classification based on CT
I. GCS 15 no focal deficits.	Grade 1 – no blood seen.
II. GCS 13–14 no focal deficits.	Grade 2 – <1 mm thick.
III. GCS 13–14 focal deficits present.	Grade 3 – >1 mm thick.
IV. GCS 7–12 irrespective of deficits.	Grade 4 – diffuse or intraventricular bleed or parenchymal extension.
V. GCS 3–6 irrespective of deficits.	

Investigations

- **Bloods:** FBC, U&E: low Na (naturiesis or SIADH) slightly more difficult to see a small SAH on CT if severely anaemic.
- **Coagulation screen:** if on anticoagulants or any suspicion of bleeding disorder, exclude low platelets.
- **ECG and CXR:** arrhythmias and pulmonary oedema possible. Dynamic T wave and ST changes may be seen but don't necessarily suggest ACS. Measure troponin and cardiology review if concerns. Obviously do not anticoagulate.
- **Non-contrast CT head:** thin cuts through base of brain shows high signal attenuation in the basal cisterns. MCA aneurysm blood in the sylvian fissure. ACOMM aneurysm causes blood in intrahemispheric fissure and frontal lobe. PCOMM/superior cerebellar artery aneurysm can cause a IIIrd nerve palsy and blood in mesial temporal lobe and basilar cistern. Blood also seen around the brainstem in prepontine, premedullary and interpeduncular cisterns as well as within ventricles. CT is 98% sensitive in the first 12 h and is over 99% in the first 6 h. **NB.** Three recent studies show that 3rd-generation brain CT scans performed within 6 h after onset of acute headache in patients with suspected aSAH reliably excludes SAH in both academic and non-academic centres, where scans are read by non-neuroradiologists. Evidence suggests that LP is not needed in these patients. Those with low GCS or unknown time of onset, where symptoms are atypical, e.g. neck pain (one case with neck pain turned out to have a cervical AVM), or >6 h from onset should be considered for LP and local expert advice taken if unsure [*BMJ* 2011;343:d4277; *Stroke* 2012;43:2031; *Neurology* 2015;84:1927]. Blood on CT less clear if ↓Hb, ↓Hct. Sensitivity approaches 100% within 6 h of onset and 85% beyond 6 h. Sensitivity improves with modern scanners. Convexity SAH where blood is only seen on the convex surface is usually related to venous bleeding or venous infarction, amyloid angiopathy in elderly, PRES, vasculitis and reversible cerebral vasoconstriction syndrome.
- **Lumbar puncture with opening pressure:** (see above as CT can exclude SAH if normal in first 6 h of acute headache) if required, e.g. presentation after 6 h or atypical presentation and normal CT, then LP needs to be done at 12 h after onset (NOT BEFORE): SAH causes uniformly bloody CSF on LP with xanthochromia due to yellow bilirubin pigment from haemoglobin breakdown which is present

for up to 3–4 weeks. **Bilirubin** is degraded by light and only forms *in vivo*. Can be seen if sample held against white background such that any yellow pigment is positive test. Interpretation is variable. **Spectrophotometry** can be used to differentiate between a bloody tap and 'true' xanthochromia more objectively. Pure oxyhaemoglobin which is non-diagnostic will have a single peak, followed closely by a small bilirubin continuation and fall called the 'bilirubin shoulder'. **Red cells:** a traumatic tap may be suggested by a fall in red cell numbers in successive bottles, however, caution must be taken and this is not an absolute rule and traumatic taps can occur in those with SAH. The absolute level of RBCs must be taken and a high baseline level should still raise some suspicion of SAH. A count of <10 RBCs/mm^3 constitutes a negative tap, RBC >100/mm^3 in all tubes should be considered positive, especially if xanthochromia (bilirubin) is present. Opening pressure should be measured routinely in all LPs and if elevated one diagnosis to consider is cerebral venous sinus thrombosis and next step is CT venography or MR venography. NB: an LP is not benign and can result in a disabling low pressure headache and so should not be undertaken without reasonable suspicion despite normal CT.

- **CSF xanthochromia** (breakdown product of haem) suggests recent bleed with haemolysis and so not a bloody tap. In some centres there is restricted access as samples now go to reference laboratories. Xanthochromia can be determined visually or by spectrophotometry which is not available in some hospitals. CSF, especially if bloody, should be spun down immediately and if the supernatant is yellow (compared with water against a white background), the diagnosis of SAH is practically certain. The specimen should be stored in darkness, preferably wrapped in tinfoil because the ultraviolet components of daylight can break down bilirubin. Spectrophotometry cannot only confirm the presence of bilirubin but also exclude it. Xanthochromia is present 3 weeks after the bleed in 70% of patients, and it is still detectable at 4 weeks in 40% of patients, so there may be an argument for a late LP.
- **CT/MR angiography:** CT angiography is easily accessible, available and relatively quick and can detect aneurysms down to 1 mm (MR angiography to about 3 mm). MR angiography is more difficult in those who are unwell in terms of monitoring. Catheter angiography only needed if aneurysm not seen or more anatomical definition is needed.
- **CT/MR venography:** if cerebral venous sinus thrombosis is considered usually with a convexity bleed.
- **Catheter cerebral angiography:** gold standard. Most sensitive test to identify bleeding source and usually done by the tertiary neuroscience centre.
- **Transcranial doppler:** can detect vasospasm and delayed cerebral ischaemia in the MCA in the ITU.

Early complications of SAH
- **Rebleeding:** seen in 20% with high mortality. All interventions aim to prevent this by coiling/clipping. Rebleeding is a risk of aneurysmal SAH and much less so with AVMs or perimesencephalic bleeds.
- **Delayed cerebral ischaemia/vasospasm causing ischaemic stroke:** likely due to blood breakdown products swilling around the branches of the circle of Willis. Causes acute ischaemia and infarction which may be distant to bleeding aneurysm even on opposite side. Seen in about 30% with further resultant brain injury.
- **Obstructive hydrocephalus:** detected by CT (temporal horns dilated, blood in 4th ventricle). Refer to neurosurgeons for EVD.
- **Arrhythmias and myocardial dysfunction:** telemetry. Watch for pulmonary oedema.
- **Hyponatraemia** can be due to renal sodium loss or SIADH. Determine which using serum/urine osmolality as management differential.

- **Seizures:** manage as below.
- **Death:** from ↑ICP and coning due to massive haematoma or coning. 10–15% of patients die before hospital: 40% within the first week, and about 50% die in the first 6 months.
- **Cognitive impairment:** long term cognitive and functional issues may be seen.

Management

- **Prehospital care:** ABCs and rapid triage and transport to hospital and urgent CT. An early CT within 6 h is more sensitive than delayed imaging and is a reason to justify immediate imaging in all such patients. ITU assessment if GCS <9. Resuscitation. IV fluids usually NS. Avoid hypotonic fluids. If clearly a traumatic SAH from head injury (see topic above) then manage as per head injury and neurosurgical review for clot evacuation and monitoring for development of complications such as hydrocephalus and neurosurgical referral.
- **Bed rest.** codeine and laxative/stool softener. Antiemetics – avoid vomiting. HYDRATION and slight HYPERVOLAEMIA is suggested with 3 L/day. Low Na may well be due to renal Na loss rather than SIADH and, unless SIADH proven, fluid restriction should be avoided. Generally avoid hypotonic fluids and use NS as fluid of choice.
- **Initial:** once diagnosis made of likely aSAH then start all patients on NIMODIPINE 60 mg PO/NG 4 h for 21 days as early as possible. It reduces vasospasm and delayed cerebral ischaemic (below) neurologic deficit, cerebral infarction and mortality.
- **Rebleeding:** early intervention and management of aneurysm. In total 40% will rebleed if untreated within 4 weeks. Commonest within first 2 weeks of the SAH. A bimodal peak of the first 24–48 h and between days 7 and 10. Prevent with early angiography and aneurysm coiling or clipping.
- **Aneurysmal coiling:** preferred option with better outcomes. Interventional neuroradiologists can pack small platinum coils within the aneurysm to induce thrombosis. Note 10–15% of patients have more than one aneurysm.
- **Aneurysmal clipping:** neurosurgeons perform a craniotomy and perform microsurgical clipping of aneurysm, or management of AVM in order to prevent rebleeding.
- **Delayed cerebral ischaemia/vasospasm:** reduced flow in branches of the circle of Willis usually occurs from day 2–3 to day 14 post SAH and can lead to ischaemic stroke which may be distant to the aneurysm. It can be detected by neurological signs or by transcranial doppler showing increased velocities in circle of Willis/branches or angiography. Start NIMODIPINE early as above. Evidence for magnesium usage to prevent vasospasm is controversial. May need ITU if comatose and needs airway protection. Orotracheal intubation and mechanical ventilation if falling GCS <9 or progressive neurology. Traditionally managed also with haemodilution (target Hct 30–35%), hypertension (using vasopressors) and hypervolaemia to optimise cerebral perfusion.
- **Hydrocephalus (10%):** if acute hydrocephalus on CT due to ventricular blood then refer for EVD and maintain ICP at <20 mmHg and CPP >60 mmHg.
- **Intracranial hypertension:** hyperventilate to maintain $PaCO_2$ of 30–35 mmHg to reduce elevated ICP. MANNITOL 200 ml of 20% (20g/100ml) IV infusion over 20–30 min reduces ICP 50% peaks in effect after 90 min, and lasts 4 h. Used in ITU setting with ICP monitoring.
- **Seizures:** if occur (anticonvulsants may be given as prophylaxis) then start PHENYTOIN 20 mg/kg infusion but primary prophylaxis not usually warranted.
- **Telemetry:** risk of cardiac arrhythmias/myocardial dysfunction. May elevate troponin.
- **Hypertension:** manage BP with LABETALOL 20–40 mg IV bolus if BP >180/110 mmHg. Target SBP <140 mmHg. However, to treat and avoid ischaemia related to vasospasm

a higher BP may be preferable to improve cerebral blood flow once the aneurysm has been treated.

- **BP control and smoking cessation improve outcomes**.
- Neurological rehabilitation for any resultant brain injury.
- Take advice on screening family members for silent aneurysms.

Reference: Gray & Foëx (2015) BET 2: does a normal CT scan within 6 h rule out subarachnoid haemorrhage? *Emerg Med J*, 2015;32:898.

Cerebral hyperperfusion syndrome

- **About:** rare complication following a major increase in ipsilateral cerebral blood flow (CBF) usually seen 1–7 days following carotid reperfusion by endarterectomy or stenting. May even be seen post thrombolysis in stroke.
- **Aetiology:** damage to blood–brain barrier, severe oedema +/ – haemorrhage.
- **Risks:** Post-op HTN, recent contralateral carotid endarterectomy, high-grade stenosis with poor collateral flow.
- **Clinical:** Deterioration post CEA, drowsy, stroke like signs, seizure.
- **Investigations:** CT and MRI show ipsilateral oedema +/– haemorrhage.
- **Management:** if there is haemorrhagic transformation prognosis is poor with mortality about 50%. ITU/hyper-acute stroke unit bed, lower BP using standard agents, e.g. labetalol. Target unclear but a MAP of 110 mmHg may be considered.

11.25 Subdural haematoma

- **About:** acceleration–deceleration injury. May cause vague or focal neurology due to pressure until adaption fails and there is a large rise in ICP. If any concern then a CT head is needed especially if on any antithrombotic therapy.
- **Aetiology:** rupture/tearing of bridging veins crossing subdural space. Increased shear with larger subdural space in elderly. Mild to severe trauma. Worsened by concomitant coagulopathy or antiplatelets. Risks are falls and trauma, anticoagulants, elderly patients, dementia, alcohol abuse. Chronic persisting SDH seen more in males, older, cerebral atrophy. Risks: women > men.
- **Clinical:** confusion, headache, minimal signs, reduced GCS, IIIrd nerve palsy, coning, delirium, seizure, unsteadiness. C/L hemiparesis or hemisensory loss, dysphasia, Cheyne–Stokes respiration. Can even cause transient TIA-like symptoms, e.g. tingling, dysphasia, focal seizure.
- **Investigation:** FBC, U&E: ensure normal – low Na. Coagulation: check INR, platelets or coagulation screen if on warfarin or liver disease. **Non-contrast CT:** day 0–5: rim of hyperdense 'bright' crescent-shaped extraxial blood. Day 6–20: isodense to brain can be missed so look for midline shift or get MRI. A quarter are bilateral. Day 21+: darkens to that of CSF. Look for midline shift, obliterated IIIrd ventricle, dilation of contralateral ventricle, obstructive hydrocephalus and signs of ↑ICP. LP: avoid LP as risks of coning. SDH acts as a space occupying lesion.
- **Management:** supportive: ABC. O_2 as per BTS guidelines, IV fluids if swallow unsafe. Manage any coagulopathy. Stop all anticoagulants or antiplatelets (take advice if high risk). Consider ITU if GCS <9. **Neurosurgery:** small subdurals managed conservatively. Larger acute haematomas need craniectomy. Evacuate all with a rim >10 mm or midline shift >5 mm regardless of GCS. If GCS <9 and SDH <10 mm thick and midline shift <5 mm, then surgery indicated if GCS has dropped 2 or more points since time of injury or there are asymmetric or fixed dilated pupils and/or ICP >20 mmHg. **Chronic SDH:** over time, acute SDH can become chronic and bleeding may recur. It may take 3 months or so for things to settle. Chronic SDH managed under local anaesthetic as the usually jelly-like clot has liquefied

into a 'motor oil' consistency which is aspirated by lower risk burr-hole craniotomy without craniectomy. **Post-surgical complications:** seizures, subdural empyema, aspiration, sepsis, haemorrhagic stroke, SIADH, pneumonia.

Reference: Bullock *et al.* (2006) Surgical management of acute subdural hematomas. *Neurosurgery*, 58:S2–16.

11.26 Epidural haematoma/head trauma

- **About:** usually seen by trauma and orthopaedics rather than physicians because head injury related. Rarely non-traumatic with bleeding disorders.
- **Aetiology:** usually a tear of middle meningeal artery with bleeding. May be associated skull fracture. Can also be bleeding from veins and from fractured bone. May have rapid expansion and seen often in young where there is little room for any increase in intracranial volume. ICP rises quickly with devastating results.
- **Clinical:** trauma patients need a full top to toe survey to look for other injuries. Classically a head injury (perhaps with LOC) followed by lucid period and then sudden decline. Signs of ↑ICP. Reduced GCS, IIIrd nerve palsy, coning, delirium, seizure, headache, unsteadiness. C/L hemiparesis or hemisensory loss, Cheyne–Stokes respiration. CSF leaks: rhinorrhoea and otorrhoea can suggest skull fracture. Signs of trauma and injury: Battle's sign, panda eyes, skull lacerations or haematomas
- **Investigation:** FBC, U&E, LFT, coagulation, ABG, group and cross match. Lactate. **Non-contrast CT:** there is a hyperdense lens-shaped convexity of blood on the inner surface of the skull restricted by the suture lines of the skull. Look for midline shift and signs of ↑ICP. May be contrecoup injuries seen and subarachnoid and intraparenchymal haemorrhage. Look at bony windows for fracture. Plain X-ray/CT scan C-spine and full trauma assessment. CSF leak**: elevated glucose on dipstick. If unsure send for β₂ transferrin which is found in CSF but not in tears, saliva or nasal secretions.**
- **Management:** ABC stabilisation and urgent imaging. Caution with nasopharyngeal airway if suspected basal skull fractures. IV fluids. Resuscitation if needed. Close monitoring of GCS and pupils. If GCS <9 then ITU referral. Trauma team review. Discuss with neurosurgeons. Asymmetric pupils and coma needs IV MANNITOL 200 ml of 20% and urgent shipping to neurosurgeons for clot evacuation to lower ICP. Single or bilateral fixed dilated pupils suggests an imminent herniation syndrome and coning. Needs surgical drainage combined with drugs, hypothermia and ventilation to lower ICP and neurocritical care. Recommended to evacuate all epidural haematomas with volume >30 cm² irrespective of GCS (**www.braintrauma.org**). Pupillary abnormalities and GCS <9 should be evacuated as quickly as possible. Smaller bleeds may be managed conservatively following a period of monitoring in a neurosurgical unit with immediate access to intervention. Bleeding and haematoma expansion can occur. Ensure any other injuries are managed, e.g. long bone fractures, C-spine injuries, abdominal injuries, etc. In those rare cases of bleeding disorder being involved this needs urgent correction. CSF leaks: may settle conservatively but risk of bacterial meningitis. Steroids: avoid in traumatic brain injury. Anticonvulsants: No evidence for prophylactic use of AEDs without seizures.

Reference: Bullock *et al.* (2006) Surgical management of acute epidural hematomas. *Neurosurgery*, 58:S7–15.

11.27 Guillain–Barré syndrome

Measure FVC 6 h (caution if FVC <1.5 L and intubate when FVC is <20 ml/kg). Check ABG to look for a rise in $PaCO_2$, which occurs before any hypoxia.

- **About:** acute onset over days of weakness with areflexia and respiratory failure in some cases. Worse prognosis if preceding *Campylobacter jejuni* infection.
- **Aetiology:** possible cross-reacting autoimmune reactive T cells mediate response instigated by infectious antigen. Seen usually 7 days post *C. jejuni* infection, CMV, HIV, EBV, mycoplasma, Lyme disease, Zika fever. AIDP (acute inflammatory demyelinating polyneuropathy) commonest in West. AMAN (acute motor axonal neuropathy) seen in Asian populations (?*C. jejuni*).
- **Pathology:** most show multifocal demyelination and ↑CSF protein. Slowed conduction. Axonal variants have axonal disruption and Wallerian degeneration.

Different forms (most are demyelinating)
- **Acute inflammatory demyelinating polyneuropathy** (AIDP) (90%): various antibodies. Mortality 5%.
- **Acute motor and sensory axonal neuropathy** (AMSAN) (5%): anti-GD1a/GM1 antibodies. Post diarrhoeal *Campylobacter*. Respiratory involvement. Mortality 10–15%.
- **Acute motor axonal neuropathy** (AMAN): anti-GD1a/GM1 antibodies. Seen more commonly in Asia. Post diarrhoeal *Campylobacter*.
- **Miller–Fisher syndrome (5%):** diplopia and then ataxia, areflexia: anti-GQ1b and anti-GT1a. Needs IVIg if cannot walk.
- **Pure sensory/autonomic neuropathy**.

- **Clinical:** proximal 'ascending' weakness comes on over hours/days, usually at worst by 14 days. Sensory level or severe bowel/bladder involvement suggests a cord lesion. Symptoms peak within 4 weeks of onset. Subacute forms worsen 4–8 weeks. Beyond this diagnosis may be CIDP. Weakness moves from legs to trunk to chest and arms and head. Tingling hands/feet. Difficulty rising from a chair. A minority start in hands. Severe back pain, respiratory and swallowing weakness. Distal sensory loss. Loss of distal reflexes. Papilloedema due to ↑CSF protein. Hypertension, arrhythmias, bilateral/asymmetrical facial weakness, ptosis, ophthalmoplegia. Assess power of neck flexion/extension/shoulder abduction – correlates with diaphragmatic weakness. Some presentations may however be atypical. Reflexes may be present in early 1–2 days.
- **May not be GBS if:** Fever, Sensory level, CSF WCC > 50. Bladder involved (can be)
- **Hughes functional grading scale:** Grade 0: healthy, Grade 1: able to run, Grade 2: can walk 5 m independently, Grade 3: can walk 5 m with help, Grade 4: chair/bed bound, Grade 5: ventilated, Grade 6: death. Slow steady recovery over weeks up to 6 months is typical.

Differentials (exclude cord or cauda equina syndrome)
- **Poliomyelitis** (and similar viral illness): will give LMN weakness. Rare where immunisation is used.
- **Botulism:** flaccid paralysis, ophthalmoplegia, bulbar weakness, dry mouth, ↓BP, constipation. ▶Section 9.18.
- **Tick paralysis:** toxin within the tick. Children. Remove tick with improvement within hours. Some can worsen. Consider if recent tick exposure.
- **Acute spinal cord compression:** when signs still remain flaccid before tone increases. Sensory level, early bladder involved, pain.

- **Chronic inflammatory demyelinating polyneuropathy:** slowly progressive. Very slow velocity on NCS.
- **Acute myelopathy:** HIV, paraneoplastic. May be flaccid weakness early. But usually UMN. MRI useful.
- **Cauda equina lesion:** flaccid weakness. Pain, incontinence and saddle anaesthesia and back pain, Consider MRI.
- **Acute neuropathy:** porphyria, arsenic, thallium, organophosphates, lead. Often painful.
- **Lyme disease:** tick bite, rash.

Investigations

- **Bloods:** FBC, U&E to check K. Low Na due to SIADH can be seen.
- **ECG:** autonomic neuropathy so arrhythmias and ST/T wave changes.
- **CSF:** protein >1 g by 2nd week, 'acellular' WCC <10/mm^3. Glucose normal. If WCC >50 consider HIV, Lyme disease, polio.
- **MRI spine:** if any diagnostic doubt exclude a cord/cauda equina lesion. Will depend on pattern of weakness. GBS can cause spinal nerve root enhancement with gadolinium but this is nonspecific.
- **Nerve conduction studies:** most show demyelination (slowed nerve conduction velocities and prolonged F wave). May show axonal degeneration – worse prognosis. If very slow consider CIDP.
- **Antibody measurements** rarely useful except prognostically, e.g. anti-GD1a or anti-GQ1b found in Miller–Fisher variant.

Management

- **ABC and O$_2$** as per BTS guidelines. Respiratory support where required. Tracheal suction can cause ↓BP due to autonomic instability and so ongoing telemetry and BP monitoring, for autonomic difficulties which can lead to dysrhythmia, are required.
- **Monitor FVC to guide need for intubation.** FVC is better than negative inspiratory force or maximal expiratory pressure (*never PEFR*) at least 6 hourly for worsening but none predict intubation need well and bedside clinical review is vital. Normal FVC is 4.5 L or 70 ml/kg. HDU monitoring if FVC <1.5 L. Consider intubation FVC <1.2 L for a 65 kg person. Seen more so in those with bulbar or neck or shoulder weakness. Blood gases can be reassuring normal until late. Other factors supporting intubation are bulbar dysfunction with a need for airway protection and significant hypoxaemia due to ongoing aspiration or atelectasis. Dysautonomia is a concern in the peri-intubation period with profound hypotension.
- **Neurology consult:** before treatment. Close liaison with ITU and outreach teams should be maintained. Rapid deterioration can be seen 24–48 h. Treatment is either IVIg which is easier than plasma exchange (PLEX). Steroids not effective. In cases where response is poor a second course may be considered or PLEX tried.
- **Outcome:** 85% may have a good recovery, others are left with a degree of disability, usually monophasic but can recur and may even become progressive resembling CIDP. **Worse outcome** post-diarrhoea, ventilated, older patient, rapid onset <7 days, muscle wasting, Not given IVIg. Serum albumin < 35 g/L at 2 weeks.
- **IVIg 0.4 g/kg/day for 5 days** given within first 2 weeks. As with any blood-derived product there are issues of allergy and infection such as HIV and viral hepatitis and concerns over prions. Can give headache, malaise. **C/I** with AKI and IgA deficiency. Check IgA level first is advised but some specialists don't. Be ready to treat anaphylaxis. Take local advice. Relapse is possible in 10%. Written consent suggested.

- **Plasma exchange:** as effective as IVIg. Preferred if IgA deficiency or renal failure. Needs central venous access. Give four alternate-day exchanges over 7–10 days for a total of 200–250 ml/kg. Steroids have no benefit in GBS.
- **VTE prophylaxis:** prevent VTE with LMWH and early mobilization or IPC.
- **Ongoing rehabilitation** over weeks and months.
- **Speech and language therapy** to assess swallow safety and speech.
- **NG feeding** in the interim and PEG if delayed return of bulbar function.
- **Neuropathic pain:** carbamazepine and gabapentin and opiates as required. Amitriptyline avoided as can theoretically cause arrhythmias.
- **Laxatives** to avoid constipation from opiates and immobility.

References: Winer (2002) Treatment of Guillain–Barré syndrome. *Q J Med*, 95:717. Zhong & Cai (2007) Current perspectives on Guillain–Barré syndrome. *World J Pediatr*, 3:187.

11.28 Myasthenia gravis

- **About:** in suspected or confirmed myasthenia avoid drugs that can lead to increased weakness by checking all suitable in the BNF or equivalent. Myasthenic crisis can cause severe respiratory compromise. Precipitated by medications and acute illness.
- **Aetiology:** autoantibodies to the nicotinic acetylcholine receptor or muscle specific protein kinase (musk) protein. Complement-mediated damage of receptors and post-synaptic acetylcholine receptor.
- **Associations:** rheumatoid arthritis, pernicious anaemia, SLE. Sarcoidosis. Sjögren's disease, polymyositis, ulcerative colitis, pemphigus.
- **Clinical:** fatiguable weakness of skeletal, ocular and respiratory and bulbar musculature. Fluctuating proximal weakness worsens with exercise – fatiguability. Sustained upward gaze causes diplopia and symmetrical ptosis. Eyelid twitch response (Cogan's lid twitch) is characteristic. Normal pupils. Respiratory muscle weakness and usually matches with neck flexion weakness. Difficulty in chewing, abnormal smile, dysarthria, and dysphagia are also common. Bulbar nasal quality speech, dysphagia and risk of aspiration. Pregnancy: MG worsens in 1st trimester of pregnancy and then improves. Myasthenic crises: profound weakness leads to respiratory failure.
- **Drugs and events exacerbating weakness:** steroids, antibiotics, Phenytoin, Quinidine, Chloroquine, Verapamil, magnesium, Imipenem, Chlorpromazine. Anaesthetic agents/neuromuscular blockers: care must be taken before any anaesthesia (check *BNF*). Cardiac: beta blockers, calcium channel blockers, some antiarrhythmics, statins. Other: anticholinergic, anticonvulsants, antipsychotics, lithium. Events: acute illness, surgery or infections can worsen symptoms.
- **Differential:** Lambert–Eaton syndrome: paraneoplastic, non-fatigable. Botulism: bacterial toxin, tinned foods, mydriasis. Drug-induced myasthenia (penicillamine, aminoglycosides). Chronic progressive external ophthalmoplegia. Cholinergic crisis: excessive acetylcholinesterase inhibitors, salivation, miosis. GBS: protein and WCC LP findings. MND and myopathies.
- **Investigations:** bloods: FBC, U&E, ESR, TFTs: check K, Ca, Mg levels. Autoantibodies: acetylcholine receptor (90%), muscle specific receptor tyrosine kinase. Thymoma patients: antibody to muscle proteins ryanodine and titin. In myasthenia 10% are negative for autoantibodies. **Tensilon test:** edrophonium chloride (Tensilon). Cardiac monitor and resuscitation equipment in case of ↓HR/asystole needing atropine. EDROPHONIUM 1 mg IV test dose given and if no problems then 2 mg IV given with determination of clinical improvement in motor power. Further EDROPHONIUM 2–10 mg IV in total may be given. Particularly useful in MG patients with ocular symptoms. Onset <1 min and lasts for 5 min. Also give placebo. Ice cube test: placed over eyelid with ptosis for 1–2 min and improves ptosis. Cold

reduces activity of cholinesterase. **Repetitive nerve stimulation and single fibre electromyography** is the most sensitive test (>95%) for diagnosing MG. When a motor unit is activated, the action potentials reaching muscle fibres are not all synchronous. It is highly accurate in confirming MG by detecting 'jitter'. **MRI/CT thorax:** detect anterior mediastinum thymoma (found in 12% of patients with MG). All should be considered for thymectomy.

- **Management:** myasthenic crisis: monitor respiration: fall in FVC, a rise in CO_2 or weak neck flexion suggests respiratory muscle weakness. A fall in PO_2 may be late. May be exacerbated by bulbar weakness. Needs immediate access to intubation and ventilation so liaise closely with ITU. Steroids may worsen clinical state acutely. Stop any drug that may have exacerbated the condition and manage any other acute illness. Anticholinesterases may need to be stopped as they can cause excess secretions. PREDNISOLONE 40–80 mg/day as a single slow reducing dose may be used but can cause initial worsening so some start at smaller but less effective dose, e.g. Prednisolone 20 mg OD. Usually started under inpatient supervision. Be ready to deal with increased weakness.

- **IMMUNE MODULATION:** acute crisis use plasmapheresis or IVIg. Plasmapheresis: five sessions spread over 1–2 weeks. A fall in acetylcholinesterase receptor antibody levels correlates to clinical response. IVIg therapy is typically given at a dose of 2 g/kg *divided over 5 days*. Check for IgA deficiency. Close liaison with neurologists. Later other agents include Azathioprine, Mycophenolate and Ciclosporin.

- **PYRIDOSTIGMINE 30–60 mg orally 4 h** initially has an onset of effect in 30 min and a duration of 4 h. Long acting formulations are available for overnight. Side effects include miosis, sweating, and hypersalivation, severe weakness, ↓HR, and ↓BP.

11.29 Acute cord injury

- **About: identify** acute spinal cord or cauda equina pathology early and act quickly to prevent long-term consequences. Surgical causes might be missed despite trauma assessment in the emergency department and the patient may be admitted medically. Bilateral leg weakness can be flaccid with reduced reflexes and loss of sphincters early in both spinal and cauda equina lesion. MRI of the whole spine in those with malignant disease as other subclinical lesions may be present. Clinical pathways vary regionally so be sure to follow local protocols and referral pathways to the appropriate spinal teams where needed.

Functional anatomy: UMN becomes LMN at anterior horn cell

- UMN spinal cord starts at foramen magnum and descends within the spinal canal to lower border of L1 vertebra. There are 30 vertebrae. It carries 31 pairs of spinal nerves on either side (8 cervical nerves (but 7 vertebrae), 12 thoracic, 5 lumbar, 5 sacral, 1 coccygeal). The cord carries efferent motor and autonomic fibres to sweat glands and sphincters and afferent sensory. Cord lesions are UMN with sensory level signs and can be partial. A lesion in the cord gives weakness, increased tone, spasticity, upgoing plantars and hyperreflexia.

- LMN nerve roots exit cord and descend alongside cord in spinal canal to pass out via corresponding vertebral foramina. The cord ends as the conus medullaris with LMN spinal nerves forming the cauda equina. Cauda equina lesions are LMN mainly sensory from perianal region, saddle area and backs of legs as well as weakness, reduced tone, absent or downgoing plantars and reduced reflexes. Lesions may be bilateral or unilateral often with radicular pain. Urinary retention occurs late.

Sensory dermatomes and motor myotomes for lowest intact level localization

- **Cervical:** C2 – occiput, C3 – thyroid cartilage, C4 – suprasternal notch and spontaneous breathing, C5 – infraclavicular with shoulder shrug and biceps, C6 – thumb and elbow flexion with biceps, C7 – index finger, elbow extension triceps, C8 – little finger and finger flexion.
- **Thoracic:** T4 – nipple, T10 – umbilicus.
- **Lumbar:** L1 – inguinal region and hip flexion, L2 – medial thigh and hip flexion, L3 – medial thigh and hip adduction/knee extension, L4 – medial thigh and hip abduction/ankle dorsiflexion, L5 – web space 1st, 2nd toes and big toe extension.
- **Sacral:** S1 – lateral foot and plantar flexion, S2 – perianal and plantar flexion, S3–4 – perianal with rectal tone.

Pathology to spinal cord and cauda

Key facts: pathology at vertebral level above L1 to vertebral canal contents will cause UMN cord damage with a sensory level and LMN damage to the few roots that are waiting to exit canal lying alongside. Lesions below L1 vertebral level will affect cauda equina and roots and cause LMN and saddle distribution sensory loss.

Physical damage to vertebral column and cord

- This can be by any significant trauma, bullet, knife, shrapnel or by a tumour or haematoma or a centrally prolapsed lumbar disc. The management may be surgical decompression. Pain will usually be a key and obvious finding. A more subacute presentation with a tumour or inflammatory mass. Any lesion above L1 will damage cord and UMN, below will damage cauda and be LMN.
- Diagnostically obvious, RTA: 50%, especially if thrown from vehicle. Falls: 25% even from standing in elderly, especially at C2. Violence (especially gunshot wounds): 15%. Sports accidents: 10%, e.g. diving, rugby. Others: 5%. Increased risk: ankylosing spondylitis, cervical spondylosis, narrow spinal canal. Key issues will be to immobilise an unstable spine and ABC. If a physical cause which may need a surgical remedy then urgent imaging is needed.

Investigations

- **Trauma:** simple radiology is vital but in non-traumatic cases or where possible go straight to MRI when cord/cauda equina pathology suspected. The whole of the spine should be visualised and symptoms and signs correlated with findings. Lateral/anteroposterior and odontoid peg views of spine. Lateral view must show C7/T1 junction. CT scan head and cervical spine (especially C1/2 lesions) and may be done instead of plain films. Fractures may exist at multiple levels. MRI is better for showing bone and ligamentous injury.
- **Medical/oncological:** urgent MRI is required to diagnose and assess or exclude a mechanical cause. Infarction of the cord may show up as may inflammatory lesions and different levels of cancer involvement. Also consider FBC, ESR/CRP, ALP, myeloma screen, U&E, LFTs, HIV test, ECG (AF with vascular lesion), INR (warfarin), CXR (lung cancer/metastases/TB), B12/folate, syphilis serology, lumbar puncture.

Management (surgical referral to spinal team)

- **General:** ABCs. Manage BP and O_2, IV fluids. Skin care with 2 hourly turns to prevent pressure or neuropathic ulcers, intermittent or temporary urinary catheterisation to prevent over-distension of bladder and infection. If trauma and spine may be unstable, then spine must be immobilised using a hard collar initially and additional with sandbags. High cord lesions (above C5) with respiratory compromise may necessitate rapid sequence induction protecting C-spine.

- **MRI shows cord non-metastatic compression:** discuss with surgeons who may advise DEXAMETHASONE 10 mg IV and transfer for decompression. An extradural haematoma or abscess needs surgical review and reversal of anticoagulation or antibiotics respectively.
- **Metastatic spinal cord compression (MSCC):** ▶ Section 16.8.
- **If MRI is normal then look for a medical cause:** exclude spinal stroke – MRI DWI and gadolinium contrast, especially if AVM is in the differential. Needs LP to look for cells and protein, oligoclonal bands, HIV and consider neurology referral. Consider MRI brain if MS suspected to look for additional evidence of disseminated lesions.
- **Cauda equina lesion:** is also a surgical decompression emergency often due to a central disc prolapse below L1. Low back pain, weak legs and reduced reflexes. Saddle anaesthesia. Urgent MRI of lumbar spine and referral for surgical review. Oncology also if malignant.
- **Autonomic dysreflexia:** risk of provoking acute, uncontrolled hypertension leading to LVF, AKI, MI and cerebral haemorrhage. Spinal cord injury at or above T6. Precipitated by a strong sensory afferent input to the spinal cord. May be from bladder and bowel. Massive reflex sympathetic surge with widespread vasoconstriction below diaphragm. There is a reflex bradycardia. Pale skin with vasoconstriction and 'goose bumps' below lesion and vasodilation and sweating and nasal congestion and flushing above. Stimuli are varied from UTI to rectal exam to coitus, DVT and PE or local trauma. Treat by sitting up patient, give oral antihypertensives, IV or transdermal nitrates or oral Amlodipine and lower BP gradually. Consider catheter if retention. Manage pressure ulcers. Main issue is recognising and so take expert advice.

11.30 Acute transverse myelitis

- **About:** acute inflammation of spinal cord. Often at thoracic level. 10–20%. Some will develop MS. Urgent MRI to exclude compression.
- **Causes:** multiple sclerosis, neuromyelitis optica, infections, autoimmune or post-infectious/vaccine inflammation, vasculitis.
- **Clinical:** progressive UMN weakness over hours or days in both legs +/– hands. Back pain, sensory level, motor and sphincter deficits – urinary retention. MS often incomplete and asymmetric. Neuromyelitis optica involves 3+ cord segments with associated optic neuritis.
- **Investigations:** MRI spinal cord with gadolinium, CSF analysis. Neuromyelitis optica IgG, CXR, CRP, ESR, serum and CSF oligoclonal bands, ANA, B12, copper, HIV, Lyme disease, mycoplasma. Brain MRI – signs of MS.
- **Management:** ABC, nursing care, bladder and bowels, rehabilitation, skin care. METHYLPREDNISOLONE 1 g/d for 5 days. Plasma exchange may be considered. About one-third recover fully, one-third have some weakness and the rest no recovery.

11.31 Acute dystonic reactions

- **About:** can be quite dramatic/bizarre. Often seen in those on antipsychotics. Stop the causative drug. Commoner in males, family history of dystonia, young and with alcohol.
- **Drugs:** Erythromycin, haloperidol, metoclopramide, prochlorperazine, SSRIs, cocaine, sumatriptan, ranitidine, carbamazepine.
- **Aetiology:** nigrostriatal D2 receptor blockade, excess striatal cholinergic output. Seen within 7 days of drug.
- **Clinical:** oculogyric crises – sustained upward gaze, torticollis, tongue protrusion, trismus. Sustained contractions of facial muscles, neck, trunk, pelvis, extremities,

larynx. Everything else is normal, e.g. cognition, consciousness, vital signs. Can very rarely compromise airway with laryngeal/pharyngeal dystonia.

- **Differential:** tetanus, strychnine poisoning, hyperventilation (carpopedal spasm). Low Ca/Mg and tetany, Wilson's disease.
- **Management:** identify and stop causative drug. Reassure, explain and drug advice. May use anticholinergics. First line is PROCYCLIDINE 5–10 mg IV if severe. Otherwise PROCYCLIDINE 2.5–5 mg TDS PO until resolves. BENZATROPINE 1–2 mg slow IV or IM DIAZEPAM 2–5 mg PO/IV has been used in those who fail to respond. Give drugs up to 30 min to work.

Reference: Campbell (2001) The management of acute dystonic reactions. *Aust Prescr*, 24:19.

11.32 Acute vertigo

- Vertigo is the sensory illusion of the world moving when you are still and is caused by peripheral vestibular, and possibly central neurological, dysfunction. Sit on a chair and spin around several times with care. You will sense an unpleasant feeling of movement when you are stationary. That is vertigo and the exact historical experience you need to elicit from the patient. It is very distinct from presyncope or simple unsteadiness/disequilibrium. You need to be able to diagnose accurately to reduce unnecessary tests and referrals.
- Differentials are shown below and most cause recurrent vertigo. As with all recurrent episodic disorders, the first ever episode is the most challenging diagnostically. Stroke is a rare cause usually of a monophasic episode often with other focal lateralising neurology. Recurrent identical episodes of acute vertigo are very rarely vascular and other diagnoses should be considered first.
- Red flags suggesting central cause are a normal head impulse test, new onset (occipital) headache, any central neurological symptoms or signs, acute deafness need urgent stroke team referral. Positionally provoked vertigo is usually BPPV. Movement often makes any vertiginous symptoms worse, but in BPPV there is a very clear relationship between movement and abrupt onset.

Examination

- **ENT and neurology:** check tympanic membranes normal, no new onset deafness (rub fingers to each ear), no facial weakness, dysphagia, or dysphonia.
- **Hearing loss:** most cases suggest a peripheral cause. Very rare exception is an acute anterior inferior cerebellar artery infarct with vertigo and hearing loss.
- **Gait:** central disease usually impairs gait such that patient cannot walk unaided. Peripheral can walk unaided but with some unsteadiness and anxiety.
- **Neurology:** face/limb weakness, diplopia, objective ataxia, or sensory loss, cerebellar signs, Horner's syndrome. Check Romberg's sign. These suggest brain stem disease such as lateral medullary or cerebellar stroke or demyelination.
- **Vertigo:** peripheral disease tends to be a unidirectional nystagmus in all positions of gaze. With central the fast phase can be bidirectional or vertical.
- **Head impulse/thrust test:** positive for peripheral disease – the side to which patient turns head and there is a corrective saccade in the affected side. Sit face to face with the patient and hold the patient's head from the front. Ask patient to fixate on examiner's nose and the head is rapidly turned 10 degrees to one side and then to the other side while watching the eyes for presence or absence of any corrective movements. If turned normally the vestibular ocular reflex remains intact and eyes continue to fixate on the visual target. On affected side, the reflex fails and the eyes make a corrective saccade to re-fixate on the visual target. Sometimes the corrective saccade is easily missed so sometimes can be useful for a 3rd person to film the movements, e.g. with a smartphone for instant re-analysis. I would not do this test

if there is neck pain or any suggestion of a cervical dissection. Can follow a positive test with Unterberger test.

- **Dix–Hallpike test:** positive in BPPV, check the drug chart for ototoxic medications.
- **Unterberger stepping test:** shows which labyrinth may be dysfunctional in a peripheral vertigo. Patient stands and steps in one position for 1 min with their eyes closed. Test positive if patient rotates towards the side of the lesion. Useful only when peripheral cause suspected.

Differential investigation

- **Vestibular neuronitis and vestibular neuritis:** episodic symptoms of severe vertigo and nausea lasting several days. Subacute onset. Hearing spared. May be viral illness. No other neurology. Self-limiting but can take months. May need vestibular sedatives for a few days. Head impulse test positive. No evidence that steroids or antivirals are useful. See below for management.
- **Vestibular migraine:** vertigo may be part of a developing aura in migraine and may be followed classically by headache as well as other features of N&V which can make the diagnosis difficult. Usual precipitants. Headache is the main feature. Treat with NSAIDs. Initial episode may require imaging to exclude intracranial pathology. May require migraine prophylaxis.
- **Benign paroxysmal positional vertigo (BPPV):** transient rotatory vertigo lasts seconds to a minute precipitated by a change in head position relative to gravity (offending ear down, e.g. turning over in bed, and looking up at a high shelf). Patients experience movement sensation with nausea, vomiting and imbalance. Symptoms occur on and off over days or weeks, usually resolves in months, but may recur. Often idiopathic or post-head injury or infection. Diagnosis by Dix–Hallpike test detects posterior canal pathology. The three step (20 sec each) Epley manoeuvre or Daroff manoeuvre can be used as repositioning technique with 90% success. ENT review.
- **Ménière's disease:** older patients. Sense of fullness in ear, attacks of disabling episodic vertigo last an hour. Progressive tinnitus and low frequency hearing loss. It is progressive over years. Vestibular sedatives for acute attacks. Try a low salt diet and betahistine for prophylaxis. May consider Bendroflumethiazide. ENT referral for diagnosis, audiogram and possible surgery or other measures.
- **Brainstem/cerebellar stroke/MS:** typically cerebellar, pontine, medullary pathology. Needs MRI. Vascular syndromes, MS and such can cause a severe central vertigo. May be haemorrhagic or ischaemic stroke. Lateral medullary syndrome (PICA), labyrinthine stroke (AICA infarct) with hearing loss, brainstem lacunar stroke from pontine perforators. Refer to stroke team. Cerebellar syndrome may be found with ipsilateral signs. Feeling of disequilibrium. Ataxic. Midline lesions cause a more truncal ataxia. 'Vertebrobasilar insufficiency' is a deprecated diagnosis. Most patients with severe vertebrobasilar stenosis have few persisting symptoms.
- **Drug toxicity:** use of gentamicin, furosemide, quinine, aspirin, erythromycin or other ototoxic medications. Structures affected bilaterally so vertigo less pronounced.
- **Space occupying lesion:** acoustic neuroma is a very rare cause of acute vertigo as there is some central compensation.
- **Presyncope/faint:** feeling of disconnection, darkening of vision, feel about to pass out, usually standing, situational, provocation – fear, anxiety. No true vertigo or minimal and never the dominant symptom. Needs a cardiovascular work up – ECG, tilt table, lying standing BP.
- **Tullio phenomenon:** sound-induced vertigo and nystagmus. Hyperacusis. Can hear eye balls move. Caused by semi-circular canal dehiscence. ENT referral.

Management

- General management of acute vertigo includes correct diagnosis and management as above as well as bed rest, fluids (oral or IV if needed) and reassurance. Head movements can be particularly distressing especially with peripheral vestibular dysfunction. Vestibular sedatives, e.g. PROCHLORPERAZINE can help acutely and the sedative side effects can also promote rest. Occasionally DIAZEPAM IV or PO can be used which can suppress vestibular nucleus activity. Things tend to improve after several days with gradual return to normal function, which may take weeks for vestibular neuronitis. Activity should be promoted and helps adaptive recovery of the vestibular system. Vestibular sedatives should be weaned off as they may impair the normal compensatory mechanisms.
- Acute and chronic vertigo can lead to reduced productivity, quality of life, depression and falls/injuries.

Reference: Barraclough & Bronstein (2009) Vertigo. *BMJ*, 339:b3493.

11.33 Bell's palsy/Ramsay Hunt syndrome

- **About:** can mimic stroke but with care the diagnosis should be straightforward. Common age 15–45 years and in those with diabetes, immunocompromised, pregnancy.
- **Aetiology:** inflammation of the facial nerve within the canal. Inflammation, demyelination. Supplies muscles of facial expression, taste to front of tongue and stapedius. Likely viral (HSV-1) but mechanism poorly understood. Bilateral weakness: sarcoid, Lyme disease, botulism, GBS – refer to neurology. Slowly progressing and worsening needs malignancy excluded.
- **Clinical:** classically wake up with facial weakness and 'numbness'. Full progression peaks at 72 h. Pain behind ear, tinnitus, weak upper and lower face with weakened eye closure, difficulty raising eyebrows. Corner of mouth lower. Sensory symptoms – numb/tingling feeling though touch sensation is intact (mechanism unclear). Eye elevates on attempted eye closure (Bell's sign), hyperacusis, loss of taste on ipsilateral tongue. **Ramsay Hunt syndrome:** as Bell's palsy but painful vesicles in ear canal due to varicella. Hyperacusis and taste loss suggest lesion in temporal bone.

House–Brackmann facial nerve grading system

1. Normal: normal facial function in all areas.
2. Mild dysfunction: slight weakness on close inspection.
3. Moderate: obvious, but not disfiguring difference between two sides.
4. Moderately severe dysfunction: obvious weakness/disfigurement.
5. Severe dysfunction: only barely perceptible motion.
6. Total paralysis: loss of tone, asymmetry, no motion.

- **Investigations:** none usually. May consider FBC, U&E, glucose, ACE/Ca if sarcoid. MRI brain if pontine lesion or other CNS pathology suspected. Neurophysiological studies in selected patients.
- **Against the diagnosis:** any long tract motor/sensory signs in arm/leg, diplopia, ataxia or VI palsy or internuclear ophthalmoplegia. CNS lesions (e.g. MS, stroke, tumour) cause facial nerve palsy affecting lower face.
- **Management:** treat with steroids (balance risks of hyperglycaemia and psychosis in mild cases, lower doses/shorter courses may be given pragmatically) if within 72 h of onset – 25 mg BD for 10 days or 30 mg BD for 5 days, followed by a taper down 50/40/30/20/10 mg/d for a total of 10 days. No evidence for antivirals unless suspect Ramsay Hunt. Exceptions to steroids may be: diabetes, morbid obesity, previous steroid intolerance, and psychiatric disorders. Pregnant women should be treated

on an individualised basis. **Eye care is key:** wear glasses, artificial tears, tape lid and eye patch at night, ask patient to physically close eyelids with fingers during day at times. Give eye lubricating drops. If severe then refer ophthalmology for tarsorraphy and botox to upper lid to aid closure. 70% full recovery, 15% partial, 15% residual signs. If at 6 weeks there is poor resolution ENT referral. **Ramsay Hunt syndrome:** give ACICLOVIR +/− STEROIDS. Prognosis is worse.

Reference: Clinical Practice Guideline Summary: Bell's Palsy. AAO-HNS Bulletin, 2013.

 Acute demyelination

- **About:** usually seen as part of multiple sclerosis. Rarer types include acute disseminated encephalomyelitis (ADEM), neuromyelitis optica (NMO).
- **Aetiology:** flare up of existing MS or *de novo* presentation. Effects depend upon how much myelin involved and if partial or total. Stress, fatigue, infection and heat can exacerbate neurology.
- **Clinical: 'clinically isolated syndrome'** (CIS) is one of the MS disease courses with a first episode of neurologic symptoms that lasts at least 24 h and is caused by inflammation or demyelination. In itself it cannot substantiate a diagnosis of MS. **Optic neuritis** – altered colour vision, blind spots, blurred/complete visual loss. **Cerebellum** and its connects – vertigo, nystagmus, ipsilateral cerebellar signs. **Brainstem** – ataxia, rubral tremor, VI nerve palsy or INO with diplopia, vertigo, nausea, vomiting, hiccough, swallowing. **Subcortical white matter** – C/L weakness and sensory signs, dysarthria. Rarely dysphasia. **Cord** – transverse myelitis. Shock-like sensation on flexing neck (L'hermitte's symptom), tingling, weakness, sphincter disturbance.
- **Differential: ADEM** – single episode, multiple lesions, seizures, reduced GCS. Post vaccination/viral. MRI – multiple enhancing CNS lesions. **MS** – single CIS and later relapsing recurring lesions. May be primary or secondarily progressive. **Progressive multifocal leucoencephalopathy** JC virus in immunosuppressed, AIDS (CD4 50–100), Natalizumab, Rituximab. **Stroke disease** – multiple subcortical lesions, diabetic, HTN – consider CADASIL. **Rare:** other rarer leucodystrophies. **NMO** – transverse myelitis affecting 3+ levels with optic neuritis. High cervical lesions can affect respiration. Needs steroids. NMO (aquaporin 4) antibody.
- **Investigations:** FBC, U&E, CRP, sepsis screen. Urinalysis. CXR. HIV test. NMO antibody if needed. CT scan is useful but generally shows subcortical hypodensity.
- **MRI head and spine:** preferred in defining size, location, number and acuteness and aetiology of lesions (e.g. MS patients do have strokes). MRI may not always be needed if typical clinical relapse in known relapsing remitting disease and so fairly good diagnostic certainty. MS shows round or ovoid lesions in the periventricular and corpus callosum, which may have been clinically silent. Best seen on T2 and FLAIR sequences. Acute plaques enhance with gadolinium as rings. Linear Dawson's fingers perpendicular to ventricles. Older lesions may be seen in brainstem and cerebellum or cervical cord. **CSF:** increased IgG and oligoclonal bands in CSF not found in serum. CSF analysis to exclude any infective cause particularly before considering steroids if diagnostic uncertainty.
- **Management:** any individual who experiences an acute episode (including optic neuritis) sufficient to cause distressing symptoms or an increased limitation on activities should be offered steroids. Consider METHYLPREDNISOLONE 500 mg OD PO for 5 days. NICE recommends no more than 3 courses/year and steroids should last no longer than 3 weeks. Those not treated should improve and admission needed only if unable to manage at home. Steroids do not reduce disability and can have adverse effects on weight, BP, bones and diabetes. Neurology review needed for disease modifying therapies (DMTs). ADEM and NMO also treated with steroids

and potentially plasmapheresis. Rehabilitation and specialist MS neurologist review (now 13+ agents available) and neuro-rehabilitation to help manage and offer advice on catheters and other issues. MS prognosis worse if motor rather than sensory symptoms and high number and volume of lesions on brain MRI and younger age of onset.

Reference: NICE (2014), CG186: Multiple sclerosis in adults: management.

11.35 Acute peripheral mononeuropathy

- **About:** usually either vascular or pressure. Occasionally toxic. Weakness is LMN with fasciculations, wasting, areflexia.
- **Patterns: mononeuropathy:** flaccid weakness or sensory loss in distribution of a single peripheral nerve. **Mononeuritis multiplex:** multiple mononeuropathies. **Polyneuropathy:** often length related and so start distally. GBS, AIDP, CIDP.
- **Aetiology:** nerves require nutrients, e.g. B12 and folate. Vulnerable to toxins, e.g. chemotherapeutic agents, amiodarone, lead, alcohol. Metabolic: diabetes.
- **Causes: trauma:** pressure impairs vascular supply and damages nerve. **Vascular:** HTN, DM, acute onset. **Motor:** porphyria, lead, diphtheria, GBS/CIDP, drugs. **Sensory:** alcohol, DM, hypothyroid, uraemia, sarcoid, paraneoplastic, B12 deficiency, amyloid.

Acute peripheral neuropathies

- **Radial nerve:** wrist drop. Pressure on nerve as wraps around humerus and often lies between skin and bone and can be damaged and awareness reduced, e.g. anaesthetised by alcohol excess or perioperative with arm resting on edge. Median and ulnar nerve intact.
- **Median nerve:** carpal tunnel syndrome pain in hand and arm worst at night.
- **Ulnar nerve:** weakness of small muscles of the hand.
- **Common peroneal nerve:** high stepping gait. Look for a history of extrinsic compression at neck of fibula. Sensory to lateral calf. Sensation to space between 1st and 2nd toe. Spares the 5th toe. Reflexes, plantars and ankle jerk normal. Differentiate from L5 lesion (backpain with sensory loss outer thigh to buttocks with prolapse at L4/5). If unsure get spine imaging. Worldwide commonest cause is leprosy. Also diabetes.
- **Facial nerve (VII):** see Bell's palsy and Ramsay Hunt syndrome ▶ Section 11.33.
- **III/IV/VI:** causes diplopia. Painful IIIrd nerve suggests SOL/aneurysm and needs urgent attention.

- **Investigations:** none needed if clear cause, e.g. trauma. FBC, U&E, ESR, B12, folate, TFT, glucose, ferritin iron, PPE, HIV.
- **Management:** often conservative. Treat any pressure palsy. Manage any diabetes. Often resolves after several weeks. Consider splinting in neutral position, ensuring mobility passively continued to prevent stiffness.

11.36 Motor neurone disease (amyotrophic lateral sclerosis)

- **About:** slow insidious onset with UMN/LMN signs. May present acutely with weakness or aspiration. Look in mouth.
- **Clinical:** aged 40+ (sometimes younger). Progressive weakness over weeks or longer. Mixed UMN/LMN in arms and legs in the same areas with florid fasciculations, wasting, hyperreflexia, **no diplopia or sensory loss or sphincter involvement**. Bulbar palsy. Sphincters preserved. Wasting fasciculation especially in hands, legs and tongue. Muscle wasting causes weight loss. Look in the mouth! Wasted fasciculating tongue. Exaggerated jaw jerk.
- **Investigations:** EMG. May need MRI head and spine.
- **Differential:** multifocal motor neuropathy with conduction block affecting males in 40s, Cervical spondylosis.

- **Management:** supportive. Ventilatory assistance in some. PEG tube can help. Palliation. RILUZOLE adds 2–3 months to life expectancy of 2 years from diagnosis. Course can be unpredictable. Death average 2 years from diagnosis.

11.37 Dementias

- **About:** a global loss of brain function, of memory, personality, decision making, speech, walking, eating. Eventual weight loss and frailty. Some can coexist – AD and vascular.
- **Definition:** acquired and persistent compromise in multiple cognitive domains that is severe enough to interfere with everyday functioning. There is usual an insidious and progressive decline.
- **Assessments:** MMSE, the MoCA, AMTS. **Investigations:** FBC, U&E, LFTs, glucose, B12, TFT, ECG. EEG and CSF not usually needed. CT/MRI to exclude mimics and can localise atrophy. Syphilis serology and HIV test as needed.

Causes

- **Alzheimer dementia (AD):** commonest. 5–10% of age >70. Extracellular amyloid (tau) plaques and intracellular neurofibrillary tangles. Progressive short term memories. Remembers distant events not recent ones. Then visuospatial and language affected. Increasing immobility. Ends up bed bound, akinetic and mute. Death from infection and frailty. Most sporadic, rarely genetic. Risk: trisomy 21, low educational attainment, head injury. MRI: atrophy of hippocampus and medial temporal lobes. Treat cholinesterase inhibitors, memantine. Carers support with ADLs.
- **Vascular dementia:** step-wise progressive decline of cognition in a patient with stroke disease. Dyspraxic gait, incontinence. May be associated with AD. Risks – HTN, smoker, lipids. CT/MRI severe white matter disease. Cholinesterase inhibitors may help.
- **Lewy body dementia:** age >70. Dementia with hallucinations, Parkinsonism, REM sleep disorder. MRI may show hippocampal atrophy. Trial of Madopar from Parkinsonism and cholinesterase inhibitors for cognition.
- **Frontotemporal dementia:** manifest as altered behaviour with disinhibition and rigid thinking. Others with primary progressive aphasia. Alien limb phenomena. Seen in those aged 40–60. Gross atrophy of frontal and temporal lobes seen on MRI. Treat with SSRI, neuroleptics.
- **Normal pressure hydrocephalus:** reduced cognition, dementia, dyspraxic gait, urinary incontinence. Falls, confusion. CT/MRI degree of hydrocephalus is out of proportion to any expected ventriculomegaly due to simple atrophy. T2 FLAIR shows periventricular hyperintensity. LP and CSF removal of 30–50 ml of CSF can result in improved gait and mentation but very subjective and false positives and negatives. Needs expert review to decide need for shunting. Improvement with CSF removal does not guarantee improvement with shunting.
- **HIV dementia:** gradual onset of dementia. Need low threshold for detection and testing. Atrophy on MRI. Check HIV and CD4. Consider HAART.
- **Creutzfeldt–Jakob disease: sporadic form:** middle aged, rapid decline, myoclonic jerks, typical EEG and MRI findings as progresses. Elevated CSF protein 14-3-3.

11.38 Acute hydrocephalus and shunts

- **About:** hydrocephalus is an excessive accumulation of cerebrospinal fluid (CSF) within the head caused by a disturbance of formation, flow or absorption. CSF volume 120–150 ml. Body produces 500 ml/day from choroid plexus. Travels from lateral ventricles via 3rd ventricle via aqueduct into 4th ventricle and out via foramen of Magendie and Luschka. Into subarachnoid space. CSF production falls as ICP rises and compensation (stabilisation of hydrocephalus at a new steady state) may occur through transventricular absorption of CSF.

- **Types: communicating:** CSF flow is unimpeded due to obstruction to CSF reabsorption. **Obstructive:** there is a partial or total occlusion to CSF flow somewhere in the normal pathway. The proximal cavities are distended. There is a pressure differential. LP can result in herniation and should be avoided. **Normal pressure hydrocephalus:** signs of enlarged ventricles on imaging, ICP seems normal.
- **Acute causes in adults: communicating:** haemorrhage, meningitis, SAH, head injury, idiopathic, cerebral venous sinus thrombosis. **Non-communicating:** tumour, colloid cyst, mass, haemorrhage, posterior fossa infarct/bleed/tumour.
- **Clinical:** symptoms of raised ICP (▶Section 11.39), slowing of mental capacity, unsteadiness, incontinence, drowsiness, headaches. Gait dyspraxia, dementia, rarely papilloedema. May also be symptoms of causes, e.g. sarcoid, TB, meningitis, malignancy.
- **Investigations:** CT: shows distended ventricles proximal to obstructed system. Enlargement of the temporal horns (best indicator). The temporal and frontal horns dilate first, often asymmetrically. CT also can show periventricular oedema or "lucency". If 3rd ventricle dilated there will be outward bowing of the lateral walls. Assess the size of the fourth ventricle – if large, this suggests a communicating hydrocephalus, whereas a relatively small 4th ventricle implies obstructive hydrocephalus that might be best treated by endoscopic 3rd ventriculostomy rather than a ventriculo-peritoneal shunt. MRI shows distended system and oedema around the ventricles. MRI may also show the site and cause of blockage if not apparent on CT. Transependymal oedema, or periventricular oozing, may be visible as high T2. **NB:** LPs if needed can be performed only in cases of communicating hydrocephalus.
- **Management: medical:** ACETAZOLAMIDE reduces CSF. MANNITOL *in extremis*. Consider urgent neurosurgical referral for ventriculo-peritoneal (VP) shunt. Alternatives for obstruction are endoscopic 3rd ventriculostomy. Shunts have a valve which drains if CSF pressure >10 mmHg. The shunt is normally inserted through a burrhole in the right parieto-occipital region and the valve will usually sit behind the right ear.
- **Shunt blockage:** drowsiness is by far the best clinical predictor of VP shunt block. Headache and vomiting are less predictive of acute shunt block. Other symptoms reported are seizures, abdominal pseudocyst, syringomyelia, cranial nerve palsies, and hemiparesis. Causes include choroid plexus, red cells, tumour cells, or a high CSF protein concentration. Infection is always a concern. Wherever possible CT scan findings should be interpreted in the context of previous imaging. NB: not all cases of proven shunt blockage present with an increase in ventricle size. Take neurosurgical advice.

Reference: Hydrocephalus and shunts: what the neurologist should know. *J Neurol Neurosurg Psychiatry*, 2002;73:i17–i22.

11.39 Managing raised intracranial pressure

The brain and CSF and blood are all contained within a rigid bony box. ICP will increase linearly with added volume with some compensation until a point where ICP rise becomes exponential.

- **About:** ↑ICP can lead to coning and death. Needs rapid diagnosis and treatment. CPP = MAP – ICP (or CVP if greater). Remember pressure on the diencephalon and consciousness structures only to rise to that which impairs venous drainage before symptoms of coma are caused.

- **Aetiology: excess soft tissue:** benign/malignant/primary/metastatic tumour, cerebral oedema (vasogenic/cytotoxic), brain (DKA, the non-ketotic hyperosmolar state, and low Na), abscess. **Excess CSF:** hydrocephalus (obstructive or communicating), e.g. idiopathic intracranial hypertension, cerebral venous thrombosis, SAH with impaired ventricular drainage. **Excess blood:** haematoma (ICH/SDH/EDH/SAH), vasodilation (↑PCO_2).
- **Clinical:** triad: headache, papilloedema and vomiting often after waking is considered indicative of ↑ICP. The headache is worse with coughing, sneezing, recumbency or exertion. papilloedema: if fundi can be seen. Mydriatics can confuse eye signs and best avoided. Papilloedema usually indicates ↑pressure. However, ↑ICP may fail to cause papilloedema if the subarachnoid sleeve around the optic nerve does not communicate with the subarachnoid space. Progressive coma: fall in GCS, pupillary dilation, Cheyne–Stokes respiration, ↓HR, hypertension and additional signs with herniation syndromes. If you see a SOL don't stop there because metastases can be multiple so look at all the slices pre- and post-contrast, always look for an SDH, subarachnoid blood and check no early signs of hydrocephalus.
- **Investigations:** FBC, U&E: may show anaemia and suggest pathology. LFTs – liver failure, alcoholism. CXR: may show a lung tumour or sarcoidosis or TB. Lactate, ABG – sepsis, acidosis. CT brain +/– contrast: IV contrast is usually given (ensure IV access) if radiology identify a SOL during initial CT. CT may show haemorrhage or tumour and vasogenic or cytotoxic oedema. May be signs of herniation. Cerebral oedema alone may be due to DKA, traumatic injury, Reye's syndrome, low Na, fulminant hepatic encephalopathy, encephalitis and other toxic/metabolic insults.
- **Non-contrast CT** may show obstructive hydrocephalus with enlarged temporal horns and trans-ependymal oedema as low density margins of the ventricles which can resemble small vessel disease. Measurement of ICP can be by direct invasive measures in a neurological ICU by inserting a probe into ventricles. ▶ Section 11.39.

Herniation syndromes
- **Anterior/sub-falcine herniation:** unilateral pressure from above and laterally pushing down and medially pushes the cingulate gyrus under the falx and can nip the contralateral anterior cerebral artery and cause infarction. Usually a superior frontoparietal cortical space occupying lesion or SDH/EDH. Coma usually, leg weakness, abulia.
- **Trans-tentorial herniation:** compresses IIIrd nerve (ipsilateral), stretching VIth nerve. Posterior cerebral artery (C/L hemianopia), cerebral peduncle (C/L hemiparesis); posterior midbrain: bilateral ptosis, upward gaze; reticular activating system: coma, medulla: HTN and ↓HR.
- **Uncal herniation:** uncus is displaced medially and inferiorly over the free edge of the tentorium cerebelli. Usually due to a mass inferiorly in the cerebral hemisphere in the temporal lobe. Indentation of the contralateral cerebral peduncle, known as Kernohan's notch, causes ipsilateral hemiparesis, which falsely localizes the symptoms to the other side. **Clinical:** coma, ipsilateral IIIrd nerve palsy, ipsilateral hemiparesis.
- **Kernohan's notch weakness:** Fascinatingly rare but does occur. A high cerebral SOL forces the brain down and laterally and compresses the opposite motor fibres in the cerebral peduncle against the tentorium causing a notch and this pressure therefore causes an ipsilateral rather than contralateral weakness to the SOL. E.g. R SDH with R hemiparesis.
- **Tonsillar herniation:** compression of the medulla (apnoea and death), compressed PICA (lateral medullary syndrome). Cushing reflex – raised BP + bradycardia.

Emergency management of raised ICP

- **Decide whether treatment is appropriate:** with a massive cerebral injury (infarct or haemorrhage or tumour) and clear evidence of ↑ICP then outcome is likely to be poor and palliation may be more appropriate. Take expert advice. Ensure oxygenation, treat fever, manage BP and elevate the head of the bed. Hypothermia is sometimes used. Monitor blood sugar and attempt glucose control between 5 and 15 mmol/L but with close monitoring and avoidance of hypoglycaemia.
- **Look for definitive plans:** external ventricular drainage for hydrocephalus, burr holes or craniectomy for large SDH/EDH, hemicraniectomy for malignant MCA, and sub-occipital craniectomy for cerebellar bleed, tumour debulking by surgery or radiotherapy. Use medical measures to buy time to allow transfer to a neurosurgical centre.
- **Ensure SaO₂ 94–98%:** intubation and hyperventilation to lower $PaCO_2$ <4.0 kPa reduces ICP. Use PROPOFOL, MIDAZOLAM and MORPHINE.
- **MANNITOL** 0.25–2 g/kg IV infusion over 30–60 minutes which can be repeated.
- **DEXAMETHASONE 8 mg stat IV and 6 mg 4 h PO/IV** if tumour with vasogenic oedema. Steroids also for suspected bacterial or TB meningitis with antimicrobials. Steroids should be avoided with ischaemic or haemorrhagic stroke or head trauma.
- **Avoid ↓BP:** if SBP <100 mmHg consider inotropes/vasopressors to maintain brain perfusion. Cerebral autoregulation is impaired and so BP needs to be supported.
- **Infections:** treat if any suspicion of meningitis, encephalitis. Get an LP if safe.
- **Lumbar puncture:** removal of CSF may be dangerous if, for example, there is a large supratentorial mass lesion or hydrocephalus but it can be diagnostic and therapeutic (e.g. idiopathic intracranial hypertension) if there is communicating hydrocephalus but must only be done after imaging excludes a lesion that could precipitate a herniation syndrome. Take expert advice if unsure.

11.40 Cerebral oedema

- **Vasogenic:** vascular permeability of blood–brain barrier, e.g. tumour (steroids potentially useful). Increased permeability of capillary endothelial cells, tumour, abscess, around a haemorrhage, contusion, meningitis. The neurons and glia are relatively normal in appearance. May respond to steroids. On CT the grey–white matter differentiation is maintained and the oedema involves white matter, extending in finger-like fashion.
- **Cytotoxic:** 'cell death', e.g. ischaemic stroke. Failure of the normal homeostatic mechanisms that maintain cell size: neurons, glia, and endothelial cells swell. Due to cellular energy (ATP) failure. Hypoxic ischaemic/infarction, osmolar injury, some toxins; part of the secondary injury sequence following head trauma. Does not respond to steroids. BBB remains intact.
- **Interstitial or transependymal:** characterised by an increase in the water content of the periventricular white matter. Seen with obstruction of CSF flow, e.g. hydrocephalus.

11.41 Neurosurgical options

Procedures

- **Burr-holes:** hole through skull which may be done under local anaesthetic to drain extradural haematoma or chronic SDH. Can allow placement of drains or monitoring equipment.
- **Craniectomy:** removal of part of the skull, e.g. hemicraniectomy for malignant MCA syndrome or sub-occipital craniectomy for cerebellar strokes or SOLs. Needs General anaesthesia.

- **Clipping aneurysms:** neurosurgeon places a clip across the base of aneurysm. Requires craniotomy. Hospital stay at least 2–3 days. Higher risk of complications than coiling.
- **Coiling aneurysms:** neuro-interventionalist (neuroradiologist or neurosurgeon or neurologist) packs detachable platinum coils into the aneurysms to induce thrombosis. Usually done via catheters inserted via femoral artery. Studies have shown that patients with a ruptured aneurysm tend to do better in the long term after a coiling procedure. Hospital stay shorter.
- **Biopsy:** may be indicated to get tissue samples of areas within the brain that are suspicious for tumours or infections. A simple biopsy may be done for easy to access lesions. Stereotactic biopsy may be needed for deep-seated lesions, multiple lesions, or lesions in a surgically poor candidate who cannot tolerate anaesthesia.
- **Debulking tumours:** those that cannot be resected completely a palliative debulking can take place to slow progression and symptoms.

12 Rheumatological emergencies

12.1 Septic arthritis

- **About:** infected joint can become a permanently painful and destroyed joint. Involve orthopaedic team and microbiology immediately.
- **Aetiology:** destruction of cartilage begins within 48 h due to pressure, proteases and cytokines from macrophages, bacteria and inflammatory cells.
- **Microbiology:** *Staph. aureus*, streptococci, gonococci, Gram negatives, Lyme disease, salmonella (sickle cell). Viral – hepatitis B, parvovirus B19, and lymphocytic choriomeningitis viruses. Propionibacterium acnes can cause post-op shoulder septic arthritis.
- **Risks:** immunosuppressed, RA, age >80, prosthetic joints, recent steroid joint injections, diabetes. Sickle cell, IV drug user, gonococcus, cellulitis, ulcers.
- **Clinical:** new joint pain/swelling or increase in usual pain, erythema. Immobility (held in maximal position of comfort), systemic fever. Knee 50%, hip 22% and shoulder. Also ankles, wrists, elbow, PIPs and DIPs. Also sternoclavicular and sacroiliac joints in generally decreasing frequency. Note that concurrent immunosuppression can dampen clinical findings.
- **Differential:** gout, pseudogout, fracture, reactive arthritis, osteoarthritis. RA itself does not give this presentation but it can have secondary infection. Crystal deposition uncommon in RA affected joints. Gonococcus – rash, sexually active. Lyme disease affects knee. Polyarticular – *Haemophilus*, gonococcus, meningococcus.
- **Investigations:** FBC: ↑WCC, ↑ESR, ↑CRP, U&E, LFT, bone, urate, glucose, blood culture, CXR. Joint aspiration: relieves pressure and pain in a tense effusion. Turbid pus with ↑WBC, predominantly neutrophils. Send aspirate for Gram stain, microscopy for crystals and culture. Consider urethral culture for gonococcus or skin lesion if STD likely. Plain X-rays to look for bony changes. Ultrasonography: can detect effusions and synovial changes. MRI can show bone and joint destruction and osteomyelitis. Radionuclide leucocyte scans can detect inflammation.
- **Management:** urgent consult with orthopaedics as requires joint aspiration especially if prosthesis. This will relieve pressure and pain and provide microbiological information. FLUCLOXACILLIN IV. MRSA positive consider VANCOMYCIN or TEICOPLANIN IV penicillin allergic. Add GENTAMICIN IV if coliforms are likely. If *N. gonorrhoea* then CEFTRIAXONE IV/IM OD. High risk MRSA consider VANCOMYCIN IV (adjusted to renal function).
- **Contact consultant microbiologist** if risk factors for, or evidence of, MRSA colonisation or infection or HIV positive patient. Orthopaedic review as arthroscopy or open surgery may be required. Prosthetic joint infections: needs urgent microbiologist and orthopaedic review. Empirical therapy is usually not indicated unless patient is septic. Later physiotherapy and rehabilitation may be required.

12.2 Osteomyelitis

- **About:** infection of bone which can rapidly lead to pain, deformity and chronic disease if not treated. Differing picture in adults and children. Association with sickle cell disease and salmonella infection. Infection either haematogenous or direct from local wound sepsis.
- **Adult disease:** 60% are due to *Staph. aureus*, enterobacter or streptococcus. In older adults the vertebral bodies are more likely to be infected, due to changes in

blood flow with spinal osteomyelitis. TB still remains prevalent in certain groups. Risks: open fractures, prostheses, diabetes, diabetic foot, alcoholism, AIDS, immunosuppression. Sickle cell, IV drug abuse – blood spread to vertebrae, chronic steroids.
- **Clinical:** toxic, febrile and rigors, localised bone pain – long bone or spine, foot, tenderness, warmth and swelling. Children can have just vague symptoms for weeks.
- **Investigations:** plain X-ray: unreliable (will take 2–4 weeks for demineralization of bone). CT or MRI or USS or three-phase bone scan. MRI modality of choice and will show early oedema. Blood cultures +positive in 50% of cases of acute osteomyelitis. FBC: ↑ESR, ↑WCC, ↑CRP. Obtain pus by open surgery or needle aspiration. Bone biopsy for culture and histology.
- **Differential:** synovitis, trauma and fracture, bone cancer, sickle cell crisis.
- **Management:** rapid diagnosis and orthopaedic and microbiology liaison to choose optimal antimicrobial therapy. Acute osteomyelitis: FLUCLOXACILLIN IV +/– FUSIDIC ACID PO. Penicillin allergy: TEICOPLANIN IV + FUSIDIC ACID PO. Duration of therapy: usually 4–6 weeks (minimum 2 weeks IV). High risk of MRSA add VANCOMYCIN IV. Discuss with microbiology. Surgical: debridement and removal of necrotic tissue and drainage of any abscess or collections. Replacement of dead space with tissue flaps or bone grafts. Internal/external fixation. Amputation may be needed. Sickle cell disease: *Staph. aureus* and salmonella often involved organisms.

12.3 Reactive arthritis

- **About:** inflamed joint but sterile joint aspirate. Infection may be a trigger.
- **Aetiology:** salmonella, chlamydial, shigella, campylobacter. Others may be post viral e.g. hepatitis B, parvovirus B19, hepatitis C, rubella, HIV, EBV. Post streptococcal with glomerulonephritis and vasculitis.
- **Clinical:** co-existing urethritis, conjunctivitis, diarrhoeal illness, males > females. Balanitis, keratoderma blennorrhagica (soles of feet). Large joints, knee, sacroiliitis, fever, malaise.
- **Investigations:** joint aspirate excludes infection and crystals. ↑WCC, ↑ESR, ↑CRP. Urethral swab. Stool for culture. Consider HIV test.
- **Management:** rest joint, NSAIDs, intra-articular steroids. Treat urethritis. Rheumatology review.

12.4 Acute gout and pseudogout

Always aspirate any red hot painful joint to exclude septic arthritis, send Gram stain, culture and microscopy for crystals.

- **About:** 20% population ↑uric acid, 20% develop gout. Uric acid is product of purine metabolism. Humans lack uricase. 90% of the uric acid filtered at the glomerulus is taken up in proximal convoluted tubule. Pseudogout due to calcium pyrophosphate deposits (CPPDs).
- **Aetiology:** monosodium urate (MSU) crystallizes in joint. Causes local inflammatory response.
- **Risks:** obese, thiazides, low dose aspirin (<3 g/day), Ciclosporin. Fructose syrup. Renal disease, Myelo/lymphoproliferative, psoriasis, alcohol, red meat. Rare purine enzyme defects (Lesch–Nyhan syndrome), glycogen storage disease. Pseudogout seen with haemochromatosis, hyperparathyroidism, Wilson's disease, alkaptonuria.

- **Clinical:** red hot swollen painful joint, often 1st toe (podagra), ankle or knee onset age 40–60 usually. Pain often overnight. Fever, malaise. Attack usually lasts 1–2 weeks. Over time develops gouty tophi and microtophi in joints. Gout affects men more and in older women affects joints damaged by OA, e.g. knees or DIP joints with Heberden nodes. Clinically similar. Pseudogout common in elderly women and affects the knee or wrist.
- **Differential:** bacterial infection, soft tissue injury or fracture, sarcoidosis, and CPPD arthropathy (pseudogout).
- **Investigations:** U&E, LFTs, FBC, ↑ESR and CRP, TFT, calcium. Glucose, lipid. **Urate:** elevated level. Levels may fall during a flare. Upper limit is 420 µmol/L in males; 360 µmol/L in females. Gout rare if levels <360 µmol/L **Joint aspiration:** MSU crystals – intracellular needle-shaped crystals with strong negative birefringence is diagnostic. Taken from aspiration of joint, bursa or tophus. CPPD crystals show rhomboidal, weakly positively birefringent crystals. Always send for Gram stain and culture of the fluid. May be elevated WCC. **Plain films** may be needed if fracture is a concern or erosive arthritis in chronic gout. **Haemochromatosis:** transferrin saturation is increased (50–100%) and serum ferritin is substantially elevated (>1.1 to 7.4 µmol/L (90–600 mg/dL or 900–6000 mcg/L).
- **Management:** lifestyle: hydration, obesity. Reduce red meat and alcohol, high fructose corn syrup. **Acute gout/pseudogout:** joint aspiration can reduce pain. NSAIDs may be tried first if no contraindication. Early active mobilisation is important. COLCHICINE 1 mg stat PO then 0.5 mg 4 h (max dose of 6 mg taken or diarrhoea). A low dose COLCHICINE 0.5 mg 12 h may be given for weeks with allopurinol. Lastly a short course of PREDNISOLONE 10–20 mg OD may be considered for a week or more.
- **Prevention:** urate lowering therapy for repeated severe gout attacks with target urate <300–360 µmol/L. Do not start until 1 month after acute attack has settled and give along with NSAID/Colchicine for 2–4 weeks. ALLOPURINOL 100 mg/day increasing slowly over weeks to 300–600 mg/day to lower urate. Alternatives: FEBUXOSTAT 40–80 mg OD. Continue urate lowering therapy for 6 months at least. LOSARTAN may help to lower uric acid. **Never use ALLOPURINOL/FEBUXOSTAT if on Azathioprine or Ciclosporin as may result in fatal pancytopenia.**

12.5 Rheumatoid arthritis

- **About:** known patient with RA and acute flare up. In older patients can cause immobility – 'off legs'.
- **Clinical:** painful joint(s). Usually warm and tender to touch or squeeze. Involves wrists, MCP, PIP, ankles, etc. Morning stiffness. Rarely red hot joint. Active synovitis. Specialists may assess disease activity score.
- **Investigations:** ↑WCC/ESR/CRP. U&E. Aspirate joint for infection/crystals. Exclude infection before steroids. Rheumatoid factor, anti-CCP rise may come years before clinical manifestations.
- **Management:** rest but maintain some mobility. NSAIDs and other methods such as applying heat/cold can ease stiffness or pain. Consider low dose PREDNISOLONE 20 mg OD and assessment of other DMARDs, e.g. methotrexate, sulfasalazine. May consider IM depot of steroids. Very severe flares with systemic complications may need IV METHYLPREDNISOLONE. Rheumatological review when possible. Steroids often used to bridge the onset of action of DMARD to suppress disease progression. Consider bisphosphonate and calcium 1 g/day and vitamin D 800 U/day.

Trauma and fractures in elderly

The patient who is confused, demented or comatose may easily have undiagnosed fractures or other trauma as they do not communicate their pain well. Traditional signs such as bony tenderness become redundant. Have a very low threshold for X-ray and examine head to toe front and back. Take heed of therapist or nurses mentioning pain, deformity or swelling.

 Proximal femoral fracture

- **About:** not uncommon in older population who may be confused and delirious. Screen for in any older patient who falls. Mortality 10% in first month.
- **Aetiology:** trauma, osteoporosis, females, some may be pathological – tumour.
- **Clinical:** pain in the hip following fall, shortened and externally rotated. Pain on mobilising, bruising, agitation, delirium. Check skin integrity and detail co-morbidities.
- **Investigations:** FBC, U&E, Ca, LFTs, INR if on warfarin, CXR, ECG – any medical cause of fall. AP pelvis and lateral X-ray hip and orthopaedic review. MRI preferred or CT pelvis if unsure. Fractures may be intracapsular or extracapsular. CT head if any associated head trauma or neurology.
- **Management:** is based on multidisciplinary working – surgeons, geriatricians, nurses, therapists. Identify and manage both the cause of the fall and any co-morbidities such as anaemia, anticoagulation, volume depletion, electrolyte imbalance, uncontrolled diabetes, uncontrolled heart failure, correctable cardiac arrhythmia or ischaemia, acute chest infection, exacerbation of chronic chest conditions so as not to delay surgery. Ensure analgesia (Paracetamol +/– Codeine), hydration, nutrition, skin care. Thromboprophylaxis.
- **Surgical management:** schedule hip fracture surgery on a planned trauma list same day if possible. Perform replacement arthroplasty (hemiarthroplasty or total hip replacement) in patients with a displaced intracapsular fracture. Offer total hip replacements to those with a displaced intracapsular fracture who were able to walk independently out of doors with no more than the use of a stick, who are not cognitively impaired and are medically fit for anaesthesia and the procedure. Use extramedullary implants such as a sliding hip screw in preference to an intramedullary nail in patients with trochanteric fractures above and including the lesser trochanter. Surgery and fixation or total hip replacement improves pain control and mobility and outcome compared with non-operative approach. Mobilise day after surgery. Transfuse any bleeding. Adequate analgesia but avoid opiate/ codeine toxicity. Operate on patients with the aim to allow them to fully weight bear (without restriction) in the immediate post-operative period. In high risk patients, e.g. end stage dementia, a non-operative approach may be justified. Long term convalescence. Outcome poor.
- **Complications:** avascular necrosis, pneumonia, skin lesions, anaemia, hyponatraemia/SIADH, UTI.

References: NICE (2011) CG124: Hip fracture: management.

 Fractured pubic ramus

- **About:** pelvic fractures range in severity from low energy, relatively benign injuries to life threatening, unstable fractures. Those at the more benign end often come to medicine for management of pain and rehabilitation. They must first be reviewed by those specialised in trauma and orthopaedics especially to exclude other injuries. Fractures of pubic rami with insignificant or minimal trauma can be a presentation of osteoporosis. They are common in the older generation and often missed. A fracture of a pubic ramus is the commonest fracture of the pelvis. They are stable fractures and managed conservatively.

- **Risks:** women 5× men. Dementia, delirium, osteoporosis.
- **Investigations:** FBC, U&E, Ca, plain X-ray, ECG, CT may be useful.
- **Management:** patients require adequate analgesia and mobilisation as tolerated. VTE is a risk as is continence and loss of confidence and these patients may need prolonged rehabilitation and many will end up in placement. Be careful with those on anticoagulation as pelvic bleeds can be severe and the Hb can drop. Consider Ca/vitamin D and bisphosphonate. Falls assessment. Such a fracture has been shown to reduce long term survival.

13 Ophthalmological emergencies

Introduction

Ophthalmological problems are best dealt with by ophthalmic urgent care. They have the skills and equipment to perform a comprehensive eye examination. The most important part of any eye exam is detecting reversible reductions in vision. An assessment of acuity must always be made. The red eye and the blind eye are easy enough to diagnose. It is surprising how patients with structural brains lesions do not appreciate their hemianopia even when gross. Occasionally a red eye can be associated with systemic disease. The headache and painful IIIrd nerve signifying an expanding saccular aneurysm about to rupture is an important diagnosis not to miss. Horner's syndrome is a useful sign in stroke medicine and apical lung tumours. Those with suspected amaurosis fugax (transient monocular blindness) need an antiplatelet and referral to TIA services. Giant cell arteritis (GCA) mustn't be missed – steroids must be started to preserve vision in the unaffected eye to prevent complete blindness.

13.1 Acute visual loss

Check ESR and CRP if GCA suspected and consider starting high dose steroids.

Causes

- **Arteritic anterior ischaemic optic neuropathy:** arteritic 'inflammatory' AION usually due to GCA. Occlusion of posterior ciliary artery which supplies optic nerve. Usually painless. ↑ESR/CRP. Aged >50. Temporal artery tenderness. Headache, jaw claudication. Usually unilateral but may proceed to complete visual loss in both eyes. Afferent pupillary defect. Start steroids: PREDNISOLONE 1 mg/kg if suspected. ▶ Section 13.4 on GCA below.
- **Non-arteritic anterior ischaemic optic neuropathy:** atherosclerotic or thromboembolic occlusion of posterior ciliary artery which supplies optic nerve. Usually painless, associated with arteriosclerotic vascular disease, older males. Usually unilateral but may proceed to complete visual loss in both eyes. Atrial fibrillation. Main issue is differential from GCA. Afferent pupillary defect. Treat as for stroke disease. Echo for embolic source. ECG for AF. Carotid doppler may show plaques or stenosis on affected side; assess and manage vascular risk factors.
- **Central retinal artery occlusion:** sudden severe visual loss in seconds. Afferent pupillary defect. May be complete or affect branches. Retina is pale and white with a cherry-coloured spot at macula. Associated with vascular risk factors. If seen within first hour, sudden pressure and release to the globe may dislodge embolism or propel it peripherally. Refer all patients who present with retinal artery occlusion within 24 hours of the symptoms to ophthalmologist to attempt dislodging the embolus causing the occlusion. After 24 hours from onset refer them to an ophthalmologist within one week who may refer on to TIA clinic. Should have carotid dopplers and ESR/CRP to exclude GCA. Give steroids immediately if GCA suspected. IV thrombolysis has been trialled and looks promising but awaits further evidence. A recent review suggests that a clinical trial of early systemic fibrinolytic therapy for CRAO is warranted within a 4.5 h window and that conservative treatments are futile and may be harmful. [*JAMA Neurol* 2015;72:1148.]
- **Central/branch retinal vein occlusion** (CRVO/BRVO): sudden or gradual painless visual loss in seconds. Afferent pupillary defect. May be complete or affect branches. Fundi - Retina is red with haemorrhage with bloody venous infarction and engorged

dilated retinal veins. Associated with HTN, DM, atherosclerosis, and glaucoma are major risk factors for the development of CRVO/BRVO in older patients. Others are vasculitis and thrombophilia. If seen within first hour sudden pressure and release to the globe may dislodge embolism or propel it peripherally. Several trials support the use of vascular endothelial growth factor (VEGF) inhibitors and intravitreal corticosteroids for the treatment of macular oedema in CRVO and BRVO. A fluorescein angiogram shows delayed filling in venous phase. Rare causes: Behçet's syndrome, antiphospholipid syndrome, and protein C deficiency, sarcoidosis

- **Retinal detachment:** painless progressive visual loss depending on retinal area detached. If macula affected then central vision is lost. May see floaters and describe flashes of light. Fundoscopy shows pigmented cells in vitreous. Retinal detachment or break. In retinal detachment, the inner sensory retina detaches from the underlying pigmented epithelium of the retina. Patients also describe a shadow or curtain that comes across their field of vision. The most common cause of retinal detachment is a tear or hole in the retina that may be secondary to a posterior vitreous detachment or an ocular trauma.
- **Corneal ulcer:** severe pain, red eye and visual loss (see Red eye, ▶Section 13.2).
- **Acute angle closure glaucoma:** PAIN + RED EYE + VISUAL LOSS (see Red eye, ▶Section 13.2).
- **Occipital stroke:** may give only clinical finding as visual loss. Haemorrhagic or infarction. May give homonymous hemianopia but bilateral strokes may occur depending on aetiology. ▶Section 11.19. Bilateral occipital lesions. Anton's syndrome: blind patient maintains they can see. A form of visual anosognosia.
- **Occipital/parietal/temporal tumour:** visual loss and hemianopia progressive +/− headache.
- **Optic neuritis:** eye movements may be painful. May be seen as a first presentation of multiple sclerosis or NMO. Often young and more commonly female. Monocular blindness comes on over hours so more subacute than acute. Afferent pupillary defect. Vision worse with heat. Variable defects and scotomas. Altered colour perception initially. Optic disc may be normal or swollen. Some recovery over 2–6 weeks with residual temporal pallor. Discuss high dose IV methylprednisolone with neurology.
- **Vitreous haemorrhage:** may be due to proliferative retinopathy. Blood may obscure retina and loss of red reflex and afferent pupillary defect.
- **Pituitary apoplexy:** sudden headache and visual loss and possible IIIrd nerve palsy. Steroids for acute pituitary insufficiency and urgent neurosurgical decompression if vision affected (▶Section 5.9).

13.2   Red eye

Consider urgent ophthalmic referral for severe ocular pain, photophobia, sudden reduction in vision, coloured halos around point of light, proptosis or smaller pupil in affected eye. Any involvement of cornea or visual loss or glaucoma or orbital cellulitis or severe symptoms needs ophthalmic review.

- Patients with a red eye should go straight to eye casualty but may be misdirected to the general take. Watch for acute angle closure glaucoma in older patients where the presentation can be unclear.
- **Allergic conjunctivitis:** allergic (history and other features of atopy). Conjunctiva is red and injected and there may be a discharge and anything from tingling to pain. Vision is normal. Cornea normal. Consider local steroids.
- **Bacterial conjunctivitis:** vision is normal. Cornea normal. Red conjunctiva, swollen eyelids, more purulent discharge. Vision may be reduced. Gritty eye. Good hand

hygiene. Treat with CHLORAMPHENICOL 0.5% one drop at least 2 h. Continue for 48 h post resolution. Occasionally due to gonorrhoea where it is very severe with discharge and chemosis, preauricular node enlargement. Needs topical penicillin.

- **Viral conjunctivitis:** epidemics common. Painful red eye with watery exudate and conjunctiva can be bilateral. Vision is normal. Cornea normal. Eyelids can be swollen. Preauricular node. Good hand hygiene. May consider treatment with CHLORAMPHENICOL 0.5% if bacterial infection in differential. Can also be due to chlamydia.
- **Acute anterior uveitis** (iritis): red eye + pain + visual loss. Both redness, tearing and ocular pain on palpation over the sclera and involvement of the anterior chamber which can blur vision. Vessels dilated around the cornea. Pupil constricted, keratic precipitates and hypopyon in anterior chamber. Ophthalmic referral. Check CRP/ ESR, ANA, RF, etc. Associated with ankylosing spondylitis (HLA-B27), inflammatory bowel disease, sarcoid, tuberculosis, syphilis, toxoplasmosis, Behçet's syndrome, etc. Management for inflammatory causes is topical steroids with cyclopentolate 1%.
- **Corneal ulcer/abrasion:** red eye + intense pain + visual loss. Corneal defect on fluorescein staining. Needs ophthalmology and ACICLOVIR ointment 5/day for 2 weeks if HSV considered.
- **Acute angle closure glaucoma:** unilateral red eye + pain + visual loss. Halos around lights. Emergency and patients have an acute elevation in intraocular pressure. Mid dilated pupil. IOP >45 mmHg. Aged >50. May have systemic symptoms of N&V even abdominal symptoms. Seen later in day/evening as pupils dilate. Exam shows narrow anterior chamber and needs urgent ophthalmic referral. Give ACETAZOLAMIDE 250–500 mg IV over 10 min (check for contraindications) and pilocarpine 4% drops to constrict pupil.
- **Subconjunctival haemorrhage:** common, painless, may be associated with trauma or simple coughing and exacerbated by anticoagulants (check INR if on warfarin). Conservative management.
- **Orbital cellulitis:** Needs a low threshold for IV antibiotics. Take expert help. Monitor visual acuity. (▶ Section 18.3).
- **Ophthalmic herpes zoster or simplex:** inflammation of the cornea. May be due to HSV. Pain, foreign body sensation and photophobia and lacrimation. HSV ulcer shows up with fluorescein zoster rash over eye. Can affect cornea. Needs ophthalmic review. ACICLOVIR 800 mg 5/d + ACICLOVIR 3% ointment applied 5/d.

13.3 Neuro-ophthalmology

- **Advice:** CT is excellent for detecting bleed. MRI can positively confirm stroke or other lesion, e.g. plaque. MR angiography for aneurysms. Always check visual acuity with some form of quantitative assessment that can be repeated. Snellen chart if available. Take expert advice early if unsure. Much acute neurology is vascular and stroke or neurology team may be helpful. Important diagnoses are ↑ICP, acute hydrocephalus, large SOLs, pituitary apoplexy and expanding aneurysms. Large posterior communicating aneurysms may not be seen on non-contrast CT.

Differential
- **Horner's syndrome:** disruption of sympathetic tract from ipsilateral thalamus through brainstem, cervical cord, thorax and lung apex along carotid artery to the eye. Small miosed pupil with mild ptosis. Three main diagnoses are lateral medullary syndrome, apical lung tumour and carotid dissection. Needs MRI/MR angiography brain +/− CT chest.
- **Surgical IIIrd nerve lesion:** ptosis with dilated pupil down and out. Can be incomplete and milder versions. Concern is a posterior communicating aneurysmal expansion with pressure on IIIrd nerve as a signs of impending rupture and catastrophic SAH. Needs urgent CTA/MRA and/or urgent neurosurgical consult.

- **Stroke IIIrd nerve lesion:** ptosis with dilated pupil down and C/L hemiparesis seen with Weber's syndrome and medial midbrain infarction often affects thalamus too. Needs MRI/MRA.
- **Medical IIIrd nerve:** ptosis with non-dilated pupil down and out and less severe variants. Damage to vasa nervorum supplying core of nerve. Pupillary fibres on nerve surface and unaffected. Needs work up for vascular disease. Diabetes, HTN and rarer causes of ischaemic neuropathy. Can be managed as outpatient with MRI and vascular work up, start antiplatelet. Ophthalmic support.
- **Parinaud's syndrome:** lesion dorsal midbrain affecting IVth nerve with inability to look up. Confirm with MRI.
- **Internuclear ophthalmoplegia:** damage to the medial longitudinal fasciculus and the connections that yoke the eyes together between IIIrd and VIth nerve nuclei for lateral gaze. Failure to adduct with nystagmus in abducting eye. Usually seen in MS and stroke. Needs MRI. 'Can't add'.
- **Diplopia:** monocular diplopia is an eye rather than neurology issue. Binocular diplopia always consider orbital and intracranial issues affecting III/IV and VI and their connections with MLF. Exclude compressive lesion and orbital pathology, e.g. Graves' disease. Look for other localising signs to help, e.g. VI and VII suggests pontine lesion. C/L hemiparesis and IIIrd is midbrain. MRI is test of most use and if normal may simply be a cranial neuropathy which can be worked up with risk factors – DM, HTN and sarcoid, B12, folate etc., but can be often idiopathic and settle conservatively. Consider also Wernicke's–Korsakoff syndrome and need for urgent PABRINEX IV 2 pairs of vials TDS for 3–5 days if suspected.
- **Intermittent diplopia:** suggests myasthenia gravis with fatigability. Associated ptosis. Needs Tensilon test and neurology follow up.
- **Bitemporal visual loss:** may be asymmetrical. Always consider pituitary apoplexy and/or tumour and need for IV HYDROCORTISONE and neurosurgical referral.
- **Homonymous hemianopia:** will be a stroke or SOL. Needs CT/MRI brain.
- **Ophthalmoplegic migraine:** recurrent episodes of headache and associated symptoms and diplopia which resolves. Initial events need full work up.
- **Retinal migraine:** recurrent episodes of headache and associated visual symptoms – fortification spectra, scotomas, bright lights, complete monocular blindness. Initial events need full work up to exclude occipital lobe lesion, e.g. MRI.
- **Papilloedema:** optic nerve oedema. ↑ICP, idiopathic intracranial hypertension, SOL, tumours, SDH, EDH, SAH, AVM, hydrocephalus. Needs CT head.
- **Optic neuritis:** acute visual loss. Idiopathic, MS, viral, TB, sarcoid, visual loss over hours/days. (▶Section 13.1).

13.4 Giant cell (temporal) arteritis

- **About:** inflammation of small and mid-sized arteries with occlusion/infarction. Occluded posterior ciliary arteries causing an anterior ischaemic optic neuropathy (AION). Atypical cases occur and can be a diagnostic challenge. Treat first and get TAB/USS and expert opinion later. Delayed treatment can result in complete blindness.
- **Aetiology:** Commoner in females. Superficial temporal, posterior ciliary and ophthalmic arteries. Immune attack to the internal elastic lamina of the vessel wall. Large vessel disease can show aortic inflammation on PET scanning.
- **Pathology:** Granulomatous infiltration, Disruption of the internal elastic lamina, Proliferation of the intima, Occlusion of the lumen.
- **Clinical:** headache, jaw and tongue claudication (pain when chewing). Temporal artery tender and pulseless. Transient or permanent monocular visual loss. Systemic symptoms, e.g. weight loss, malaise, fever. PMR – pain over shoulders, proximal

weakness. Fundoscopy: white optic disc oedema with splinter haemorrhages at disc margin.

- **Differential:** migraine, TIA, non-arteritic AION. Optic neuritis, causes of sudden monocular blindness.
- **Investigation: FBC:** normocytic normochromic anaemia. **B12 folate ferritin:** normal (or ferritin elevated with CRP). **ESR:** elevated >50 mm/h (classically >100 mm/h). **CRP:** elevated. **ALP:** elevated. **Temporal artery biopsy** (TAB): needed within 7–14 days of starting steroids. **MRI:** T1 + gadolinium may show increased wall thickness and mural inflammation. **Temporal artery Ultrasound:** shows increased diameter of the TA and hypoechoic wall thickening (halo). Resolves with corticosteroid treatment. May be an alternative to TAB.
- **American College of Rheumatology classification criteria:** 3/5 five criteria for diagnosis of GCA: sensitivity of 93.5% specificity of 91.2% (1) Age 50 years or older. (2) New onset localised headache. (3) Temporal artery tenderness or decreased temporal artery pulse. (4) ESR >50 mm/h. (5) TAB showing mononuclear infiltration or granulomatous inflammation.
- **Management:** if suspicion then high dose steroids started immediately to avoid any residual visual loss: PREDNISOLONE 1 mg/kg usually. Higher doses may sometimes be used. **Steroids:** reduce slowly over 18 months titrated to clinical response and ESR/CRP. Steroid-sparing agents may be used. Start bone protection. TAB organised urgently and may help adjust therapy. A negative biopsy does not entirely exclude GCA as 'skip lesions'. Consider ASPIRIN 75 mg OD and PPI as well as good BP and vascular risk factor management. TIA/stroke seen in these patients.

14 Toxicology emergencies

Basic advice

- All patients suspected of taking a deliberate overdose need a psychiatric evaluation before being discharged, if they abscond or attempt to discharge against advice seek urgent help from your senior and/or psychiatric service.
- Toxicology is continuously changing. In the UK, up to date and expert online support is available at **Toxbase** which can be accessed from NHS computers. Advice can be sought at the National Poisons Information Service. Also consult local guidelines and experts for help. Similar local and national systems exist in other countries.
- Most overdoses have stabilised by 12 hours; however, delayed toxicity may be seen with aspirin, paracetamol, iron, paraquat, TCAs, co-phenotrope and overdoses of modified release preparations. All need admission.
- Death following overdose is thankfully rare but can be further reduced with ABC management, early access to ITU if needed and airway protection, ventilatory support, arrhythmias, electrolyte, acid–base, seizure and psychosis management and sedation as needed. Some will need antidotes, bowel irrigation and dialysis. Identify these.

14.1 ▶ Reduce absorption or increase excretion/elimination of toxins

Action	Comments
Gastric lavage *Only if highly toxic overdose taken within last hour and airway protected*	Rarely used now. Airway protection needed to avoid aspiration. Intubated with anaesthetist at hand. Ensure O_2 and suction at hand. Place patient in left lateral head down position. Raise foot of bed. **Not if corrosive agents or petroleum products** which can cause a chemical pneumonitis and ARDS if aspirated. Lubricated size 36–40 FG stomach tube inserted and attached to a funnel. Listen over stomach for injected air or aspirate gastric juices. If intubated then concerns about being in the trachea are unwarranted. Pour in 300 ml aliquots and then allow aspirate to come out. Massage over stomach to help tablets out. Finish with 50 g of activated charcoal.
Activated charcoal *Binds materials by van der Waal's forces or London dispersion force*	High degree of microporosity; 1 g surface area >500 m². Consider when less than 1–2 h since tablets taken. Tablets are toxic and can bind. Activated charcoal is estimated to reduce absorption of some substances by up to 60%. It remains within the GI tract and eliminates the toxin in faeces. May require laxative to aid passage. Best taken by cooperative patient or if not then consider administration via NG tube. For drug overdose or poisoning: 50–100 g of activated charcoal is given at first (usually 1 g/kg). Unless a patient has an intact or protected airway, the administration of charcoal is contraindicated. Does not bind *iron, lithium, methanol or ethylene glycol.*
Multi-dose activated charcoal	Give 50–100 g of activated charcoal, then repeated dose 2–4 h equal to 12.5 g/h. Interrupts enteroenteric, enterogastric, enterohepatic circulation of drugs, e.g. carbamazepine, dapsone, phenobarbital, quinine, or theophylline toxicity.

Action	Comments
Whole bowel irrigation (WBI)	Nonabsorbable polyethylene glycol (PEG) is given via NG tube into bowel. About 0.5–2 L/h. Useful for body packers, sustained release formulations. Does not cause fluid shifts. Administer until clear effluent from bowels.
Haemodialysis	For substances **not heavily protein bound:** alcohol, dabigatran, salicylates, lithium, ethanol, ethylene glycol, valproate, methanol, theophylline, carbamazepine.
Haemoperfusion	Carbamazepine, paraquat, theophylline, barbiturates, lipid soluble drugs.
Intralipid therapy	Intravenous fat emulsion (IFE), in the form of Intralipid 20%, is for life-threatening arrhythmias/cardiac arrest caused by lipid-soluble drugs especially local anaesthetics. ▶ Section 14.3 for more.
Urinary alkalinisation	Used in salicylate toxicity. Aim is to alkalinise blood and urine to 'trap' ionized salicylate, keep it out of the brain, and enhance urinary elimination. Salicylate toxicity, ▶ Section 14.31 for more. Hypokalaemia, ▶ Section 5.4 is the most common complication. Alkalotic tetany occurs occasionally, but hypocalcaemia is rare.

14.2 ▶ Supportive management of specific issues

Problems	Management
Acute anxiety or agitation	Consider **DIAZEPAM IV 5–20 mg, LORAZEPAM 1–4 mg IV/IM, HALOPERIDOL 0.5–5 mg IM** (not if seizure). Use smallest dose in elderly.
Airway	Recovery position (lowermost leg straight and the upper leg flexed) nasopharyngeal airway if comatose. Assess for intubation and ventilation if loss of gag/cough reflex or drop in GCS <9. Pulse oximetry and ABG.
Arrhythmias: *treat any hypoxia, acidosis or hypokalaemia*	**Bradycardia:** ATROPINE 0.5–1 mg IV (max 3 mg), adrenaline, isoprenaline, ventricular pacing, calcium (not with digoxin). High dose insulin–glucose therapy for beta-blockers, CCBs, glucagon. Digibind for digoxin overdose. **Sinus tachycardia:** treat cause. Beta-blockade may be considered. **TdP:** IV magnesium, pacing. Cardiology review. **VT:** Digibind for DIGOXIN overdose. IV NaHCO₃ for TCA/MAOI. Overdrive pacing, DC shock. Hypokalaemia, ▶ Section 5.4.
Coma and respiratory depression	Look for opiate or TCA toxicity and consider NALOXONE or flumazenil (not if risk of seizure). Enlist help of ITU especially if GCS <9 or any airway compromise, e.g. angioedema or loss of gag reflex or cough. Place in recovery position – lower leg straight, upper flexed. Low threshold to CT head/LP if any concerns of other intracranial pathology. Coma worsened by any drug combined with alcohol/other sedatives. Give thiamine and NALOXONE for obtunded.
Delayed toxicity	Paracetamol: day 3: liver/renal failure. Also iron and paraquat.
Hypertension	May respond to DIAZEPAM if agitated. Treat pain, catheter for acute urinary retention. Consider IV Nitrates or Nitroprusside or PO Amlodipine. ▶ Section 3.21.

Problems	Management
Hyperthermia	Fans, IV fluids and NG fluids, iced baths, **IV DANTROLENE 1 mg/kg IV** (max 10 mg/kg). **CHLORPROMAZINE 25 mg IM** to stop shivering. Paralysis + tube and ventilate.
Hypocalcaemia	Ethylene glycol, CCB overdose, CALCIUM GLUCONATE IV less irritant to $CaCl_2$ but either acceptable. Give $1-2 \times 10$ ml ampoules of 10% calcium gluconate/chloride in 100 ml of G5 over 10 minutes.
Hypoglycaemia	Excluded in all patients with confusion, coma, delirium, by rapid bedside glucose testing. Consider GLUCAGON 1 mg IM/SC but if no response within minutes then 20–50 ml 50% GLUCOSE IV or equivalent must be given. With longer-acting insulins and the sulphonylureas treat for 24–48 h with 10% Glucose. Octreotide for sulphonylurea-induced hypoglycaemia.
Hypotension	Raise foot of bed, get patient supine. Should be managed with fluid resuscitation and/or inotropes/vasopressors depending on cause, e.g. CCB/TCA/beta-blocker with negative inotropic effect, ACEI with vasodilation, hypovolaemia needs IV fluids.
Hypothermia	Rewarming blankets. Watch for vasodilation induced ↓BP. Give warmed IV and NG/PO fluids at 37°C. Warmed humidified oxygen by face mask.
Hypoxia	Give O_2 as per BTS guidelines; target 94–98% in most and 88–92% in COPD. (Sats mislead with CO poisoning.)
Metabolic acidosis	Look for cause and manage. Check lactate, glucose, ABG, anion gap and osmolar gap if high anion gap. May need IV $NaHCO_3$.
Nausea/vomiting	Check patient has no signs of bowel obstruction. Exclude constipation, infection. Check U&E, FBC, Ca. Consider **METOCLOPRAMIDE 10 mg IV/PO, CYCLIZINE 50 mg IV/PO 8 h, ONDANSETRON 8 mg PO/IV BD**. IV fluids. PABRINEX IV paired vials TDS for 1–2 days if chronic, e.g. hyperemesis, etc.
Oliguria	Often pre-renal so hydrate to aim for urine output (aiming for 35–50 ml/h). Exclude urinary obstruction. Catheter.
Rhabdomyolysis	Pressure necrosis of muscle on hard surface in sedated patient or due to drugs or heat or muscle spasm. ↑CK, muscle pain. Compartment syndrome needing fasciotomy. AKI seen ↑↑CK >6000 U but sometimes lower. Good hydration, e.g. 0.9% NS IV 500 ml/h Initially to encourage urine output titrated to avoid overload. Alkalinise urine with $NaHCO_3$ infusion. Diuretics, e.g. Furosemide or Mannitol may enhance urine output. Treat any hyperkalaemia. Treat severe symptomatic hypocalcaemia.
Seizures	ABC, LORAZEPAM 1–4 mg IV, DIAZEPAM 5–20 mg IV/PR.
Urinary alkalinisation	Chlorpropamide, methotrexate, chlorophenoxy herbicides. See Salicylate overdose for details, ▶ Section 14.31.

Determine history

Paramedics will often bring information from setting – tablets taken, how many, when, empty bottles or packets and the circumstances. Was there a suicide note, was alcohol or other drugs taken? What are patient's co-morbidities? Does patient have capacity? Patients may abuse their own drugs or often those of others. It is sensible to always screen for paracetamol and salicylate as these are common and for paracetamol early treatment may be life saving. Patients also do not always tell the truth especially if they do want to die.

Specific clinical signs

Clinical signs and possible causes

- **Pink rosy colour:** cyanide, carbon monoxide.
- **Breath:** bitter almonds with cyanide, acetone with DKA, peanut smell with certain rodenticides, pear drops smell with chloral hydrate.
- **Nausea, vomiting:** paracetamol, opiates, NSAIDs, iron, salicylates.
- **Bullae:** TCAs, barbiturates.
- **Small pupils:** opiates, GHB, pontine bleed, cholinergic syndrome (insecticides), organophosphates.
- **Large pupils:** cocaine, TCAs, amphetamines, anticholinergic, adrenergic syndrome, atropine, 'belladonna', phenothiazines, hypoxia, hypothermia.
- **Nystagmus:** anticonvulsants, needle tracks, heroin.
- **Tinnitus:** salicylates.
- **Severe HTN:** cocaine, amphetamines, adrenergic syndrome.
- **Bradycardia:** digoxin, beta-blockers, CCBs, amiodarone, organophosphates, TCA, cyanide.
- **Tachycardia:** anticholinergic, salicylates, theophylline, sympathomimetics, anxiety, adrenergic syndrome.
- **Arrhythmias:** digoxin, TCAs, phenothiazines, anticholinergics.
- **Hypoglycaemia:** insulin, sulphonylurea, meglitinides, alcohol, quinine, salicylates. (Not metformin.)
- **Hyperglycaemia:** organophosphates, theophyllines, MAOIs.
- **Hyperventilation:** salicylates, metabolic acidosis (alcohols), renal failure.
- **Renal failure:** salicylates, paraquat, ethylene glycol.
- **Hyperthermia:** serotonin syndrome, cocaine, ecstasy, salicylates, MAOIs, TCAs, theophylline, strychnine, malignant hyperthermia, neuroleptic malignant syndrome.
- **Hypothermia:** sedation/alcohol, phenothiazines, barbiturates.
- **RUQ pain/jaundice:** paracetamol poisoning, organic solvents, iron toxicity.
- **Abdominal pain:** iron poisoning, lead toxicity, NSAIDs.
- **Seizures:** mefenamic acid, TCAs, opioids, theophylline, cocaine, alcohol, amphetamines.
- **Rhabdomyolysis:** amphetamines, neuroleptics.
- **Acute hearing loss:** aminoglycosides, chloroquine, high-dose loop diuretics, chemotherapeutic agents.
- **Chest pain:** cocaine, carbon monoxide.
- **Oral ulcers:** corrosives, paraquat.
- **Elevated osmolar gap:** acetone, mannitol, methanol, acetone, ethanol, ethylene glycol.
- **Metabolic acidosis:** cyanide, hydrogen sulphide, isoniazid, metformin, NRTIs, iron.
- **Raised anion gap metabolic acidosis:** ethylene glycol, diethylene glycol, methanol, NSAIDs, toluene, salicylates.
- **Lactic acidosis:** ethylene glycol, cyanide, carbon monoxide, toluene, salicylates.
- **Dystonia:** metoclopramide, neuroleptics.
- **Blindness:** methanol, quinine.
- **Polyuria:** lithium toxicity, high glucose, low K, high Ca.

Toxidromes

Anti-cholinergic syndrome 'dry, dilated and delirious'	Central acetylcholine blockade central and peripheral. Dry flushed skin and mouth, mydriasis, delirium, fever, sinus ↑HR, ↓bowel sounds, functional ileus, urinary retention, hypertension, hyperthermia, tremulousness, and myoclonic jerking. **Causes:** antihistamines, antipsychotics, antidepressants, ATROPINE-like drugs, belladonna and other plant-derived agents. **Management:** supportive, IV DIAZEPAM for seizures. IV fluids, ECG monitoring. Beta-blockers for ↑HR. Catheterisation for retention.
Cholinergic syndrome 'wet and weak' Saliva ++, urine +, resp fluid ++, diarrhoea +	**Excess acetylcholine** at central and peripheral acetylcholine receptors. May be due to ↓breakdown of acetylcholine by acetylcholinesterase. Seen with sarin/organophosphate poisoning and carbamate pesticides. Excess medications for myasthenia or dementia. Flaccid paralysis, respiratory failure, increased sweating, hypertension, urination, diarrhoea, salivation, ↓HR, copious bronchial secretions, seizures. **DUMPSS** diarrhoea, urination, miosis, paralysis, seizure, secretion. **Management:** ABCs. O₂ give antimuscarinic drugs like ATROPINE IV and PRALIDOXIME. Intubation and ventilation if not improving. Atropine blocks muscarinic sites. Pralidoxime blocks muscarinic and nicotinic sites. Supportive.
Opioid syndrome	Small pinpoint pupils, comatose, ↓HR and ↓BP, constipation, itch. Respiratory depression. **Management:** supportive. Reverse with NALOXONE. O₂ as per BTS guidelines. Watch ABG. May need intubation and repeated NALOXONE.
Serotonin syndrome	Excess CNS serotonin, ↑HR, shivering, sweating, mydriasis, diarrhoea, myoclonic jerks, ↑reflexes, clonus, ↑temp. Agitation, metabolic acidosis, rhabdomyolysis. DIC, AKI, seizures. **Cause:** antidepressants (SSRIs and SNRIs) and opioids, TCAs, MAOIs, lithium. **Management: DIAZEPAM** IV for seizures and agitation and can affect muscle tone. IV fluids. Supportive. Cyproheptadine. Should settle once causative drug stopped. Give O₂ as per BTS guidelines.
Adrenergic	Agitation, sweating, HTN, ↑temp, dilated pupils, seizures, ↑HR.

Investigations for overdose

Problems	Comments
Basic	FBC, U&E, LFT, Mg, Ca, glucose – all should have these.
Toxins	Salicylate, paracetamol levels on all deliberate overdoses. Can measure digoxin, theophylline, alcohol, ethylene glycol, lithium, TCA, barbiturates, benzodiazepine, paraquat, cocaine, opiates, amphetamine, cannabinoids as needed.
Coagulation screen	Any bleeding, petechiae, DIC. Warfarin – INR, heparin – APTT, prothrombin time.
ECG	All – especially ↑HR, ↓HR, digoxin. Look for long QT.

Problems	Comments
CXR	Any breathlessness or suspected lung disease.
Urine	Ethylene glycol toxicity with calcium oxalate crystalluria.
CT head +/– LP	History unclear or coma, signs of meningitis, encephalitis, SAH.
ABG (VBG)	Metabolic acidosis with ethylene glycol, methanol – salicylates. Renal/liver/RF. ABG for suspected RF.
Anion gap metabolic acidosis	$(Na + K) - (Cl + HCO_3) = 10–14$. If >14 consider toxicity due to ethanol, methanol, ethylene glycol, metformin, cyanide, isoniazid, salicylates.
Osmolar gap	Calculate lab measured osmolality = $2 \times (Na + K) +$ glucose + urea. Gap usually <10. If >10 then consider ethanol, methanol, ethylene glycol.

14.3 Intralipid therapy

- Expanding use for cardiac arrest due to local anaesthetics and any lipid-soluble drugs. Intravenous fat emulsion (IFE), in the form of Intralipid 20% is for life-threatening arrhythmias/cardiac arrest caused by lipid-soluble drugs, especially local anaesthetics. May be used in toxicity from CCBs, haloperidol, TCAs, lipophilic beta-blockers. Use only under senior guidance adhering to local policies.
- **Administration.** Lipid emulsion 20% at 1.5 ml/kg IV in 1 min followed by an infusion of 0.25 ml/kg/min for 30–60 min. **In a 70 kg patient** – take a 500 ml bag of Intralipid 20% and a 50 ml syringe, draw up 100 ml and give stat. Attach the Intralipid bag to an IV administration set (macrodrip) and run it IV over the next 15 min. Repeat 100 ml bolus if spontaneous circulation has not returned. Maximum total dose of 10 ml/kg is recommended in first 30 min, i.e. 700 ml. Continue CPR to aid circulation. Further information at www.lipidrescue.com.

14.4 (High dose) Insulin–glucose euglycaemic therapy

- May be used for beta-blocker and calcium channel blocker toxicity. Monitored closely HIET is safe, and adverse events are predictable, uncommon, and easily managed. Insulin increases glucose and lactate uptake by myocardial cells and improves function without increased oxygen demand.
- Insulin promotes excitation–contraction coupling and contractility. It may be best used adjunctively with other measures such as catecholamines, for two reasons. First, insulin-mediated inotropy is not catecholamine-mediated, and is not affected by beta-blockers. Secondly, although insulin appears to improve myocardial contractility, it has no chronotropic effect and may cause vasodilation. Side-effects: hypoglycaemia, hypokalaemia, hypomagnesaemia, hypophosphataemia.
- **Give** 10% IV GLUCOSE with loading bolus of 0.5–1 U/kg INSULIN then INSULIN at 1–10 U/kg/h (higher doses may be given according to clinical response). Used in an ITU/HDU setting with close monitoring. Very large doses of insulin have been given with few side-effects as long as blood glucose and other electrolytes maintained.

14.5 Amphetamine ('speed') and 3,4 MDMA ('ecstasy') toxicity

- **Various types:** methamphetamine ('crystal meth' or 'ice') and 3,4 methylene-dioxymethamphetamine ('ecstasy') all cause increased presynaptic noradrenaline, dopamine. Increased serotonin release.
- **Clinical:** euphoria, psychosis, violence, dilated pupils, ↑HR, ↑BP. ↑Temp, anorexia, bruxism, sweating.
- **Complications:** seizures, cerebral oedema, DIC, liver failure, AKI and rhabdomyolysis.
- **Investigations:** FBC, U&E ↓Na (MDMA due to SIADH), LFT, Mg, Ca, ↑CK, glucose, lactate. ECG. CT head +/– LP if fever, meningism, coma, confusion, suspected cerebral oedema, infection.
- **Management:** if ingestion recent then activated CHARCOAL may be used. Huge amounts, e.g. body packing for drug trafficking, consider whole bowel irrigation. **Supportive:** ITU review if GCS <9. ABC, O₂ as per BTS guidelines. ECG monitoring. **Hyperthermia:** external cooling. May consider DANTROLENE 1 mg/kg IV (max 10 mg/kg). If **low BP:** give IV crystalloid if normonatraemic and euvolaemic or hypovolaemic. Fluids may be delayed until results back where ecstasy-reduced SIADH may be suspected. MDMA-associated SIADH usually responds to fluid restriction. If comatose these patients should receive hypertonic saline solution to correct a portion of the metabolic imbalance rapidly. **Agitation:** consider DIAZEPAM 10–20 mg IV. **Seizures:** manage as per status epilepticus with IV LORAZEPAM 2–4 mg.

14.6 Beta-blocker toxicity

- **About:** widely used drugs. Competitively blocks β1 and β2 adrenoceptors.
- **Aetiology:** glucagon activates adenyl cyclase increasing cAMP. Bypasses beta adrenoceptor.
- **Clinical:** bradycardia-related low BP. Bronchospasm. Worsening LVF, shock.
- **Investigations:** FBC, U&E, LFT, Mg, Ca, glucose, lactate. ECG: heart blocks and ↓HR, QT changes.
- **Management:** supportive: ABC/O₂, HDU if severe, close monitoring, IV crystalloid, telemetry. Consider gastric lavage if very early presentation. Bronchospasm – SALBUTAMOL neb. Severe bradycardia: ATROPINE 0.5–1 mg up to 3 mg IV and/or temporary pacing may be needed.
- **If hypotension/shock then consider first line** inotropes, e.g. ADRENALINE. If response poor consider GLUCAGON 2–10 mg slow IV in G5 over 10 min followed by infusion 1–5 mg/h. An alternative is **insulin–glucose euglycaemic therapy:** ▶Section 14.4.
- **Intra-aortic balloon pumping** has been used for circulatory support.
- **Intralipid therapy** should be considered if fat soluble beta-blocker. ▶Section 14.3.

References: Engebretsen *et al.* (2011) High-dose insulin therapy in beta-blocker and calcium channel-blocker poisoning. *Clin Toxicol*, 49:277. Shepherd (2006) Treatment of poisoning caused by beta-adrenergic and calcium-channel blockers. *Am J Health Pharmacy*, 63:1828.

14.7 Benzodiazepine toxicity

- **About:** seen with Diazepam, Clonazepam, Temazepam. Used as sedatives and anxiolytics. Accidental overdose with IV procedural sedation. Exacerbated with alcohol or other sedatives.
- **Clinical:** drowsiness and coma. If coma (GCS <10) look for other drugs or pathology. Pupils may be partially dilated, ataxia, dysarthria. Higher risk where combined with other sedation, alcohol, underlying chest disease and elderly.

- **Investigations:** FBC, U&E, LFT, Mg, Ca, glucose, lactate. ECG. ABG if comatose or low saturations or breathless.
- **Management:** supportive: ABCs. Within 1 h activated charcoal may be given. Most overdoses are 'slept off'. Give O_2 as per BTS guidelines. Recovery position (lower leg straight, upper leg flexed) and nasopharyngeal airway if needed. IV fluids. Severe respiratory depression and GCS <9 and concerns about the airway/cough/gag reflex: FLUMAZENIL 200 mcg (0.2 mg) over 15 sec and then 100–300 mcg repeated doses (0.1–0.3 mg) might be given (max dose of 3 mg). There is a risk of lowering seizure threshold, especially in a mixed overdose with other drugs that also lower seizure threshold, e.g. alcohol, TCAs. Lone overdoses will rarely need ITU. Most are stable <24 h depending on severity of overdose.

14.8 Calcium channel blocker toxicity

- **About:** occasionally lethal so do not underestimate seriousness, admit CCU/ITU and give IV calcium. Take advice.
- **Aetiology:** CCB block Ca influx into myocardial/vascular tissues via L-type channels. Amlodipine and Nifedipine overdose cause ↑HR and ↓BP. Verapamil and Diltiazem cause ↓HR and ↓BP, ↑glucose, circulatory collapse, cardiac arrest, cardiogenic shock.
- **Investigations:** FBC, U&E, LFT, Mg, Ca, ECG:↓HR.
- **Management:** give calcium (see below), supportive: ABC, O_2, ECG monitoring. Best on CCU or ITU/HDU. Give 500–1000 ml IV crystalloids. Treat ↓HR with IV ATROPINE 0.5–1 mg (max 3mg). Cardiac pacing if needed. Whole bowel irrigation with PEG and activated charcoal can reduce absorption of sustained-release verapamil.
- **Immediate:** CALCIUM GLUCONATE 10–20 ml 10% IV over 5–10 min for ↓BP. Aim for mild high Ca – monitor for 12h+ with modified release preparations. Persisting ↓BP/shock. Consider ADRENALINE 2–10 mcg/min or ISOPRENALINE 5 mcg/min or GLUCAGON 2–10 mg slow IV in G5 over 10 min followed by infusion 1–5 mg/h. If this fails consider **insulin–glucose euglycaemic therapy** (▶ Section 14.4). **Intra-aortic balloon pumping** has been used for circulatory support. Cardiac pacing may be considered for persisting significant ↓HR-induced ↓BP.
- **Other steps:** intralipid therapy: may have a role for verapamil and diltiazem, unclear for dihydropyridines. If there is acidosis consider IV $NaHCO_3$.

References: Engebretsen *et al.* (2011) High-dose insulin therapy in beta-blocker and calcium channel-blocker poisoning. *Clin Toxicol*, 49:277. Shepherd (2006) Treatment of poisoning caused by beta-adrenergic and calcium-channel blockers. *Am J Health Pharmacy*, 63:1828.

14.9 Sodium valproate toxicity

- **About:** commonly used and generally safe anticonvulsant. Valproate-induced hyperammonaemic encephalopathy (VIHE) may be seen without overdose.
- **Clinical:** progressive delirium and coma, hypotension, respiratory depression, increased seizure frequency (VIHE).
- **Investigations:** as for coma. FBC, U&E, LFTS, glucose, ECG, CT head, serum valproate, EEG (VIHE) shows continuous generalised slowing, theta and delta activity, triphasic waves. Blood ammonia elevated.
- **Management:** ABC, stop valproate, supportive. Multidose activated charcoal +/– WBI may be considered if early. Try NALOXONE. IV L-CARNITINE may be helpful when there is hyperammonaemia, hepatotoxicity, and coma. Treat until improves. Severe cases consider haemodialysis.

14.10 Carbon monoxide toxicity

- **Note: Pulse oximetry will be falsely normal and fail to report severe hypoxia.** If you suspect CO you must check ABG and CO-Hb levels. CO is an odourless, colourless gas, formed by the incomplete combustion of fossil fuels such as in exhaust fumes. Accidental – poorly ventilated faulty home heating. Low dose toxicity may be subtle in its presentation, e.g. flu-like illness. Cold spell where gas/solid fuel home/water heating used, changes to home heating or ventilation.
- **Aetiology:** CO binds avidly to Hb with $\times$ 240 times more affinity than does O_2. Saturation probes treat CO-Hb as O_2-Hb giving a false normal SaO_2. Normal CO-Hb is 3–5% with levels up to 10% in smokers. Result is tissue hypoxia and metabolic acidosis. The result is leftward shift in O_2-Hb dissociation curve. Causes myocardial and cerebral hypoxia and cerebral oedema.
- **Clinical:** drowsiness, flu-like illness, headache, fatigue, breathlessness, coma and death. Pink rosy colouration.
- **Investigations:** FBC, U&E, LFT, lactate. Only an ABG will show hypoxia. Troponin. ECG. CXR. Measure CO-Hb specifically if diagnosis considered. Patients get O_2 en route and so hospital CO-Hb may not represent prior levels or the extent and severity of any hypoxia. Severe when CO-Hb >10%.
- **Differential:** excess opiates, sedatives, alcohol. Stroke/SDH/SOL.
- **Management:** remove source: open windows, switch off heating/car engine. Supportive: O_2 sat probe unreliable. Check ABG. Give 100% O_2 via tight-fitting mask unless COPD and Type 2 RF and if so consider ventilation. 100% O_2 will reduce half-life of CO from 4 h to 40 min. Give O_2 12 L/min via CPAP mask for at least 6 h until CO-Hb is less than 5%; may be needed for 12–24 h.
- **Severe cases:** (when CO-Hb >10% or ECG shows ischaemia or signs of cerebral oedema) cause fitting and cardiorespiratory arrest. Prone to cerebral oedema so do neurological observations. Patients may need IV MANNITOL. Risk of long term neuropsychiatric damage, Parkinsonism and cerebellar symptoms. Indications for hyperbaric O_2 (HBO) at 3.0 atm pressure for 60 min and repeated as per local protocol (reduces CO half-life to 20 min) are: CO-Hb >40%, coma, neurological or psychiatric problems, ECG changes, e.g. ST depression, T wave changes, arrhythmias, pregnancy (fetal CO-Hb is to the left of mother's). Transporting patients to a distant hyperbaric chamber can be hazardous and difficult and the role of hyperbaric O_2 is controversial. Take early expert advice.

14.11 Cocaine toxicity

- **Always:** ask about usage if considered as a factor with HTN, chest pain, stroke. It is a CNS stimulant derived from the leaves of the coca plant.
- **Aetiology:** blocks reuptake of dopamine, serotonin and noradrenaline. Chronic usage may actually accelerate atherosclerosis. Pleasure from raising dopamine levels in the mesolimbic reward centres.
- **Administration:** snorted and absorbed via well-vascularised tissues lining the nose – causes localised vasoconstriction and eventual damage to the nasal mucosa. Smoked or taken IV give a rapid response but a shorter high than snorting. Rubbed on gums or small amounts taken orally, or as a suppository. Cocaine-induced chest pain usually due to spasm and generally not treated with thrombolysis. Users often have coexisting atherosclerotic disease and so are actually more prone to spasm.
- **Clinical:** chest pain, neurology from ischaemic or haemorrhagic stroke, aortic dissection, ↑↑BP, ↑HR, ↑temp, euphoria/psychotic, mydriasis. Chronic – myocarditis, atherosclerosis.

- **Investigations:** FBC, U&E, LFT, troponin at baseline and 12 h. CXR cardiomegaly. ECG: ischaemia or look for STEMI, LVH. CT head if any neurology.
- **Management:** O_2 as per BTS guidance. IV fluids. Suspected ACS with ST elevation necessitates primary PCI. Thrombolysis avoided especially where markedly hypertensive. Consider GTN 2 sprays (800 mcg) or GTN 500 mcg tablet SL. If chest pain persists then IV GTN 1–10 mg/h prior to PCI. Avoid beta-blockade, which will cause HTN due to unopposed alpha effects. Hyperthermia is a side-effect of cocaine and should be treated with fluids, cooling and DANTROLENE. Agitation: DIAZEPAM 1–5 mg PO/IV. Avoid haloperidol and phenothiazines which lower fit threshold.

14.12 Local anaesthetic toxicity

- **Source:** usage of lidocaine, bupivacaine overdose (accidental or deliberate).
- **Aetiology:** local anaesthetics block open Na channels.
- **Clinical:** tingling lips, blurred vision, tinnitus, respiratory depression, seizure, coma, arrhythmias, hypotension, cardiac arrest.
- **Management:** ABC. Severe toxicity consider INTRALIPID therapy (▶Section 14.3).

14.13 Cyanide toxicity

- **Source:** inhaled smoke contains hydrogen cyanide and CO which can kill. Confirmation of cyanide poisoning is a process which currently takes days. Empiric treatment with hydroxocobalamin is central to the treatment algorithms.
- **Aetiology:** accidental exposure, e.g. chemical industry. Suicide or homicide attempt. Inhaled smoke from burning of plastics/foam. Excess nitroprusside infusion. Binds mitochondrial cytochrome a3, blocks oxidative phosphorylation.
- **Clinical:** in lethal overdoses death is usually pre-hospital. Survival to hospital bodes well. Evidence of smoke inhalation, cherry-red skin colour, breath smell of bitter almonds. Chest pain and dyspnoea, seizures, coma.
- **Investigation:** FBC, U&E, LFT, CXR, ECG. Lactate increased. ABG: metabolic acidosis, elevated venous oxygen saturation.
- **Management:** supportive: ABC and respiratory support with high flow O_2. ITU if high EWS. DICOBALT EDETATE 300 mg IV over 1 min followed by 50 ml of 50% GLUCOSE, but only if severe toxicity confirmed because it is itself very toxic. Otherwise, Cyanokit – HYDROXOCOBALAMIN 5 g IV over 15 min repeated to a total of 10 g; it combines to form cyanocobalamin. **Side-effects:** BP rise, anaphylaxis, rash, chest tightness. Also give Sodium thiosulphate (25 ml of 50% solution), which enhances the conversion of cyanide to thiocyanate, which is renally excreted.

14.14 Digoxin toxicity

Do not give IV Calcium for hyperkalaemia in setting of digoxin toxicity.

- **About:** deliberate and accidental overdose. Lethal dose = 10 mg (adult) and 4 mg (child). Well absorbed orally. Half-life 30–40 h, with peak toxicity at 6 h and death at 6–12 h post ingestion. Do not give calcium. Those with ↑K need Fab. ↑K >5.5 mmol/L suggests fatal toxicity. Correct low K and low Mg.
- **Aetiology:** blocks Na/K ATPase pump: ↑intracellular Ca reduces AV conduction. Causes ↓HR, ↑vagal tone, automaticity, and hyperkalaemia.
- **Clinical:** N&V, yellow vision, abdominal pain. ↓HR, AV block, SVT (with AV block), AF, VT and even VF.
- **Investigations:** bloods: FBC, U&E, calcium, digoxin level. U&E: K >5.5 mmol/L suggests 90% untreated fatal toxicity. Serial ECGs: monitor for symptomatic ↓HR, CHB, VT, VF, AF, MAT.

- **Management:** supportive: admit for CCU monitoring: can lead to low BP, arrhythmias, cardiac arrest. ATROPINE 0.5–1 mg IV (max 3 mg) for AV block. Gastric lavage if seen within 1 h. Give activated charcoal if within 1 h of ingestion in cooperative patient. Repeated dosing may be helpful. Manage low K with replacement. Manage high K with $NaHCO_3$ and/or INSULIN/GLUCOSE. Give MAGNESIUM 2 g (8 mmol) over 10 min IV and consider LIDOCAINE 50–100 mg IV for refractory VT/VF. DIGOXIN immune Fab: given where adult dose >10 mg ingested, serious life-threatening arrhythmias, DIGOXIN level >15 nmol/ml (12 ng/ml), K >5 mmol/L. Note: each Digibind vial will bind approximately 0.5 mg of DIGOXIN (or digitoxin), so multiple vials will need to be given in a significant overdose, e.g. 10 mg DIGOXIN taken. You will have to summon as much as possible, e.g. 20 vials. It is expensive and not always stocked. Contact Pharmacy and Poisons Advisory Service for nearest stores. If renal failure, then plasmapheresis may be needed to clear digoxin–Fab complexes. In a cardiac arrest continue to give multiple vials of this for up to 30 min as resuscitation continues.

14.15 Ethanol (C_2H_5OH) toxicity

- **About:** ethanol is metabolised to acetaldehyde by alcohol dehydrogenase and then to acetate by acetaldehyde dehydrogenase found in liver mitochondria. Significant toxicity in overdose and mixed with other sedatives. Found in mouthwashes, hand-washes, antiseptics. Ingested alcohol is almost totally absorbed within 1 h.
- **Clinical:** small amounts cause mild incoordination, euphoria and reduced reaction time. Moderate amounts lead to a cerebellar-type ataxia, dysarthria and even diplopia, sweating and ↑HR. Disinhibition, aggression and resulting violence and accidents. Severe overdose: coma, respiratory depression and aspiration and death.
- **Investigations:** FBC, U&E, LFTs, GGT, PTT. Chronic usage – elevated GGT and macrocytosis. ABG: acute intake can cause a metabolic acidosis. Ethanol levels: mild: <150 mg/dL, moderate: 150–300 mg/dL, severe: 300–500 mg/dL.
- **Complications:** coma, aspiration, head injury (low threshold for CT if concerns), hypoglycaemia. Alcoholic ketoacidosis, lactic acidosis, AKI, rhabdomyolysis.
- **Management:** supportive: ABC, give sufficient O_2 as per BTS guidance. ITU if high EWS. Rapid gastric uptake renders lavage and charcoal unhelpful. Neuro-observations and physiological monitoring (O_2 sats, BP, HR, blood glucose). Most are slept off in recovery position with close monitoring, but some require intubation and ventilation for severe respiratory depression. IV NS to ensure hydration. PABRINEX IV paired vials TDS for 1–2 days should be given in chronic alcoholics. Hypoglycaemia may be seen and should be treated with 10% GLUCOSE IV. Benzodiazepines: LORAZEPAM 2–4 mg IV or DIAZEPAM 5–10 mg IV for seizures. Haemodialysis with blood ethanol levels >4 g/L (400 mg/dL) or severe metabolic acidosis pH <7.0–7.1. Most patients have stabilised by 12 h. Later referral to community addiction teams.

14.16 Ethylene glycol toxicity

- **About:** antifreeze and used to bulk alcohol drinks. Co-administration with alcohol may reduce toxicity. Its metabolite glycolate/oxalate is main toxicity.
- **Aetiology:** metabolised to harmful metabolites by alcohol dehydrogenase at 4–12 h post ingestion. Progressive anion gap metabolic acidosis. Formation of oxalic acid with tissue deposition of calcium oxalate crystals.
- **Clinical:** 0–4 h 'drunk'; 4–12 h CNS depression/coma, acidotic breathing, aspiration, seizures, cerebral oedema; 12–24 h low/high BP, tachycardia, CCF, ARDS; 24–72 h AKI with oxalate crystals.
- **Investigations:** ABG: ↑anion gap >12 mmol, ↓pH, ↓HCO_3 (anion gap = [Na] + [K]) − ([Cl] + [HCO_3]) U&E, LFT, FBC, ABG. ↓Ca, glucose. pH <7.3. Osmolar gap >10 mOsm/L.

Lactate and ketones mildly elevated. Calcium oxalate crystalluria. Ethylene glycol levels: >500 mg/L (8 mmol/L) is severe.
- **Management:** supportive: ABC, O_2. IV fluids. ITU if GCS <9. Treat: evidence of ingestion or suspicion + metabolic disturbance – osmolar gap >10 mmol/dL, arterial pH <7.3, raised anion gap metabolic acidosis.
- **Antidotes:** FOMEPIZOLE and ETHANOL (▶Section 22.3 for drug formulary). Consider IV Calcium for **severe** symptomatic hypocalcemia (may ↑calcium oxalate crystals). **Acidosis:** correct with IV NaHCO$_3$. **Seizures:** standard treatment. **Haemodialysis:** if pH <7.25, AKI, ethylene glycol levels >500 mg/L. Continue until metabolism corrected and serum levels of ethylene glycol. Monitor for cerebral oedema.

Reference: Brent (2009) Fomepizole for ethylene glycol and methanol poisoning. *New Engl J Med*, 360:2216.

Methanol toxicity

- **About:** methanol 10 ml can cause blindness, 30 ml death. Metabolised to formaldehyde then formate. Use with alcohol may reduce toxicity.
- **Clinical:** latent period 0–12 h 'drunk'. Toxicity symptoms >12 h. Coma, abdominal pain, acidotic breathing, ↑HR, death. Dilated pupils, early optic disc oedema/ blindness. Later polyneuropathy, tremors, rigidity, spasticity. Parkinsonism with mild dementia.
- **Investigations:** ABG: ↑anion gap >12 mmol, ↓pH, ↓HCO$^-_3$. Anion gap = ([Na] + [K]) − ([Cl] + [HCO$_3$]), U&E, LFT, FBC, Ca, glucose. pH <7.3. Osmolar gap >10 mOsm/L. Lactate and ketones. AKI. Serum methanol >500 mg/L severe poisoning. Serum formate ≥11–12 mmol/L associated with visual/CNS sequelae. CT/MRI head: bilateral putaminal haemorrhagic necrosis, ↑amylase.
- **Management:** ABC, O_2. IV fluids. Airways protection. ITU if low GCS. Treat when: evidence of ingestion or suspicion + metabolic disturbance – osmolar gap >10 mmol/dL, arterial pH <7.3, raised anion gap metabolic acidosis.
- **Antidotes:** 1st line: FOMEPIZOLE; 2nd line: ETHANOL. Alcohol dehydrogenase has a 20-fold greater preference for ethanol than methanol. NB: Alcohol is a CNS depressant. FOLINIC ACID (LEUCOVORIN) 1 mg/kg then FOLIC ACID 1 mg/kg QDS until acidosis resolves may help prevent ocular toxicity. **Acidosis:** correct with IV sodium bicarbonate. **Seizures:** standard treatment.
- **Haemodialysis:** removes formate/methanol. Indicated if pH <7.25, AKI, continue until metabolism corrected and serum levels of methanol undetectable. Monitor for cerebral oedema.

Reference: Brent (2009) Fomepizole for ethylene glycol and methanol poisoning. *New Engl J Med*, 360:2216.

14.18 Gamma hydroxybutyrate (GHB) toxicity

- **About:** white powder, dissolved in water forms an odourless, colourless liquid. Abused as a date rape drug or sleep aid or by bodybuilders. Effects enhanced with alcohol/other drugs and unpredictable
- **Aetiology:** stimulates release of GH. It is a GABA agonist. Gamma butyrolactone (GBL) is a similar drug with similar effects.
- **Clinical:** euphoria, miosis, agitation, violence, amnesia, low BP, low HR, myoclonus. Rapid LOC with coma and then recovery after 2–4 h.
- **Investigations:** FBC, U&E, ABG as needed. Toxicology screen.
- **Management:** supportive: ABC and O_2 as per BTS guidelines. ITU if high EWS. IV fluids, mechanical ventilation 6–8 h then recovers rapidly.

14.19 Insulin toxicity

- **About:** deliberate or accidental. Insulin given IV/SC/IM causes hypoglycaemia (no effect orally). Long acting insulins last >24 h.
- **Clinical:** hypoglycaemic: confusion, tremor, hunger, panic, altered behaviour, confusion, coma, violence, agitation, amnesia.
- **Investigations:** blood sugar every 30–60 min and with symptoms. Check FBC, U&E (K falls) and LFTs. Check C-peptide (not elevated if exogenous insulin).
- **Management:** manage coma, support airway basic ABC, consider IV glucose 10–20% (with 20 mmol/L K) infusion to maintain blood glucose at >4 mmol/L. New long acting insulins with significant overdose need an ongoing infusion. Surgical removal of insulin injection site has been used for overdose of long acting insulin.

Reference: Eldred *et al.* (2013). Problem based review: the patient who has taken an overdose of long-acting insulin analogue. *Acute Med*, 12:167.

14.20 Iron (ferrous sulphate) toxicity

- **About:** often taken accidentally. Doses <60 mg/kg unlikely to be toxic. Higher doses toxic particularly for children. Delayed presentation can be fatal.
- **Clinical:** minor: N&V, dyspepsia to haematemesis, rectal bleeding, melena. Major: cardiovascular collapse, Kussmaul's breathing, hepatorenal failure. After 48 h: hepatocellular necrosis can occur. Later liver fibrosis and scarring.
- **Investigations:** iron level at 4 h, lactate, ECG, FBC, U&E – AKI, LFTs. Abdominal X-ray – KUB: radio-opaque iron tablets seen suggest trying WBI. ABG/VBG: metabolic acidosis (↑anion gap). Monitor for liver injury: ↑LFTs, prothrombin time, hypoglycaemia.
- **Management** (early action can be lifesaving): supportive: ABCs, resuscitate, IV crystalloids. ITU if high EWS. **Assess risk:** ingested dose 20–60 mg/kg will give GI effects, 60–120 mg/kg systemic toxicity. Dose >120 mg/kg is potentially lethal. Act quickly. **Perform WBI:** those with radio-opacities on KUB until the opacities clear or for amounts taken >60 mg/kg. Surgical or endoscopic removal for significant overdoses. If coma or shock start IV DESFERRIOXAMINE 15 mg/kg/h (up to 80 mg/kg in 24 h) Toxic levels >90 μmol/L at 4–6 h post ingestion especially if metabolic acidosis or altered mental state can be lifesaving. If severe toxicity expected from amount ingested then treat before the result of the serum-iron measurement.

14.21 Lithium toxicity

- **About:** used for bipolar affective disorders. No protein binding. Toxicity with dehydration or use of diuretics. Most cases due to reduced excretion of the drug. Precipitants of toxicity: dehydration, worsening renal function, infections, diuretics or NSAIDs, deliberate overdoses can have delayed effects.
- **Clinical:** acute toxicity: tremor, dysarthria, confusion, delirium, seizures, coma, death. Polyuria, polydipsia due to nephrogenic diabetes insipidus (NDI). Chronic toxicity: encephalopathy/coma, neuropathy, cerebellar dysfunction.
- **Investigations:** FBC, U&E: high Na due to NDI. ECG: T wave flattening, U waves, long QT, sepsis screen. Lithium levels at 6+ h: therapeutic range 0.6–1.2 mmol/L. Toxic symptoms >2.0 mmol/L, coma 3.0 mmol/L, massive overdose >5.0 mmol/L. CT head if diagnosis unclear.
- **Complications:** truncal, gait ataxia, nystagmus, short-term memory loss and dementia. SILENT – syndrome of irreversible lithium-effectuated neurotoxicity.
- **Management:** ABC, IV fluids to adequately resuscitate, measure I/O, avoid diuretics and NSAIDs. Supportive: rehydration to manage NDI which can take weeks to

recover. WBI: consider oral PEG solution if <2 h from acute ingestion in sustained release drug. Haemodialysis: important as can significantly lower lithium levels but may need repeated. Consider if comatose, ataxia, seizures.

14.22 Monoamine oxidase inhibitors toxicity

- **About:** caution as severe toxicity in overdose and risk of drug interactions.
- **Clinical:** euphoria, restless, pyrexia, seizures, opisthotonos, rhabdomyolysis and coma. May be delayed 12–24 h. BP can be high or low.
- **Investigations:** watch FBC, U&E, CRP, CK.
- **Management:** IV crystalloid for low BP. DIAZEPAM 5–20 mg IV for agitation. DANTROLENE 1 mg/kg IV for malignant hyperpyrexia.

14.23 Neuroleptics toxicity

- **About:** block dopamine D2 receptors. Haloperidol, sulpiride, or new agents: amisulpiride, olanzapine, quetiapine, risperidone.
- **Clinical:** ↓BP, ↓GCS, respiratory depression, hyper/hypothermia, seizures, rhabdomyolysis, acute dystonias.
- **Investigations:** FBC, U&E, CK. **ECG:** long QT, TdP.
- **Management:** stop drug. IV fluids, pressor agents for low BP. Correct acidosis with IV NaHCO₃. Consider IV MAGNESIUM or overdrive pacing for TdP.

14.24 Direct (novel) oral anticoagulants toxicity

- **About:** thrombin inhibitor (TI) and factor Xa inhibitors (XaI). Used in non-valvular AF and VTE prophylaxis and treatment. Dabigatran (TI) has a half-life of about 12–14 h. Others: apixaban, rivaroxaban (both XaI).
- **Clinical:** when was last dose taken? Look for evidence of bleeding. Hypotension, shock, melena, haematuria. Retroperitoneal bleed, psoas, intramuscular, intradermal blood.
- **Investigations:** FBC, clotting screen. U&E, LFTs. Cross match if bleeding suspected.
- **Management:** apply direct pressure to halt bleeding. Surgical input as needed. Transfuse and support. Half-life short and wears off after 24 h but bleed risk may continue for several days especially if impaired renal function. Activated charcoal may be given if medication dose recently taken. Apixaban or rivaroxaban reversal: PCC is given. Discuss FFP with haematologist. Dabigatran reversal PRAXBIND (idarucizumab) 5 g IV may be used for. Guidelines changing so take expert advice.

14.25 Non-steroidal anti-inflammatory drugs (NSAIDs) toxicity

- **About:** accidental and deliberate overdose. Ibuprofen and mefenamic acid.
- **Clinical:** gastric irritation. Abdominal pain. Mefenamic acid can cause seizures. AKI and metabolic acidosis. Low GCS, nystagmus and ↑HR rarely seen.
- **Investigations:** FBC: anaemia with gastritis, U&E: AKI. ABG: low HCO⁻₃ and metabolic acidosis (associated with ibuprofen overdoses).
- **Management:** give ABC, supportive, ACTIVATED CHARCOAL 50 g PO if more than 10 tablets in past 1–2 h. Seizures: ABC, O₂. Recovery position. Manage as per status epilepticus (▶Section 11.16). **Gastritis:** oral PPI if symptoms. Manage upper GI haemorrhage (▶Section 6.4). **Discharge:** most medically fit for discharge by 12 h if stable except in significant mefenamic acid or phenylbutazone poisoning, a 24-hour post ingestion observation is advised due to the increased risk of complications.

14.26 Opioid/opiate toxicity

- **About:** those with chronic opiate dependence – palliative care, chronic pain or addiction need **very small doses of NALOXONE**. Toxicity – accidental/ deliberate HEROIN (DIAMORPHINE) overdose. Also seen medically with CODEINE, DIAMORPHINE and MORPHINE. Have a very low threshold to giving NALOXONE.
- **Aetiology:** opiates bind to kappa and mu CNS opioid receptors.
- **Clinical:** coma, respiratory depression. Small pupils. Abuse – needle marks. Cardiac effects, e.g. QRS widening, arrhythmias and heart block with dextropropoxyphene. Look for transdermal skin patches of opiate medications.
- **Investigations:** check paracetamol/salicylate levels, toxicology screen. Blood glucose, U&E, FBC, ABG, LFTs, CXR. CT head if coma diagnosis unclear.
- **Management:** supportive: ABC, O_2. HDU area. Recovery position. If airway unsafe consider intubation and ventilation especially if GCS <8 and not rapidly responsive to NALOXONE. Consider other causes of coma – check glucose and CT head. Remove transdermal opiate patches: can be easily missed in those with fentanyl and other patches which can be forgotten. Monitor for return of symptoms, e.g. pain.
- **Opiate overdose in opiate naïve patient:** NALOXONE 0.4 mg (400 mcg) IV in 10 ml 0.9% NS IV. Repeat up to 2 mg in total. Consider infusion if helps. Give 2/3rds of the dose needed to wake the patient as an infusion. IM NALOXONE has been used. Drug abusers may become agitated with NALOXONE-induced withdrawal (see below). No response after 10 mg of NALOXONE then search for an alternative diagnosis. Effect – enlarging pupils, improving respiratory rate and GCS.
- **Opiate overdose with chronic opiate dependence:** (terminal care, long term usage or addiction) reduce opiate induced respiratory depression without causing pain or harmful cytokine release. Give NALOXONE 40–100 mcg. Make up 100 mcg in 10 ml NS and give slowly. Repeated up to 400 mcg (0.4 mg) then review. Note: tramadol and naloxone: excess tramadol can cause respiratory depression and seizure. NALOXONE will give some improvement.

References: Stage One: Warning risk of distress and death from inappropriate doses of NALOXONE in patients on long-term opioid/opiate treatment (Nov 2014). NHS/PSA/W/2014/016. NHS England.

14.27 Organophosphate/carbamates toxicity

- **About:** OPs used as agricultural chemicals. Similar to nerve agent sarin. Carbamates have similar effects.
- **Aetiology:** both bind to an active site of acetylcholinesterase and inhibit the functionality of this enzyme by means of steric inhibition. Therefore unable to break down acetylcholine. There is excess acetylcholine in synapses and neuromuscular junctions. Causes muscarinic and nicotinic symptoms. Excess bronchial secretions and respiratory muscle weakness causes respiratory failure. Also bind erythrocyte cholinesterase which can be measured.
- **Clinical** ('wet and weak'): acute: bradycardia may be missing, N&V, colic, diarrhoea, sweating, rhinorrhoea, bronchorrhoea, miosis, generalised weakness, fasciculation, weak respiratory muscles, respiratory failure.
- **Intermediate syndrome:** within 96 h with all-over weakness needing respiratory support. Recovers within 3 weeks. OP-induced delayed polyneuropathy (OPIDN): at 1–3 weeks with distal symmetrical flaccid weakness and tingling wrist and foot drop.
- **Investigations:** low erythrocyte cholinesterase activity (better guide than serum cholinesterase activity). FBC, U&E, CXR: oedema, consolidation. ABG: Type I RF. ECG: prolonged QTc interval.

- **Management:** general: decontamination. Protective clothing. Remove their clothes and wash skin with soap and water. Irrigate eyes, remove contact lenses. OPs can penetrate latex – use locally advised kit. Contaminated clothing is hazardous waste.
- **Supportive:** ABC. O_2. High dependency area. If doubtful then ATROPINE 1 mg IV with skin flushing and marked increased HR makes OP toxicity unlikely. Intubate and ventilate if hypoxia despite high FIO_2. Give adequate ATROPINE 2–3 mg IV and repeat doubling dose every 5 min (3 mg, 6 mg, 12 mg and so on) until drying of bronchial secretions and hypoxia improves, HR >80 beats/min, SBP >80 mmHg. Consider ATROPINE infusion at about 5 mg/h. Watch for development of intermediate syndrome with progressive weakness over 72 h with respiratory muscle weakness. TdP should be treated (▶Section 3.13). $MgSO_4$ may be beneficial. PRALIDOXIME (2-PAM) 1–2 g slow IV in 30 min reactivates acetylcholinesterase and is given for nicotinic (weakness) symptoms. Seizures: managed with LORAZEPAM 2–4 mg IV/IM or DIAZEPAM 5–10 mg IV as per seizure section (▶Section 11.16).

14.28 Paracetamol (acetaminophen) toxicity

- **About:** liver failure/death in those who present late or are inadequately treated. Hepatotoxicity unlikely if *N*-ACETYLCYSTEINE (PARVOLEX) started <8–10 h after ingestion. Toxic adult doses start at 16–20 × 500 mg tablets (10 g) in any 24-hour period (max dose 4 g/d or >150 mg/kg in 1 hr).
- **Pathophysiology:** paracetamol converted to highly toxic metabolite (*N*-acetyl-*p*-benzo-quinone imine (NAPQI)) by hepatic cytochrome P450 2E1 (CYP2E1). Causes liver/renal failure. NAPQI inactivated by glutathione but rapidly consumed in overdose. Low glutathione: chronic alcoholics, starvation/fasting. Enzyme-inducing drugs (e.g. carbamazepine, phenytoin, barbiturates, St John's wort, isoniazid, and rifampicin), AIDS, cystic fibrosis, and other liver disease. Low BMI, urinalysis positive for ketones, low serum urea concentration. These factors no longer play a part in dosing algorithm.
- **Clinical history 1–24 h:** no symptoms. Nausea, vomiting. 24–72 h: RUQ pain/discomfort. ↑AST, ↑PTT 72–96 h: hepatic necrosis and fulminant liver failure, jaundice, coagulopathy, delirium, encephalopathy, death. Consideration for transplantation. 4 days – 2 weeks: resolution or death. Post-transplant recovery.
- **Investigations:** paracetamol (and salicylate) level: 4 h or later post ingestion. FBC, U&E, LFTs and baseline PT at baseline and then at least daily. ↑↑ALT >1000 IU/L severe liver damage. ↑Lactate, ↑PT useful prognostically. Watch for AKI.
- **Management:** activated charcoal if dose of paracetamol >150 mg/kg was taken <1 h. If unable to establish position on treatment graph, e.g. if overdose timing uncertain or unknown or staggered overdose or history unclear, then start NAC immediately in all patients at potential risk. Concern if >12 g or 150 mg/kg taken in past 24 h period and even less if high risk. The threshold for treatment has been lowered to a 4 h paracetamol level of 100 mg/L by MHRA.
- **MHRA(UK) Guidance 2014:** all patients with a timed plasma paracetamol level on or above a single treatment line joining points of 100 mg/L at 4 h and 15 mg/L at 15 h after ingestion should receive NAC based on a new treatment nomogram, regardless of risk factors (see figure below). Where there is doubt over the timing of paracetamol ingestion including when ingestion has occurred over a period of 1 h or more – 'staggered overdose' – NAC should be given without delay (the nomogram

should not be used). Administer the initial dose of NAC as an infusion over 60 min to minimise the risk of common dose-related adverse reactions; hypersensitivity is no longer a contraindication to treatment with NAC (www.gov.uk/drug-safety-update/treating-paracetamol-overdose-with-intravenous-acetylcysteine-new-guidance).

- **Able to establish position on the treatment graph:** follow nomogram. The threshold for treatment has been lowered to a 4 h paracetamol level of 100 mg/L by MHRA. Determine if patient is above or below the treatment line. Treat those on or above the treatment line with NAC.
- **Presenting 8+ h following ingestion >150 mg/kg or with symptoms of toxicity:** treat any late presenters with evident liver disease or symptoms immediately with NAC. Do not wait for levels but give NAC prior to results. Assess paracetamol level and time post overdose on the graph and use to guide treatment. At >16 h post ingestion, interpret paracetamol concentrations with caution – most patients in this group with any detected paracetamol should be treated. Have a low threshold for considering paracetamol toxicity and giving NAC in all with acute unexplained liver failure.
- **IV NAC:** NAC can cause rash, angioedema, wheeze, ↓BP in 1–2% usually in first 2 h. Harm recorded when non-immunological adverse reactions to NAC are interpreted as anaphylaxis and NAC is withheld. Treat but should be continued at a slower rate where needed. Give CHLORPHENAMINE 10 mg IV/IM. Occasionally, bronchodilators are required (e.g. nebulised salbutamol 5 mg) and, rarely, IM ADRENALINE and IV HYDROCORTISONE for severe ↓BP. If cannot take NAC then consider oral METHIONINE but this can be hard to obtain out of hours and may not be in stock. If for some reason NAC or methionine cannot be given, then haemodialysis may be considered. In the USA oral NAC is used: consists of a loading dose of 140 mg/kg orally and maintenance dose of 70 mg/kg every 4 h for 17 doses. Induces nausea or vomiting in more than 50% of patients but is inexpensive and easier to give. Safer than IV administration. There is no evidence of any difference in efficacy (Green *et al.*, 2013). Take expert advice if unable to take NAC.

N-Acetylcysteine (NAC) administration

- Bag 1 NAC 150 mg/kg in 200 ml 5% Glucose over 1 h (now over 1 h)
- Bag 2 NAC 50 mg/kg in 500 ml 5% Glucose over 4 h
- Bag 3 NAC 100 mg/kg in 1 L 5% Glucose over 16 h

- **Acute liver failure:** escalate any significant sign of liver failure as early as possible with the regional liver centres. Monitor for coagulation, encephalopathy, hypoglycaemia, oliguria, thrombocytopenia, acidosis, cerebral oedema.
- **Orthotopic liver transplant:** may be the only hope of survival with hyperacute liver failure following paracetamol. Criteria below are used in UK. Do not wait for criteria to be met before picking up telephone. Some are transferred and may settle. Post recovery: for those who recover they must be seen by psychiatry prior to discharge. Pregnant: should be treated same as non-pregnant. Paracetamol and NAC cross placenta. No evidence of teratogenicity. Fetus protected by treating mother.
- **King's College criteria for liver transplant:** paracetamol-induced liver failure: an arterial pH <7.3 at 24 h after ingestion OR a PT >100 sec OR creatinine >300 µmol/L. Grade III or IV hepatic encephalopathy. Discuss with local liver centre long before this stage is reached.

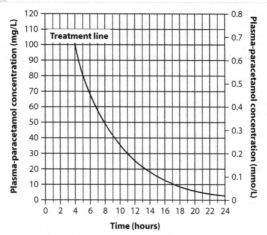

Time (hours)

Nomogram for paracetamol overdose. Treat those with a timed overdose level above or on the line. Reproduced from the MHRA 2014 with permission.

References: Bateman (2011) Management of paracetamol poisoning. *BMJ*, 342:d2218. Green *et al*. (2013) Oral and IV acetylcysteine for treatment of acetaminophen toxicity: a systematic review and meta-analysis. *West J Emerg Med*, 14:218.

14.29 Paraquat toxicity

- **Aetiology:** fatal with dose >6 g. Pulmonary–renal syndrome. Possibly formation of superoxides and free radicals.
- **Clinical:** mucosal ulceration, vomiting, diarrhoea. alveolitis, AKI. Oesophageal perforation, mediastinitis. CCF, RF.
- **Investigations:** U&E: AKI. CXR: ARDS with oedema and fibrosis. ABG: Type 1 RF and metabolic acidosis. Check paraquat levels.
- **Management:** ABC, give sufficient O_2 to match a saturation of 92%. Excess O_2 may be harmful. Eventually Type 1 RF occurs and increased FiO_2 will be needed. Remove any contaminated clothing and wash from skin or mucous membranes. Give ACTIVATED CHARCOAL 50 g PO/NG and get early expert advice. Extracorporeal removal by prolonged haemodialysis or haemoperfusion have been used until paraquat levels are undetected. IV fluids to force diuresis. Consider cyclophosphamide and steroids. Salicylates may also be of benefit. Lung transplantation has failed whenever used.
  Prognosis: dose >6 g is fatal, 1.5–6 g mortality is 60–70%, and <1.5 g is rarely fatal.

14.30 Chloroquine/quinine toxicity

- **About:** quinine used to treat malaria and nocturnal cramps. Toxic on retinal photoreceptor cells with spasm/vasoconstriction. Sodium channel blockers.
- **Clinical:** quinine: partial or complete blindness, tinnitus, N&V, headache, fatigue. Tremor, ataxia, coma, respiratory depression, arrhythmias, low BP, cardiac arrest. Chloroquine: low BP, cardiac failure, agitation, seizures, arrhythmias, cardiac arrest.
- **Investigation:** ECG: widened QRS and prolonged QTc with both, risk of VT, TdP and VF.

- **Management:** ABC, MULTIDOSE ACTIVATED CHARCOAL 50 g PO/NG and gastric lavage if early presentation. Correct K. **↓HR:** ATROPINE 0.5–1 mg slow IV (max 3 mg) which may be repeated, or transvenous pacing. Give IV NaHCO₃ if QRS >120 msec, aiming for a pH of 7.45–7.55. Early ventilation and DIAZEPAM may help with chloroquine. Overdrive pacing for VT (TdP) (magnesium not effective).

14.31 Salicylate toxicity

- **Aetiology:** weak acid uncouples oxidative phosphorylation leading to hyperthermia. Classically a mixed respiratory alkalosis and then metabolic acidosis. Calculate toxic doses per bodyweight of patient: mild > 150 mg/kg, moderate >250 mg/kg, severe >500 mg/kg taken.
- **Clinical:** dehydration, low K and a progressive metabolic acidosis occur late. N&V and tinnitus, vertigo, hyperventilation, ↑HR. Agitation, delirium, hallucinations, convulsions, lethargy, and stupor may occur. Hyperthermia is sign of severe toxicity, especially in young children. Dyspnoea due to 'noncardiogenic' pulmonary oedema. Risks: elderly and young, CNS involvement, metabolic acidosis, hyperpyrexia, pulmonary oedema, salicylate >700 mg/L (5.1 mmol/L).
- **Investigations:** U&E: ↓K and AKI, FBC, coag: coagulopathy, LFT, ↑lactate, ABG – mixed picture. ↓Glucose, CXR if breathless. Salicylate level at 2 h post ingestion if symptoms and at 4 h if no symptoms. A level >500 mg/L is severe and above 700 mg/L (5.1 mmol/L) is very severe and life threatening. Check ECG – arrhythmias, hypokalaemia.
- **Management:** gastric lavage if >500 mg/kg taken (with airway protection). If <1 h from ingestion +/– then MDAC 50 g PO/NG stat repeated within 2–3 h of ingestion. Consider WBI with PEG if significant overdose. Promote diuresis with IV fluids 3–4 L/day. 10% Glucose IV if hypoglycaemia. May need potassium – it is important to ensure normokalaemia to allow acid–base correction.
- **Urinary alkalinisation:** *May be used for salicylates >500 mg/L (3.6 mmol/L): Aim is to achieve urine pH 7.5–8.5:* IV 1 L 1.26% NaHCO₃ with 40 mmol KCl over 4 h repeated as needed up to 4 L/day. Consider haemodialysis with salicylate levels >700–900 mg/L or with seizures, severe acidosis pH <7.2, AKI, ARDS, coma, CCF, non-cardiogenic pulmonary oedema. Watch for hypokalaemia. Alkalotic tetany may occur but hypocalcaemia is rare.

14.32 SSRI/SNRI toxicity

- **About:** selective serotonin (noradrenaline) reuptake inhibitor drugs. ↑CNS serotonin – serotonin syndrome. Less toxic than TCAs. SSRI / SNRI, e.g. fluoxetine, citalopram and venlafaxine.
- **Clinical: SSRI:** N&V, tremor, prolonged QTc, serotonergic syndromes. **SNRI:** ↑HR, tremor, agitation, ↑QRS and QTc duration, arrhythmia, seizures, coma. **Mirtazapine:** drowsiness, NV.
- **Investigations:** U&E, LFT, FBC, CK, glucose, coagulation. Monitor ECG: long QT, TdP with citalopram.
- **Management:** ABC, IV fluids, respiratory support if needed. Agitation/seizures: IV Lorazepam or Diazepam. Manage hyperthermia. Activated charcoal 50 g PO if <1 h from overdose and 10+ tablets taken. Manage TdP with IV magnesium. Long QT/ wide QRS give 250 ml 1.26% NaHCO₃, monitor CK for rhabdomyolysis, DIC, ARDS. Severe serotonin syndrome: usually medically stable by 12 h.

14.33 Tricyclic antidepressant toxicity

- **About:** amitriptyline and first generation drugs very toxic. Avoid or controlled access in those at high risk of suicide.
- **Aetiology:** anticholinergic toxidrome, adrenergic blockade. Inhibition of NA and 5HT reuptake. Blockade of fast Na channels in myocardial cells (quinidine-like membrane-stabilising effects). Block K channels. Histamine receptor blockers.
- **Clinical:** ↑HR, dilated pupils, urinary retention, hyperreflexia, ↓BP, seizures, coma, arrhythmias, prolonged QRS duration, metabolic acidosis.
- **Investigations:** FBC, ABG: hypoxia, hypercarbia, metabolic acidosis. Paracetamol, salicylate levels. ECG changes suggest toxicity and Na channel blockade with QRS >120 msec, R wave >3 mm in aVr, prolonged QT, Brugada appearance and LBBB/ RBBB. CT head if seizure/coma to exclude other brain pathology.
- **Management:** supportive: ABCs. Correct ↓BP, hypoxia, acidosis, IV fluids, CCU/ITU monitoring. If <1–2 h and >10 tablets consider lavage +/− activated CHARCOAL 50 g PO/NG if >10 tablets. Manage seizures with IV LORAZEPAM 2–4 mg or DIAZEPAM 5–10 mg. *Avoid Phenytoin which may be arrhythmogenic.* Monitor ECG: QRS >140 msec, VT, TdP, VF, heart block in CCU/ITU. Antiarrhythmics avoided generally other than MgSO₄ for TdP. Coma may persist 1–2 days and wake up with agitation/hallucinations.
- **VT:** CCU bed, overdrive pacing / IV MgSO₄ / lidocaine. If QRS >120 msec or ↓BP or arrhythmias give 50 ml 8.4% NaHCO₃ IV and repeat if needed. ↑pH helps to ↑protein binding, ↓QRS interval, stabilises arrhythmias, ↑BP. TCA are highly protein bound so haemodialysis not useful. Psychiatry assessment. Final: consider IV Glucagon, inotropes for persisting ↓BP. Cardiac arrest: consider prolonged resuscitation. Intralipid emulsion 'lipid rescue' as TCAs are lipid soluble.

14.34 Theophylline toxicity

- **Aetiology:** used to treat asthma/COPD. Narrow therapeutic window. Inhibits phosphodiesterase with elevated cAMP and adrenergic stimulation.
- **Clinical:** nausea, severe vomiting, abdominal pain, ↑HR, seizures.
- **Investigations:** ABG: metabolic acidosis. Low K, phosphate, Mg. Low/high Ca, hyperglycaemia. Check levels: range 10–20 mcg/ml, toxic levels >20 mcg/ml. ECG and telemetry: all arrhythmias, AF/atrial flutter/SVT/VT/VF.
- **Management:** stop any oral or IV theophyllines. ABC, give O₂ as per BTS guidelines. Manage seizures: LORAZEPAM 2–4 mg IV (▶Section 11.16). (May need ITU). Limit absorption: multidose activated charcoal (MDAC) is important to help elimination of theophylline. Gastric lavage may be considered if taken within 1 h of a significant amount or sustained-release preparation. WBI in patients with exposure to theophylline preparations due to enterohepatic circulation of drug. Manage hypokalaemia: cautious correction of low K. Arrhythmias: consider beta-blockers (usually C/I for asthma/COPD) or disopyramide suggested for ventricular arrhythmias.

14.35 Body packers ('mules')

- **About:** a normal abdominal X-ray does not rule out body packing, a non-contrast abdominopelvic CT scan must be performed to confirm/refute the diagnosis. Drugs usually wrapped in some latex condom, balloon or finger of a latex glove. Nowadays more sophisticated with multilayered latex. May be 1–200 found. Usually heroin and cocaine but also amphetamine, ecstasy and marijuana. Each packet holds 3–15 g of the drug. Total carried may be 1 kg. Each packet of heroin, cocaine or amphetamine contains a potentially life-threatening dose of the drug.

- **Clinical:** heroin OD causes coma, miosis, respiratory depression or apnoea and is treatable. Cocaine and amphetamine OD with pupil dilatation, diaphoresis, ↑HR, hypertension, seizure and coma, MI, VF, symptoms of small bowel obstruction or perforation.
- **Classification** (I, II, III are radiolucent, IV is radiopaque): Type I: loosely packed cocaine covered by two to four layers of condoms or other latex-like material; this type has the highest risk for leakage/rupture. Type II: tightly packed cocaine powder or paste covered in multiple layers of tubular latex. Type III: tightly packed cocaine powder or paste covered by aluminium foil. Type IV: dense cocaine paste is placed into a device, condensed and hardened and packaged in tough tubular latex covered with coloured paraffin or fibreglass. Least likely to cause problems.
- **Investigations:** FBC, U&E, LFT, ECG. Usually but not always seen on abdominal X-ray or by abdominal USS. Abdominal/pelvic CT scan is imaging of choice – Hounsfield unit of 219 and heroin 520.
- **Management:** endoscopy avoided with risk of perforation of packages. If there are symptoms suggesting perforation or obstruction then urgent surgery is advocated. Total/whole bowel irrigation with PEG may be given. Laxatives (avoid oil-based laxatives). Close observation and detection and management of any related drug toxicities. Cocaine overdose is fatal in 60%. Follow local policies regarding involvement of police.

References: Kelly *et al.* (2007) Contemporary management of drug packers. *World J Emerg Surg*, 2:9. Pinto *et al.* (2014) Radiological and practical aspects of body packing. *Br J Radiol*, 87:20130500.

14.36 Cannabis toxicity

- **About:** from plant *Cannabis sativa*. IV usage more toxic. Smoked (effects within 10–20 min) or ingested (effects 1–2 h) or IV.
- **Clinical:** euphoria/ psychosis, drowsiness, visual distortions, HTN, ↑HR. IV cannabis – ↓BP and AKI, watery diarrhoea, pulmonary oedema, DIC.
- **Investigations:** urine toxicology: positive for several days. U&E: AKI.
- **Management:** supportive. Consider DIAZEPAM 5–20 mg IV for aggression. Start IV NS at 250 ml/h for low BP. Serious poisoning rare. Resolves quickly.

14.37 Sulphonylurea toxicity

- **Examples:** gliclazide, glipizide (short acting) chlorpropamide (long acting). Short acting less harmful.
- **Clinical:** mild to severe hypoglycaemia. **Investigations:** U&E, LFT. Low glucose (confirm lab glucose).
- **Management:** 10% glucose infusion with OCTREOTIDE 50 mcg IV. $NaHCO_3$ to alkalinise the urine reduces the half-life of chlorpropamide.

14.38 Methaemoglobinaemia

- **Aetiology:** methaemoglobin (MetHb) unable to bind O_2 as iron in Fe^{3+} state.
- **Causes:** Dapsone, Primaquine and other drugs, nitrites. Can be inherited.
- **Clinical:** blue breathless patient, chocolate coloured blood.
- **Investigations:** low SpO_2 with a fairly normal PaO_2.
- **Management:** ↑MetHb level on ABG. If >30% then give METHYLTHIONINIUM (methylene blue) 1–2 mg/kg over 5 min. May be repeated after 30–60 mins.

14.39 Phenobarbital toxicity

- **Clinical:** sedation, coma, ↓HR, low BP. **Investigations:** CT head if unsure.
- **Management:** supportive care. Urinary alkalinisation to pH 7.5–8 and multiple doses of activated charcoal can enhance the elimination.

14.40 Carbamazepine toxicity

- **About:** enzyme inducer. Toxicity with enzyme inhibitors.
- **Clinical:** drowsy, ataxia, confusion, nystagmus, TEN/SJS.
- **Investigations:** ECG: arrhythmias.
- **Management:** supportive, repeat dosing of activated charcoal and WBI is important. Haemoperfusion may be necessary if end-organ toxicity becomes evident. Serious harm very rare. WBI requires 1.5–2 L/h (20–30 ml/min) of PEG. NaHCO₃ if QRS >100 msec due to carbamazepine toxicity and sodium channel blockade.

14.41 Lead, arsenic, mercury, thallium (heavy metal) toxicity

- **Toxic metals** include lead, mercury, and cadmium. Other metals, e.g. iron, used in physiology but may be toxic in excess. Some, e.g. radioactive metals like polonium, are toxic due to emitting particles. Acute toxicity usually industrial. Take expert help. Similar clinically to lead.
- **Clinical:** mixed picture of nausea, vomiting, dehydration, abdo pain, hepatotoxicity, pancreatitis, seizure, Fanconi syndrome, acute encephalopathy, neuropathies, e.g. foot drop, gout in suspicious setting. Thallium: painful sensory neuropathy and alopecia. Arsenic: clinical signs of pancytopenia.
- **Investigations:** FBC: (lead) anaemia and basophilic stippling on blood film. U&E, AKI/ATN, ECG, metabolic acidosis. LFTs, amylase, lactate. If suspicious measure whole blood lead in lead free tube. Urine spot test for arsenic and 24 h urine collection for total arsenic excretion.
- **Management:** lead, mercury, arsenic, thallium. Remove source. WBI with PEG may help. Chelation therapy (IV EDTA). Chelating agents – BAL (British Anti Lewisite) or DMSA (2,3-dimethylenediaminetetracetic acid) on expert advice. Thallium needs Prussian Blue. Arsenic may need dialysis and BAL.

15 Medical emergencies in pregnancy

15.1 Medical problems in pregnancy

- **About:** the call to the obstetric unit for medical issues can be intimidating to even the most accomplished doctor. This is a collection of a few basic facts and principles to help you. As ever, if unsure of what you are doing then get help. This is to deal mainly with acute and on-call questions. Pregnancy is covered within resuscitation, asthma and DVT/pulmonary embolism and headache sections.

- **General principles:** most women in pregnancy are healthy. Those with known or anticipated medical disorders require expert care which is really the preserve of the obstetric team liaising with medical specialists as needed. Communication is key. Medical disorders can be considered in terms of disorders caused by the pregnancy and pre-existing disorders exacerbated by the effects of the pregnancy, e.g. heart disease, asthma, immune disorders, clotting disorders, epilepsy. It is important to involve senior members of the obstetric team when making any significant management plans that can affect the pregnancy.

Medical advice on managing pregnant patients

- There are two (or sometimes more) patients.
- Give folate prior to conception and in the first trimester.
- Tachypnoea or ↑HR must not be ignored.
- A pink Venflon is useless in a sick pregnant patient.
- Ectopic pregnancy can be atypical, e.g. 'fainting, D&V'.
- ALP (placental) rises in 3rd trimester.
- CXR: safe (3 days background radiation) but shield fetus.
- Avoid prescribing in 1st trimester unless proven safety.

- Avoid NSAIDs, ACEIs, ARBs, trimethoprim, warfarin.
- For anticoagulation use LMWH or IV heparin.
- Consider diagnosing PE by diagnosing a DVT first.
- For hyperemesis don't forget thiamine (give Pabrinex).
- You can use salbutamol, steroids and magnesium for asthma.
- Magnesium for preventing eclamptic seizures.
- Accidental magnesium overdose can be fatal. Give IV calcium gluconate.
- Maximum cardiac at 14 weeks and just following delivery.

15.2 Pharmacology in pregnancy

Sources of prescribing advice in UK

- *BNF* or your local equivalent. National Teratology Information Service (NTIS) in Newcastle – call 0191 2321525 (5944 urgent Monday to Friday 17.00–20.00); 08448920111 – emergency 24 h advice line for poisoning/chemical exposure in pregnancy.
- Websites: http://toxbase.org; http://toxnet.nlm.nih.gov; www.ukmi.nhs.uk. Also consult with local obstetric medicine team. The safety of any drug used in pregnancy must be checked with manufacturer's data sheet or *BNF*.
- **Known or potential teratogens to stop/avoid:** ACEIs, AT2 blockers, NSAIDs, statins, cigarette smoking, cocaine, warfarin, fluconazole, isotretinoin (Accutane), lithium, misoprostol, penicillamine, tetracyclines, doxycycline, thalidomide, valproic acid, cyclophosphamide, mycophenolate, sirolimus.
- **Some possible teratogens:** alcohol binge drinking, carbamazepine, colchicine, disulfiram, ergotamine, glucocorticoids (benefits often outweigh risks), lead, metronidazole, primidone, quinine (suicidal doses), streptomycin, vitamin A (high doses), zidovudine (AZT).

- **Drugs to avoid when breastfeeding:** chloramphenicol, metronidazole, nitrofurantoin and sulphonamides (haemolysis with G6PD deficiency), tetracycline (stains teeth and bones), lithium, antineoplastics and immunosuppressants, psychotropic drugs (relative).
- **Drugs which can be used acutely in pregnancy:** heparin and LMWH, ampicillin, cephalosporins, clindamycin, erythromycin, gentamicin, paracetamol (acetaminophen), folate, pyridoxine, thyroxine, steroids, salbutamol, aspirin, magnesium, anticholinergic inhalers, theophyllines, lorazepam, diazepam, phenytoin. Give usual doses of GTN, IV nitrates, furosemide, morphine, calcium blocker, mechanical support, e.g. IABP, LVAD, Digoxin, beta-blockers.

15.3 Amniotic fluid embolism

- **About:** amniotic fluid (fetal cells, hair, or other debris) enters maternal circulation. Causes cardiac arrest/shock in labour/caesarean or within 30 min post-partum. Resembles anaphylaxis.
- **Aetiology:** usually during labour but also abortion and trauma. Fetal squamous cells found in the maternal pulmonary circulation. These are also found in well patients. Possibly complement activation.
- **Clinical:** acutely dyspnoeic with ↓BP and hypoxia, cough, seizures, cardiac arrest. Coagulopathy or severe haemorrhage.
- **Investigations: ABG:** Type 1 RF. **CXR:** pulmonary oedema. **ECG:** non-specific. **Coagulation** screen: coagulopathy.
- **Management:** as per cardiac arrest (▶Section 1.2). CPR, ABCs, intubate and ventilate. Manage with IV fluids for ↓BP. Invasive monitoring and exclude alternative diagnoses. Manage any coagulopathy. Haemodialysis with plasmapheresis for AKI. Steroids if immune-mediated mechanism suspected.

15.4 Hypertension in pregnancy

- Hypertension during pregnancy carries risks of increased perinatal mortality, preterm birth and low birth weight.
- Pre-eclampsia and gestational hypertension come on later in pregnancy.
- Pre-existing hypertension can be discovered at initial contact.
- ACE inhibitors and ARB drugs are teratogenic and contraindicated in pregnancy.

Degree	Values
Mild	DBP 90–99 mmHg and SBP 140–149 mmHg
Moderate	DBP 100–109 mmHg and SBP 150–159 mmHg
Severe	DBP >110 mmHg and SBP >160 mmHg

HTN in pregnancy (BP >140/90 mmHg, 2 readings seated 6 h apart)

- Gestational (pregnancy-induced) HTN (new onset but minimal proteinuria).
- Pre-eclampsia and eclampsia (new hypertension with proteinuria).
- Chronic hypertension (renal disease, primary/essential hypertension).
- Pre-eclampsia superimposed on chronic hypertension.

15.5 Eclampsia and pre-eclampsia

- **About:** reported frequencies from 2 to 7% of all pregnancies after 20 weeks. Not all can be anticipated by finding hypertension and proteinuria. Pre-eclampsia toxaemia (PET): after 20 weeks + BP >140/90 mmHg + proteinuria >300 mg/24 h. Severe = PET + end organ damage.
- **Note:** low-dose ASPIRIN helps prevent pre-eclampsia in high-risk women.
- **Risk factors: moderate risk factors:** 1st pregnancy, age >40 years, pregnancy interval >10 years, BMI >35 kg/m^2 at first visit, family history of pre-eclampsia, multiple pregnancy. **High risk factors** (give ASPIRIN 75 mg OD from 12 weeks): HTN during previous pregnancy, CKD, APL, T1DM, T2DM, chronic hypertension.
- **Clinical: pre-eclampsia:** severe headache, severe pain just below ribs, epigastric or hypochondrial (hepatic congestion/liver capsule stretching). Is baby moving normally (fetal wellbeing)? Visual problems such as blurring or vomiting, flashing before eyes, sudden swelling of face, hands or feet. Disorientated, hyperreflexia, clonus, stroke and cerebral oedema. **Severe pre-eclampsia:** severe headache, visual problems, papilloedema, clonus >3 beats. Liver tenderness. **Eclampsia:** grand-mal seizures last 60+ sec preceded by facial twitching. There is generalised muscle contraction. May be coma and period of hyperventilation.
- **Complications: stroke:** ischaemic or haemorrhagic get CT head, manage BP, ASPIRIN where indicated. Exclude cerebral venous thrombosis and SAH. **HELLP:** platelets <100 × 10^9/L, haemolysis (↑LDH), elevated LFTs. Fatal in 2%. **AKI** (acute cortical or tubular necrosis): fall in GFR, elevated creatinine, urea. Oliguria, proteinuria >5 g/24 h. **Others:** fetal growth retardation, fetal death, placental abruption, ARDS, hepatic infarction, DIC.

Investigations

- **FBC:** low platelet count (HELLP syndrome). Anaemia due to microangiopathic haemolysis (schistocytes, burr cells) or physiological haemodilution of pregnancy. **U&E:** AKI: renal dysfunction (late), ↑urate in eclampsia. **LFTs:** ↑AST/ALT, mild: increase LDH or bilirubin. Low haptoglobin levels with haemolysis. **Clotting:** (not routinely if platelets >100 × 10^9/L). MSU to exclude UTI as cause of protein. **Fetal assessment:** fetal HR, USS for growth, CTGs. Maternal: cervical assessment (depending on gestation). **CT head:** arrange post seizure to exclude haemorrhage or other pathology. **Prevention: ASPIRIN 75 mg started at 12 weeks treatment** to reduce risk of PET. Moderate but consistent reductions in PET, preterm delivery and serious outcomes. Start in those at high risk – hypertensive disease during a previous pregnancy, CKD, systemic lupus erythematosus or antiphospholipid syndrome, type 1 or type 2 diabetes, chronic hypertension.

Management

- **Antihypertensives in pregnancy:** the following are acceptable: methyldopa, labetalol, clonidine, prazosin, doxazosin, nifedipine. **HTN:** mild consider LABETALOL PO and monitor closely to keep BP <150/80–100 mmHg. In more severe cases consider LABETALOL IV/PO, HYDRALAZINE slow IV 5–10 mg diluted in 10 ml NaCl 0.9%. NIFEDIPINE PO.
- **Eclamptic seizures or severe pre-eclampsia: IV MAGNESIUM SULPHATE 4 g IV over 5 min, followed by infusion of 1 g/h for 24 h.** Further dose of 2–4 g given over 5 min if recurrent seizures. Monitor urine output, reflexes and respiratory rate. Ongoing seizures managed as per status epilepticus (▶ Section 11.16). **Delivery:** recommended but timing depends on gestational age and fetal maturity and risk to mother of continuing the pregnancy. Obstetrician may give steroids to improve lung maturity if delivery planned within 1 week.

- **Gestational hypertension:** avoid ACEIs, ARBs. Give **ASPIRIN 75 mg** from 12 weeks. Consider α-methyldopa, hydralazine, labetalol and nifedipine. Diuretics avoided.
- **Chronic hypertension:** stop ACEIs, ARBs. Switch to safer drugs in pregnancy. Give ASPIRIN from 12 weeks. Ensure underlying causes excluded, Consider α-methyldopa, hydralazine, labetalol and nifedipine (avoid sublingual as it can cause sudden ↓BP). Diuretics avoided.
- Warfarin, ACE inhibitors and AT2 blockers are absolutely contraindicated in pregnancy. Diuretics are not contraindicated but are generally avoided.

Reference: NICE (2010) CG107: Hypertension in pregnancy.

15.6 Diabetes in pregnancy

- **Target BM:** fasting glucose <5.3 mmol/L. 1 h glucose <7.8 mmol/L. 2 h glucose <6.4 mmol/L.
- Test urgently for ketonaemia if diabetic or unwell, to exclude diabetic ketoacidosis.
- Reducing HbA1c level towards 48 mmol/mol (6.5%) is likely to reduce congenital malformations in baby.
- Avoid pregnancy if HbA1c level >86 mmol/mol (10%) because of the associated risks.
- Use isophane or long acting insulins. Avoid ACE inhibitors, ARB, stop statins.

15.7 Acute hepatobiliary disease in pregnancy

Liver disease is rare in pregnancy. The liver or spleen is not usually palpable. AST, ALT, GGT, bilirubin, LDH, PT, PTT are normal. ALP, WBC, fibrinogen, caeruloplasmin, alpha and beta globulins, AFP are elevated. There are reduced levels of Hb, albumin, gammaglobulins, uric acid, urea, total protein, and antithrombin III concentrations. Management of liver disease in pregnancy requires collaboration between obstetricians and gastroenterologists/hepatologists.

Cause of abnormal LFTs in pregnancy by trimester

Use the gestational age of the pregnancy as the best guide to the differential diagnosis of liver disease in the pregnant woman	
All stages	Consider viral or drug-induced hepatitis, gallstone disease, or malignancy or Budd–Chiari in the differential diagnosis of abnormal liver tests in any of the trimesters of pregnancy.
First trimester	**Hyperemesis gravidarum.** AST <1000 U. **Viral hepatitis.**
Second trimester	**Cholestasis of pregnancy** – early delivery should be considered when possible. **Portal hypertension and variceal bleeding** usually occur in the second trimester as the intravascular volume expands, or occurs at delivery. **Viral hepatitis** can occur.
Third trimester	**Pre-eclampsia** related (HELLP) in 2nd half of pregnancy, usually 3rd trimester. **Acute viral hepatitis** – can occur at any time in pregnancy but most severe in 3rd trimester.
Post-partum	Acute fatty liver of pregnancy, HELLP syndrome, Budd–Chiari syndrome.

15.8 Diagnoses and management of liver disease in pregnancy

Chronic liver disease	**Chronic hepatitis B/C, autoimmune hepatitis, Wilson's disease, PBC, cirrhosis** present throughout the pregnancy, variable course from patient to patient. PBC compatible with normal pregnancy. Primary sclerosing cholangitis pregnancy rare but monitor closely. AIH: fetal death is seen. Use of azathioprine may be harmful. Wilson disease – higher risk of fetal loss. Trientine may be teratogenic.
Cirrhosis and portal hypertension	Portal hypertension leads to increased risk of variceal bleeding, liver failure and encephalopathy, jaundice, splenic artery aneurysm. Screen pregnant women with cirrhosis for varices from 2nd trimester and start on beta-blockers if indicated. Avoid vasopressin.
Hyperemesis gravidarum	Severe N&V. Elevated AST <1000 U. Resolves by week 20, rarely can persist. Management supportive, fluids, nutrition, thiamine.
Cholestasis of pregnancy or obstetric cholestasis	Usually seen 2nd trimester. and may cause jaundice. Ursodeoxycholic acid is safe. Common especially Asian/Chilean origin. ↑risk of prematurity and stillbirth. Severe pruritus (no rash) often worse at night, palms and soles. Jaundice. ↑AST <1000U. ↑ALP ×4. GGT may be normal. Biopsy: cholestasis. Check LFTs every 1–2 weeks. If worsening escalate and consider other diagnosis. Check postnatal resolution of pruritus and LFTs. Topical emollients are safe. URSODEOXYCHOLIC ACID or COLESTYRAMINE improve pruritus and liver function. If PTT prolonged then VITAMIN K is indicated. Long term risk of gallstones, cholecystitis, pancreatitis, diarrhoea, steatorrhea. Recurs in subsequent pregnancies.
HELLP *Usually 27–36 weeks and post-partum*	Pre-eclampsia spectrum. Definition (1) PET findings: BP >140/90 mmHg + proteinuria + >20 weeks; (2) haemolysis, ↑LFTs, ↓platelets. **Clinical:** often well, ↑BP may not be present. C/O epigastric pain, N&V, jaundice. No liver failure. Eclampsia with seizures or coma. **Investigations:** FBC: ↓Hb, ↓plt <100 × 10⁹/L, WCC normal. ↑LDH >600 U/L (haemolysis). Smear: schistocytes and burr cells. LFT: ↑AST, ↑GGT. Liver USS normal. Urate normal. PT normal. Proteinuria >300 mg/24 h. Urine dipstick >1+. **Management:** vaginal delivery if >34th gestational week or the fetal and/or maternal conditions deteriorate. Higher maternal and perinatal morbidity and mortality rates.
Acute fatty liver of pregnancy *Raised PT, ↓fibrinogen, ↓ATIII, liver failure differentiate from HELLP*	Potentially lethal liver failure seen at the end of pregnancy. 1 in 20 000, death 1.8%. Mitochondrial cytopathy. Increased incidence with LCHAD deficiency. **Clinical:** last trimester with jaundice, malaise, abdominal pain, nausea and upper GI bleed. AKI with oliguria, uraemia, hypoglycaemic episodes. Fulminant liver failure: jaundice, encephalopathy, coagulopathy. Pancreatitis. Diagnostic criteria: in absence of other diagnosis – need >5 of: (1) vomiting, abdominal pain, encephalopathy, bilirubin >14, glucose <4 mmol/L; (2) urate >340, WCC >11, ascites/bright liver US, AST/ALT >42; (3) creatinine >150 μmol/L, PT >14 s, microvesicular steatosis on biopsy. **Investigations:** FBC, U&E: anaemia, AKI, ↑urate. **LFTs:** conjugated hyperbilirubinaemia, ↑AST, ↑ALT, ↑PT. Clotting: look for DIC: ↑PT, ↓fibrinogen, ↓antithrombin levels. Amylase increased if pancreatitis. USS/CT abdomen may be normal or show increased echogenicity. Biopsy usually not done due to coagulopathy. Hepatitis viral serology and other differentials. **Differential:** HELLP, viral, drug/toxin induced hepatitis. **Management:** delivery of the fetus irrespective of gestational age within 24 h of diagnosis by induction or caesarean section. Correct coagulopathy. Manage as fulminant hepatic failure. Plasma exchange seems to help. Prognosis for those who survive is usually excellent.

Hepatic infarct haematoma and rupture	Seen with HELLP, AFLP, TTP, HUS or pre-eclampsia. Subcapsular haemorrhage with hepatic rupture with death of mother and fetus. Fever, shock, RUQ pain, haemoperitoneum. CT infarct left lobe. Rupture seen more in HELLP. Best managed surgically by a trauma team as liver lacerations. Prompt delivery and ITU care.
Acute viral liver disease Take expert advice	Acute viral infection – HSV, CMV, HEV. HSV infection – IV ACICLOVIR, thus not requiring early delivery. The natural course of acute hepatitis A or B is not altered in the pregnant woman, and interruption of the pregnancy or early delivery is not indicated. Acute hepatitis B in the second or third trimester may pose a risk for transmission to the baby, and immunization with hepatitis B immunoglobulin (HBIG) and hepatitis B vaccine at birth is advocated. Chronic hepatitis B or C requires no therapy in pregnancy, but poses a risk of transmission to the offspring. Take advice. HCV 5–10% risk of vertical transmission.
Gallstones	Pregnancy increases biliary sludge and gallstones which may resolve after delivery. If possible, acute cholecystitis is best managed medically in the first and third trimesters, when the risk of premature delivery prompted by surgery is greater than in the second trimester. Choledocholithiasis can be managed with ERCP (shield fetus and restrict fluoroscopy time) which may be necessary in the management of symptomatic common bile duct stones leading to cholecystitis or pancreatitis.
Budd–Chiari syndrome	Cause of acute liver failure. Seen any time. May need transplant.

References: Lee & Brady (2009) Liver disease in pregnancy. *World J Gastroenterol*, 15:897. Riely (1999) Liver disease in the pregnant patient. *Am J Gastroenterol*, 94:1728.

15.9 Pulmonary embolism and pregnancy

- **About** PE is a leading cause of pregnancy-related death usually due to extensive iliac vein thrombosis. Risks extend from early pregnancy to 4–6 weeks postpartum. ▸ Section 4.17.
- **Clinical diagnosis** difficult if signs subtle because signs and symptoms resemble physiological changes of pregnancy. The tests are imperfect and must be gauged with clinical findings. D-dimer is often mildly elevated and so a raised value must be corroborated with other investigations. Involve senior obstetricians, radiologists and respiratory team urgently if patient compromised or peri-arrest. If clinically likely **treat as such with LMWH or IV heparin** whilst tests awaited.
- **The RCOG** has published a new guide increasing the number of those who should get VTE prophylaxis during and after pregnancy (April 2015). High risk women should be considered for prophylactic **LMWH from 28 weeks and will usually require prophylactic LMWH for 6 weeks postnatal with a risk reassessment.** Risks include obesity (BMI >30), age >35, parity ≥3, smoker, gross varicose veins, current pre-eclampsia, immobility, e.g. paraplegia, family history of unprovoked or oestrogenic-provoked VTE in first-degree relative, low-risk thrombophilia, multiple pregnancy, IVF/assisted reproduction. Consult with obstetrics/haematology to advise on VTE prophylaxis.
- **Investigations:** you should do a CXR. It is appropriate and may identify and rule out other pathology (PTX, effusion, consolidation, pneumonia, cancer) and involves a tiny radiation dose and the fetus can be shielded. Useful evidence from **USS doppler of leg veins for a DVT** (ask radiologist to screen from calf veins to inferior vena caval bifurcation as there are often large pelvic thrombi) will indicate a need for anticoagulation without radiation. **Echocardiogram** may show right heart changes. The **perfusion (Q) only part of V/Q scanning** may be used. **CTPA**

may be considered, especially where there has been preceding lung disease. The theoretical concern is CTPA irradiating pregnant breast tissue with long-term breast cancer risks, but misdiagnosis kills mother and fetus and the radiation risk is small compared with the risk of misdiagnosis and not treating. If there is diagnostic suspicion and Q scan and echo/doppler equivocal/unhelpful then CTPA.

- **Standard treatment is LMWH. Warfarin is contraindicated. IV heparin preferred if imminent delivery being contemplated and should be stopped 4–6 h before.** In extreme situations thrombolysis, and catheter and surgical embolectomy have been performed. Take local expert advice because protocols vary. Manage with obstetric input at all stages. After delivery warfarin can be started and is safe in breastfeeding. Continue anticoagulation for at least 6–12 weeks post-delivery.

15.10 Acute severe asthma in pregnancy

- **Pregnancy:** treat very actively as in non-pregnant. Asthma can kill mother and child. Real risk is under treatment.
- **In pregnancy:** Asthma in 1/3 improves, 1/3 worsens and 1/3 no change. Always continue medications to ensure good asthma control.
- **Uncontrolled asthma** is associated with many maternal and fetal complications, including hyperemesis, hypertension, pre-eclampsia, vaginal haemorrhage, complicated labour, fetal growth restriction, preterm birth, increased perinatal mortality, and neonatal hypoxia.
- **Must stop smoking.** Take anti-asthma drugs (safe to use in pregnancy and during breastfeeding). Give standard therapy as needed. Leukotriene antagonists may be continued in women who have demonstrated significant improvement in asthma control with these agents prior to pregnancy not achievable with other medications.
- **In labour:** if anaesthesia is required, regional blockade is preferable to general anaesthesia. Prostaglandin E2 may safely be used for labour inductions. However, use prostaglandin F2α with extreme caution in women with asthma because of the risk of inducing bronchoconstriction. Women receiving steroid tablets at a dose exceeding PREDNISOLONE 7.5 mg per day for more than 2 weeks prior to delivery should receive parenteral HYDROCORTISONE 100 mg 6–8 hourly during labour.

15.11 Status epilepticus in pregnancy

- **About:** women with epilepsy should be delivered in a consultant-led maternity unit and one to one midwifery care given during labour. Low threshold for epidural anaesthesia. Anti-epilepsy drug medication should be continued during labour and post-natally with neurology input. An elective caesarean section should be considered if there have been frequent tonic–clonic or prolonged complex partial seizures towards the end of pregnancy. Valproate is generally avoided as an anticonvulsant in pregnancy. All women should be given folate 5 mg OD.
- **Status epilepticus** (▶Sections 11.16 and 11.17) (exclude eclampsia, BP, urine, platelets, LFTs and get obstetric help to assess mother/fetus): establish the ABCs, and check vital signs, including oxygenation. Maternal airway and oxygenation should be maintained at all times. Intraosseous or venous access should be in SVC distribution. If seizures associated with eclampsia then use IV MgSO₄. If seizure persists give LORAZEPAM 2–4 mg IV or DIAZEPAM as per usual protocol. Consider PHENYTOIN 20 mg/kg IV. Check laboratory findings, including electrolytes, anti-epilepsy drug levels, glucose, and toxicology screen. If signs of fetal distress consider urgent delivery.
- **Juvenile myoclonic epilepsy:** first line are Valproate and Lamotrigine. However, in fertile females valproate avoided due to fears of teratogenicity and side effects.

- **Delivery should be expedited following a seizure during labour**, and neonatal expertise should be available. Needs CT with appropriate precautions to exclude intracranial pathology if fits are atypical or symptoms or signs suggest new pathology or worsening baseline pathology.
- **Possible causes of first fit in pregnancy:** idiopathic, eclampsia, sagittal vein thrombosis, anti-phospholipid syndrome, infarction, intracerebral haemorrhage, thrombotic thrombocytopenic purpura, amniotic fluid embolism, gestational epilepsy, alcohol withdrawal, brain tumour, SAH, vasculitis and other causes.
- **Pregnancy/eclampsia:** MAGNESIUM 16 mmol (4 g) over 20 min and then 1 g/h for 24 h in addition to LORAZEPAM and get obstetric help. If seizures continue then load with anticonvulsant. Choice will depend if patient already taking anti-epilepsy drug. Neurology consult.

15.12 Cardiac disease in pregnancy

- **About:** pregnancy is a cardiac stress test with increased cardiac output at week 20. Therefore subclinical cardiac disease, e.g. rheumatic mitral stenosis may present acutely. Main issue nowadays is maternal congenital heart disease especially in those with Eisenmenger's syndrome. There is a drop in SVR with pregnancy so in those with R–L shunts this favours increased right to left shunting and so reduced pulmonary oxygenation of blood which can worsen cyanosis and hypoxia.
- **Management:** LMWH in those at enhanced risk of VTE. The optimal delivery is vaginal with appropriate anaesthetic support and low dose epidural. Oxytocin is generally avoided. General postpartum complications are badly tolerated in those with Eisenmenger's. Those with murmurs or known cardiac disease must be managed during pregnancy by specialists.

15.13 Inflammatory bowel disease and pregnancy

- **About:** IBD if inactive does not affect fertility. Complications such as fetal loss and infertility are seen in active disease. Good effective treatment is therefore important. IBD should be well controlled prior to trying for pregnancy.
- **Drugs:** aminosalicylates, steroids and azathioprine may be used and do not affect conception or pregnancy. Methotrexate is contraindicated at conception in both partners and in pregnancy. Mycophenolate and ciclosporin are also avoided.

16 Oncological emergencies

16.1 Malignancy-related hypercalcaemia

- **About:** causes polyuria and dehydration and delirium. Seen in 10–20% of all adults with cancer. Also see ▶Section 5.5.
- **Causes:** solid tumours, such as lung or breast cancer tumours. Multiple myeloma and other haematological malignancies.
- **Aetiology: PTH-related peptide** increases renal calcium reabsorption. Humoral hypercalcaemia due to circulating tumour secreted factors. Osteolytic hypercalcaemia due to primary or secondary bone lesions.
- **Clinical:** severe dehydration, bone pain, anorexia, N&V. Signs of underlying malignancy.
- **Investigations:** FBC, ↑urea, ↑creatinine, ↑Ca, PTH, PTH-related peptide, CXR. Serum immunoglobulins, Bence–Jones protein, skeletal survey.
- **Management:** palliate selected patients. If severe, rehydrate with 3–6 L NS over 24 h. Close watch on renal function and level of calcium and cardiac status. Once rehydrated repeat calcium and consider renal function before PAMIDRONATE 30–90 mg IV or ZOLEDRONATE 4 mg IV infusion over 15 min. Also see Hypercalcaemia, ▶Section 5.5 for further detail.

16.2 Tumour lysis syndrome

- **About:** seen with treatment of chemosensitive malignancies and death of neoplastic cells. Potential AKI, seizures and arrhythmias.
- **Aetiology:** seen with bulky tumours, high turnover, chemosensitive. Cell death causes ↑↑LDH, ↑uric acid, pre-chemotherapy or impaired renal function.
- **Chemotherapy for malignancies:** acute leukaemias (ALL, AML, APML, CLL/CML with blast crisis). High-grade non-Hodgkin lymphomas, Burkitt's lymphoma. Breast cancer, small cell lung cancer, sarcomas.
- **Clinical:** vague, lethargy, N&V. Carpopedal spasm (low Ca), seizure, arrhythmias (high K).
- **Investigations:** FBC: watch Hb, WCC and platelets. U&E: AKI, ↑urea, ↑creatinine. Cell lysis: ↑uric acid, ↑LDH, ↑phosphate, ↑K and low Ca. ↑CRP: increase can suggest infection/inflammation/malignancy. ECG and telemetry to detect effects of high K. ↑lactate, ABG: ↑anion gap metabolic acidosis. Coagulation screen: rarely a coagulopathy can develop such as DIC.
- **Management:** prevent with hydration with IV fluids if needed. Central line if needed (4–5 L per day). Cardiac monitoring for ↑K. Standard replacement for K/Ca/Mg. Monitoring bloods 2–3 times daily for 48–72 h after chemotherapy initiation. Hyperuricaemia: ALLOPURINOL 300 mg 8 h (reduce if CKD/AKI) started prior to treatment or RASBURICASE. Some patients with renal impairment may need to be on dialysis prior to the initiation of therapy. Urinary alkalinisation with NaHCO₃ to maintain a urine pH >7.0 can help clearance of uric acid.

16.3 Hyperviscosity syndrome

- **About:** increased plasma viscosity due to increased cells (red and white cells) or large proteins, e.g. immunoglobulins.
- **Causes:** Waldenstrom's macroglobulinaemia, myeloma (increased IgM, IgA, IgG), immunoglobulin M (IgM) paraproteins. Leukaemias (WCC >100), myeloproliferative diseases, polycythaemia and thrombocytosis. Eisenmenger's syndrome.

- **Clinical:** visual disturbances, bleeding (GI bleeds, mucous membranes, epistaxis, retinal haemorrhage), neurological manifestations, e.g. stroke/TIA, vertigo and hearing loss.
- **Investigations:** FBC, U&Es, LFT, ESR, Ca. PPE: monoclonal band, urinary Bence–Jones protein. CT brain: if stroke/TIA, CXR: if breathless.
- **Management:** ABC, IV access and ensure well hydrated, treat infection. Treat the underlying condition. Acutely may consider phlebotomy with simultaneous infusion of isovolaemic fluid for RBC/WCC excess. **Plasma exchange** is the gold standard treatment.

16.4 Brain tumour

- **About:** primary or secondary. Variation in behaviour – some benign, others grow slowly over years, some very rapid. Histology can help plan treatment.
- **Causes:** primary: usually single (primary CNS lymphoma often multifocal). Metastatic: single or multiple (10 times commoner than primary). Most are intradural. Leptomeningeal disease with adenocarcinomas.
- **Risk: primary brain:** radiation, HIV/AIDS, genetics – von Hippel–Lindau disease, tuberous sclerosis, Li–Fraumeni syndrome, and neurofibromatosis. **Secondary:** smoker and lung cancer, breast lumps, skin melanoma, renal mass, haematuria, etc.
- **Differential:** stroke (ischaemic and haemorrhagic), abscess, inflammatory, infection, PML.
- **Clinical:** seizures, morning headache, vomiting, ↑ICP, papilloedema, cognitive, behavioural changes. Focal neurology dependent on site, e.g. weakness, cerebellar signs, hemianopia, personality change. May present as stroke, e.g. with subcortical hypodensity or with a haemorrhage. Leptomeningeal spread more insidious with cranial nerve palsies, headache.
- **Signs of an extracranial primary malignancy:** lung: weight loss, cough, hoarseness, Horner's syndrome. Breast lump, Paget's disease of nipple, localised nodes. Testicular mass. Haematuria, renal mass: renal cell tumour. Anaemia: gastrointestinal primary. Skin pigmentation: look for melanoma.
- **Investigations: bloods:** FBC: anaemia from gut malignancy. U&E, LFT, Ca, ALP: liver metastases. **CT brain + contrast:** usually a well demarcated hypodense lesion which enhances with ring appearance often sited at grey–white matter border, or even within the dura, with associated vasogenic oedema. In adults most are in the cerebral hemispheres with a minority in the posterior fossa. Look for hydrocephalus. Melanomas, renal cell carcinomas, lung tumours and choriocarcinomas and anticoagulated tend to bleed. **MRI head with gadolinium:** FLAIR, T1 and T2 with contrast can confirm lesion. **CXR:** lung tumour or lung metastases. **CT chest abdomen pelvis** for primary malignancy. **PET scan:** specialist use only. **Brain biopsy:** to confirm histology at open craniotomy or CT-guided stereotactic techniques. **LP:** generally avoided especially with a large SOL and oedema and risk of brain herniation.
- **Metastatic tumours** (64/100 000 pa): lung cancer, renal cell cancer, colonic tumour. Melanoma, breast cancer, testicular tumours/choriocarcinoma.
- **Primary tumours** (10 per 100 000 per year): **gliomas:** Grade IV: glioblastoma multiforme is aggressive (high grade), Grade III: anaplastic astrocytomas (high grade), Grade II: astrocytoma, Grade I: pilocytic. Oligodendrogliomas: anaplastic oligodendroglioma (high grade). **Ependymal:** lining of ventricles: anaplastic ependymoma (high grade). **Others:** medulloblastomas (posterior fossa in children), meningiomas (falx, sphenoid, skull base, resection usual), pituitary tumours, craniopharyngiomas, vestibular schwannomas, CNS lymphoma: HIV, deep in brain, cause seizures, multiple.

- **Management:** will depend on age, morbidities and underlying health status as well as the nature of the tumour, its size and its responsiveness to surgery or radiotherapy and patient choice. Determine primary if possible – for some metastatic tumours the primary is elusive.
- **Steroids:** symptoms of ↑ICP and oedema – usually DEXAMETHASONE 10 mg IV stat or po depending on symptoms. Then a dose per day of 4–24 mg usually in divided doses depending on extent of oedema and symptoms. Lower doses may be equally effective as higher. Start with 4 mg TDS IV/PO. Don't give doses after 5 pm as will cause insomnia. The only exception is where primary brain lymphoma is suspected when it is preferable to do a brain biopsy first. If falling GCS: consider IV MANNITOL. ▶ Section 11.4.
- **Acute obstructive hydrocephalus.** Discuss with neurosurgeons for external ventricular drainage. Mannitol if decompensating.
- **Seizures:** consider starting PHENYTOIN OD or IV if needed if there has been any seizure-like activity.
- **Surgery:** removal of a solitary metastasis may be superior to radiation/steroids alone.
- **Management: referral to a neuro-oncology MDT:** oncology, neuroradiologists, neurosurgeons, palliative care and specialist nurses.
- **Surgery:** some tumours can be removed and cured or survival improved, e.g. meningioma, pituitary, solitary lesions. More difficult if brainstem or language or sensorimotor areas or basal ganglia. Palliative surgical resection or debulking of the primary or secondary tumour.
- **Whole Brain Radiotherapy:** 30 Gy in 10 fractions in 2 weeks. Usually for low grade tumours. But no improved survival; causes cognitive decline.
- **Chemotherapy:** possibly useful, e.g. primary cerebral lymphoma or small cell lung cancer, non-Hodgkin's lymphoma and germ cell tumours. Maybe combined with radiotherapy. Median prognosis is 6 months and depends on primary.

16.5 Neutropenic sepsis

- **About:** temp >38°C for 1 h or single reading >38.5°C with signs or symptoms of sepsis + neutrophil count <0.5 × 10⁹/L. Mortality increases significantly once neutrophil count <0.5–1.0 × 10⁹/L. Those on steroids/immunosuppression and the elderly may not mount a febrile response.
- **Microbiology:** Gram +ve infections via indwelling lines. Invasive *Aspergillus* and *Candida* infections. Gram –ve sepsis from enteric organisms as well.
- **Causes of neutropenia:** bone marrow suppression 1–2 weeks post chemotherapy would be commonest. Carbimazole or propylthiouracil cause agranulocytosis, infection. Idiosyncratic drug reaction (check all new drugs): azathioprine and allopurinol. Malignant bone marrow infiltration, SLE, RA, splenic sequestration. Benign ethnic neutropenia is seen in those of African and Middle Eastern descent.
- **Clinical:** care because may be septic but no fever. Usually temp >37.5°C, diarrhoea, malaise. Sore throat, cough, sputum, dysuria, ↓BP, ↑HR, oliguria, rigors after flushing a central line. Inspect mouth, skin and perineum for infection. Defer rectal examination until antibiotics given. Look for other infections, e.g. herpes zoster. Look for tenderness or erythema around cannula/central line sites. Chronic neutropenia causes chronic sinusitis and mouth ulcers.
- **Investigations:** FBC, blood film, U&Es, LFTs and ESR, CRP. Lactate. Urine dipstick and culture. Culture Hickman lines, blood, urine, sputum, stool. Baseline CXR in all especially if any chest signs or symptoms. Additional: folate, B12, iron and ferritin, LFTs, ANA and anti-dsDNA antibodies and rheumatoid factor and TFTs. CT chest/abdomen and pelvis or USS: abdominal candidiasis and other infections. Viral infection suspected: HSV or VZV – send glass slide touched against opened lesion

and allowed to air dry. Transport in a slide carrier (vesicular skin lesion kit). Swabs and blood for viral PCR and send serum (clotted blood) for IgG and IgM. Send EDTA blood for CMV PCR. Fungal infection suspected: EDTA blood for *Aspergillus* and *Candida* PCR.

Management

- **ABC** and high flow O₂ if shocked and resuscitate as for sepsis. Start IV fluids. Isolate and reverse barrier nursing and good handwashing. If patient completely well then observe and take blood cultures. Manage sepsis (▶Section 2.21). Do not remove central venous access devices as part of the initial empiric management of suspected neutropenic sepsis – take advice.
- **Give O₂ as per BTS guidelines.** ABG if hypoxic. Adhere to local policies. Liaise with microbiologist/haematologist/oncologist. Different groups to consider in terms of risk. Guidance here refers to highest risk group who are immunocompromised, neutropenic and possibly septic. Temperature control with tepid sponging and PARACETAMOL 1 g PO 6 h or NSAIDs can be used (check renal function).
- **Antimicrobials:** give TAZOCIN 4.5 g 8 h IV to all patients with unresponsive fever unless alternative cause of fever is likely. Some give GENTAMICIN 5 mg/kg OD only if fever persists, others give it first line with Tazocin. Take local advice. Reassess at 48 h and switch to oral antibiotics if better. Consider stopping antibiotics after 3 days fever free if all markers show improvement and count >500/mm³. If fever persists and central line *in situ* add IV VANCOMYCIN 1–1.5 g 12 h for suspected line sepsis to cover MRSA or coagulase-negative staphylococcal sepsis. Penicillin allergy consider MEROPENEM 1 g 8 h. Low risk patients may get CIPROFLOXACIN 750 mg 12 h OR CO-AMOXICLAV 625 mg 8 h. Take ongoing specialist advice. Persisting symptoms may lead to consideration of AMPHOTERICIN IV based on microbiological advice. Consider CO-TRIMOXAZOLE if pneumocystis considered. Oral ACICLOVIR and oral FLUCONAZOLE for prophylaxis may be indicated depending on local policies. If there is evidence of active HSV or VZV infection then give ACICLOVIR 5 mg/kg 8 h IV for HSV and 10 mg/kg 8 h IV for VZV infection.
- **Colony stimulating growth factors** (G-CSF, GM-CSF) may be considered in cytotoxic therapy induced neutropenia. Discuss with haematologist.
- **Autoimmune neutropenia** may require steroids, high dose IVIg and G-CSF – arrange urgent haematological assessment.

Reference: NICE (2012) CG151: Neutropenic sepsis.

16.6 Malignant superior vena caval obstruction

- **Malignant causes:** lung cancer, metastases, lymphoma, testicular, breast, thrombosis from malignancy.
- **Non-malignant causes:** mediastinal fibrosis: histoplasmosis, TB, sarcoid. Thrombosis: central line/pacemaker/AICD leads. Compression from thoracic aortic aneurysms. Behçet's syndrome, fibrosis from radiation.
- **Clinical:** breathless, oedema of face and neck, headache and sensation of fullness. Cough, haemoptysis, weight loss, dilated veins in upper chest and neck. Horner's syndrome, effusion, clubbing, hoarseness. Phrenic nerve palsy with raised hemidiaphragm. Lymphadenopathy, testicular mass, hepatosplenomegaly. Cerebral or laryngeal oedema suggests a poor prognosis. ↑SVC pressure can even lead to oesophageal varices and bleeding. Pemberton's sign: high mediastinal mass which plugs off the thoracic outlet when arms raised above head for 1 minute – facial flushing, engorged veins, stridor, ↑JVP.
- **Investigations:** FBC, U&Es, LFT, ESR, CRP, Ca, CXR: tumour mass, hilar lymphadenopathy, fibrosis, TB. CT +/– biopsy chest, bronchoscopy, sputum cytology, staging and biopsies.

- **Management** ABC, O_2 as per BTS guidelines. Airways management, remove central venous lines if cause. Steroids: if malignancy consider DEXAMETHASONE 8 mg stat PO then 4 mg PO qds. Exception would be where lymphoma suspected where haematology advice should be taken first. Consider PPI, e.g. LANSOPRAZOLE. Diuretics: have been given for malignant causes unresponsive to other options. Endovascular stenting indicated for an extrinsic compressive cause and this also helps non-malignant/fibrotic causes. The rare downside of stenting is that the sudden improved venous return can lead to pulmonary oedema. Anticoagulation: may need anticoagulation at least for VTE prophylaxis. Full anticoagulation if the obstruction is thrombotic. Radiotherapy: may be considered for sensitive tumours. Chemotherapy: for chemosensitive tumours, e.g. small cell lung cancer or lymphoma.

16.7 Severe nausea and vomiting

- **About:** may be single cause or multifactorial.
- **Causes to screen for:** constipation/bowel obstruction, dehydration and uraemia – check output, opiates, chemotherapy (what drug, when taken), radiotherapy, brain tumour and ↑ICP, oesophageal obstruction, gastric outlet obstruction.
- **Investigations:** FBC, U&E, amylase, Ca, CT head where indicated, erect CXR, AXR/CT if obstruction considered.
- **Management:** IV fluids, rehydration. Record strict I/O and consider weighing. Hold any chemotherapy/biological therapies until senior advice taken.
- **Consider an antiemetic:** ONDANSETRON 8 mg PO/IV BD (needs laxative), CYCLIZINE 150 mg/day via a syringe driver. Others – DEXAMETHASONE 4–8 mg PO BD IV dose *Others:* HALOPERIDOL 1–2 mg PO TDS/QDS, LORAZEPAM 0.5 mg S/L maximum 2 mg in 24 h.

16.8 Malignant spinal cord compression

- **About:** malignant compression of the contents of the dural sac (spinal cord or cauda equina). Back pain seen in 90% with known malignancy warrants urgent investigations. 5% of lethal malignancies show signs of spinal cord compression.
- **Aetiology:** there is little space for lesions lying in the canal to expand without compressing neural structures. Malignant usually extradural cord compression compromises vascular supply to the cord. Tumour, usually within the vertebral body, enlarges. Compression results in oedema, venous congestion, and demyelination. Cord ends L1, cauda below. Cord is UMN, cauda is LMN.
- **Levels:** 70% thoracic, 20% lumbosacral and 10% cervical.
- **Cancers:** lung, prostate, breast, renal cell, myeloma, colorectal, lymphoma. Primary tumours: ependymomas, astrocytomas, haemangioblastomas.
- **Clinical:** may have a known malignancy or this may be the presentation. Progressive worsening back pain, paralysis, sensory loss and sphincter dysfunction. Localised tenderness can help localise lesion, radicular pain. Tone flaccid initially. If cord then tone increases + spasticity, extensor plantars and sensory level. Up-going plantar reflex suggests significant cord compression. **Cauda equina damage:** saddle anaesthesia, loss of sphincters, lax anal tone with asymmetrical or bilateral LMN leg weakness. Electric shock sensation (L'hermitte's sign) with flexion suggests cord involvement.
- **Investigation:** bloods: FBC, U&Es, ESR, Ca, PSA, CRP, CXR, myeloma screen. MRI scan of entire spine +/– gadolinium: 25% have multiple lesions. If MRI not available or contraindicated then obtain plain films and discuss CT imaging. Abdominal CT: to help find primary if unknown. Histology: if unknown cancer then obtaining histology is of paramount importance. Plain films may show bony changes, e.g.

'erosion of pedicle', 'bone lesions'. Bladder scan: retention >150 ml may suggest neurological damage.

- **Management** (liaise quickly and closely with oncology, radiology and spinal surgery teams): until stability of spine known, patient should lie flat with neutral spine alignment. 'Log rolling' when required for pressure relief and toileting. Manage pain, catheterise if urinary retention. Malignant spinal cord compression median survival is now 6 months. Discuss with oncology/haem/surgeons. Urgent imaging if neurological signs. May need surgery or radiotherapy. DEXAMETHASONE 16 mg IV/PO daily in divided dose until treated then reduce (hold steroids until biopsy taken if significant suspicion of lymphoma and discuss urgently with haematology). A PPI is given with steroids for gastroprotection, e.g. LANSOPRAZOLE. Consider referral to local spinal surgery team: surgery may be considered if single compressive lesion, unknown primary or other areas to biopsy, radio-resistant tumour, progressions despite radiotherapy, bone compression or vertebral collapse in patient with good performance status. If there are none of these but there are spinal metastases then radiation without surgery should be considered. Emergency radiotherapy (same day) for those with radiosensitive tumours such as lymphoma, myeloma, small cell lung cancer, seminoma, neuroblastoma and Ewing's sarcoma. If a patient has complete paraplegia with loss of sphincter control for more than 48 h, radiotherapy is unlikely to improve neurological function but can palliate pain, e.g. in breast, prostate, myeloma. This may not be given same day. Benefits may take weeks. Surgeons prefer not to operate post radiotherapy as wound healing impaired. Ongoing: review steroid dose and side effects. Review pain control, need for a catheter (if appropriate). VTE prophylaxis, mood, nutrition, palliation, etc.

17 Miscellaneous emergencies

17.1 Abnormal gaits

Walking a patient is an excellent test of neurological, cardiorespiratory and locomotor systems as well as cognition, vision and safety. Getting patients up to both examine and assess their ability and their safety for discharge is a key tool in acute medicine. Done on the post take round it can shorten length of stay. It starts rehab.

Gait description

- **Hemiplegic:** flexed arm, extended straight leg. circumduction gait.
- **Spastic diplegia:** scissors type walking. Increased tone. Seen with MS, cerebral palsy.
- **Proximal myopathy:** waddling gait. Movement initiated by trunk to swing leg forward.
- **Parkinsonism:** flexed slow hesitant freezing gait. No arm movement. Associated signs.
- **Cerebellar:** unsteady ataxic usually worse on one side unless central lesion. Nystagmus and other signs.
- **Dorsal column:** high stepping foot slapping. Falls with eyes closed. Sensory neuropathy.
- **Foot drop:** has to lift foot higher, may rotate pelvis.
- **Dyspraxic:** slow, small steps, unsteady. Small vessel stroke disease.
- **Antalgic:** painful slow usually hip pain.

17.2 Falls with no altered consciousness

Wards have policies to reduce falls – ensure these are in place and being adhered to. Most are reported on Datix for audit. The most effective fall prevention strategies involve multidisciplinary interventions targeting identified risk factors.

- The price of our bipedal upright posture is the risk of falls. A fall is defined as inadvertently coming to rest on the ground or other lower level without loss of consciousness (otherwise the issue is syncope) and other than as a consequence of sudden onset of paralysis, epileptic seizure, excess alcohol intake. The diagnosis may be masked if there is a head injury and amnesia post fall. Try to get as much information and witness statements. It may be due to walking on an uneven surface, slips on snow and ice or trips on a rug or the cat. A patient letting themselves slowly to the ground is a fall. Falls without syncope can be for a variety of reasons: awareness and some degree of self-protection are intact so injuries may be less severe. Causes are usually related to poor gait be they musculoskeletal or neurological or sensory – neuropathy or blindness as well as medication and acute illnesses, e.g. UTI and most are often multifactorial. Frequent fallers are those with 2 or more in a 6-month period.
- We can prevent falls by simply not allowing patients to walk, but the immobility and cost in terms of reduced independence and function and quality of life is very high. We need to aim to prevent falls and learn to reduce falls risk (it can never be eliminated) where possible. Anyone can fall but in most cases it is the frail elderly and so is a well-developed geriatric specialty. The risk of falls can cause huge loss of confidence and fear of mobilisation which can be doubly disabling. Falls themselves can cause significant trauma especially fractures, e.g. neck of femur, wrist, forearm, vertebral, femur, pelvis, humerus as well as head injury and SDH and even ruptured spleens. Post fall all patients need a top to toe trauma assessment and radiology/ CT head where fractures or head injury suspected. May need to involve trauma and orthopaedics team.

- Taking referral/answering bleep: how is the patient now? Observations? Why and how did the fall happen? Any head or other injury? If so, what is GCS? Any bony pain: hip, back pain, wrist, etc.? What were the events of fall: ↓? BP, chest pain, breathless, confusion?

On arrival

- **Review all information:** see GP, ambulance and ED notes, review observations and medication. Mechanical fall, i.e. simple trip with clear consciousness. Medical fall – patient unwell or presyncopal or faint or hypoglycaemia or confused prior? Assess any obvious injury: fracture or head injury and arrange imaging as needed. Colles fractures suggest consciousness and outstretched hand. Analgesia and orthopaedic review for fracture. CT head if any persisting neurology. General examination especially for low BP. Neurological observations if head injury or seizure occurred. Document findings – anticoagulants increase risk of SDH and haematomas. ECG and telemetry and regular observations best on CCU if any suggestion of arrhythmia or vascular cause.

- **Secondary trauma:** exclude SDH, ICH, ruptured spleen, fractures. Non-displaced hip fracture may be missed and not all have classical leg shortening and external rotation. Repeat exams may be needed. Pain may not be noted until attempts to mobilise. Initial trauma surveys can miss things so have a low threshold to repeat examination and imaging if there is evidence or suspicion of possible problems. Do not get distracted by the secondary trauma and so forget about the primary cause of syncope. Special attention to those needing frequent toileting and those with delirium.

- **Practical environmental steps to reducing falls risk.** Frames surrounding toilets and raised toilet seats. Availability of chairs of varying heights to suit patients with different heights. Access to walking aids out of hours to ensure safe mobility and transfers. Chair raisers to suit the height of patients. Supply of approved slippers for patients. Bars along walls to assist and support those patients who are frail in walking independently. Access to appropriate bed rails to support patients who may be at risk of rolling or slipping out of bed.

- **Needs therapy assessment:** occupational therapy and physiotherapy can often do a comprehensive assessment of footwear, gait, safety awareness, home environment and help give a plan to reduce falls risk. For some, rehabilitation may help and nutrition is important in others. Loss of muscle bulk can be helped with enrolling in exercise programmes incorporating gait and balance training. Others may need walking aids and other devices to reduce risk. Syncope inducing medications stopped. Those at risk of fractures with osteoporosis may be started on Bisphosphonate + Calcium and Vitamin D. Other issues may be correcting vision, e.g. cataract removal or new glasses may help or avoid wearing wrong glasses when doing stairs. A very holistic and forensic approach is needed. A home visit may help to identify and manage hazards and risks. Stairs are risky – consider additional stair rail, assisted supervised usage, stairlift or downstairs living.

- **Long term:** may consider referral to localised falls clinic. Discussing falls risk realistically with patient and family key. For those with possible syncope further tests such as tilt table or telemetry may be considered. Pacing may be helpful with cardioinhibitory syncope.

17.3 Fat embolism

- **About:** consider if recent fracture with sudden dyspnoea (may not be a PE). A skin rash or new neurology. Consider in sickling crisis chest syndrome.
- **Aetiology:** fat enters the venous circulation and passes into the systemic circulation. Results in vascular occlusion and release of inflammatory mediators. Fat

from marrow from long bone (femur usually) or pelvis fractures. Also lipid infusions, recent steroid administration.

- **Causes:** blunt trauma, bone fractures, acute pancreatitis, and sickle cell crisis. Decompression sickness. Parenteral lipid infusion.
- **Clinical:** acute dyspnoea, ↑HR, febrile. Type 1 RF, petechiae, confusion, delirium. Coma, retinal haemorrhages with fatty lesions.
- **Investigations:** FBC: ↓platelets, Hb and fibrinogen. Urinalysis: fat globules in the urine are common after trauma. CXR: infiltrates. ABG: hypoxia and Type 1 RF. U&E: AKI. CT chest: ARDS picture, infiltrates. CT head: diffuse white-matter petechial haemorrhages.
- **Management:** ABC and give O_2 as per BTS guidelines. Supportive, oxygenation, circulatory support.

17.4 Air embolism

- **About:** air within the circulation results in obstructive shock.
- **Aetiology:** air sucked into negative pressure venous circulation above right atrium. Enters heart and with loss of pumping effectiveness and sudden death. Any operative procedure where the exposed site is >5 cm above right atrium.
- **Causes:** surgical procedures, e.g. neurosurgery or ENT where patients sit upright. Back street abortion – air accidentally injected into pelvic venous plexuses. Penetrating chest injuries with bronchopulmonary venous fistulae. Central venous catheterisation, especially with loss of connections.
- **Clinical:** most episodes are clinically silent or result in mild, transient ↓BP. Acute dyspnoea, chest pain, agitation or disorientation.
- **Investigations:** ABG: hypoxia, hypo/hypercarbia, respiratory and/or metabolic acidosis. **ECG:** ↑HR, ST / T changes of ischaemia. CXR: oligaemia.
- **Management:** give 100% O_2. Fluid resuscitation. Clamp/remove any central line entry point. Put patient head down and left lateral decubitus (on left side with head down) to trap the air in ventricle and not in right ventricular outflow tract.

17.5 Refeeding syndrome

- **About:** potential fatal metabolic consequence of rapidly providing calories enterally or parenterally to severely malnourished patients.
- **Physiology:** feeding leads cellular metabolism to switch from catabolism to anabolism. Insulin is released and causes glycogen, fat and protein synthesis and cellular uptake of potassium, phosphate, and magnesium as well as water causing ↓phosphate, ↓magnesium, ↓potassium.
- **At risk patients have one or more of the following:** BMI <16 kg/m², unintentional weight loss >15% in the past 3–6 months, little or no nutritional intake for >10 days, low levels of potassium, phosphate, or magnesium before feeding. Or the patient has two or more of the following: BMI <18.5, unintentional weight loss >10% in the past 3–6 months, little or no nutritional intake for >5 days, history of alcohol misuse or drugs, including insulin, chemotherapy, antacids, or diuretics.
- **Management:** refeeding should be started at a low level of energy replacement. Vitamin supplementation should also be started with refeeding and continued for at least 10 days. Bloods should be checked and dietetic input needed.

Reference: NICE (2006) CG32: Nutritional support for adults.

17.6 Accidental hypothermia

- **About:** drop in core body temp below 35°C. Elderly at highest risk. Core temperature <32°C is moderate, <28°C is severe. Ask why – did hypoxia or cardiac arrest precede hypothermia? With cardiac arrest do not stop resuscitation until patients are warm and 'dead'.

- **Aetiology:** body heat generated by basal metabolic rate and muscle activity. Heat lost to environment by conduction, convection and evaporation. Hypothalamus manages temperature. Core temperature set at 37 +/− 0.5°C. Peripheral vasoconstriction and shivering are normal response.
- **Risks:** falls, stroke, sepsis, confusion, hypothyroidism, patient with dementia and wandering. Alcohol, phenothiazines, immersion in water. Suicide attempt. Those found in cold water may do better than those in warm water.
- **Clinical:** mild ataxia, confusion and dehydration, ↓HR, ↓BP. AF common when temp <32°C. Confusion and lack of awareness so no attempt is made to reduce heat loss. Severe (<28°C) coma, absent pupillary responses and corneal reflex, cardiac standstill. Seen with stroke or falls patients incapacitated in a cold environment. Rectal probes inserted 15 cm but may be 0.5–1°C above core.
- **Investigation:** FBC: ↑haematocrit and ↑urea/creatinine from dehydration. U&E: ↑↑↑K >10 mmol/L is not associated with survival and is considered a marker of hypoxia before cooling. Lactate and pH less reliable. ↑Cardiac troponin if any ACS/MI. ECG: arrhythmias, e.g. CHB, AF, VT/VF, ectopics. The height of the Osborn/J wave is roughly proportional to the degree of hypothermia. **Arterial/venous blood gases:** ↓pH, ↓HCO$_3$, ↑lactate. TFT: ↑TSH, ↓T4 as hypothyroidism can cause hypothermia. Cortisol/short synacthen: low threshold for suspecting hypoadrenalism. **Amylase:** ↑ in pancreatitis which may be subclinical. Toxicology screen: overdose, e.g. opiate, benzodiazepine. Carboxyhaemoglobin: carbon monoxide poisoning. **CT head:** if comatose or focal neurology.
- **Differential:** stroke or any brain injury – consider urgent CT. (Intentional ?) drug overdose – alcohol, opiates, benzodiazepines, etc. Myxoedema coma, hypoglycaemia (▶Section 11.4 on page).
- **Management: ABCs and give O$_2$ as per BTS guidelines.** Consider urinary catheter to detect oliguria/anuria. Always use a low reading rectal thermometer. Axillary, tympanic and oral temperatures can all be misleading. Full monitoring and resuscitation facilities must be available as patient may develop VF and need defibrillation. Use warm blankets and warm drinks if able and not severe – beware excess vasodilation which can drop BP. Cardiac monitoring and repeated bloods in severe cases. **Get IV access** and give IV fluids warmed to 38–42°C and several litres of crystalloid may be needed due to cold diuresis and then vasodilation on warming which, if excessive with ↓BP, can be treated with VASOPRESSIN. Consider rarities of hypopituitary, hypoadrenalism and/or hypothyroidism. Consider IV HYDROCORTISONE, IV GLUCOSE/THIAMINE/NALOXONE.

Classification

- **Hypothermia I:** conscious, shivering, core 35–32°C – warm area, warm clothing, warm sweet drinks, and active movement where possible.
- **Hypothermia II:** impaired consciousness, not shivering, core <32–28°C. Needs cardiac monitoring, rest to avoid arrhythmias, horizontal position and immobilization, full-body insulation, active external and minimally invasive rewarming techniques (warm environment; chemical, electrical, or forced-air heating packs or blankets; warm parenteral fluids). IV NS warmed to 43.0°C. Warm peritoneal lavage and dialysis.
- **Hypothermia III:** unconscious, not shivering, vital signs present. Core <28–24°C. Hypothermia II + manage airway. Consider transferring to a centre that offers ECMO or cardiopulmonary bypass if there is cardiac instability that is refractory to medical management.
- **Hypothermia IV:** no vital signs. Core <24°C. Hypothermia II + III plus CPR and up to three doses of adrenaline (epinephrine) 1 mg IV or IO and defibrillation, with further dosing guided by clinical response; rewarming with ECMO or cardiopulmonary

bypass (if available) or CPR with active external and alternative internal rewarming. Mechanical chest compression device may be used as resuscitation can be prolonged. Hypothermic patients in cardiac arrest should be resuscitated until they have a normal core temperature >32°C. Central line insertion should be cautious as arrhythmias occur easily.

Reference: Brown *et al.* (2012) Accidental hypothermia. *N Engl J Med*, 367:1930.

17.7 Malignant hyperpyrexia

- **About:** previous uneventful anaesthesia does not preclude malignant hyperpyrexia. Usually precipitated by drugs in those genetically susceptible.
- **Aetiology:** autosomal dominant 1 in 20 000. Genetic defect, e.g. ryanodine receptor on 19q13. Rises in cell calcium causes rigidity and rhabdomyolysis.
- **Causes:** all inhalational agents except nitrous oxide: Halothane, Methoxyflurane, Suxamethonium.
- **Clinical:** onset within 1 h of drug administration. Masseter muscle spasm an early sign. Hyperpyrexia >40°C, ↑HR, muscle stiffness. Monitoring: elevation of end-tidal CO_2 is early, sensitive and specific sign of malignant hyperpyrexia.
- **Investigation:** FBC: ↑WCC. ↑Glucose possible. Coagulation: monitor for DIC. U&E: ↑K. AKI from dehydration or myoglobinuria, ↑CK, phosphate. Watch for complications: AKI due to rhabdomyolysis, arrhythmias, ↑K. ABG: ↑lactic acidosis.
- **Management:** ABC, high FiO_2 initially and then O_2 as per BTS guidelines and reassess after ABG. Telemetry for ↑K. Try cooling and allow heat loss. Tepid sponging, fans, avoid paracetamol/salicylates. Genetic counselling as familial. Acute anaesthetic management: stop causative drug immediately and stop surgery if possible. Do not waste time securing another anaesthetic machine, use an Ambu bag and an O_2 cylinder initially. Hyperventilate the patient with 100% O_2 at 10 L/min via a clean breathing circuit. Otherwise maintain anaesthesia with IV agents such as propofol until surgery is completed. Cooling management – cool IV fluids and ice packs. DANTROLENE 1 mg/kg bolus then repeat doses of 1 mg/kg (max 10 mg/kg) until the HR, rise in CO_2 production and pyrexia start to subside.

17.8 Acute rhabdomyolysis

- **About:** muscle damage can lead to AKI. Damage to striated muscle can lead to myoglobinuria. Plasma myoglobin levels exceed protein binding. Precipitates in the tubules can lead to AKI, renal vasoconstriction and direct nephrotoxicity.
- **Causes:** trauma/crush injuries, high voltage electrical injury, near drowning. Falls and lying on floor for prolonged periods, severe exercise. Neuroleptic malignant syndrome (NMS), malignant hyperthermia. Cocaine/heroin use, amphetamines, ketamine, LSD. Generalised seizures, alcohol, methanol, ethylene glycol, carbon monoxide. Ischaemic limb with muscle necrosis, polymyositis, viral myositis – influenza. HIV, Coxsackie, echovirus, statins +/– fibrates, hypo-/hyperthyroidism. Snake bites with action of phospholipases, compartment syndrome. Muscle genetic disorders – carnitine deficiency, caffeine, aspirin. Low K, hypophosphataemia, diabetic ketoacidosis and HHS. Sepsis with bacterial infections, MI or myocarditis can raise CKMB.
- **Clinical:** muscle pain and weakness. Muscles hard and tender especially when crush injury. Dark urine – burgundy coloured or dark tea. Cause may be apparent, e.g. trauma. Evidence of trauma or falls or prolonged immobility. Family history might suggest genetic cause. Drug history – neuroleptics. Fever, increased tone, neuroleptic malignant syndrome.
- **Investigations:** FBC: ↑WCC. U&E: ↑urea, ↑creatinine. Tissue damage: ↑K, ↑CK, ↑urate, ↑myoglobin, phosphate, myoglobinuria. ABG: metabolic acidosis. Coagulation

screen: DIC. MRI detects muscle damage. ECG and ↑cardiac troponin if myocardial injury suspected.

- **Complications:** ↑↑K, hypovolaemic shock, AKI. DIC, sepsis, death.
- **Management:** supportive, ABCs, IV fluids, watch and treat high K. Risk of AKI low if CK <15 000–20 000 units/L. CK >60 000 units/L is predictive of AKI and death. **Early hydration** (even prior to hospitalisation) with NS. Goal is a good diuresis (200–300 ml/h). Carefully monitor for fluid overload, particularly in elderly/ CCF. FUROSEMIDE can enhance diuresis if overloaded. **Alkalinisation of urine:** enhances myoglobin solubility. Target urine pH >6.5 with IV NaHCO$_3$ where CK >6000. Consider **dialysis** in AKI or refractory hyperkalaemia or fluid overload. MANNITOL 200 ml of 20% (20 g/100 ml) IV over 30–60 min and can be repeated to enhance diuresis, renal vasodilator and free radical scavenger. **Treat DIC** with FFP, cryoprecipitate, and platelet transfusions. BROMOCRIPTINE or DANTROLENE in the case of neuroleptic malignant syndrome. **Fasciotomy** for any compartment syndrome. Revascularisation for limb ischaemia.

17.9   Painful leg

- **Taking referral/answering bleep:** painful since when? Was there trauma or fall? Is patient mobile on it? Any redness, shortened and externally rotated? Pyrexia? Normal observations? Why is patient in hospital? Anticoagulants – ?haematoma.

Differentials

- **Trauma – soft tissue injury – bruising and swelling.** Rest, ice, elevate. Severe trauma can cause rhabdomyolysis and compartment syndrome. Follow appropriate criteria, e.g. Ottawa guidance for ankle pain. Bony tenderness should warrant suspicion if fracture. Experience in older patient is to reasonably assume any patient with leg pain warrants exclusion of pelvic/hip fracture or long bone fracture as clinical signs can be reduced and difficult in confused/dementia patients.
- **Deep vein thrombosis:** warm, dilated veins, swollen, calf tender, ↑D-dimers. Important diagnosis as can rapidly kill if missed and untreated. If suspected begin treatment immediately.
- **Compartment syndrome:** post trauma or fracture or ischaemic limb needs fasciotomy. Distal ischaemia and reduced pulses. Surgical emergency.
- **Haematoma:** trauma +/− excessive anticoagulants and muscle haematoma. Check clotting. Reverse warfarin or stop heparin or manage bleeding disorder.
- **Inflammation:** acute gout or pseudogout or septic arthritis: red-hot joint with effusion. Aspirate joint.
- **Osteomyelitis:** acute or chronic bony pain, sickle cell. May be associated soft tissue infection, e.g. diabetic foot. Sciatica – pain radiating down leg corresponding to disc lesion. Limited straight leg raising.
- **Cellulitis:** usually a newly warm red tender leg starting distally and moving proximally. Bilateral cellulitis should make one question diagnosis. Florid red legs may be chronic and cool to the touch. Check for diabetes and skin infection entry points. Emollients for dry skin. Antibiotics for confirmed cellulitis.
- **Rheumatoid arthritis:** can affect the knee as a tender warm joint with synovial thickening and may have an effusion. Rarely acutely inflamed. Patient has clinical features of rheumatoid arthritis. Check ESR/CRP and serology. Must aspirate knee if joint sepsis suspected.
- **Lymphoedema:** unilateral swollen leg may be painful. Look for evidence of malignancy if new. Check nodes at groin. Pyoderma gangrenosum – may be seen with bowel disease and presents as a painful non-healing violaceous rash with ulceration. Needs management of underlying condition. Dermatological referral.
- **Necrotising fasciitis:** hard woody feeling, intense pain, gas bubbles below skin, margin which is moving. Needs urgent surgery.

- **Acute ischaemic limb:** mottled, pale, painful, pulseless, perishing with cold. A vascular emergency.
- **Paget's Disease:** Bone pain, warm, deformed. Older males. Raised ALP. Plain X-ray changes. Bone scan increased uptake. Consider new Bisphosphonates.
- **On arrival:** check general observations, EWS and review notes. Examine legs: front and back for tenderness, red – possible cellulitis. Tender muscles: suspect rhabdomyolysis – check CK and statin usage or other causes. Recent trauma/ischaemia and pain – compartment syndrome which will need urgent surgical decompression. Recent fall – even something trivial can cause a fracture. Fractured neck of femurs have few signs if undisplaced. Check for pubic bone fracture. Any doubts X-ray. Acute gout can cause a painful large toe – check urate. Tender erythematous. Calf – always consider DVT and D-dimer may help, but may need USS leg veins. Start LMWH treatment whilst you get doppler if DVT suspected.

17.10 Acute limb ischaemia

- **About:** early action may preserve life and limb, either thrombotic occlusion or embolic. May be acute on chronic background of limb ischaemia. Rarely severe venous thrombosis can lead to ischaemia.
- **Clinical:** limb is pale, painful, pulseless, paraesthesia, perishing with cold. May be background of shortening claudication distance. Leriche syndrome with associated buttock pain and impotence. Often co-existing vasculopathies – stroke, TIA, MI.
- **Aetiology: local atherosclerotic stenosis:** HTN, smoking, diabetes, male, age, cholesterol. **Embolic** AF is a common embolic source. On heparin? HITT must not be missed – check for falling platelets. LV thrombus from MI, cardiac murmurs, aortic aneurysm. Young heavy smokers consider Buerger's disease. Rare also arteritis.
- **Investigation:** FBC: WCC, platelets (↓platelets with HITT). Coagulation screen. U&E: AKI, hyperkalaemia, glucose, troponin. CXR: cardiomegaly. ECG: AF, MI. Doppler ultrasound: can give evidence of flow and flow rates. Angiography: evidence of thrombus.
- **Ankle/brachial BP:** ABPI 0.6–0.9 with claudication. Resting ischaemia with ABPI 0.3–0.6. Tissue loss if <0.3.
- **Management: vascular surgical emergency.** Refer quickly and meantime **ABC**, oxygen as per BTS guidelines and reassess after ABG. Get IV access and start 1 L NS. **Analgesia:** MORPHINE 5–10 mg IV + CYCLIZINE 50 mg IV. Watch for respiratory depression. **Senior vascular surgical review:** mottled white leg with skin petechiae with hard painful muscles is beyond salvage and may need amputation or palliation. Consider co-morbidities. An acute white cold leg without advanced changes then vascular surgeons need to decide whether to preserve the limb or not. Active treatment which can be angiography initially with plan for thrombolysis, embolectomy or angioplasty, or even arterial bypass. **Heparinisation/thrombolysis/embolectomy:** consider heparin 5000 units IV bolus and then 1000 units/h with APTT 2–2.5. Embolectomy can be done under local anaesthesia. Compartment syndrome may require fasciotomies to be done. Warfarin should be considered post-operatively.
- **Long term:** smoking prevention, control vascular risks.
- **Amputation** finally is indicated if all options are futile. Must be done at a level high/proximal enough to allow for stump healing to sustain a prosthesis.
- **Sympathectomy:** in some cases consider percutaneous lumbar sympathectomy which requires CT guidance.
- **Gabapentin for ongoing pain can be helpful.**
- Rare cases of leg ischaemia due to **severe venous thrombosis** can be treated by elevation, starting heparin and providing analgesia.
- **Complications:** death in 20%, limb loss, ARDS, pneumonia, sepsis, rhabdomyolysis, hyperkalaemia, AKI.

17.11 Abdominal aortic aneurysm

- **About:** an AAA is defined as aortic diameter increasing by 50%, therefore >3 cm. Those >5.5 cm need surgical repair, the rest are monitored. Most begin below the renal artery and extend down as far as the iliac arteries. Mortality risk of elective surgery is 6% and emergency surgery 50%.

- **Aetiology:** chronic inflammatory process with loss of smooth muscle. May be a genetic basis leading to a weakness in the wall. A reduction in elastin and collagen is seen and may be a factor. Shape can be fusiform or saccular. Wall tension increases with increasing radius so increasing risk of rupture.

- **Risk factors:** smoking, increasing age, male ×5, increased height and BMI. Connective tissue disorders. A family history is a risk factor. Risk factors for rupture: female ×3, smoking, low FEV_1.

- **Clinical:** think AAA if abdominal/back pain + ↓BP and/or a pulsatile expansile mass. An aortoenteral fistula may cause an upper GI bleed (fistula between the AAA and the 4th part of duodenum. Distal clot embolisation leading to limb ischaemia.

- **Investigations:** FBC, U&E, amylase, LFTs, group and cross-match 6+ units. USS abdomen – identifies and measures AAA. Can see mural thrombus – this may be done in ED as a focused assessment with sonography, and if the aorta appears dilated (>3 cm) in an unstable patient then assume leaking AAA and resuscitate and call vascular surgeons. Any bleeding is retroperitoneal. Emergency choice is CT scan which can aid the decision for surgery.

- **Acute management:** ABC and urgent resuscitation if needed. Get good IV access fast. Group and cross-match 6–8 units. Fast bleep vascular surgeons. Emergency repair has grim prognosis. Abdominal muscles contract splints aneurysm. This is reversed with anaesthesia with subsequent ↓BP. Laparotomy and aorta cross-clamped above the leak. Mortality and complications including MI, renal failure, coagulopathy are common.

- **Elective repair:** no survival benefits for operating with stable AAA <5.5 cm. Operate elective surgery AAA >5.5 cm. Midline incision, aorta cross-clamped, heparinised. Dacron graft used. May be trouser graft if iliacs included. Enclosed in aneurysmal sac. AAA >5.5 cm have an almost 10% 1 year risk of rupture.

- **Endovascular aneurysm repair** (EVAR) can repair the aneurysm by endovascular stenting which avoids a laparotomy and cross-clamping can be done on selective cases via the femoral artery.

18 Dermatological emergencies

18.1 Introduction

- **Rashes that kill:** there are several rashes which must be diagnosed because early treatment may be lifesaving. The spreading urticaria and erythema that may suggest anaphylaxis along with wheeze, hypotension. The non-blanching purpuric rash of meningococcaemia with possible meningitis. The rapidly advancing all consuming, painful, red, hot necrotising fasciitis which spreads in hours. The slower advancing red, hot, tender cellulitis or erysipelas which can result in systemic sepsis.
- **Other life threatening rashes** include pemphigus vulgaris, toxic epidermal necrolysis (milder form called Stevens–Johnson syndrome (SJS)), erythema multiforme major, drug rash with eosinophilia and systemic symptoms (DRESS) syndrome, toxic shock syndrome (TSS).

18.2 Toxic epidermal necrolysis/Stevens–Johnson syndrome

- **About:** involves skin as well as mucous membranes – mouth, genitals, vagina, eyes. **TEN is a more severe form of SJS.** Ask about drugs within the preceding 2 months as a reaction may be delayed.
- **Aetiology:** idiopathic – worse prognosis than drug-induced. Drug-induced – sulphonamides, cephalosporins, antibiotics, anticonvulsants. Commoner with HIV and in slow drug acetylators.
- **Clinical:** preceding flu-like illness with myalgia, fever in recent days. Milder: erythema, target lesions, blistering on skin and oral/genital mucosa. Spreading tender erythema and confluent blistering rash followed by loss of sheets of epidermis. Pain may be severe. Involves skin and oral/genital mucosa. Detachment of the skin and mucosal epidermis. Progressive exfoliation. Recovery may lead to scarring, altered pigmentation and loss of sweating. Positive Nikolsky sign when slight lateral pressure to the epidermal surface slips upper layers away from lower.
- **Differential:** staphylococcal scalded skin syndrome (seen in children and mucosa spared). Toxic shock syndrome, phototoxic skin reactions. Drug reaction with eosinophilia.

Prognostic severity factors for toxic epidermal necrolysis
- Age >40 years +1, HR >120 +1, cancer or haematological malignancy +1.
- Involved body surface area >10% +1, urea >10 mmol/L +1, HCO_3^- <20 mmol/L +1.
- Blood glucose level >14 mmol/L +1.
- Mortality rates: 0–1 = 3%, 2 = 12%, 3 = 35%, 4 = 58%, 5 or more = 90%.

- **Investigation:** bloods: FBC, U&Es, LFT, CRP. Blood cultures, urine culture, CXR if febrile. Skin biopsy: necrotic keratinocytes with full thickness epithelial necrosis and sheets of epidermal detachment helps differentiate from staphylococcal scalded skin syndrome.
- **Management** (urgently speak with dermatologist): stop all possible drug causes, early detection. Optimise hydration. Watch input/output. Low threshold for starting antibiotics or antivirals for any superinfection. Transfer to burns unit. Supportive – fluid balance and nutrition, avoid hypothermia. Some may consider IVIG but **steroids/immune suppression not indicated.** Appropriate bedding – Clinitron mattress, avoid IV lines to reduce sepsis. Fluid/nutrition orally or via NG tube. Eye care to avoid scarring. VTE prophylaxis.

18.3 Cellulitis/erysipelas, bites, surgery

- **About:** beware over-treating chronic bilateral usually cold or warm mildly tender red legs. It's possible, but unusual, for cellulitis to be symmetrical. It may be chronic changes. Always look and feel all cases yourself. Unwrap bandages. Look at CRP, etc. Distal skin integrity key and simple emollients can soften dry eczematous legs.
- **Organism:** cellulitis mostly due to β-haemolytic streptococci. Often initially slow to respond to therapy or may worsen initially due to toxins produced by group A strep. and other local tissue factors. Less common *Staph. aureus* and MRSA.
- **Clinical:** subcutaneous skin infection. Red, very painful swelling often of a limb. Pyrexia and malaise. Inguinal nodes. Look for the point of entry – dry cracked skin between toes or insect bite or trauma. Look at heels and back of legs.
- **Diagnosis:** erysipelas is more superficial than cellulitis, and is typically more raised and demarcated but may have systemic symptoms of fever, malaise. Treat the same.
- **Mild–moderate cellulitis:** non-severe – afebrile and systemically well and no osteomyelitis. Give FLUCLOXACILLIN 500 mg 6 h PO for 7–14 days. If penicillin allergic then CLARITHROMYCIN 500 mg 12 h IV/PO for 7–14 days.
- **Severe cellulitis:** FLUCLOXACILLIN 1 g 6 h IV/PO until patient shows clinical improvement, no sepsis and tolerating oral intake then switch to oral therapy. Outpatients consider CEFTRIAXONE 2 g IV OD. Penicillin allergy TEICOPLANIN 6 mg/kg IV 12 h × 3 loading doses then 6 mg/kg OD.
- **Orbital cellulitis (serious infection):** has various causes and may be associated with serious complications including visual loss. Prompt diagnosis and proper management are essential. Unless very mild needs admission and CT + contrast and monitor function and IV antibiotic therapy. CO-AMOXICLAV 1.2 g 8 h IV or treat as severe cellulitis as above. Fungal infection requires IV antifungal therapy along with surgical debridement.
- **Soft tissue infection and MRSA positive:** consider VANCOMYCIN 1–1.5 g 12 h or TEICOPLANIN 6 mg/kg IV 12 h × 3 loading doses then 6 mg/kg OD.
- **Leg ulcers, pressure sores:** treat with antibiotics only if demarcated cellulitis or systemic infection observed. Refer to the cellulitis guidelines above. Wound cleaning and skin. Discuss with tissue viability specialist.
- **Animal bites/human bites:** CO-AMOXICLAV 625 mg PO or CO-AMOXICLAV 1.2 g 8 h IV if severe. Penicillin allergy DOXYCYCLINE 100 mg 12 h PO + METRONIDAZOLE 400 mg 8 h PO. Severe human bites, take advice. Duration: 7 days. Human bites consider HBV, HIV and tetanus risks too. Review at 24 h especially if near a joint.
- **Following clean surgery:** *mild/moderate:* FLUCLOXACILLIN PO/IV doses as for cellulitis. *Severe:* BENZYLPENICILLIN 1.2–2.4 g 6 h IV + FLUCLOXACILLIN 1 g 6 h IV.
- **Impetigo:** *mild:* MUPIROCIN 2% ointment 8 h or FUSIDIC ACID 2% cream 8 h. *Moderate* FLUCLOXACILLIN 500 mg 6 h PO.
- **Erysipelas:** *mild:* AMOXICILLIN 500 mg 8 h PO or severe BENZYLPENICILLIN 1.2–2.4 g 4–6 h IV.
- **Periodontal abscess/dental infections:** AMOXICILLIN 500 mg 8 h PO + METRONIDAZOLE 400 mg 8 h PO. Alternatively CO-AMOXICLAV 1.2 g 8 h IV. Should be accompanied by drainage and removal of source of infection.

18.4 Erythroderma (exfoliative dermatitis)

- **About:** erythema on >90% of the skin. Several causes. Determine underlying cause but 25% are idiopathic. Commoner in males.
- **Causes:** dermatitis (atopic, contact and seborrhoeic types). Drug eruptions. Cutaneous T-cell lymphoma, idiopathic. HIV infection, pityriasis rubra pilaris, toxic shock syndrome.

- **Clinical:** scaling erythematous dermatitis with erythroderma and heat/fluid loss. Risks of hypothermia, heart failure, fluid/electrolyte imbalance. Capillary leak syndrome may cause cutaneous oedema and acute lung injury.
- **Differential** (see causes): cellulitis, cutaneous T-cell lymphoma.
- **Investigation:** FBC: ↑ WCC. U&Es: AKI, ↑CRP, ESR. LFTs: low albumin. Skin biopsy may be required. Increased serum IgE.
- **Management:** detect and treat any underlying cause. Bed rest, keep warm, bland emollients. Fluid and electrolyte management. Manage hypoalbuminaemia. Erythrodermic pustular psoriasis treated with systemic steroids. NB. Withdrawal of systemic steroids can trigger erythrodermic pustular psoriasis. Consider HDU care and close monitoring for those with capillary leak syndrome.

18.5 Severe (erythrodermic/pustular) psoriasis

- **About:** extensive psoriasis affecting more than 80% body surface area and generalised pustular psoriasis. Prior history of psoriasis.
- **Clinical:** widespread severe erythema with pustules which coalesce to form lakes of pus. Fever.
- **Investigation:** FBC: ↑WCC. U&Es: AKI, ↑CRP.
- **Management:** admit, hydration, emollients and oral weekly Methotrexate 5–7.5 mg/week. Monitor for neutropenia and hepatotoxicity should be monitored closely. Other choices are Ciclosporin and biological agents, e.g. infliximab. Retinoids are first line for severe pustular psoriasis. Antibiotics for any bacterial infection. Take dermatology advice. The use of potent or very potent corticosteroids in psoriasis can result in rebound relapse, development of generalised pustular psoriasis, and local and systemic toxicity.

18.6 Necrotising fasciitis

- **About:** surgical emergency – minutes matter because infection proceeds rapidly and lethally. Consider if extremely painful cellulitis with a hard woody feel. Early diagnosis can be life and limb saving. Often polymicrobial 75%.
- **Aetiology:** usually group A β-haemolytic streptococci but can be aerobic, anaerobic, or mixed. Diabetics, arterial and venous vascular disease. Can follow mild trauma. Rate of spread relates directly to the thickness of the subcutaneous layer. Necrotising fasciitis moves rapidly along the fascial plane.
- **Clinical:** severe localised pain, myalgia, malaise, fever. Localised defined erythema. Crepitus and surgical emphysema from gas-forming bacteria in the soft tissue. Blistering and hardening. Mark out limits of erythema.
- **Differential:** cellulitis, pyoderma gangrenosum.
- **Investigation:** FBC: ↑WCC, ↑ESR, ↑CRP. U&Es: AKI, ↑K. Plain X-ray of affected area may show gas in soft tissues. MRI/CT: may be used to detect soft tissue infection, however, surgery should not be delayed for confirmatory radiology if clinical suspicion high. **Needle aspirate:** at edge of lesion and Gram stain can help. Finger test: suspected area infiltrated with local anaesthesia and a 2 cm incision is made in the skin down to the deep fascia. Bleeding should be evident. A lack of bleeding suggests necrotising fasciitis. May just see dirty fluid. More extensive surgery should follow. Assess Laboratory Risk Indicator for Necrotizing Fasciitis (LRINEC) score; see online.
- **Management:** ABC, high flow O_2 to get saturation – 100% unless severe COPD. Resuscitation. IV fluids (needs may be high with capillary leak) and antibiotics and immediate surgical consult. Complications include AKI, sepsis, limb loss, toxic shock, so no time to delay. Immediate surgery with extensive wide debridement can decrease mortality: once diagnosed patient requires burns unit or trauma unit

transfer to those with experience in extensive debridement and reconstructive
surgery. Amputation may be needed. Hyperbaric O_2 where facilities available.
IV CLINDAMYCIN – as well as antimicrobial effect it is a potent suppressor of bacterial
toxin synthesis. May be combined with IV BENZYLPENICILLIN 1.2–2.4 g 4–6 h and
GENTAMICIN IV. Liaise closely with microbiology.

 ## Other important rashes for acute physicians

Time	Comments
Erythema multiforme	Erythematous tender target lesions usually on arms and legs and mucosa. Causes are HSV, EBV, sulphonamides, anticonvulsants, *Mycoplasma* infection, SLE, PAN, HIV, WG, carcinoma, lymphoma. Can help with diagnosis of systemic disease.
Pyoderma gangrenosum	Painful single or multiple ulcers with violaceous borders anywhere from face to limbs. Patient usually unwell. Look for IBD, RA, myeloma, MGUS, leukaemia, lymphoma, PBC. Idiopathic in 20%. Management with potent topical steroids or 0.1% tacrolimus ointment.
Lupus pernio	Reddish brown dermal papules on the face and elsewhere. Consider sarcoid – may have CXR changes or ↑calcium.
Erythema nodosum	Red roundish raised nodules seen on the shins. Streptococcal infection, TB, sarcoid, IBD, penicillin, etc.

19 General management

19.1 Enteral feeding

- **Screening adults:** the MUST tool is a five-step screening tool to identify those who are malnourished, at risk of malnutrition (undernutrition), or obese. It also includes management guidelines which can be used to develop a care plan. See risk calculator at www.bapen.org.uk/
- **Before:** commencing nutrition always consider the risks of *refeeding syndrome* and screen the patient. Enteral feeding is used where there is a functioning GI tract but some physical reason (e.g. acute stroke or MND, or facial or ENT surgery) that prevents normal swallowing. The enteral route is always preferable to the parenteral route if possible. It is important to note that directly feeding the stomach does not necessarily prevent aspiration as gastric contents can reflux and enter the lungs if there are poor protective reflexes and an inability to cough.
- **Nasogastric tube:** commonly used but uncomfortable and can cause nasal trauma. Easily dislodged and only used as a temporary feeding measure for up to several weeks. If there is a clearly defined time for which swallowing will not be possible then best to replace with better option. Where outcome is unpredictable and survival unsure it may be used for several weeks, e.g. acute stroke. It is important that these are placed properly and local guidelines followed.
- **Never events:** NG tubes can be accidentally placed in bronchi and feed given – this is regarded as a never event (▶ Section 19.9). To show the tip is in gastric lumen an aspirate is obtained and checked for <pH 4 and if any doubt a CXR should show the NG tube in the **midline in the thorax and then passing down below the diaphragm.** Usual distance from nose to oesophageal junction is about 40 cm.
- **Percutaneous endoscopic gastrostomy (PEG):** medium to long term need for on-going enteral feeding. There is no decrease in risk of aspiration pneumonia with placement of gastric or post-pyloric feeding tube and there might be increased risk. There is no evidence that PEG feeding improves nutritional markers or decreases the risk for pressure ulcer formation or improves healing of ulcers in a demented patient. PEG tubes do not appear to contribute to comfort at the end of life. Performed by gastroenterologists at endoscopy and involves a puncture from abdominal surface through to the gastric lumen. Risks are real and include infection, peritonitis, sepsis, haemorrhage and displacement and the risks of sedation. Other intra-abdominal organs can be punctured. A fibrous fistulous tract forms over about 10–14 days after which replacement of any tube can be undertaken.
- **Percutaneous endoscopic jejunostomy (PEJ):** same as a PEG but tube advanced beyond pylorus.
- **Radiologically inserted gastrostomy:** ideal where there is a medium to long term need for on-going enteral feeding and the patient, for whatever reason, does not tolerate endoscopy. Performed by radiologists under fluoroscopy and involves a puncture from abdominal surface through to the gastric lumen. Complications and principles similar to PEG.
- **Needle catheter jejunostomy:** fine catheter inserted into jejunum at laparotomy and brought externally through a puncture in the abdominal wall.
- **Enteral feeding regimen:** with a simple polymeric diet consisting of protein and fat and carbohydrate containing essential minerals and vitamins. In those with small bowel disease a more elemental diet may be given such that proteins are given more as amino acids and fats as medium chain triglycerides.

19.2 Parenteral feeding

- **Assess for risk of refeeding syndrome.** Parenteral route really only used where the GI tract is non-functional. Higher risk of complications than enteral feeding, particularly sepsis. In terms of feeding it is much less physiological. Not usually considered when needed for less than 1 week. Several routes.
- **Peripheral venous line:** used with low osmolality feeding as it soon causes thrombophlebitis. The lines are 20 cm in length and can be used for up to 5 days.
- **Peripheral inserted central catheter (PICC):** a 60 cm catheter inserted in the antecubital fossa. The distal end lies within central veins. Hyperosmolar solutions may be used. Thrombophlebitis is less. These can last up to a month and may be inserted before a central venous line is considered.
- **Central venous line:** feeding via jugular/subclavian or femoral line using a silicone catheter. The infraclavicular subclavian route is often preferred and is most practical. A skin tunnel is usually created. The complications are the same as those of inserting any central line here and include infection, haemorrhage, arterial puncture and pneumothorax. Catheter-related sepsis should always be considered if any signs of infection. This will require IV antibiotics and removal of the line.
- **Different preparations:** of feed are given depending if central or peripheral access, but all attempt to give about 3 L of feed over 24 h containing between 1700 and 2250 calories with sufficient protein, glucose, lipid, electrolytes, vitamins, water, and fat soluble and trace elements. Steroid and heparin and insulin may also be given. The feeds are usually prepared by pharmacy in liaison with the dietitian and intensivists. These patients are normally on the HDU/ITU or surgical wards.
- **Parenteral feeding:** requires frequent monitoring and daily U&Es and glucose, and 2–3 times per week FBC, LFTs, Ca, P, Mg, Zn and glycerides. Monitor nutritional status. Any signs of sepsis requires FBC, CRP, blood cultures and assessment for chest or UTI. Take advice from seniors and microbiology as to management of the catheter. If that is the presumed or proven source then it will need to be removed.

Nutritional support and feeding regimens

Needs	Information	Comment
Water	Usually 2–3 L/day	Increased if other losses, e.g. urinary, GI, fistulas
Energy	1750–2400 kcal/day	Titrated to needs
Protein	10–15 g/day of nitrogen in about 90 g of protein	More in severely catabolic states, e.g. burns
Minerals	Na 100 mmol/day, K 60–90 mmol/day, Ca, Mg	Increased K needed with some GI losses
Trace elements	Selenium, iodide, fluoride, iron, zinc, manganese and chromium	Increased for enteral as uptake not 100%
Vitamins	Give all fat and water soluble as per minimal daily requirements (not covered here)	Increased for enteral as uptake not 100%. VITAMIN K added to parenteral feeds

19.3 Pain management

- Successfully managing pain requires some knowledge of analgesia. Become familiar with a core group of medications. The team looking after a patient should certainly work with the hospital pain team. The perception of pain is multifactorial and often

- subjective and personal and varies with cause, depression, fears as to causation and control, and often cultural and social issues.
- Some patients are stoical and will accept mild to occasional moderate pain if explained without recourse to analgesia. Others will want all discomfort minimised. All effective analgesics carry side effects and these need to be weighed up with their usage. Paracetamol within normal dose range is probably the safest but only appropriate as a single agent for mild pain but can be combined with stronger medications.
- Pain is feared by patients and the experience will vary between those with post-operative pain control and those with pain related to a chronic disease or malignancy. Pain control must be appropriate and proportionate. Be aware of the WHO analgesic ladder which you ascend, but manage pain based on severity. Don't forget to consider specific management of fear, anxiety and depression which may well be pain multipliers. Anxiety may be based on mistaken fears which can be addressed. Addiction to opioids when used for pain control is very rare indeed.

19.4 WHO pain ladder

- **Mild:** PARACETAMOL 1 g IV/PO 6–8 hourly if not controlled then step up. SE: liver/renal failure with overdose. Avoid in liver failure.
- **Moderate:** PARACETAMOL 1 g 6–8 hourly + CODEINE 30–60 mg 6–8 hourly or IBUPROFEN 400 mg 8 hourly. VOLTAROL (DICLOFENAC) 50 mg 8 h or slow release 75 mg (max 150 mg daily) PO/PR in 2–3 divided doses. VOLTAROL 100 mg suppository PR. Caution with NSAIDs in those with impaired renal function as can cause AKI. TRAMADOL 50–100 mg 4–6 hourly is another possibility; even mild opiates can cause delirium in the elderly.
- **Severe:** strong opioid, e.g. MORPHINE 5 mg 4 hourly PO and then calculate the daily requirement and give as a long acting agent, e.g. MORPHINE if pain is ongoing or likely to worsen. Others include IV or SC DIAMORPHINE +/– non-opioid, +/– adjuvant

Managing specific pain syndromes

- **Acute MI/ACS:** NITRATES, DIAMORPHINE 2.5–5 mg IV or MORPHINE 5–10 mg IV, PCI/thrombolysis/CABG.
- **Acute abdomen:** IV MORPHINE 5–10 mg + IV CYCLIZINE 50 mg.
- **Bone fracture:** IV MORPHINE 5–10 mg + IV CYCLIZINE 50 mg.
- **Bone pain, inflammation pain:** NSAIDs, e.g. DICLOFENAC 50 mg 8 h or IBUPROFEN 400–600 mg 8 h. Bisphosphonates can help in some forms of bone pain, e.g. myeloma, Paget's disease, especially with high Ca. Try IV PAMIDRONATE or ZOLEDRONATE.
- **Headache of malignancy:** DEXAMETHASONE and radiotherapy and codeine may help if cerebral oedema.
- **Ischaemic pain:** NSAIDs, ketamine, MORPHINE.
- **Liver metastases:** steroids.
- **Localised pain:** analgesic infiltration, e.g. lidocaine or nerve root blocks.
- **Metastatic bone disease:** osteolytic metastases and bone pain with breast cancer or myeloma. Bisphosphonates, e.g. PAMIDRONATE 60–90 mg IV every 4 weeks, NSAIDs, MORPHINE.
- **Neuropathic pain:** gabapentin, amitriptyline often given at night, pregabalin, steroids and radiotherapy may be useful in malignancy-related neuropathic pain, shingles, trigeminal neuralgia.
- **Non-specific:** (e.g. back pain): TENS machine, acupuncture.

- **Renal colic:** consider VOLTAROL 50 mg tds PO/PR or DICLOFENAC 75 mg OD PO/PR. A second dose can be given after a minimum of 30 min if necessary. Alternative is MORPHINE 5–10 mg IV + CYCLIZINE 50 mg IV.

19.5 ▶ Using opiates and other analgesics

- When prescribing opiates the **drug, dose and frequency and route of administration** should be written clearly. If it is as part of a prescription then the dose must also be spelt out. When pain is expected to be temporary, e.g. post-op or for some other reason, it is wise to time limit the drug so that it is reviewed days or weeks later, so that it does not continue indefinitely if not required.
- Weak opiates are often effective both short and long term. However, with dehydration and renal failure they can become toxic, especially in the elderly, and caution must be taken. Always consider codeine as a cause of reduced awareness and delirium and coma and consider a trial of NALOXONE if unclear. The other main side effects are constipation and a laxative should be added. They may also cause N&V and are often combined with an antiemetic. DIAMORPHINE in reasonable concentrations can be given along with METOCLOPRAMIDE, CYCLIZINE or HALOPERIDOL in a syringe driver. Myoclonus may also be seen.
- Strong opiates include MORPHINE, DIAMORPHINE and FENTANYL. They should be commenced at low starting doses: MORPHINE 5 mg every 4–6 h which can be given orally or IM or IV or SC. DIAMORPHINE 2.5 mg can be given parenterally only. Both should be increased as needed and titrated to pain.
- Fentanyl is often used transdermally and may be preferred with renal dysfunction and when there are difficulties with oral formulations. However, at times it may accumulate and lead to confusion and coma and the patch should be removed and analgesia needs assessed. With oral medications there is a simple feedback loop. If the medication causes coma then no more medications are taken and the patient recovers until able to swallow the next dose. With parenteral and transdermal routes this pseudo-safety feedback loop does not exist and extra care must be taken.
- MORPHINE comes as either a faster-acting immediate release formulation which works in minutes and covers about 4 h. Can be started as MORPHINE 5 mg 4–6 hourly. Once MORPHINE need is estimated a longer-acting once-daily controlled release formulation can be used. Additional immediate release MORPHINE should be available for breakthrough pain. Patient dose varies with tolerance and renal function and patients may take anywhere from 10 to 5000 mg of MORPHINE per day. Pethidine is sometimes used but has a very short $t_{1/2}$.

MORPHINE Oral (mg/day)	MORPHINE SC, IM, IV (mg/day)	Fentanyl Patch (mcg/h)	DIAMORPHINE SC (mg/day)	Oxycodone Oral (mg/day)	Oxycodone SC (mg/day)
30	15	12 patch	10	15	10
60	30	12–25 patch	20	30	15
90	45	25 patch	30	45	20
180	90	50 patch	60	90	45
270	140	75 patch	90	130	70
360	180	100 patch	120	180	90

Equivalence to MORPHINE 10 mg PO = MORPHINE 5 mg SC/IV/IM = DIAMORPHINE 3 mg IM/IV/SC = CODEINE 100 mg PO = DIHYDROCODEINE 100 mg PO = TRAMADOL 100 mg PO = OXYCODONE 6.6 mg PO. Great care must be taken – doses shown are for 24 h. For medications just for 4–6 h these need to be divided into their individual dose.

NSAIDs

Very useful for acute and chronic pain management, but chronic usage can lead to peptic ulcer disease and renal impairment. Best avoided in anyone with CKD, or PUD, or low platelets, or bleeding, or in acute illness, as can precipitate AKI. If there is dyspepsia then adding a PPI may be useful. Side effects limit usage in the elderly. Commonly used formulations include IBUPROFEN and DICLOFENAC.

Neuropathic pain

Most anticonvulsants and TCAs have action against neuropathic pain. Examples include GABAPENTIN and AMITRIPTYLINE and CARBAMAZEPINE. Specialists may use pregabalin, ketamine.

19.6 Venous thromboembolism prevention

All patients should be screened for their risk of DVT/PE and managed according to NICE guidance with mechanical or pharmacological agents after a full risk assessment. Avoid pharmacological VTE prophylaxis if the patient has any risk factor for bleeding and the risk of bleeding outweighs the risk of VTE.

Patients who are at increased risk of VTE
Medical or surgical or trauma patients
- Mobility significantly reduced for 3+ days or expected to have ongoing reduced mobility relative to normal state plus any VTE risk factor (see below).
- If total anaesthetic + surgical time >90 min or if surgery involves pelvis or lower limb and total anaesthetic + surgical time >60 min.
- If acute surgical admission with inflammatory or intra-abdominal condition.
- Significant reduction in mobility or any VTE risk factor present (see below).

VTE risk factors
- Active cancer or cancer treatment or obesity (BMI >30 kg/m^2).
- Age >60 years, critical care admission, dehydration, known thrombophilias.
- One or more significant medical co-morbidities (e.g. heart disease; metabolic, endocrine or respiratory pathologies; acute infectious diseases; inflammatory conditions).
- Personal history or first-degree relative with a history of VTE.
- Use of HRT or oestrogen-containing contraceptive therapy.
- Varicose veins with phlebitis.

Patients who are at risk of bleeding
- Active bleeding, acquired bleeding disorders (such as ALF).
- Concurrent use of anticoagulants (such as warfarin with INR >2).
- LP/epidural/spinal anaesthesia <4 h ago or expected within the next 12 h.
- Acute stroke or uncontrolled systolic hypertension (>230/120 mmHg).
- Thrombocytopenia (platelets <75 × 10^9/L).
- Untreated inherited bleeding disorders (such as haemophilia or von Willebrand's disease).

Choice of method
- **Mechanical VTE prophylaxis:** anti-embolism stockings (thigh or knee length), foot impulse devices, intermittent pneumatic compression devices (thigh or knee length).

- **Pharmacological VTE prophylaxis:** most trusts use LMWH, however, doses need to be adjusted if there is renal failure. Alternatives include fondaparinux. Dabigatran, rivaroxaban and apixaban have been used in elective hip and knee surgery. Follow local policies.

- **Stroke patients:** there is no fixed standard and practices vary between centres. Compression devices are recommended for the first 30 days. Some centres use LMWH, in some patients with severe disability and at high risk of VTE even in haemorrhagic strokes. LMWH may still be considered after the acute period. Follow local guidance. Balance against risks of haemorrhage.

- **Pregnancy or up to 6 weeks postpartum:** VTE prophylaxis if undergoing caesarean section or if any of the following risk factors: expected to have significantly reduced mobility for 3 or more days; active cancer or cancer treatment; age >35 years; critical care admission, dehydration, excess blood loss or blood transfusion; known thrombophilias; obesity (pre-pregnancy or early pregnancy BMI >30 kg/m²); significant medical co-morbidity (such as heart disease, metabolic, endocrine or respiratory pathologies, acute infectious diseases or inflammatory conditions); personal history or first-degree relative with history of VTE; pregnancy-related risk factor, including ovarian hyperstimulation, hyperemesis gravidarum, multiple pregnancy, pre-eclampsia; varicose veins with phlebitis.

Reference: NICE (2010) CG92: Venous thromboembolism: reducing the risk. RCOG (2015) Reducing the risk of venous thromboembolism during pregnancy and the puerperium: Green-top Guideline No. 37a – *please use this new guidance to risk assess pregnant or post-partum patients.*

19.7 Duties of a doctor

- Good advice is given by the GMC. Doctors need to be satisfied that they have consent from a patient, or other valid authority, before undertaking any examination or investigation, providing treatment, or involving patients in teaching and research. The GMC has very useful guidance on the duties of a doctor. Patients must be able to trust doctors. To justify that trust you must show respect for human life and you must: always make the care of your patient your first concern and protect and promote the health of patients and the public. Provide a good standard of practice and care. Keep your professional knowledge and skills up to date. Recognise and work within the limits of your competence. Work with colleagues in the ways that best serve patients' interests.

- Treat patients as individuals and respect their dignity: treat patients politely and considerately. Respect patients' right to confidentiality. Work in partnership with patients: listen to patients and respond to their concerns and preferences. Give patients the information they want or need in a way they can understand. Respect patients' right to reach decisions with you about their treatment and care. Support patients in caring for themselves to improve and maintain their health. Be honest and open and act with integrity. Act without delay if you have good reason to believe that you or a colleague may be putting patients at risk. Never discriminate unfairly against patients or colleagues. Never abuse your patients' trust in you or the public's trust in the profession. You are personally accountable for your professional practice and must always be prepared to justify your decisions and actions.

Reference: For *Good Medical Practice* document see: www.gmc-uk.org/static/documents/content/GMP.pdf.

19.8 Medical errors, harm and duty of candour

- 'To err is human' is true. We all make errors, the question is how we prevent errors, especially those that can cause patient harm, and what we do when we realise that an error has occurred. Errors by definition are unintentional. Multiple issues – health systems are complex, interconnected and multitasking, with lots of competing priorities, and different levels of knowledge and experience. One of the commonest sources of error is with medication. Avoid writing up drugs on rounds, sit down and do it later when not distracted. Always examine the drug chart as well as the patient on all hospital rounds. It is impossible here to go into the complete list of medical errors, but there are a list of events which should 'never occur'. These are called **'never events' and are listed below**.

- When clinical errors result in clinical harm, alert your consultant immediately. Immediately reduce any possible further harm done. Take advice. Be honest about errors with everyone involved – the patient, their family, others in the team, your boss. Document everything, fully. Say sorry when things have gone wrong. That one word may make trouble simply disappear. It may hurt to say it, but say it. Sorry does not in itself admit blame or liability. Once you start to focus on an error the responsibility rarely lands on one set of shoulders. There may be educational and training issues, work issues, responsibility issues. Most errors occur as several events conspired to happen together and a mistake that would have been caught any day was able to perpetuate itself through until real harm had occurred. It has become clear that a simple blame culture does little to perpetuate change and improve things. In many cases, but not all, the error could have happened to most of us and the only differentiating factor has been bad luck. Many systems seem set up to allow failure and blaming a scapegoat is, sadly, still a part of healthcare culture which we must try to change.

19.9 Never events – events that should 'never' occur

The NHS has defined a list of never events. Systems and practices should be enabled to prevent these. All need thorough investigation.

• Maladministration of potassium-containing solutions.	• Falls from unrestricted windows.
• Wrong route of administration of chemotherapy.	• Transfusion of ABO-incompatible blood components.
• Wrong route of administration of oral/enteral treatment.	• Transplantation of ABO or HLA-incompatible organs.
• Maladministration of insulin.	• Misplaced naso- or oro-gastric tubes.
• Severe scalding of patients.	• Wrong gas administered.
• Overdose of Midazolam during conscious sedation.	• Failure to monitor and respond to O_2 saturation.
• Opioid overdose of an opioid-naive patient.	• Air embolism.
• Suicide using non-collapsible rails.	• Misidentification of patients.
• Entrapment in bed rails.	• Inappropriate administration of daily oral methotrexate.
• Escape of a transferred prisoner.	

19.10 Risk management and risk register

- Acute medicine clinicians should play a fundamental role in risk management. All NHS organisations should have a risk management framework, which provides assurance to the Board that appropriate processes are in place to manage corporate and operational risks effectively; recommending procedures for the effective identification, prioritisation, treatment and management of risks to minimise or maximise the effect of an uncertain event or set of events on the delivery of objectives; ensuring a cohesive approach to the governance of risk; identifying risk management resources; and establishing risk management as an integral part of the NHS culture.

- Risks to patient safety and care should be identified and the risk mitigated against. All risks should have a risk owner and an action owner who mitigates the risk and updates those involved on the progress of this. Risks are assessed using a score of 1–5 for harm if it occurs and a score of 1–5 in terms of likelihood, and a resultant product value obtained. Risks over a certain value are escalated for further action. Risks and issues often get confused and a useful way of remembering the difference is: *risks* are things that might happen and stop us achieving objectives, e.g. safe surgery or otherwise impact on the success of the organization; *issues* are things that have happened, were not planned and require management action.

- Each trust has a risk register which should contain as a minimum a risk reference; risk owner, risk description, ratings of likelihood and impact (for both current and after actions), risk proximity, action plans, action owner for each action, and completion date for each action.

 ## Duty of candour

- The principle of the duty of candour is that care organisations have a general duty to act in an open and transparent way in relation to care provided to patients. This is an entirely new requirement from the CQC (UK). Organisations will have to ensure they have systems in place to capture notifiable safety incidents and processes to inform the patient and provide support. A "notifiable safety incident" means any unintended or unexpected incident that occurred in respect of a service user during the provision of a regulated activity that, in the reasonable opinion of a healthcare professional, could result in, or appears to have resulted in:

  (a) the death of the service user, where the death relates directly to the incident rather than to the natural course of the service user's illness or underlying condition, or

  (b) moderate or severe harm, or prolonged psychological harm.

- The Organisation must, as soon as possible after becoming aware that a notifiable safety incident has occurred, inform the patient (or their representative) and provide reasonable support to him/her in relation to the incident. This is followed by written notification of the incident with an apology and details of further enquiries into the incident that are to be undertaken.

- Provide support to the patient to ensure that the patient understands the discussions (this may include providing emotional support). Keep a written record of all discussions and correspondence. The consultant must be involved and will be key in ensuring this is done.

 ## Discharging patients safely

- Discharging patients safely is a skill developed through knowledge and experience and is really a decision for the registrar or above. Beds are always tight and pressures mean you can only admit the sickest patients if you discharge other patients.

- Before admitting a person ask why: is being onsite going to mitigate some anticipated risk, what is the natural history here, what are the risks? Often there are social and medical reasons. Is admission to a busy, noisy potentially infectious assessment area in the patient's best interest?

- Your hospital should have ambulatory care clinics that can do blood tests, monitor symptoms and continue investigations. Patients should not have to sleep in hospital to have an urgent test done – this is irrational and uneconomical. Patients are admitted only if there is no alternative. Hospitals are sources of new infections, strange environments that will cause significant new cognitive challenges leading to falls and overmedication of elderly patients, with insomnia from their agitated neighbours. Admission means packages of care are terminated that can be time-consuming to reinstate. Many expect an oasis of peace, quiet and relaxation but this is just not possible on a busy acute assessment unit.

- In terms of hospital admission there is often an 'illusion of safety'. Patients are often placed overnight onto busy wards far from the doctors on take with 2 trained nurses and a healthcare assistant serving 25 or more patients. The patient may be in a side room. If the patient develops a problem it may take time for them to raise help (if the call buzzer is out of reach perhaps) and even longer for the nurse to alert the medical team in another part of the hospital and have them attend.

- The medical team have to prioritise their ill patients in the emergency department with ward patients and this adds to delays. In some instances it is better to let stable, mobile and able patients go home, where they will have 1 to 1 care from a sensible spouse or carers who can call 999 and have an emergency ambulance attending within minutes, providing very solid basic medical care if the need arises. This is obviously not appropriate for those with a STEMI or acute severe asthma, but for some patients with less severe conditions it certainly bears consideration.

- The bottom line is that for some patients their own bed at home will be a safer, quieter, more relaxing environment for healing and improvement than a hospital bed. So when sending patients home with their particular illness you need to have a sensible understanding of the natural history of the disease and its expected behaviour. I ask myself – what is the most reasonable worst-case scenario and can I mitigate against it in any way?

- Before you do a discharge check that the patient wants to go home. Make sure they know to come back via 999 if there are any problems – make this very clear to the patient and it helps if family support this. Ensure that you have documented a thorough assessment, including what you have told the patient, and make sure all are happy and agree. Do not do this if the patient is sick and lives very distant from the hospital or is alone or has cognitive or mental health issues, or there is a lack of family support or a general reluctance for the plan.

- An elderly man has new confusion and all the signs and tests point quite clearly to a UTI causing acute delirium. You explain that admission might worsen the confusion and agitation. He is mobile and safe with supervision. Patient goes home on oral antibiotics, family member volunteers to sleep over at their house to give some support and provide close supervision on the stairs and give him his medication and meals. They liaise with the GP. He is reassessed by phone call from intermediate care or the GP to check improvement and has slept well and taken his antibiotics and is improving. In the admission scenario the disorientated patient climbed over cotsides and fell from bed and has a fractured hip and SDH. Non-admission is good when it can happen but it might be just too difficult and the daughter in this scenario may have other responsibilities, but consider it. The most fundamental question is did I put the welfare and wishes of the patient first?

- An elderly gentleman with advanced dementia has mild haematuria from an advanced bladder cancer; he is sent in and seen in ED. Devoted staff from his nursing home attend and are happy to have him back for palliation and end of life care if needed. No family. You feel discharge back to nursing home from ED with community palliative services is in best interests. You stop the aspirin for secondary prevention. You feel vulnerable without family agreement. You get a rapid second

opinion from a geriatrician who agrees plan in best interests. Discharge from
ED enabled.

19.13 Self-discharge

- An informed competent patient should be able to refuse admission with no
  prejudice to ongoing care. Patients can absolutely decline what we consider best
  care. Is there a second best way – ambulatory care or a rapid outpatient clinic? Is
  sleeping in the hospital really needed? If that is the only way to rapidly access a
  service then you need to think how to change your services.
- Hospitals are not prisons and patients (who have capacity until proven otherwise)
  do have a right to leave at any time. It would be good if they told us why and even
  told us they were going but some will just go. Most of the time it is frustrating but
  harmless. Doctors have a duty of care, however, sometimes patients who have
  on-going needs do decide to leave. It is important to define why they need to stay –
  are they at risk of arrhythmias or do they need urgent tests? Try to find out why – can
  the patient leave and do whatever they deem important and come back? The need
  to leave may be entirely understandable and so try to be reasonable and flexible in
  your approach, but do negotiate a reasonable level of co-operation. Can they come
  to ambulatory care next day? If the patient decides to leave against advice and there
  is a risk they will come to serious harm, then explain and document any potential
  complications that you have explained to the patient. If you feel there is significant
  risk of harm but the patient has the capacity to appreciate this, then all you can do
  is document conversations and advice given. If concerned then take senior advice.
  It would be wise to ring the GP then or next morning who may call and visit with the
  patient. There may be a change of heart.
- Families can help but you need consent to discuss. Most hospitals have a standard
  form, but even if the patient refuses to cooperate then both you and nursing staff
  should record contemporaneous notes over what was said and what happened
  and any advice given. Always make it clear they can and should come back, even
  though that may mean via A&E if any more problems or a change of mind. **Always
  do a discharge letter to document the events and keep in it any advice and
  make sure the GP is made aware**. Problems arise when you suspect that there is
  impaired capacity. You might consider that the patient is suffering from a temporary
  capacity issue due to acute delirium (alcohol withdrawal, sepsis, hypoxia, etc.) or has
  chronic problems (e.g. dementia), and in these cases you should take senior advice.
  It might be very reasonable to restrain the patient in such a case, either physically
  or with sedation, but this should be done with senior (preferably consultant) advice
  and using hospital staff or even the police if needed, usually under common law
  initially. At all times you must be able to prove that you acted in the best interests of
  the patient. If a septic patient leaves and dies you may be blamed for your inaction
  and have to answer in a coroner's court. If the patient does leave and you have not
  been able to restrain them then involve hospital security and police. Be seen to be
  doing all possible to protect the patient. The care of the patient must always be your
  main focus.

19.14 Suicidal patients

- Suicidal patients who perhaps came in with an overdose should not be allowed to
  discharge against advice without senior involvement. Involve psychiatry. Take senior
  advice immediately. If they go you should involve police. Involve the GP. It is rare
  but it does happen that overdose patients leave the hospital and finish their lives by
  some other means. You must act.

- All patients admitted with an attempted suicide must be seen by the psychiatry team or equivalent prior to discharge. Senior advice must be taken if there is any attempt to abscond or self-discharge, or if they leave the premises which will usually mean police involvement. These are some of the risk factors for those who go on to commit suicide. Note that most people who commit suicide have seen a doctor in the preceding month.

Factors to screen for increasing suicide risk
- A history of depression and substance abuse or borderline personality disorder.
- Age >45 years, living alone.
- Gender: men try more lethal means, women try more often.
- Marital status: never married, divorced, widowed, recently separated.
- Extensive and detailed plans or plans using highly lethal means.
- Family history of suicide, still expressing a wish to die, recent job loss.
- Puerperal, chronic painful illness.
- Recent loss of loved one or the anniversary of the loss.
- Previous suicide attempts – this is one of the best predictors.
- Gay/lesbian youth, Caucasian youth, impulsive or reckless behaviour.

Assessment: ask about suicidal ideation: where concerned, always ask patients about suicide and their intentions. Do they feel life is worth living? Have they thought of ending it? Most patients will discuss. It is very rare, but the person committed to suicide will say whatever gets them out of hospital. Older, single men with financial worries and job loss are one group of concern and you should take experienced advice regardless of what they say. **Management:** check your local policy, but anyone with a suicide attempt or suicidal ideation should have a psychiatric evaluation before discharge. Patients may even try to self-discharge. Get immediate help from psychiatry and take senior advice.

19.15 Common law and Mental Health Act

- When the patient is unconscious or lacks capacity, common law allows the doctor to act in the patient's best interests. This may enable urgent detention against the patient's will to allow further assessment and treatment when a delay would result in immediate potential harm to the patient, and where there is no time for a more measured approach to be used. In A&E common law is used. It allows life-saving surgery or sedation and detention to give IV antibiotics for confusion due to sepsis, meningitis or to treat hypoglycaemia, etc. When time is available then admit patient and use the Mental Health Act.

Mental Health Act
- **Section 5(2):** allows either a ward doctor to detain a patient for a mental health assessment on ward for 72 h and form H1 is completed and the duty psychiatry team should be informed. The patient should have a mental health assessment at earliest opportunity. Seek support from on-call psychiatry and the appropriate consultant. It is sometimes called a 'holding power'. During the 72 hours the person would be assessed for Section 2 or 3.
- **Section 5(4):** Nursing staff can use this to detain a patient if a doctor is not available and this is valid for up to 6 hrs. Complete form H2. If the doctor/approved clinician has not arrived within 4 hours the duty consultant should be contacted by the Clinical Team Leader/Senior Nurse on-call and should attend.
- The Mental Health Act does not allow you to treat physical conditions against their will but only the mental health issues, unless the physical cause is the cause of the mental issues. However, you may consider doing so if capacity is uncertain and

you have the defence of patient's best interests. Take advice. Otherwise the Mental Capacity Act 2005 is used.

19.16 Mental capacity

An assessment of capacity is decision and time specific. Patients are only lacking capacity for the particular question asked. Assume capacity to make the decision in question until proven otherwise. The Mental Capacity Act Code of Practice describes a test of capacity you can use to decide whether a person is able to make that decision. An assessment that a person lacks capacity to make a decision must never be based simply on their age or their appearance, assumptions about their condition or any aspect of their behaviour. The risks and benefits should be discussed in detail to satisfy the questions below. In many cases the loss of capacity is partial, it may also be temporary and it may change over time. It can be useful to repeat the assessment on a 'better' day. There are several things to consider when assessing if a person can make a decision:

- Do they understand the decision and why they need to make it?
- Can they understand, use and weigh up the relevant information?
- Can they communicate the decision (talking, sign language, etc.)?
- Could professional (speech and language therapist) help be useful?
- Is a more thorough assessment required, e.g. doctor or other expert?
- See Chapter 4 of the Code of Practice.

19.17 Managing opiate addicts

- **Note:** do not initiate methadone or buprenorphine treatment without advice and without arranging continuation of treatment on discharge with addiction services.
- **About:** usual GMC responsibilities for doctors apply and a non-judgemental approach should be followed. The clinician must treat the drug misuser but should determine the impact of their drug misuse on other individuals, especially dependent children, and child protection policies followed. Heroin users are the largest single group. Opiate substitution prevents people dropping out of treatment – suppresses illicit use of heroin, reduces crime, reduces the risk of blood-borne virus transmission, reduces risk of death. Addicts have increased risk of viral hepatitis, bacterial endocarditis, HIV, tuberculosis, septicaemia, pneumonia, deep vein thrombosis, pulmonary emboli, abscesses and dental disease. Only in exceptional circumstances should the decision be made to offer substitute medication without specialist advice being sought, e.g. a drug misuser presenting with opioid withdrawal in late pregnancy, a patient with serious concomitant physical or psychiatric illness where withdrawal is complicating the clinical problems, someone who is opioid dependent and demonstrating withdrawal. Indeed, in such circumstances it is vital that the doctor fulfils their responsibilities by ensuring adequate assessment and appropriate management that facilitates the retention of the patient in treatment.
- *Treat any emergency or acute problem first.* Take history including dosage, route of administration, time last used, and check for injecting sites. Take appropriate screen for opiate drugs to confirm/deny. **Assessment:** general examination, including IV sites, local and systemic sequelae of injecting. Urinalysis for illicit drugs (with consent) should be undertaken. In pregnancy, prescribing should be supervised by a specialist in maternity management.
- **Clinical:** look for and document evidence of **opiate withdrawal syndrome:** drug craving, anxiety, drug seeking (6 h), yawning, sweating, running nose, lacrimation

(8 h), dilated pupils, goose skin, tremors, hot/cold flushes, aching bones/muscles, loss of appetite, abdominal cramps and irritability (12 h), insomnia, hypertension, N&V, diarrhoea, febrile, fetal position. Opiate-dependent individuals undergoing opiate withdrawal syndrome may present to relieve the distressing symptoms of opiate withdrawal whilst in hospital. Do not give in to undue pressure to prescribe immediately. Take time to assess the patient. But they may not, if experiencing withdrawal symptoms, be able to cooperate with staff. Look for objective signs of opioid withdrawal. A negative urine test for opioids makes addiction unlikely.

- **Prescribing (take senior advice first – SpR and above):** do not feel pressurised to prescribe. Methadone and buprenorphine are both approved for the treatment and prevention of withdrawals from opioids but this must only be prescribed following liaison with the community drug team. Methadone is preferred. Optimal doses for most people lie between 40 and 120 mg, but will depend upon size, gender, age, other health problems and metabolic clearance rates. Same care as in prescribing any opiate. Do not give methadone if heroin has been taken in past 8 h or methadone in past 24 h. NEVER give more than 10 mg (methadone mixture 1 mg/1 ml) as an initial dose to patients not receiving a methadone prescription in the community and do not exceed more than 40 mg of methadone in the first 24 h period. NEVER give methadone to a patient already intoxicated with opioids or other drugs including alcohol. Treat opioid overdose with standard resuscitation techniques and with the use of naloxone. Naloxone is given 0.4–2.0 mg parenterally (IV/IM/SC) and this can be repeated after every 5 min, up to a maximum dose of 10 mg. It is important to remember the $t_{1/2}$ of naloxone is much shorter than methadone and other opioids. **Managing opiate withdrawal**. May need LOPERAMIDE (diarrhoea) 4 mg stat followed by 2 mg after each loose stool (max 16 mg daily), METOCLOPRAMIDE (N&V) 10 mg tds or PROCHLORPERAZINE 5 mg tds oral or 12.5 mg IM 12 hourly. MEBEVERINE (stomach cramps) 135 mg tds, DIAZEPAM (agitation/anxiety) 5–10 mg tds, ZOPICLONE (insomnia) 7.5 mg nocte, NSAIDs, paracetamol.

19.18 Driving and disease

The law is quite clear. If a patient has a condition that impairs their ability and makes them unsafe to drive then the doctor has a duty to inform the patient and the patient is legally obliged to inform and follow the advice of the DVLA (Driver and Vehicle Licensing Agency). Ultimately it is the DVLA who will determine if the patient can retain their driving licence. All driving advice given (or advice not to drive) should be documented in the notes. Licences are normally issued valid until age 70 years unless restricted to a shorter duration for medical reasons as indicated above. There is no upper limit but after age 70 renewal is necessary every 3 years. All licence applications require a medical self-declaration by the applicant. This guidance is for a private car or motorcycle. **For those with a licence to drive a bus, coach or lorry, all must inform the DVLA because there are more stringent restrictions**. See www.dvla.org.uk for more information and in particular for the DVLA document entitled 'Fitness to drive', which can be obtained online. If you have any concerns you can ring the DVLA medical advisors. When assessing a patient consider if they would be in full control of the car at all times, e.g. can they do an emergency stop? For borderline cases there are driver assessment centres. Car modifications can allow a disabled patient to drive to the necessary standard. Advise the patient to also inform their car insurers.

Quick guide for private car drivers only (bus, coach, lorry drivers must inform DVLA)

Always check the DVLA website (www.dvla.org.uk) as specific advice changes at times.

Condition	Private car	Coach, lorry, bus drivers should inform DVLA
TIA	Drive after 28 days	No driving for 1 year
Multiple TIAs	No driving for 3 months	No driving for 1 year
Stroke (fully recovered)	Drive after 28 days if recovery with no impairment to driving ability	No driving for 1 year
Stroke	Not to drive – decision to be made by DVLA if residual neurology affecting ability to drive	Not to drive – decision to be made by DVLA if residual neurology affecting ability to drive
First seizure or suspected seizure	Can drive after 6 months – should be seen at seizure clinic	Restricted for a minimum of 5 years – neurology review
Epilepsy	No driving for 1 year	No driving
Unexplained LOC	Restricted for 6 months	Restricted for 12 months
Vasovagal syncope	No restriction	No restriction
Visual field defect	No driving until formal assessment	No driving until formal assessment
Angina	No driving if angina whilst driving	No driving if symptoms
ACS	No driving for 1 week if successful angioplasty, or else for 1 month and EF >0.4	No driving for 6 weeks
Angioplasty	No driving for 1 week	No driving for 6 weeks
Pacemaker	No driving for 1 week	No driving for 6 weeks
CABG	No driving for 4 weeks – inform DVLA	No driving for 3 months; EF >0.4
AICD	No driving for 6–12 months (see guidance)	No driving – inform DVLA
Hypertension	No restriction	Must maintain resting BP <180/100 mmHg or else inform DVLA
Head injury/bleed	No driving for 6–12 months – inform DVLA	Inform DVLA
Incapacitating arrhythmia	No driving until 4 weeks after controlled	Controlled for 3 months and LVEF >40%
AAA >6 cm	Inform DVLA if >6 cm	Inform DVLA
Brain aneurysm	Inform DVLA	Inform DVLA
Post-surgery	At doctor's discretion about pain and ability – need to be in complete control of vehicle	At doctor's discretion about pain and ability – need to be in complete control of vehicle
Diabetes and insulin/ hypo-glycaemics	Need to be aware of hypos. Two or more hypos needing help of another person in past 12 months is a bar to driving – inform DVLA	Full hypo awareness. Regular monitoring. One episode of hypo needing help in past 12 months stop driving and inform DVLA

19.19 Do not attempt cardiopulmonary resuscitation (DNACPR)

- DNACPR as in other issues around dying is a polarising and emotive concept. There are strongly held beliefs by those who would not want it and those who feel they or a loved one would be being denied a beneficial life saving therapy. Many don't want to discuss it and find that upsetting. However, the law is clear. We must discuss it with the patient unless distress is likely to be severe or they lack capacity. If there is no DNACPR in place then medico-legally you are obliged to initiate resuscitation.
- CPR and defibrillation was designed to prolong good quality of life in those with easily reversible causes, e.g. VF due to a STEMI which is shockable, giving the patient many good years ahead, or a post traumatic tension PTX with instant improvement. It was not to interfere in the natural death of an elderly frail patient with co-morbidities from frailty, bronchopneumonia and stroke. Our role is, fundamentally, to prolong life and not to prolong death/dying. We should find out what the patient wants and do that if possible, legal and reasonable.
- To avoid inappropriate "unnatural" CPR we need to always discuss with the patient, but if this is not possible then with those important to them or next of kin. This has been clearly stipulated legally to include ringing relatives at 3 am if needed. It is about the patient's "right to life". You must discuss, achieve consensus if possible. Ultimately DNACPR is a decision for the healthcare team caring for the patient. Document well if there is disagreement and get a second opinion to support your view. If no one is contactable despite reasonable attempts and the patient lacks capacity and time is short then share the decision with the team, e.g. senior nursing staff or colleagues – at least a phone call. Consult others.
- **New guidance:** "Decisions relating to CPR" from BMA/RCN/UK Resuscitation council 2016 3rd edition (1st revision) states that "if the healthcare team is as certain that a person is dying of an underlying disease or catastrophic event and CPR would not start the heart and breathing for a sustained period then CPR should not be attempted". This is not the default position and is for extreme time critical situations and family should always be consulted about the healthcare decision. Doctors must avoid unilateral signing of DNACPR forms without attempting dialogue with patient, family or the wider healthcare team.

19.20 End of life care

- End of life care is one of the most challenging aspects of current medicine when the increasing expectations of contemporary medical practice come up against the realities of the limitations of medical science. Medicine is fundamentally about care, adding quality to life and reducing suffering. We must strive to prolong life but not to prolong and draw out an unpleasant death. Withdrawal of medical care and supportive management often happens at a time when discussions with the patient are not possible. It is important to involve close family. Keep them informed at all stages. It is difficult and input from colleagues can be helpful and reassuring when decisions are difficult. Newer strategies such as AMBER (www.ambercarebundle.org) try to pre-empt palliation and involve the patient and close family in discussing end of life care much earlier and need to be promoted to optimise such care.
- If the patient has a well-defined terminal illness then the natural history of the disease will be helpful. In some the natural history is less clear, such as stroke or sepsis complicating mild dementia. However, be cautious especially with acute deteriorations which may have simple remedies, e.g. UTI, hypoglycaemia, opiate toxicity and it can be reasonable to trial therapy for 24–48 h. Many malignancies and advanced dementia and other neurodegenerative diseases, heart failure and

often chronic lung disease are terminal illnesses with high morbidity and mortality. Some patients are dying due to a multitude of age-related issues which lead to frailty, weight loss, immobility and becoming progressively bed bound and often succumbing to chest infections.

- Before an end of life pathway is instituted, make sure you are completely up to date on the patient's letters and notes. If unsure get the GP patient record faxed over. Be well briefed before you talk to family. When you do make sure you get the right family – record names of those involved in discussions, it is always best to find out first what they know because they may have additional information for you or tell you things not recorded. Discover what they have been told. What are their expectations? Some issues have been discussed in the recent NICE end of life guidance (December 2015) on which the following is based. EOL decisions on new frail older patients should be avoided based on a snapshot initial assessment which may not reflect the true state but on sequential assessments over several days.

- **Recognising when a person may be in the last days of life:** it can be difficult to be certain that a person is dying. Experienced clinical judgment is needed to manage any uncertainty. If dying, assess person's physiological, psychological, social and spiritual needs, current clinical signs and symptoms, medical history and the clinical context, including underlying diagnoses, the person's goals and wishes and views of those important to the person about future care.

- **Monitor for clinical changes:** agitation, Cheyne–Stokes breathing, deterioration in level of consciousness, mottled skin, noisy respiratory secretions and progressive weight loss, increasing fatigue and loss of appetite. Observe reduced communication, deteriorating mobility or performance status, or social withdrawal. Improvements could indicate that the person may be stabilising or recovering.

- **Investigations:** avoid if unlikely to affect care in the last few days of life unless there is a clinical need to do so with clear benefits.

- **Multidisciplinary:** interprofessional discussions and information sharing is key and issues discussed. Monitor at least every 24 h and update the person's care plan. Include a second/senior opinion when there is uncertainty about optimal management.

- **Communication is key.** With family, other staff and when possible with the patient. Establish the communication needs and expectations of people who may be entering their last days of life. Ask if they would like a person important to them to be present when making decisions about their care. Assess their current level of understanding that they may be nearing death. Assess cognitive status and if they have any specific speech, language or other communication needs. How much information would they like to have about their prognosis? Respect cultural, religious, social or spiritual needs or preferences.

- **Consent:** healthcare professionals caring for adults at the end of life need to take into consideration the person's current mental capacity to communicate and actively participate in their end of life care.

- **Information:** provide where possible information about prognosis (unless they do not wish to be informed), explaining any uncertainty and how this will be managed, but avoiding false optimism. Discuss fears and anxieties, and invite questions about their care in the last days of life. Offer further discussions. Discuss any advanced decisions or wishes. Ensure well documented. Discuss any personal goals and wishes, preferred care setting, current and anticipated care needs, including: preferences for symptom management and needs for care after death, if any are specified. Ensure appropriate revisions and updates as time passes. If it is not possible to meet the wishes of a dying person explain the reason why to the person and those important to them.

- **Maintaining hydration:** support the dying person to drink if they wish to and are able to. Address any difficulties. Offer frequent care of the mouth and lips to the dying person as part of standard care, with cleaning of teeth or dentures, if they would like. Offer frequent sips of fluid. Monitor hydration status. Assess if appropriate or desirable to start clinically assisted hydration, respecting the person's wishes and preferences. It may give some symptoms relief. It may, however, cause problems – overload, local oedema, pain and may prolong life or extend the dying process. Discuss with the dying person or those important to them before starting clinically assisted hydration. Factors to consider are culture, religious beliefs, wishes, their level of consciousness, ability to swallow, evidence of thirst, risk of pulmonary oedema and the possibility that even temporary recovery is possible. Consider a trial of hydration if there is belief that it may help and keep under review. When stopping hydration and nutrition there is a lot to be said for sharing the plan and getting a second opinion or that the consensus of the healthcare team have been consulted and content with any end of life care.

- **Pharmacological interventions:** can be helpful to manage breathlessness, agitation, insomnia, pain. Discuss the balance in benefits and harms of any medicines offered. Decide on the most effective route; avoid IM, so give either SC or IV injections. Consider using a syringe pump to deliver medicines for continuous symptom control if more than 2 or 3 doses of any 'as required' medicines have been given within 24 h. New drugs should be started with the lowest effective dose and titrated as clinically indicated. Regularly reassess, at least daily, the dying person's symptoms during treatment to inform appropriate titration of medicine. Get specialist input where needed.
- **Breathlessness:** treat cause, e.g. heart failure, bronchospasm. Consider an opioid or a benzodiazepine or both.
- **Nausea and vomiting:** treat a treatable cause if possible. If obstructive bowel disorders in patients who have nausea or vomiting, consider: hyoscine butylbromide or octreotide if the symptoms do not improve within 24 h of starting hyoscine.
- **Anxiety, delirium and agitation:** explore causes. Look for unrelieved pain or a full bladder or rectum. Treat any medical cause. Consider a trial of a benzodiazepine to manage anxiety or agitation or antipsychotic medicine to manage delirium or agitation. Seek advice if unsure.
- **Managing noisy respiratory secretions:** look for cause. Consider atropine or glycopyrronium bromide or hyoscine butylbromide or hyoscine hydrobromide. Monitor for improvements every 4–12 h. Watch for side effects, e.g. delirium, agitation or excessive sedation when using atropine or hyoscine hydrobromide. Consider changing or stopping medicine if unacceptable side effects, such as dry mouth, urinary retention, delirium, agitation and unwanted levels of sedation, persist.

Reference: NICE (2015) NG31: Care of dying adults in the last days of life.

19.21 Palliative care drugs

Review symptoms at least every 24 h and adjust and record accordingly. Syringe driver useful as needle can be placed subcutaneously especially when unconscious, dysphagia, vomiting, confused. All IV or SC drugs to be given by a standard calibrated syringe pump. Consult local guidance. MORPHINE is the most important drug for controlling pain and breathlessness and is given MORPHINE 5–10 mg every 4 h (low dose 2.5 mg if opiate naïve, renal dysfunction). If significant renal impairment transdermal FENTANYL recommended as 72 h patches. These agents may have a dual effect, e.g. respiratory depression as well as reducing dyspnoea or pain. The prime aim should be always to reduce suffering.

Symptom	Management
Breathlessness	MORPHINE SULPHATE 2.5–5 mg SC 4 h. If 2 or more doses in 24 h then MORPHINE 5–10 mg in syringe driver. MIDAZOLAM 2.5 mg stat SC and if ongoing then MIDAZOLAM 5–10 mg/24 h. MORPHINE and MIDAZOLAM can be combined.
Pain	MORPHINE 2.5–5 mg SC 4 h to start. Escalate to MORPHINE 10 mg IV SC via syringe pump over 24 h. Increase dose to match pain relief. Those already on opiates need an increased dose adequate for their needs. Addiction is not an issue in EOL care. Excess MORPHINE can be managed with small amounts of NALOXONE for partial reversal. See *Section 22.3* for Drug formulary. SC MORPHINE dose is half the oral MORPHINE dose. SC DIAMORPHINE dose is one-third oral MORPHINE dose. Prescribe ORAMORPH or SC opiates for breakthrough pain.
Nausea and vomiting	HALOPERIDOL 0.5–1 mg SC PRN up to 10 mg/day. Ongoing need HALOPERIDOL infusion 2.5–5 mg SC over 24 h. LEVOMEPROMAZINE 12.5–25 mg SC stat or PRN. Ongoing symptoms consider LEVOMEPROMAZINE infusion 50 mg/day. CYCLIZINE 50 mg 8 h PO/SC. Ongoing symptoms CYCLIZINE 150 mg/day by infusion if needed. Alternative: ONDANSETRON 8 mg PO/IV BD (may need laxative).
Restless agitation	MIDAZOLAM 2.5–5 mg SC PRN repeated at 30 min if remains symptomatic. If 2 or more doses given in a day consider MIDAZOLAM 10 mg SC/24 h via syringe driver. Exclude pain, full bladder, full rectum, anxiety, breathlessness.
Psychosis	HALOPERIDOL 1.5 mg stat and then 0.5–1 mg S/C PRN up to 10 mg per day. If continues, consider HALOPERIDOL infusion 3 mg/24 h. LEVOMEPROMAZINE 12.5–25 mg S/C PRN 2-hourly or given as 50 mg in a syringe driver over 24 h.
Respiratory secretions	GLYCOPYRRONIUM 200 mcg SC 4 h. If >2 doses in 24 h then start infusion of 1.2 mg over 24 h.
Gastric distension	DOMPERIDONE 10 mg 8 h which is a prokinetic and may aid gastric emptying.
Bowel obstruction	HYOSCINE butylbromide 60–120 mg/24 h SC. Octreotide can reduce bowel secretions.

Considerations in the dying patient

- Reduce or stop non-essential usual primary and secondary prevention medications, e.g. statin, aspirin, antihypertensives, etc.
- Retain only drugs for symptom control, e.g. a diuretic to avoid pulmonary oedema if fluid intake continues. Judge each case individually.
- Stop inappropriate investigations. Remove cardiac monitors and O_2 sats and stop blood tests. Stop EWS-type observations.
- Monitor for pain, agitation, distress, skin lesions, bowels, bladder, nausea, vomiting and manage those.
- Stop IV or SC fluids if these are futile treatments because they tend only to prolong death rather than life.
- Oral fluids and mouth care for care and symptom support as part of EOL care.
- Ensure DNACPR (do not attempt CPR) and any escalation policy is completed and has been communicated to the nursing staff.
- Ensure family are aware and up to date on the status of the patient.
- Any religious or spiritual needs or cultural expectations of care of the body after death which will be handled by the bereavement office.
- Ensure death certification and any referral to coroner is done as early as possible after death and liaise with the bereavement office.

- GP should be made aware through local arrangements rather than reading local obituary columns.

6 'Cs' of end of life care
- Communication with patient and family and GP and others as appropriate.
- Consent – involving the patient in determining their care.
- Compassionate care at all times.
- Control of symptoms – see below.
- Culture – respect religious and cultural views and expectations.
- Clear documentation of plan and discussions and handovers.

Roles and responsibilities after death

Introduction
- The diagnosis of death has been formalised by the Academy of Medical Royal Colleges (2008) paper *A code of practice for the diagnosis and confirmation of death* which should be read.
- The definition of death should be regarded as *the irreversible loss of the capacity for consciousness, combined with irreversible loss of the capacity to breathe*. This may be secondary to a wide range of underlying problems in the body, for example, cardiac arrest. The irreversible cessation of brain stem function, whether due to intra/ extracranial events will produce this clinical state and therefore irreversible loss of function of the brain stem equates with the death of the individual and allows the diagnosis of death.
- Loss of the capacity for consciousness does not equal death. Patients in the vegetative state have also lost this capacity. Those declared dead by virtue of irreversible cessation of brain stem function do not breathe unaided. This also means that even if the body of the deceased remains on respiratory support, the loss of integrated biological function will inevitably lead to deterioration and organ necrosis within a short time.

Diagnosing death
- During the day or when on call you may well be called to see patients who have died to 'certify' them' as dead. These are usually patients who have had unsuccessful attempts at resuscitation or who have died and who are not for resuscitation. In some, such as those on care plans for the dying and palliation, the death will have been expected, in others it may not have been.
- Diagnosing death is rarely an urgent request but one should seek to certify as soon as convenient so that the patient can be moved off the ward to the morgue. Check that family have been informed – they will rarely need to speak to a doctor unless the death is entirely unexpected. If you do have to speak to the family then it is best to set aside some time and find a convenient space to talk to them, preferably with nursing staff to hand. Any contentious issues should be escalated to the responsible consultant to liaise with the family in normal hours.
- **In practice, attend the patient and listen and auscultate the chest for 5 min** to show absence of continued cardiorespiratory arrest, the absence of the pupillary responses to light, of the corneal reflexes, and of any motor response to supra-orbital pressure, should be confirmed and the time of death is recorded as the time at which these criteria are fulfilled. Document your findings and ensure accurately timed and dated and signed and GMC number. Additional comments, e.g. RIP and religious comments are not needed.

- **Nurses:** the nurses prepare the body which usually involves closing eyes and mouth. Pumps and syringe drivers are removed but the actual lines are left *in situ*. Orifices are packed with cotton wool. The patient is wrapped in a sheet. The porters will usually come with a special trolley to bring the patient to the mortuary. Often the nurses will close the curtains on adjacent beds whilst this occurs.

Brainstem death

- Mainly an ITU issue in ventilated patients in whom withdrawal of support is being considered. Reversible causes of persisting unconsciousness must be excluded. There should be no doubt as to the cause of irreversible brain damage, so when the cause is unclear brain stem testing cannot be undertaken. One must try to exclude any potentially reversible causes of coma – exclude depressant drugs – narcotics, hypnotics and tranquillizers. Consider hypothermia, renal or hepatic failure.
- Time may be allowed for drug excretion. Naloxone and Flumazenil given as indicated. Body temperature should be >34°C before testing. Glucose and electrolytes should be normalised. K <2 mmol/L or Na >160 mmol/L or <115 mmol/L and Mg and phosphate should be corrected. Hypothyroidism and Addison's disease should be treated. Neuromuscular blockers stopped. In a trauma patient C-spine should be imaged to exclude high-cord lesion causing apnoea.

Testing for absence of brain stem reflexes: consultant and a doctor registered for at least 5 years

- Pupils are fixed and do not respond to sharp changes in light intensity.
- No corneal reflex.
- Absent oculo-vestibular reflexes – no eye movements with slow injection of 50 ml of ice cold water over 1 min into each external auditory meatus in turn.
- No motor responses within the cranial nerve distribution can be elicited by adequate stimulation of any somatic area.
- No motor response can be elicited within the cranial nerve or somatic distribution in response to supra-orbital pressure.
- No cough reflex response to bronchial stimulation by a suction catheter placed down the trachea to the carina, or gag response to stimulation of the posterior pharynx with a spatula.
- Hypercarbia – apnoea test.

19.23 ▶ Death certification

- Even if you are the person who certified the patient as deceased you cannot do the death certificate unless you personally attended the patient within the past 14 days. Prompt and accurate certification of death is essential. The death certificate provides legal evidence of the fact and cause of death, which has legal and statistical importance and enables the death to be formally registered. Only then can the family make arrangements for cremation/burial of the body. As a new doctor the 'Bereavement office' will be calling on your services frequently and it is wise to work well with them. They have little flexibility and the death certificate should be done as soon as is reasonably possible – you are required by law to do so. Death certification can be done by an F1 or above, but it is important that you take advice from senior members of the team. You are legally responsible for the delivery of the death certificate to the registrar, but the bereavement office staff will often do this and usually it is the family who bring it to the registrar.

Information requested as part of death certification

- **Patient's age at death:** work it out from the notes and check it is correct.
- **Place of death:** record the precise place of death (e.g. typically the name of the hospital and ward or the address of a private house or, for deaths elsewhere, the locality). This may not be the same as the place where you are completing the certificate. It is particularly important that the relative or other person responsible for registering the death is directed to the Registrar of Births and Deaths for the sub-district where the death occurred, unless (from 1st April 1977) they have decided to make a declaration of the details to be registered before another registrar.
- **When last seen alive by me:** record the date when you last saw the deceased alive, irrespective of whether any other medical practitioner saw the person alive subsequently.
- **Information from post-mortem:** you should indicate whether the information you give about the cause of death takes account of a post-mortem. Such information can be valuable for epidemiological purposes. If a post-mortem has been done, circle option 1. If information may be available later, do not delay the issue of your certificate, circle option 2 and tick statement B on the reverse of the certificate. The registrar will then send you a form for return to the Registrar General giving the results of the post-mortem. If a post-mortem is not being held, circle option 3.
- **Seen after death** (only one option can be circled): you should indicate, by circling option a, b or c, whether you or another medical practitioner saw the deceased after death.

Ask the bereavement office staff to check your work – it can save you lots of problems if there are issues or simple mistakes or typographical errors.

When to refer a death to the coroner

You should refer when any of the following occur. In hospital the bereavement office staff will usually assist with this. You may speak to the coroner or their officer who will advise. Occasionally the staff may ask for a written referral which is faxed over. Follow local policy.

- The cause of death is unknown or it cannot readily be certified as being due to natural causes.
- The deceased was not attended by the doctor during his last illness or was not seen within 14 days or viewed after death.
- There are any suspicious circumstances or history of violence.
- The death may be linked to an accident (whenever it occurred).
- There is any question of self-neglect or neglect by others.
- The death has occurred or the illness arisen during or shortly after detention in police or prison custody (includes voluntary attendance at a police station).
- The deceased was detained under the Mental Health Act.
- The death is linked with an abortion.
- The death might have been contributed to by the actions of the deceased (such as a history of drug or solvent abuse, self-injury or overdose).
- Death could be due to industrial disease or related to the deceased's employment.
- The death occurred during an operation or before full recovery from the effects of an anaesthetic or was in any way related to the anaesthetic (in any event a death within 24 h should normally be referred).
- Death related to a medical procedure or treatment whether invasive or not.
- The death may be due to lack of medical care.
- There are any other unusual or disturbing features to the case.

- Death within 24 h of admission to hospital (unless admission was purely for terminal care).
- It may be wise to report any death where there is an allegation of medical mismanagement or care issues.

Cause of death

This section of the certificate is divided into Parts I and II. Part I is used to show the immediate cause of death and any underlying cause or causes. Part II should be used for any significant condition or disease that contributed to the death but which is not part of the sequence leading directly to death. State the cause or causes of death accurately to the best of your knowledge and belief. It is wise to take senior advice routinely especially if unsure or any doubts. **Underlying cause of death:** consider the main causal sequence of conditions leading to death. State the disease or condition that led directly to death on the first line [I(a)] and work your way back until you reach the Underlying Cause of Death, which initiated the chain of events leading ultimately to death. **The lowermost completed line in Part I should therefore contain the Underlying Cause of Death.** Sometimes there are apparently two distinct conditions leading to death. If there is no way of choosing between them, they should be entered on the same line indicating in brackets that they are joint causes of death, e.g. ischaemic heart disease and chronic bronchitis. 'Smoking' may be included if accompanied by a medical cause of death. Do not use the following as the single sole cause of death, e.g. *asphyxia, debility, respiratory arrest, asthenia, exhaustion, shock, brain failure, heart failure, syncope, cachexia, hepatic failure, uraemia, cardiac arrest, hepatorenal failure, vagal inhibition, cardiac failure, kidney failure, vasovagal attack, coma, renal failure, ventricular failure, liver failure*. These are clinical syndromes which need pathological explanation as to why they occurred. Old age or senility, although acceptable, should not be used as the only cause of death in Part I unless a more specific cause of death cannot be given and the deceased was aged 70 or over. **Part II:** should be used when one or more conditions have contributed to death but are not part of the main causal sequence leading to death. It should not be used to list all conditions present at death. In some cases you can put an interval as to the diagnosis of each in hours, days, months or years before the death occurred. In Part I and II, you should give information about clinical interventions, procedures or drugs that may have led to adverse effects, e.g. warfarin-induced bleeds, etc.

Example of acceptable entries

I(a): cerebral metastases, I(b): squamous cell lung cancer, I(c): smoking.

I(a): respiratory failure, I(b): lobar pneumonia, I(c): squamous cell lung cancer.

II: Type 2 diabetes mellitus.

Employment-related death: if you believe that the death may have been due to (or contributed to) the employment undertaken at any time by the deceased, you should indicate this. Tick the appropriate box on the front of the certificate and then report it to the coroner.

Sign the form: you must sign the certificate and add your qualifications, address and the date. It would greatly assist the registrar if you could also PRINT YOUR NAME IN BLOCK CAPITAL LETTERS. If the death occurred in hospital, the name of the consultant who was responsible for the care of the patient must also be given. Have you remembered your signature, notice to informant, counterfoil? Even now I always get bereavement office staff to check through what I have done. They might spot simple errors, which could cause problems for the family in getting the patient registered.

It is so easy to get a date wrong and this can halt a funeral or a cremation ceremony. The bereavement office staff are experts and will help to prevent any problems.

19.24 Managing inpatients with pressure sores and ulcers

Adults at high risk usually have multiple risk factors and should be assessed **within 6 h of admission** by nursing teams and then daily during inpatient stay (e.g. limited mobility, nutritional deficiency, inability to reposition themselves, significant cognitive impairment). Encourage high risk adults at risk to change their position frequently at least every 4 h. Offer a nutritional assessment if intake is inadequate. Document the surface area and depth of all pressure ulcers in adults (transparency tracing or a photograph). Use **high-specification foam mattresses**. If not sufficient to redistribute pressure, consider the use of a dynamic support surface. Assess the seating needs of adults who have a pressure ulcer who are sitting for prolonged periods. High specification foam or equivalent for those who use a wheelchair or sit for prolonged periods and who have a pressure ulcer. Consider debridement if necrotic tissue and tolerated. Consider systemic antibiotics if there is clinical evidence of systemic sepsis, spreading cellulitis or underlying osteomyelitis. Take local antimicrobial advice. Try to develop strategies for heel ulcers to offset pressure. (NICE (2014) CG179: Pressure ulcers: prevention and management).

- **Category/Stage I:** non-blanchable redness of intact skin usually over a bony prominence. May be painful, firmer or softer, or warmer or cooler than adjacent tissue.
- **Category/Stage II:** partial thickness skin loss or blister. Shallow open ulcer with a red/pink wound bed, without slough.
- **Category/Stage III:** full thickness skin loss (fat visible), bone, tendon, or muscle are not exposed.
- **Category/Stage IV:** full thickness tissue loss (muscle/bone visible).

19.25 Rehabilitation, function and discharge

- Rehabilitation is an active process in which an attempt is made to improve a patient's level of functional ability to manage their own personal needs – eating, washing, dressing, transferring, toileting, mobility, shopping, working and independence. One needs an 'acute rehabable pathology', e.g. acute stroke, UTI, infection, fracture, where the natural processes of healing and repair will deliver gains in strength, dexterity, cognition, etc., that therapists can exploit to regain natural functional return to live as independent a life as possible. Pathologies such as progressive cancer and dementia or simply ageing respond poorly to rehabilitation. Rehabilitation requires a patient who is willing to cooperate and focus on the tasks. The clinician can start the process with simply encouraging sitting out of bed and activity because, to paraphrase a wise orthopod, "Bed rest is rehabilitation for the coffin".
- Getting a patient out of bed on Day 1 if appropriate will reduce length of stay, reduce risk of VTE, enable more normal bowel and bladder function and normal eating and drinking. Transfers are an important concept to describe the process by which we, in our daily lives, move our bottoms from one surface to another. In the most dependent this may be by hoist or, in those with some abilities, using aids such as rota stands, boards and other devices. A patient who can transfer their weight from a bed to a chair to a toilet has a better life than simply being bed-bound and hoisted. It is wise to get patients up and walking before discharging them. Walking is a very good screening test of cognition, vision, sensation, cardiovascular, respiratory and other neurological functions. If unsafe then ask why and involve

therapy. Patients, especially older ones, often need a functional assessment prior to discharge – can they toilet, wash and feed themselves, are they safe in a kitchen, who does the shopping, access to toilet, can they manage stairs? Consider these things and involve family early.

- Before discharge simple knowledge like getting care packages back in place is key. Does the patient live in a ground floor flat with easy access or a house with 2 flights of stairs to the bedroom/bathroom? Is there a ground floor toilet? All of this can be key. Before discharge visualise your patient's day. How do they get out of bed, wash and dress, prepare a meal, eat, shop etc.?

- A quick call to the next of kin can be hugely time saving and allow a more realistic plan. How long does rehabilitation continue – as long as it is continuing to deliver real and meaningful improvements in function that will improve quality of life. Stop rehabilitation if goals are constantly missed and build as much quality into the patient's world around their functional status, using equipment, carers, family support and optimising the environment. The key steps are to try to improve the patient and, once optimal, change the environment around them if needed. A holistic and good clinician can imagine life beyond hospital. If you don't do this they will come back.

19.26 Drains and tubes

- **Chest drains:** inserted into 4/5th intercostal pleural space to drain the pleural space of air and fluid. End inserted into water drain to ensure one-way movement of fluid/air. Inserted into the pleural space to allow removal of air or fluid. Can be thin (20 Fr) for air and in children to thick tubes (40 Fr) for blood or viscous pleural fluid in adults. Placed in the safe triangle (see ▶ Section 4.12 on pneumothorax) in 4/5th intercostal spaces in the anterior axillary or mid-axillary line. Connected to underwater one-way seal. Fluid and air can exit but not enter. Inspiration compresses the space and pleural contents should exit unless there is a leak and air continues to fill the space. Used for pneumothorax, haemothorax often as an emergency, or for a persistent/large pleural effusion. They are also commonly placed at the end of thoracic surgeries to allow for appropriate re-expansion of the lung tissue. A CXR should be obtained after any chest tube insertion to ensure appropriate placement. There is a radiopaque line on the drain which should be checked. Ensure all holes lie within chest. Respiration should cause fluid to swing and shows tube is patent and working. If air bubbles are seen in a PTX patient, then this suggests an air leak which may take a few days. Persisting leak needs specialist review. A CXR should be done for any change clinically, especially if there is a suspected blocked tube which may need to be removed and reinserted. Drains inserted for effusion can be removed when daily output <100–200 ml/d.

- **Closed suction drains:** used post-op where fluid collection and risk of infection. Kept until output <20 ml/d. The output may be blood, bile, urine or pus/exudate depending on the site and each needs a specific management of cause.

- **Gastro/jejunostomy:** Can be used to give feed or to decompress a distended upper GI tract, e.g. due to distal obstruction. **Jejunostomy tubes** are used exclusively for feeding and are usually placed to lie distal to the ligament of Treitz. Where suction is needed, keep <60 mmHg.

19.27 Surgical problems and referrals

Some surgical emergencies are included here in this text. This is to remind the physician that surgical patients can get into the medical take and surgical patients have medical problems and it is not uncommon for surgeons not to take "surgical" patients, especially if no operative intervention is foreseen. They need identifying and referral. They may benefit from medical optimisation. If it is thought that an urgent surgical procedure is needed then keep patient fasted as they may need anaesthesia. Manage fluid and electrolytes and give adequate analgesia. Issues may include decisions on managing/ reversing antithrombotic therapy, correcting electrolytes, etc. and detecting and fixing critical unresolved medical issues and pointing out critical issues and priorities in older patients with multiple pathologies and polypharmacy. Increasing evidence shows physicians can add value to perioperative surgical care especially that involving older patients. Fitness for surgery is an anaesthetic/surgical issue. It is not your job to deem fitness for surgery but only to optimise medically and ensure anaesthetists and surgeons are aware of your findings. Sometimes your role will be seeing the whole patient and identifying major issues suggesting medical and possibly surgical futility and communicating this to all. As ever take senior advice if unsure.

20 Procedures

20.1 Checks before any procedure

- The content here is to refresh memories and reinforce points to users who have been conventionally trained and are competent in these procedures. Do not perform a procedure in which you have not been trained. Get supervision if you are not competent. Generally get written consent unless dire emergency. Most invasive procedures should not take place out of hours except in an emergency.

- In terms of procedures, be aware that the only way to avoid complications is not to do any. Before you undertake a therapeutic procedure which should improve circumstances (e.g. a chest drain) or a diagnostic procedure (e.g. central line placement to measure CVP/pulmonary artery pressures), consider whether the procedure will change management significantly; can you get the information elsewhere? The information you may get might be erroneous due to failure to calibrate or other errors. Complications will happen and you can make a patient even worse, so ensure that the emergency procedure was valid and vital and could someone support or supervise you, or be doing it? Procedures are time consuming and this time might be better spent doing other things.

Questions before any procedure

(1) Is it the right patient?	(5) Is the patient anticoagulated or have a coagulopathy?
(2) Is it the right procedure?	
(3) Is it the right (or left) side?	(6) Is this the right time: can it wait until working hours?
(4) Have I the right to do it, i.e. has informed consent been obtained?	(7) Am I the right person to do this (should I get someone more skilled to do it or supervise me)?

20.2 Venepuncture

- **Equipment:** sharps bin, cannula, sterile bung and micropore tape (check for known allergies). Non-sterile gloves (check for latex allergy), alcoholic wipe 2% chlorhexidine (Clinell), tourniquet, dressing (sterile), cotton wool (sterile), trolley, syringe (10 ml), flushing agent (NS for injection).

Technique

- **Introduce self,** explain procedure and get verbal consent. Make sure that the cannula used is appropriate for indication. Choose vein and apply tourniquet above vein. Prepare skin at the selected insertion site with a med swab, wait 30 sec to allow the area to dry. Do not re-palpate the vein or touch the skin. Remove the needle guard and inspect the cannula for any faults. Hold the patient's hand/wrist/forearm using the thumb, to keep the skin taut. Do not to contaminate the site. Place the needle tip several millimetres distal to the proposed site for cannulation, with the bevel facing up and elevate the angle of the cannula to 15–25° and insert the cannula into the skin (fragile veins require a lower angle of insertion). Once the vein has been located with the needle, lower the angle for insertion. Look for back flow of blood into the cannula chamber, unless the vein is small in which case this may be delayed. Hold the cannula steady relative to the vein whilst withdrawing the needle slightly and then slowly advance the cannula. If there is any sign of swelling, haematoma, pain or resistance the vein wall may be ruptured. If so, release tourniquet or you will cause a haematoma. Remove cannula. Apply pressure with cotton wool. Otherwise, when flashback is seen along the length of the cannula the investigator or delegated person will advance the cannula until it is fully inserted into the vein. Release the skin tension and the tourniquet. Apply gloved digital pressure to the distal end of the cannula to prevent blood spillage. Remove the introducer needle and discard into an appropriate yellow sharps container. Now secure a sterile bung to the end of the cannula. Secure the cannula to the patient using a sterile dressing. Flush the cannula with a minimum of 2 ml of IV NS for injection and cap off. Check the patient feels no discomfort, and observe the cannula site for signs of swelling or redness. Ensure that you complete cannula chart and any accompanying documentation. If you fail then try again, but if you have tried several times with no success either get some help or come back to the task later. If it is an emergency then get help urgently. You cannot resuscitate a patient successfully without IV access. If you have found the cannula is intra-arterial (pulsatile, high pressure, bright red blood) then remove cannula and apply pressure over the site for 10+ minutes until haemostasis. Check distal pulses. Take senior advice if pulseless or distal ischaemia.

20.3 Chest drain insertion

- **Introduction:** ask the 'right' questions (▶ Section 20.1 above): note the use of ultrasound-guided insertion is associated with lower complication rates. Incorrect placement of a chest drain can lead to significant morbidity and even mortality. Follow local guidance. Do not attempt unless trained.
- **Indications.** (1) Pneumothorax: not all require a chest drain (▶ Section 4.12 on pneumothorax). The differential diagnosis between a PTX and a bulla requires careful radiological assessment including CT. (2) Pleural fluid: malignant pleural effusion, simple pleural effusions in ventilated patients, empyema and complicated parapneumonic pleural effusion, traumatic PTX or haemopneumothorax. (3) Postoperative: e.g. thoracotomy, oesophageal surgery, cardiothoracic surgery. The urgency of insertion will depend on the indication and degree of physiological derangement that is being caused by the substance to be drained.

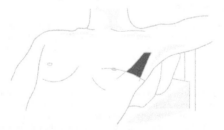

- **Procedure to insert a chest drain:** only to be done by trained or supervised persons. Done well there are 3% early complications and 8% late complications. Training reduces complications.
- **Potential complications:** incorrect placement with drain outside the pleura, in the fissure, tube kinked. Injury to intercostal vessels. Trocar must not be used as risk of spearing heart, liver and other organs. *Excessive bleeding risk*: ensure no coagulopathy – clotting screen and platelets if unsure.
- **Equipment:** aseptic pack with sterile drapes, iodine or equivalent solution. Gauze, scalpel, 2/0 silk and curved needle, 5 and 10 ml syringes. Orange and green needles, sterile gloves, chest drain (Seldinger or 'trocar' type). Chest drain bottle or bag with flutter valve.

Methods

- **Pre-procedure: informed consent** obtained and documented unless dire emergency. Check identity of the patient and the site of insertion of the chest drain. Confirm the clinical signs (percuss the chest and listen) and review the latest CXR and clinical indications. As ever, all equipment needed to insert a chest drain should be available before commencing the procedure. **Patient positioning:** as comfortably as possible because the procedure may be prolonged. Much will depend on the clinical state of the patient. If possible patient lying back at 45° with the arm on the side used flopped behind head to open up rib spaces (see figure above). Alternatively, fatigued patient may lean forward resting on some pillows on a table, as long as access to the axilla is preserved. Occasionally the procedure is done with a patient lying on their side with the affected side uppermost. In a trauma situation, or ITU, an emergency drain insertion is more likely to be performed whilst the patient is supine. **Premedication:** analgesia should be considered – MORPHINE 5 mg IM with cyclizine or MIDAZOLAM 1–5 mg IV if not hypoventilating with appropriate monitoring (pulse oximetry) and resuscitation equipment immediately available. 100% O_2 should be given to all PTX patients if appropriate as it helps resolution. **Aseptic technique:** full aseptic precautions (washed hands, gloves, gown, antiseptic preparation for the insertion site and adequate sterile field) in order to avoid wound site infection or secondary empyema.

Choice of chest drain

- Sizes 10–36Ch. Drains may be inserted via direct surgical incision (thoracostomy) or using the Seldinger technique with guide wire and dilator system. Spontaneous PTX and non-viscous effusions can be drained with relatively small calibre drains via Seldinger method. Better tolerated with less discomfort, but traumatic pneumothoracies, haemothoracies and empyemas may need larger drains, typically 26F and above. **Inserting the drain:** most placed in 4th–5th intercostal space (ICS) in the mid-axillary line – the lowest axillary hair is useful marker where present. Area known as the *safe triangle* with anterior border of latissimus dorsi, the lateral border of the pectoralis major, a line superior to the horizontal level of the nipple and an apex below the axilla as shown above. Any other placement should be discussed with a chest physician. In an apical PTX, placement in the 2nd ICS can be considered but is difficult to maintain. A specific position (identified with CT or ultrasound) may also be required for a loculated effusion. **Seldinger chest tube technique:** infiltrate with up to 10 ml of 1% lignocaine along the intended track. Remove catheter, dilator, introducer wire and introducer needle from pack and insert introducer needle into the thoracic cavity into the chosen site. Withdraw air with a syringe to confirm placement. Now thread introducer wire through needle lumen into the chest. Whilst holding wire tip and then base, remove needle leaving introducer wire running into chest. Thread dilator over introducer wire, and advance into chest, dilating a track for catheter. Remove dilator. Thread tube over the wire fully into chest ensuring side holes lie within chest cavity. Remove wire. Suture catheter in place. Attach catheter to drainage unit. *Obtain post-procedure chest X-ray.* **Rigid chest tube insertion:** infiltrate with 10–15 ml of 1% lignocaine along the intended track, make a 3–4 cm incision through skin and subcutaneous tissues between the 4th and 5th ribs, parallel to the rib margins. Continue incision through the intercostal muscles, and right down to the pleura and use dissecting forceps to bluntly dissect down to the pleura and then insert through the pleura and open the jaws widely, again parallel to the direction of the ribs. This will create a PTX if not locally present and allows the lung to fall away from the chest wall somewhat. Insert gloved sterile finger through your incision and into the thoracic cavity. Make sure you are feeling lung (or empty space) and not liver or spleen. Grasp end of chest tube with the forceps (convex angle facing down towards ribs), and insert chest tube through the hole you have made in the pleura. After tube has entered thoracic cavity, remove forceps and manually advance the tube. Clamp distal tube end with forceps and suture and tape tube in place and attach tube to drainage. *NEVER EVER USE A TROCAR TO INSERT DRAIN*. Obtain post-procedure chest X-ray for placement; tube may need to be advanced or withdrawn slightly. Need to be a bit firm but gentle. The chest tube should be placed in the pleural cavity; significant force should never be used as this risks sudden chest penetration and damage to essential intrathoracic structures. The operator should ensure controlled spreading of the intercostal muscles on the superior surface of the ribs to avoid injury to the intercostal vessels and nerves that run below the inferior border of the ribs.

The drainage system: connect to an underwater seal drainage system. This employs positive expiratory pressure and gravity to drain the pleural space. Tube is submerged at least 2 cm below water of the reservoir/collection chamber. Underwater seal acts as a one-way valve to expel air from the pleural space. Keep collection chamber below the patient at all times or air will re-accumulate in the pleural space. **Large pleural effusions:** drained in stages. Rapid shifts in pleural pressures and re-expansion can cause re-expansion pulmonary oedema, a serious complication. A limit of 1–1.5 L of fluid should be drained before the tube is clamped. If the patient starts to cough or complains of chest pain before this point is reached, drainage should be stopped and may be resumed a few hours later.

Portable valve systems can be used for patients with on-going air leaks or fluid drainage and these use a one-way flutter valve which is generally lower resistance to drainage than with conventional underwater seal units. Ambulatory systems exist.

Securing the chest drain: secure with 1/0 silk suture anchored to the skin and the drain with a suitable non-slip knot technique. This should prevent excessive travel of the drain in and out of the chest wall. The skin incision can be closed each side of the chest tube usually with one 2/0 silk suture each side. Nylon/Ethilon can be used but is more difficult to tie. Tie sutures securely. Purse string sutures should be avoided because they convert a linear wound into a circular wound which can be painful and leave an unsightly scar. **Dressings:** purpose-designed dressings should be used, i.e. *Drainfix* for small bore drains and *Mefix* for large bore drains. Excessive dressings restrict chest wall movement or cause moisture collection. Dressings should allow site inspection. Drain connections should not be covered. A tag of adhesive dressing tape can support the tube and protect it against being pulled out. Patient should be aware to look after the drain and keep the underwater bottle below the chest, avoid compressing the tube by sitting or lying on it and avoid tension on the tube.

Analgesia: ensure regular analgesia is prescribed whilst the chest drain is in place. Dressings should be changed daily for the following reasons: to enable the insertion site to be monitored for signs of infection (swab if any signs of infection), as well as to monitor for surgical emphysema, to ensure the chest drain remains well placed, and the anchor suture is intact. **Monitoring/recording:** fluid in tube should swing with respiration due to changes in intra-pleural pressure. Fluid should rise on inspiration and fall on expiration. Bubbling and swinging are both dependent on an intact underwater seal and so can only be picked up if the drain tube extends below the water level in the bottle. Ask patient to take deep breaths and cough and assess. Absence of swinging suggests drain is occluded or is no longer in the pleural space. Try flushing the drain and if no success obtain a chest X-ray to determine the underlying cause. Bubbling in the underwater seal fluid chamber generally indicates an on-going air leak which may be continuous, present on one phase of spontaneous ventilation, or only on coughing. Persistent bubbling throughout the respiratory cycle may indicate a continuing broncho-pleural air leak. Faulty connections and entrained air through the skin incision should also be assessed. If drain inserted for a fluid collection, e.g. effusion or empyema, then record volume and nature of the drain fluid recording. Drains inserted just for fluid should not bubble so the presence of this feature is abnormal and should be recorded. Any abnormal signs or complications should be referred for medical review. **Bleeding** from a drain inserted for drainage of a haemothorax (+/– PTX) needs urgent medical review. With fractured ribs most bleeding is from the intercostal vessels, which slows down as the lung reinflates. However, continued bleeding into the drain bottle is indicative of pathology that may need thoracic surgical intervention. After thoracic trauma, more than 1500 ml of blood into the bottle initially or continued bleeding of greater than 200 ml/h requires discussion with the thoracic surgeons. Small bore drains should be flushed regularly with NS; the flush should be prescribed on the Treatment Sheet and carried out by appropriately trained personnel. Full respiratory and cardiovascular observations should be carried out and documented. **Clamping chest drains:** chest tubes for PTX should not be clamped. Exceptions to this may be when the drainage bottle requires replacement or when testing the system for air leaks. Clamping a pleural drain in the presence of a continuing air leak may result in a tension PTX or possibly worsening surgical emphysema. If a chest tube is clamped it should be under the direct supervision of a respiratory physician or surgeon on a ward with experienced nursing staff. A patient with a clamped tube should not leave the specialist ward environment. Instructions should be left that if the patient becomes breathless or develops surgical emphysema, the chest tube must be unclamped immediately and the medical team alerted. In cases of PTX there is no evidence that clamping a chest drain at the time of removal is beneficial. Drains for fluid drainage can be clamped or closed to control drainage rate as necessary.

Changing the drain bottle

- When changing the drain bottle because it is full, temporary clamping of the drainage tube may be necessary to prevent entry of air into the pleural cavity. It is acceptable to clamp the tube between thumb and forefinger. This has the advantage of removing the risk of inadvertently leaving the tube clamped. Local policy should be followed with regard to asepsis and infection control. **Suction:** a patient who is free from pain and who can cough will generate a much higher pleural pressure differential than can safely be produced with suction. If a patient cannot re-inflate his own lung or a persistent air leak is preventing re-inflation, high volume, low-pressure thoracic suction in the range of 3–5 kPa (approximately 30–50 cmH$_2$O) should be used. Prescription of suction is a medical responsibility. Purpose-made low grade suction units (max 30 kPa) should be used when applying to a chest drain. Standard high volume, high-pressure suction units should not be used because of the ease with which they may lead to air stealing and hypoxaemia, the perpetuation of persistent air leaks, and possible damage to lung tissue caused by it becoming trapped in the catheter. Suction that is not working properly or is turned off without disconnecting from the drain bottle is the equivalent of a clamped drain, so when suction is no longer needed it should be disconnected from the drainage bottle. The use of suction may cause continuous bubbling from the tube; movement/swinging of fluid in the tube may not be visible. **Mobility:** if appropriate, patients should be encouraged to walk around. If the drain is on suction the patient will be restricted to the bedside. Exercise to prevent complications such as a frozen shoulder or deep venous thrombosis is essential, as are deep breathing exercises to aid re-expansion of the lung. **Removal of the chest drain:** removal of the chest drain depends on reason for insertion and clinical progress. Give adequate analgesia before removal of the chest drain. As for insertion, an aseptic technique should be used for removal and the chest drain and drainage kit disposed of appropriately. When the tube is ready to be removed, the patient should be asked to perform a valsalva manoeuvre (to ↑the pleural pressure and prevent air entering the pleural cavity) or, if that is not possible, then deep inspiration and the tube withdrawn quickly. The previously placed suture is then tied to close the hole. The operator should be able to tie sutures securely. The wound site should be checked, condition documented and an appropriate dressing applied. An X-ray should be performed following removal of the chest drain to ensure resolution. **Surgical emphysema** is the abnormal presence of air within the subcutaneous tissues with the 'Michelin man' type appearance, which may cause upper airways respiratory compromise. Its presence suggests that the drain is inadequate (too small gauge) to deal with size of air leak or occluded or misplaced. Applying suction, inserting a second drain or a larger bore tube, can improve drainage. Worsening surgical emphysema is uncomfortable, interferes with clinical examination of the patient and, at its worst, may track up to the neck and face, potentially causing airway compromise.

20.4 Central venous line insertion

- **Introduction:** ask the 'right' questions (▶ Section 20.1): possible sites: internal jugular vein, subclavian vein, femoral vein.
- **Indications.** (1) Measurement of CVP, drug administration, TPN, amiodarone, etc. (2) Administering IV fluids when peripheral access poor (poor way to give fluids quickly). (3) Insertion of Swan–Ganz catheter to measure pulmonary wedge pressures. (4) Insertion of a pacing wire, pre-operative, e.g. CABG in theatre.
- **Equipment:** central line pack, sterile drapes, sterile gloves. 5–10 ml Lidocaine 1–2%, iodine or equivalent, central line. 2×10 ml of saline/heparin flush, scalpel, 2–3×5–10 ml syringe. Green and blue needles and 100 ml bag NS.
- **Risks:** skill and luck and experience of the operator can vary as can body habitus and ease of access. Complications higher for emergency vs. elective insertion. Risks include infectious, mechanical, and thrombotic complications. Obtain chest X-ray (subclavian/internal jugular) to confirm placement and to assess for complications. Infection. Strict asepsis – hand washing, gown and gloves for all cases. Preferably in appropriate area where a sterile field can be maintained, e.g. anaesthetic room or ITU or CCU procedure room. Avoid attempts in a dimly lit general ward – those days have long gone. Catheter infections due to local site infection or via haematogenous seeding of the catheter. Use chlorhexidine skin antisepsis, selection of an optimal catheter site. Ensure daily review of the need for the catheter or removal.

Contraindications to central venous line insertion

- Severe uncorrected coagulopathy: INR >1.6, platelets $<50 \times 10^9$/L (relative contraindication). Femoral or internal jugular site is preferred with a coagulopathy because vessels can be directly compressed in the event of serious haemorrhage which may be arterial.
- There is NO safe route. Consider delaying procedure to correct coagulopathy or thrombocytopenia.
- Infected skin over the entry site, thrombosis of target vein, those unlikely to tolerate PTX or lower risk approaches to internal jugular or femoral sites may be preferred.

Potential complications of central venous line insertions

- Arterial puncture when the associated artery lies close (apply pressure and wait 5–10 min), haematoma, PTX, tension PTX, haemothorax.
- Arrhythmia, localised and systemic infection.
- Thrombotic complications: risk of venous thrombosis and embolism. Thrombosis can occur first day after cannulation. Lowest risk for thrombosis is the subclavian vein. Early removal of the catheter decreases the risk of catheter-related thrombosis.

General procedure

- Patient must be head down tilt when cannulating neck veins and head up when cannulating femoral vein to prevent air embolism. Raise bed to suitable level for yourself. Head down tilt can compromise breathless patients. Telemetry for any arrhythmias and continue O_2 saturation monitoring.

- Wash hands, asepsis. Cleanse a 15–20 cm^2 or larger area with povidone–iodine solution. Usually the right side is preferred due to more direct line to the atrium, reduces injuring the thoracic duct, is easier in the right handed operator, and dome of lung and pleura are lower than on left.

- Drape the patient with the paper/plastic drape with centre cutout provided. Estimate the length of catheter to be placed to end up with tip above right atrium. Using the blue needle, make a weal under the skin at the desired spot, and anaesthetise the subcutaneous tissue. Using the green needle, anaesthetise deeper.

- Always withdraw the plunger before injecting to detect if you are in the vein or artery to avoid intravascular injection of 1–2% **Lidocaine**. Open the pack and place the guide wire, dilator, catheter, and scalpel on the sterile drape for easy reach when needed.

- **Ultrasound guidance:** ultrasonography accurately locates the target vein, suggests venous pressure and the presence of intravascular thrombus and is strongly recommended. When using ultrasound guidance, enlist an assistant either to handle the probe or to remove it when it is no longer needed. The vein and artery appear circular and black on the ultrasound image; the vein is much more compressible when gentle pressure is applied to the skin via the probe. The needle appears echogenic and can be followed into the image of the vein. Most useful in internal jugular attempts.

- Using the 18 gauge finder needle (largest needle in the kit) and a small syringe, enter the skin at the top of the jugular triangle. Gradually advance the needle, always gently pulling back on the plunger as you progress. Look for a flashback of dark blood which indicates entrance into the vein. *Bright red or pulsatile flow should suggest carotid artery puncture. Withdraw needle and apply pressure for about 10 minutes before proceeding.* You can pierce the needle through the vein without blood, gradually withdraw; you may still get into the vein as you may have collapsed it on the way in.

- Once in the vessel, hold the needle steady and remove the syringe, holding a thumb over it, to prevent bleeding and reduce risk of embolism, and thread in the **j-tipped guide wire**. It should be a smooth process and if resistance is felt NEVER force it. Guide wire overinsertion can be dangerous. The wire needs to be advanced only far enough to maintain reliable control of the tract from the skin surface to the intravascular space.

- Watch monitor as guide wire is advanced. Ventricular ectopy indicates over-insertion and the guide wire must be withdrawn a few cm. Holding the guide wire, remove needle from skin. Make a small nick with the number 11 blade where wire enters skin with the cutting edge away from the wire. Advance dilator over guide wire with a twisting motion; there will be resistance.

- Remove dilator, holding guide wire and having some gauze 4 × 4 in your hand to apply pressure to a site that will now bleed after dilation. Place catheter over guide wire; it should advance easily. Hold guide wire at skin entrance and feed it back through distal port of central line (brown cap). When wire comes out, grab it at the end and finish advancing catheter. Remove guide wire and flush line through all 3 ports. Ensure all ports are closed.

- Now suture catheter in place via flange with holes. If more than 1–2 cm of catheter is exposed due to length, either suture the catheter down or use the snap-on flange provided in the kit. Apply a clear dressing.

- Get a chest X-ray to evaluate for line placement and complication. The tip of the catheter should be at the junction of the SVC and right atrium on chest X-ray film. New data would suggest that this is 2 cm below the superior right cardiac silhouette, which is made up by the right atrial appendage.

Internal jugular vein cannulation

- **Visualise landmarks:** locate the triangle formed by heads of sternocleidomastoid and the clavicle. Entry point is apex. Internal jugular vein runs deep to the sternocleidomastoid muscle. Use of USS is highly recommended. Place patient in head down position to prevent air embolism. In obese patients where the landmarks are not discernible, a reasonable rule of thumb is to go three finger breadths lateral from the tracheal midline, and three finger breadths up from the clavicle. Some suggest that patients turn head away from side whilst others suggest keep head in neutral midline position.
- As the head rotates away from neutral, there is an increase in both the overlap and proximity of the internal jugular vein and carotid artery which increases the risk of carotid puncture. Some advocate the use of a small gauge pilot needle to locate the internal jugular vein and an innovative technique to then stabilise it. This small gauge pilot needle may be particularly useful when patients have coagulopathy or when ultrasonography is not available. Palpate for the carotid impulse and make sure you are lateral to this. Insert the needle at the apex of the triangle and the needle should point down towards same side nipple with needle at 30° to horizontal. The vein is usually less than 1.5 cm below surface.

Subclavian vein cannulation

- Complications are higher and so this must be carried out by experienced operators only. Benefits are more comfort for longer term catheterisation than alternative sites and so can be used for dialysis or feeding. The adult subclavian vein is approximately 3–4 cm long and 1–2 cm in diameter and is a continuation of the axillary vein at the lateral border of the first rib which it crosses over and passes in front of the anterior scalene muscle. The anterior scalene muscle is approximately 10–15 mm thick and separates the subclavian vein from the subclavian artery, which runs behind. The vein continues behind medial third of clavicle where it is immobilised by small attachments to the rib and clavicle. At the medial border of the anterior scalene muscle and behind subscapularis joint, the subclavian unites with the internal jugular to form the innominate/brachiocephalic vein. The large thoracic duct on the left, and smaller lymphatic duct on the right, enter the superior margin of subclavian vein near internal jugular junction.
- **Technique:** head down position, well hydrated if possible. Place towel roll behind scapulae to pull back shoulders which brings clavicles backward. Keep patient's head in neutral position, though some teach to turn head away. Anaesthetise locally with lidocaine down to the periosteum of the clavicle. Locate subclavian vein with a 22 gauge needle and pass introducer needle parallel to retrace path. Ensure that the needle is kept very shallow to skin at no more than 10–15° from horizontal. Generally the needle is advanced medially from an entry point 1 cm below junction of middle and medial one-third of clavicle towards the posterior superior angle of the clavicle (the suprasternal notch). Advance needle aspirating. The subclavian artery, lung, and brachial plexus are all posterior to subclavian vein; if the vein is not cannulated, at least the other structures will not be hit. Once cannulated use a Seldinger technique as described above. The risk of PTX is far greater with this technique. Damage to the subclavian artery may occur; direct pressure cannot be applied to prevent bleeding. Ensure that a chest X-ray is ordered, to identify the position of the line and to exclude PTX.

Femoral vein cannulation

- The femoral vein can be used for central access. It can allow the patient to sit up slightly. The risk of infection is greater at this site. It is a useful site in patients with superior vena caval obstruction. Cardiac monitoring is not needed. The femoral vein is the continuation of the popliteal vein and accompanies the femoral artery in the femoral triangle. The femoral vein ends medial to the artery at the inguinal ligament, where it becomes the external iliac vein. Relations: nerve, artery, vein, and Y fronts – NAVY.

- **Technique:** extend the leg and abduct slightly at the hip. Adopt full asepsis. Locate the femoral artery, keep a finger on the artery and introduce a needle attached to a 10 ml syringe at 45°, 1.5 cm medial to the femoral artery pulsation, 2 cm below the inguinal ligament. Slowly advance the needle towards the head and posteriorly while gently withdrawing the plunger. When a free flow of blood appears, follow the Seldinger approach, as detailed previously. Potential complications include wound sepsis and septicaemia, deep vein thrombosis, femoral nerve or arterial damage, haematoma, arteriovenous fistula. It is certainly an easier site to control any coagulopathy as pressure can be applied.

20.5 Lumbar puncture

- **Introduction:** ask the 'right' questions (▶ Section 20.1) and also check if it is safe and if there is ↑ICP with an incipient herniation syndrome or a coagulopathy.
- **Contraindications:** incipient brain herniation syndrome suggested by seizures, GCS <13, focal neurological signs (including ocular palsies), papilloedema, pupillary dilation, impaired eye movements, coma and low HR and rising BP, older patients, HIV, recent head trauma (CT head required first). Coagulopathy, thrombocytopenia, warfarin, heparin, platelets <50 × 10^9/L. Spina bifida or skin appearances of spina bifida occulta or deformities, local infection or pressure sore, severe cardiorespiratory compromise.
- **Complications:** coning due to brain herniation, epidural haematoma with root or cauda equina compression, SAH, infection (e.g. meningitis), low pressure headache, backache, nerve palsies (e.g. diplopia from cranial nerve VI), lumbosacral nerve palsies (extremely rare), dermoid formation.
- **Patient advice:** explain procedure and reason for LP to patient. Explain complications including headache and infection. Mention that it is extremely common for a patient to experience a sharp shoot of pain down one leg and if this happens they should let the operator know and that it does not mean something has gone wrong. Explain that the needle is placed below the spinal cord and as such the needle cannot enter the spinal cord. It is almost impossible to put a needle through one of the nerve roots and the pain is typically caused by the needle touching the nerve root (e.g. like a cold drink touching an exposed nerve root in a bad tooth). Give the patient a copy of patient information sheet.
- **Preparation:** make sure you are clear what samples need to be sent and have relevant tubes ready and inform microbiologist/lab of intended procedure. Do not start without all equipment to hand including manometer. Any focal signs or suggestions of coma which could suggest ↑ICP, then a CT is needed to exclude SOL or other signs of ↑CSF pressure such as dilated third ventricles, midline shift, etc.
- ***Patient positioning is key to success:*** the patient is best positioned lying comfortably on their side, at the edge of the bed with a pillow between knees, back flexed, with the spine horizontal and perpendicular to the couch throughout its entire length. The chin should be as close to the patellae as possible in a fetal-like position. Knees and ankles should be symmetrical and together. Careful attention to positioning and explanation to patient before starting significantly increases the chance of success.
- ***Skin preparation:*** give yourself a wide sterile area. For skin preparation use **chlorhexidine or iodine aqueous solution**. It is important to use good technique for sterilizing, starting in the centre and wiping in circular motion to outside of area.
- ***Position of LP site:*** the cord ends at the lower margin of L1. The needle is usually introduced at L3/4 interspace which is indicated by a line drawn joining the tips of the iliac crests. (In adults the spinal cord usually ends at the lower border of L1 so

a needle inserted into the subarachnoid space below this level will enter the sac containing the cauda equina floating in CSF.) L3/4 interspace gives a margin of error. If unsuccessful at this level try L2/3.

Procedure

- Local anaesthetic: the skin and deeper tissues of the needle track are infiltrated. Use up to 5 ml of 2% lidocaine which should be infiltrated into the skin with a blue needle, waiting for it to take effect and then infiltrating deeper with a green needle. Continually aspirate with the syringe before injecting to ensure not in blood vessel or even CSF (e.g. in thin patient). Allow time for this to be effective. LP needle insertion: use a sharp disposable fine LP needle (e.g. gauge 22) with a stylet in position; introduce through the skin and advance through the space between the two spinous processes. The top of the bevel should always be parallel to the back (e.g. for a patient horizontal on their side, the bevel will point to the ceiling). The needle point needs to be directed slightly forwards (anteriorly). Insert to a depth of 4–7 cm; firm resistance which gives way as the ligamentum flavum is reached. Beyond this there is a slight give as the needle punctures the dura. The stylet is removed and clear CSF will drip out of the needle if this has been correctly positioned. If no fluid appears or bone is encountered, it is probable that the needle is not in the correct position. The stylet should be reinserted, the needle partially withdrawn and then advanced with a slightly different angle aiming for the umbilicus. Once in position and CSF is obtained, the stylet should be placed in the centre of the sterile trolley and kept sterile as it will need to be reinserted prior to taking the LP needle out at the end of the examination. *Failure*: commonest causes of failure are that the needle is not in the midline, the patient's back is not perpendicular to the bed (e.g. twisted at shoulders, or legs not together) or is at too great an angle with the skin. NB. If unsuccessful after 2–3 attempts, take more senior advice before giving up, or ask another more experienced doctor to try. If that is unsuccessful, X-ray screening may be used or contact a friendly anaesthetist. If LP is to evaluate presence of xanthochromia, then further attempts need to be performed at this time and not delayed by more than 2–4 h, otherwise altered blood may be found as a consequence of the 'bloody' traumatic tap and the test becomes unhelpful if xanthochromia is found. Measure opening pressure: ensure familiarity with the 3-way tap. Measure and record CSF pressure (normal <20 cmH$_2$O) using manometry and the patient lying horizontally. Sample collection: take 4 tubes and fill each with 3–5 ml (up to 40–50 ml CSF can be safely removed). Label all bottles carefully. Number them 1 to 4 in the order they were filled.
- **Routine samples:** CSF for Gram stain, microscopy and sensitivity, protein, paired sugar (blood + CSF fluoride bottles), cytology sent when indicated at least 10 ml, oligoclonal bands if demyelination suspected and also send serum sample. CSF + serum glucose important in bacterial/fungal meningitis – the CSF sugar is usually <2 mmol/L or <40% blood glucose level. Microscopy and culture: Gram stained and examined routinely for bacteria, also stains for fungi, cryptosporidium or acid-fast bacilli as requested.
- **Xanthochromia:** send 3 sequential samples for red cell count. If SAH suspected and CT negative do not perform until 12 h from headache have elapsed. Time is required to convert haemoglobin to bilirubin (xanthochromia). Bloody tap if significant RBCs; as a guide about 10 white cells/7000 red cells would normally be expected.
- **Other CSF samples:** CSF lactate: in bacterial and TB meningitis the CSF lactate >3.3 mmol/L. Lactate samples need to go the lab on ice. Inform the lab first. TB PCR can also be checked but false positives may sometimes be seen. Latex agglutination can detect *Haemophilus influenzae* B, *Strep. pneumoniae* and *Neisseria meningitidis* in >75% of affected patients. Encephalitis: samples are sent for viral PCR (e.g. HSV, VZV, CMV, etc.). ACE levels: neurosarcoid. VDRL: suspected neurosyphilis.
- **Finishing the LP:** replace the sterile stylet before removing the LP needle to reduce post-LP headache. Remove iodine with saline-soaked gauze to prevent skin rashes

or burns. Lying supine for a short period usually advocated. Hydration is sensible but does not prevent headache.

- Post-LP low pressure headache is a known complication and can be mild to severe and always occurs soon after sitting or standing – it should completely disappear on lying flat (or significantly diminish if patient already had headache prior to LP). Whilst this may settle, if it continues then the longer that treatment is delayed, the less chance of success. Analgesics are to be avoided as they may perpetuate headache. Oral caffeine does not prevent post-LP headache. An infusion of IV caffeine is the most appropriate first line management of post-LP headache (e.g. CAFFEINE 500 mg in 500 ml NS over 2 h). Persisting low pressure pain: consider blood patch – ask anaesthetists who are experienced at this.

20.6 Abdominal paracentesis

- **Introduction:** ask the 'right' questions (▶ Section 20.1): Indications: relieve ascites due to cirrhosis or malignancy – primary ovarian, colon, stomach, pancreas, lung and breast cancers, but it can also be associated with primary liver or peritoneal cancers. A diagnostic paracentesis should be performed in all cirrhotic patients with ascites who have signs and symptoms of peritoneal infection, including the development of encephalopathy, renal impairment, or peripheral leucocytosis without a precipitating factor to exclude spontaneous bacterial peritonitis (SBP).
- **Side effects:** paracentesis can cause haemorrhage, infection and may precipitate hepatorenal syndrome.
- **Relative contraindications:** coagulopathy (INR >2.0 reverse, seek advice), pregnancy, localised cellulitis, low platelets (<50), bowel obstruction.
- **Equipment:** gauze swabs, sterile dressing pack, sterile gloves, iodine or equivalent. Green and blue needles, several 5–10 ml syringes, lignocaine 1–2%. Ascitic drain and bag, adhesive dressings.
- **Investigations:** serum ascites–albumin gradient (SA–AG) >11 g/L: cirrhosis, cardiac failure, nephrotic syndrome. SA–AG <11 g/L: malignancy, TB, pancreatitis. SBP: neutrophil count of >250 cells/mm^3 empiric antibiotic therapy should be started. Check ascitic amylase if pancreatic disease suspected.

Procedure

- Obtain consent. Ask patient to micturate first. With ascites when lying supine the fluid is lowest and air-filled bowel floats to the surface. The flanks are dull and fluid filled. The safest place to go is right or left inguinal fossa just 2 cm above and medial to anterior superior iliac spine. Others suggest 2 fingerbreadths below the umbilicus in the midline. Wash hands and prepare field with iodine. Ensure sterile field and sterile gloves. Identify chosen spot. For a simple diagnostic aspiration, e.g. to detect SBP, a green needle is sufficient with appropriate asepsis. On insertion avoid inferior epigastric arteries which run in a pair just a few centimetres lateral to the midline. Apply local anaesthetic down to the point at which you can freely aspirate ascitic fluid. Remove needle and pierce skin with scalpel. Insert paracentesis catheter (Bonanno catheter) in a Z-shaped pathway at 45°, aspirating via syringe. The tip is pig tailed. Withdraw introducer whilst advancing the drain. *Patients with portal hypertensive ascites usually receive 100 ml 20% Human Albumin Solution (20 g of albumin) for each 2–3 L ascites drained.* Volume replacement is not routinely required for malignant ascites unless the patient shows ↓BP during drainage. May be reasonable to simply give 250 ml NS colloid fluid challenge if required. Send fluid for urgent cell count, microscopy, culture and sensitivity, LDH, protein and cytology. Remove drain after 6 h if cirrhosis as there is a high risk of peritonitis. Drains for malignant effusions may be left in for longer but the risk of peritonitis still exists. If SBP then consider IV CO-AMOXICLAV or TAZOCIN.

20.7 Arterial blood gas

- **Introduction:** ask the 'right' questions (▶ Section 20.1) and check both radial and ulnar arterial pulses are present.
- **Arterial blood gas kit:** 1 ml vented, pre-heparinised usually with dry lithium heparin plastic syringe. One orange or blue needle (longer needles are required for brachial and femoral artery puncture). Needle guard to prevent accidental needlestick injuries. Vent cap (for evacuation of air bubble), one biohazard-labelled plastic bag. Two 1 × 1 sterile gauze, alcohol prep pad, specimen/patient label, iodine pad. One adhesive bandage, lab form, ice.
- **Contraindications:** no absolute contraindications, mostly just extra precautions and hazards. Avoid dialysis AV shunt; mastectomy – use opposite side. Anticoagulant therapy – hold pressure on puncture site longer than normal.
- **Preparation:** introduce yourself and explain what is ordered and get informed consent. Patient cooperation helps. Check patient ID, ask patient their name, check patient ID wristband. ***Choose artery:*** select site and palpate the right and left radial arterial pulses and visualise the course of the artery. Pick strongest pulse. Radial artery is always the first choice and should be used because it provides collateral circulation. If radial pulse weak on right, move to left; if pulse on left weak, then try brachial. Brachial used as alternative site and femoral is the last choice in normal situations. Always have a fallback plan. ***Check Allen test*** using radials. In a conscious and cooperative patient simply compress ulnar and radial arteries at wrist to obliterate pulse and have patient clench and release fist until hand blanches. With radial still compressed, release pressure on ulnar artery and watch for pinkness to return. It should pink up within 10–15 sec. If patient unconscious then compress ulnar and radials and elevate hand above head, squeeze hard and release ulnar and lower hand below heart. Palpate left and right radial arteries noting maximal pulse. The one with the stronger pulse will be your site of entry.

Procedure

- Wash hands, put on gloves. Connect needle to syringe ensuring needle kept sterile and eject excess heparin and air bubbles. If using syringe with liquid heparin pull back syringe plunger to at least 1 cm^3 to give room for blood to fill syringe when puncture is made (NEVER recap needle). Stabilise the wrist in the position that gives maximal pulse (hyper-extended, using a rolled up towel if necessary) and clean chosen area with an alcohol and/or iodine wipe. Secure needle to syringe and remove cap from needle. Pierce the skin at puncture site aiming proximally and keep needle angle constant and bevel of needle up, or into the arterial flow (bevel faces the heart) and slowly advance in one plane. When the artery is punctured, blood will enter the syringe flashback. Slowly allow blood to fill syringe. If no blood appears, remove, change needles, and start again. Upon removal of the needle, hold pressure on the puncture site for at least 5 min. Pressure may need to be held longer (>5 min) if the patient is on anticoagulant therapy. ***Post puncture procedure:*** remove any air bubbles from sample and cap syringe and dispose of needle in sharps container. Roll syringe to mix heparin with sample and immediately try to lower temperature and metabolism of sample by immersing in ice and ensure rapid delivery to lab. *On lab request form indicate:* FiO$_2$, patient temperature and ventilator parameters. ***Post procedure:*** check for bleeding, movement of fingers and tingling sensation, pulse distal to puncture. If radial pulse not palpable consider an urgent vascular opinion.
- **Complications:** arterial spasm: may occur secondary to pain or anxiety. Reassure patient; explain procedure and purpose. Haematoma: leakage of blood into tissue. You possibly didn't press hard enough and long enough. Ensure using small diameter needle. Ensure proper technique in holding site for 5 min post puncture. Haemorrhage: patient receiving anticoagulant therapy or patients with known

blood coagulation disorders. Two minutes after pressure is released inspect site for bleeding, oozing or seepage of blood; continue pressure until bleeding ceases. A longer compression time is necessary. Other very rare: laceration of artery, sepsis, infection/inflammation adjacent to puncture site. Avoid sites indicating presence of infection or inflammation. Discuss with vascular surgeons any possible vascular injury. Failure: consider using femoral artery.

20.8 Nasogastric tube insertion

- **Introduction:** ask the 'right' questions (▶Section 20.1). Contraindications (or take expert advice): ENT abnormalities or infections. Suspected oesophageal stricture or pouch. Recent oesophagectomy or upper GI surgery. Recent suspected or known fractures of the base of the skull. Oesophageal varices, oesophageal perforation or oesophageal surgery. Risk of aspiration, suspected atrial–oesophageal fistula. Thrombolysed patient – delay NG insertion certainly after stroke thrombolysis.

Procedure

- NG tubes are long polyurethane or silicone tubes passed via the nose and oesophagus into the stomach. Deaths may occur due to feeding tubes displaced into the lungs causing gastric aspiration. NG tubes are most commonly inserted by nurses who are often the local experts. Sometimes done by doctors, e.g. anaesthetists in theatre. The main indications are: feeding in those, for example, with neurological disease or other cause of impaired swallowing (e.g. stroke); aspirating gastric contents (e.g. obstructed patient) which decompresses the stomach and so prevents vomiting and possible aspiration. Nasojejunal tubes are longer versions of NG tubes. They are inserted under endoscopic guidance to lie further in the jejunum and may be useful in feeding patients with pancreatitis. *Obtain consent* – verbal consent is usually sufficient. Explain the insertion procedure, together with the reasons why the tube is necessary. In some patients actions will need to be done in best interests as consent cannot be communicated.
- **Preparation:** after washing hands, prepare a trolley including gloves, local anaesthetic jelly or spray, a 60 ml syringe, pH strip, kidney tray, sticky tape and a bag to collect secretions. Determine length of NG tube to insert by external measurement from the tip of the nose to a point halfway between the xiphoid and the umbilicus distance. Usually 40–60+ cm. Better to have too long than too short – don't want the tip in the lower oesophagus. The patient should sit up. An appropriately sized tube is chosen and the tip is lubricated by smearing aqua gel or local anaesthetic gel. Anaesthetic gel is a drug so if it is used it must be prescribed, and precautions taken such as checking for allergies. The wider nostril is chosen and the tube slid down along the floor of the nasal cavity. The head should not be tilted back. Patients often gag when the tube reaches the pharynx. Asking them to swallow their saliva or a small amount of water may help to direct the tube into the oesophagus. Once in the oesophagus, it may be easy to push into the stomach. The correct intragastric position is then verified (see below). The tube is fixed to the nose/forehead using adhesive tapes. The stomach is decompressed by attaching the 60 ml syringe and aspirating its contents. Blocked tubes can be flushed open with saline or air.
- Verifying correct intragastric positioning: there are two recommended ways of confirming the tube position. These are by **pH test and X-ray**. Other methods can be inaccurate and should not be used. (1) **Measuring pH:** the NG tube is aspirated and the contents are checked using pH paper, not litmus paper. It is recommended that it is safe to feed adult patients only if the pH is <5.5. Note that taking proton pump inhibitors or H_2 receptor antagonists may alter the pH. Similarly, intake of milk can neutralise the acid. (2) **Chest X-ray:** when in doubt it is best practice to

use X-ray to check the tube's location. Patients who have swallowing problems, confused patients and those in ICU should all be given an X-ray to verify the tube's intragastric position. This involves taking a chest X-ray including the upper half of the abdomen. The tip of the tube can be seen as a white radio-opaque line and should be below the diaphragm on the left side. **Syringe test:** do not use! This test is mentioned here for historic interest only. Also known as the whoosh test, it has been shown to be an unreliable method of checking tube placement, and the NPSA has said that it *must no longer be used*. **Repeated confirmation of position:** correct intragastric positioning should be confirmed at least daily and immediately after initial placement. Before each daily feed – need to wait 1 h before testing pH. Following vomiting/coughing. Decreased O_2 saturation. If the tube is dislodged or the patient complains of discomfort. Never insert the guide wire while the NG tube is in the patient.

- **Complications:** misplaced tube and delivery of feed directly into lungs causing pneumonia/pneumonitis. Gastric possibly overfeeding with vomiting also leading to pulmonary aspiration pneumonia. Nasal trauma and local mucosal damage when NG inserted roughly or in for a prolonged time. Use lubricants. Gagging or vomiting, therefore suction should always be ready to use.

21 Normal laboratory values

21.1 Clinical chemistry values

Blood gases (breathing air at sea level)
Blood H$^+$ 35–45 nmol/L

pH	7.36–7.44
PaO_2	11.3–12.6 kPa
$PaCO_2$	4.7–6.0 kPa
Base excess	+/− 2 mmol/L
Carboxyhaemoglobin	non-smoker <2%
Carboxyhaemoglobin	smoker 3–15%

Serum values

Na	137–144 mmol/L
K	3.5–4.9 mmol/L
Cl	95–107 mmol/L
HCO$_3$	20–28 mmol/L
Anion gap	12–16 mmol/L
Urea	2.5–7.5 mmol/L
Creatinine	60–110 µmol/L
Ca	2.2–2.6 mmol/L
Phosphate	0.8–1.4 mmol/L
Serum total protein	61–76 g/L

Liver values

Albumin	37–49 g/L
Total bilirubin	1–22 µmol/L
Conjugated bilirubin	0–3.4 µmol/L
ALT	5–35 units/L
AST	1–31 units/L
ALP	45–105 units/L (over 14 years)
GGT	4–35 units/L (<50 units/L in males)
LDH	10–250 units/L

Cardiac biomarkers

CK	(males) 24–195 units/L; (females) 24–170 units/L

Others

Cu	12–26 µmol/L
Caeruloplasmin	200–350 mg/L
Al	0–10 mcg/L
Mg	0.75–1.05 mmol/L
Zn	6–25 µmol/L
Urate	(males) 0.23–0.46 mmol/L; (females) 0.19–0.36 mmol/L
Plasma lactate	0.6–1.8 mmol/L
Plasma ammonia	12–55 µmol/L
Serum ACE	25–82 units /L

Fasting plasma glucose	3.0–6.0 mmol/L
HbA1c	3.8–6.4%
Fructosamine	<285 μmol/L
Serum amylase	60–180 units/L
Plasma osmolality	278–305 mOsm/kg

Lipids and lipoproteins: assess overall lifetime risk

Serum cholesterol	<5.2 mmol/L
Serum LDL cholesterol	<3.36 mmol/L
Serum HDL cholesterol	>0.55 mmol/L
Fasting serum TG	0.45–1.69 mmol/L

Serum tumour markers

α-fetoprotein	<10 kunits/L
Carcinoembryonic antigen	<10 mcg/L
Neuron-specific enolase	<12 mcg/L
Prostate-specific antigen	(males >40) <4 mcg/L; (males <40) <2 mcg/L
hCG	<5 units/L
CA125	<35 units/ml
CA19-9	<33 units/ml

Cerebrospinal fluid

Opening pressure	50–180 mmH$_2$O
Total protein	0.15–0.45 g/L
Albumin	0.066–0.442 g/L
Chloride	116–122 mmol/L
Glucose	3.3–4.4 mmol/L
CSF lactate	1–2 mmol/L
Cell count	lymphocytes 60–70%; monocytes 30–50%; neutrophils: none
IgG/ALB	<0.26
IgG index	<0.88

Urine

Albumin/creatinine ratio (untimed specimen)	(males) <3.5 mg/mmol; (females) <2.5 mg/mmol
GFR	70–140 ml/min
Total protein	<0.2 g/24 h
Albumin	<30 mg/24 h
Ca	2.5–7.5 mmol/24 h
Urobilinogen	1.7–5.9 μmol/24 h
Coproporphyrin	<300 nmol/24 h
Uroporphyrin	6–24 nmol/24 h
Δ-aminolevulinate	8–53 μmol/24 h
5-hydroxyindoleacetic acid	10–47 μmol/24 h
Osmolality	350–1000 mOsmol/kg

21.2 Haematology values

Full blood count

Haemoglobin	(males) 13.0–18.0 g/dL;
	(females) 11.5–16.5 g/dL
Haematocrit	(males) 0.40–0.52;
	(females) 0.36–0.47
MCV	80–96 fL
MCH	28–32 pg
MCHC	32–35 g/dL
White cell count	4–11 × 10⁹/L
White cell differential	(× 10⁹/L)
neutrophils	1.5–7
lymphocytes	1.5–4
monocytes	0–0.8
eosinophils	0.04–0.4
basophils	0–0.1
platelet count	150–400
reticulocyte count	25–85 OR 0.5–2.4%
ESR	<50 years: (males) 0–15 mm/1st hour;
	(females) 0–20 mm/1st hour
	>50 years: (males) 0–20 mm/1st hour;
	(females) 0–30 mm/1st hour
Plasma viscosity	1.50–1.72 mPa/sec

Coagulation screen

Prothrombin time	11.5–15.5 sec
INR	<1.4
APTT	30–40 sec
Fibrinogen	1.8–5.4 g/L
Bleeding time	3–8 min

Coagulation factors

Factors II, V, VII, VIII, IX, X, XI, XII	50–150 IU/dL
Factor V Leiden, vWF	45–150 IU/dL
vWF antigen	50–150 IU/dL
Protein C	0–135 IU/dL
Protein S	80–120 IU/dL
Antithrombin III	80–120 IU/dL
Activated protein C resistance	2.12–4.0
Fibrin degradation products	<100 mg/L
D-dimer screen	<0.5 mg/L

Haematinics

Serum iron	12–30 µmol/L
Serum iron-binding capacity	45–75 µmol/L
Serum ferritin	15–300 mcg/L
Serum transferrin	2.0–4.0 g/L

Serum B12	160–760 ng/L
Serum haptoglobin	0.13–1.63 g/L
Serum folate	2.0–11.0 mcg/L
Red cell folate	160–640 mcg/L

Haemoglobin electrophoresis

Haemoglobin A	>95%
Haemoglobin A2	2–3%
Haemoglobin F	<2%

21.3 CSF values

	Normal	Bacterial meningitis	Viral meningitis	TB meningitis	GBS	SAH
CSF	Clear and colourless	Cloudy and turbid	Normal	Normal/cloudy	Normal	Blood stained
WCC	0–5 × 10⁶ per litre Lφ	↑Nφ	↑Lφ	↑Lφ	Normal	Normal
RCC	0–10 × 10⁶ per litre	Normal	Normal	Normal	Normal	Very high 'hundreds'
Protein	0.2–0.4 g/L	High/very high	Normal/high	High, very high	High by week 2	Normal, high
Glucose	3.3–4.4 mmol/L	Low	Normal/low	Very low	Normal	Normal/low

Lφ = lymphocytes, Nφ = neutrophils. Bloody tap you can allow 1 white cell for 500–1000 red cells.

22 Emergency drugs (use with *BNF*)

22.1 Prescribing and side effects abbreviations

Indications are in italic
SE: side effects
CI: contraindications

Route
IM = intramuscular
IO = intraosseous
IV = intravenous
PO = oral
SC = subcutaneous

Frequency
OD = once per day (no time specified)
OM = once in the morning
ON = once at night
BD = twice per day (12 h)
TDS/TID = three times per day (every 8 h)
QDS/QID = four times per day (every 6 h)

Code for side effects
APX = anaphylaxis
C = constipation
D = diarrhoea, F = fever
H = headache, N = nausea
R = rash, SEIZ = seizures
V = vomiting

Drug calculations
1 g = 1000 mg
0.1 g = 100 mg
1 mg = 1000 mcg (microgram)
0.1 mg = 100 mcg
1 L = 1000 ml
E.g. DIGOXIN 0.125 mg = 125 mcg

Digoxin is almost always prescribed in microgram (mcg) and an equivalent dose in milligrams is 1000× times the dose and lethal. Microgram should be written in full – the symbol μg must never be used in a prescription.

22.2 Antibiotic prescribing advice

In certain cases, for example, a septic patient, you must ensure that the first dose of the appropriate antibiotic(s) is given WITHIN ONE HOUR. It is not enough to write it up. Check availability of that drug on that ward, and check nurses understand urgency of delivering drug to patient. This is especially true for these conditions: suspected bacterial meningitis, septic arthritis, neutropenic sepsis, severe sepsis (of any cause), and also HSV encephalitis.

- **Penicillin allergy:** penicillins are life-saving antimicrobials and patients should not be labelled 'penicillin-allergic' without careful consideration. Nausea, vomiting or diarrhoea do not, by themselves, constitute an allergic reaction. They are not a contraindication for penicillin use. Anaphylaxis related to histamine release occurs about 30–60 min after administration of a penicillin; symptoms may include erythema or pruritus, angioedema, ↓BP or shock, urticaria, wheezing, rhinitis. Patients with a history of immediate hypersensitivity/anaphylaxis to penicillin should NOT receive a cephalosporin. TAKING A RELIABLE HISTORY IS VERY IMPORTANT.
- ERTAPENEM or MEROPENEM is recommended as an alternative to penicillin for some severe infections. However, if there is a history of an anaphylactic reaction, or an accelerated allergic reaction DO NOT prescribe these drugs. Please discuss alternative antibiotics with a microbiologist. Remember, penicillins (and cephalosporins) can also be nephrotoxic (as they can induce an interstitial nephritis).

- **Definite Penicillin allergy** – the following **must not be given:** Amoxicillin, Augmentin (Co-amoxiclav), Benzylpenicillin (Penicillin G), Flucloxacillin, Phenoxymethylpenicillin (Penicillin V), Piperacillin/tazobactam (Tazocin), Pivmecillinam, Temocillin.
- **WARNING:** this is a quick look-up guide for drugs with which you should be familiar and in no way replaces the *BNF*. All drugs should be checked in the *BNF* for safety of use in pregnancy, breastfeeding and renal and liver failure. Allergy is such an obvious contraindication that it is not mentioned. All allergies should be documented.

22.3 Commonly used and emergency drugs

ABCIXIMAB (REOPRO) (monoclonal Ab antiplatelet activity). *ACS/PCI*: ABCIXIMAB* 250 mcg/kg IV bolus over 1 min 10–60 min before the start of PCI, followed by a continuous IV infusion of ABCIXIMAB* 125 ng/kg/min (max 10 mcg/min) for 12 h. **SE:** bleed, low platelets, N, V, H, F, alveolar haem, ARDS, low BP. **Caution:** risk of bleeding complications or imminent surgery, e.g. CABG. Specialist use only – prescribe under senior cardiology direction. *Note: caution as units here are microgram and nanograms.

(N) ACETYL CYSTEINE (PARVOLEX or NAC) (replenishes glutathione). *Paracetamol toxicity*: N-ACETYL CYSTEINE = NAC G5 = 5% GLUCOSE. **Bag 1:** NAC 150 mg/kg in 200 ml G5 IV over 1 h. **Bag 2:** NAC 50 mg/kg in 500 ml G5 IV over 4 h. **Bag 3:** NAC 100 mg/kg in 1 L G5 over 16 h. Total NAC dose given is 300 mg/kg in 21 h. NB. First bag now over 1 h to reduce risk of reactions. **SE:** low K, anaphylactoid reaction (N, V, R, flushing, urticaria, itching, wheeze) more common if given too quickly. Slow and continue if possible with CHLORPHENAMINE 10 mg IV/IM. Use plasma levels and treatment line to judge therapy. Do not stop treatment due to SE without senior discussion. May continue NAC at dose rate of 3rd bag if any liver damage (INR >2) or AST >1000 until normalise. Take hepatology advice.

ACICLOVIR (inhibits DNA polymerase in infected cells only). *HSV/VZV infections (not CMV/EBV). Non-genital/genital*: ACICLOVIR 200–400 mg 5/d PO for 5 d. (10 d if genital). *Higher dose/longer course in HIV and immunocompromised. Severe infection*: ACICLOVIR 10 mg/kg IV 8 h for 5 d or more. *HSV encephalitis*: ACICLOVIR 10 mg/kg IV 8 h × 21 d until CSF PCR negative. *Age >16 with chickenpox or shingles*: ACICLOVIR 800 mg PO 5/d for 7 d given as early as possible. **SE:** N, V, R, H, abdo pain, confusion (IV), phlebitis. Hepatotoxicity, AKI, SEIZ. Confirm CSF negative for HSV before stopping treatment for HSV encephalitis. Reduced dose in renal failure. Ensure well hydrated to prevent AKI. Give over 1 h in 0.9% NS.

ACTIVATED CHARCOAL (binds with a surface area of 1000 m²/g). *Single dose*: ACTIVATED CHARCOAL 50–100 g (1 g/kg) PO/NG in 250 ml water PO/NG given if within 1 h of toxin ingestion (2 h with aspirin, opiate, TCA). May need to give IV antiemetic. *Multidose activated charcoal (MDAC) for carbamazepine, dapsone, quinine, theophylline ingestion*: ACTIVATED CHARCOAL 50 g (1 g/kg) PO/NG in 250 ml water then 12.5 g/h. MDAC interrupts enterohepatic recirculation and is vital. Control N&V with IV ONDANSETRON in order to perform MDAC treatment. **SE:** black stools, pneumonitis if aspirated, constipation (give with laxative), N&V (give with antiemetic). *Other drugs that bind*: methotrexate, benzodiazepine, phenobarbital.

ADENOSINE (nucleoside – blocks purine A2 receptors). *Terminates re-entrant SVTs, e.g. AVNRT/AVRT/atrial flutter*: if on dipyridamole, cardiac transplant or via central line start low with: ADENOSINE 1–3 mg fast IV over 1–3 sec then 20 ml NS bolus (use a 3-way tap). Usual dose ADENOSINE 6 mg fast IV with 20 ml NS bolus – watch ECG; if fails then ADENOSINE 12 mg fast IV with a 20 ml NS bolus (use a 3-way tap) watch ECG. **SE:** low BP, flushing, breathless, angina, H, palpitations, transient asystole, bronchospasm, SEIZ. **Cautions:** warn that transient unpleasant symptoms may occur. Aminophylline or theophylline may reduce effect of adenosine. Avoid in asthmatics, heart block, pregnancy. In those with asthma/COPD and narrow complex tachycardia then IV Verapamil may be preferred.

ADRENALINE (EPINEPHRINE) (α and β agonist can cause peripheral vasodilation (a β2 effect) or vasoconstriction (an α effect); as the dose increases α effects dominate). With all inotropes start low and up titrate to response. Adrenaline increases HR and stroke volume and SVR at higher doses. *Cardiac arrest*: ADRENALINE 1 mg (1 in 10 000) IV/IO given as 10 ml mini-jet every 3–5 min (ALS). *Anaphylaxis*: ADRENALINE 0.5 ml = 0.5 mg of 1 in 1000 IM. Give into anterolateral aspect of muscle bulk of the middle third of the thigh in adults. May be repeated at 5 min intervals depending on HR/BP. *Bradycardia*: ADRENALINE 2–10 mcg/min IV. Titrate to response. Closely monitor and titrate dose. Overdose may cause fatal arrhythmias. **SE:** N, V, overdose can cause fatal arrhythmias, lactic acidosis. **Caution:** IHD, severe angina, HOCM, stroke, arrhythmias. Telemetry and resus equipment needed. IV usage only for cardiac arrest and in exceptional circumstances in an ITU setting under close observation.

ALBUMIN (human albumin solution (HAS)). *Ascites, hepatorenal syndrome, plasma exchange*: 500 ml HAS 4.5–5% (20 g albumin), or 100 ml 20% HAS (20 g albumin). Usually issued from blood bank on named patient basis. 20% albumin is hyperoncotic and can expand up to 400 ml within 25 min and so rapid administration can cause overload and CCF so care must be taken.

ALENDRONATE (bisphosphonate). *Postmenopausal osteoporosis, Paget's disease, bone metastasis, breast cancer*: ALENDRONATE 10 mg OD or 70 mg once weekly. (Take with glass of water and remain standing or sit up on empty stomach for 30 min before any other intake.) Not on going to bed. **SE:** N, V, D, H, oesophageal ulceration, stress fractures. Patients need calcium and vitamin D supplement if not replete. Osteonecrosis of the jaw may be seen in cancer patients (get dental assessment first).

ALLOPURINOL (xanthine oxidase inhibitor). Not for acute gout. *Gout prevention*: (2+ attacks): ALLOPURINOL 100–300 mg OD with food. Reduce dose if renal impairment. Use lowest dose to keep uric acid <6 mg/dL. *Tumour lysis syndrome*: ALLOPURINOL 100–300 mg 8 h. **SE:** acute gout, N, V, R, AKI, risk of SJS or TEN (Asian HLA-B*5801 allele), liver toxicity, gynaecomastia. **Cautions:** ↑INR in those on Warfarin. An NSAID or low dose of Colchicine 0.5 mg 12 h can be given for a month initially along with Allopurinol 100 mg to prevent acute attacks. *Severe fatal toxicity with Azathioprine or Ciclosporin.*

ALTEPLASE. *PE with haemodynamic compromise under expert guidance*: ALTEPLASE 10 mg over 2 min then 90 mg over 2 h. Max 1.5 mg/kg for those weighing <65 kg. *STEMI (within 12 h of symptoms onset)*: ALTEPLASE 15 mg IV bolus followed by 0.75 mg/kg (max 50 mg) IV over 30 min and then 0.5 mg/kg (max 35 mg) IV over 60 min. If weight >67 kg give 15 mg/50 mg/35 mg. *Ischaemic stroke*: ALTEPLASE 0.9 mg/kg (max dose 90 mg) with 10% bolus and 90% over 60 min. **Interactions:** other antithrombotics ↑bleeding risk. **SE:** low BP, bleeding; mild ↓BP may need IV fluids and leg raising, bleeding, anaphylaxis, angioneurotic oedema, tongue swelling with alteplase especially if on

ACEI. **Cautions:** anaphylaxis, active bleeding, anticoagulation, varices, aortic dissection, cavitating lung disease, heavy vaginal bleeding, stroke disease (take specialist advice), active peptic ulcer disease, anaemia suggesting occult bleeding, recent surgery, recent trauma, severe hypertension, pericarditis, any haemorrhagic stroke, active bleeding, trauma, malignancy.

AMILORIDE (K-retaining diuretic). *CCF*: AMILORIDE 2.5–10 mg OD PO. **SE:** high K, low BP, GI upset, low Na. Watch for lithium toxicity.

AMINOPHYLLINE/THEOPHYLLINE (phosphodiesterase inhibitor). *Asthma, COPD, bronchospasm*: loading dose: AMINOPHYLLINE 250–500 mg (max 5 mg/kg) then infusion over 20 min in 100 ml NS or G5 (no loading dose if on aminophylline or theophylline already). *Maintenance dose*: AMINOPHYLLINE 500–750 mg in 500 ml over 24 h (0.5 mg/kg/h), adjust as per levels. Smokers need higher dose; elderly or CCF smaller dose, e.g. long term oral dosing: sustained release THEOPHYLLINE 175–500 mg PO BD. **SE:** N, V, restlessness, insomnia, serious arrhythmias, convulsions. **Cautions:** monitor plasma levels. Aim for serum levels of 10–20 mg/L. Wait until 4–6 h after infusion started. Stop infusion and wait 15 min and then take level. **Interactions:** Ciprofloxacin, Macrolides, oral contraception, Cimetidine can lead to theophylline toxicity. Enzyme inducers reduce levels. Levels increased by cardiac disease, hepatic disease or concurrent administration of hepatic enzyme inhibitors. Decreased by smoking and hepatic enzyme inducers.

AMIODARONE. It is irritant and extravasation can be serious, so use central access where possible. *Cardiac arrest*: AMIODARONE 300 mg IV/IO with 20 ml flush (G5) preferably via central line or large Venflon and flush. *Stable tachycardia/chemical cardioversion*: AMIODARONE 300 mg diluted in 250 ml of 5% dextrose and run through a new, proximal cannula, in a large peripheral vein, e.g. antecubital fossa. If initial bolus is unsuccessful then an infusion of 900 mg over the following 23 h may be commenced. This should always be administered through a central cannula, e.g. PICC line, femoral or neck line. This should be diluted in a 500 ml bag of 5% dextrose over 23 h. **SE:** N, V, low BP, ↓HR, thrombophlebitis, photosensitivity, thyroid dysfunction, alveolitis, TdP. Extravasation causes tissue damage. Follow local treatment policies. Ensure peripheral IV lines are working and flush after usage. **Caution:** Amiodarone should not be used in individuals with TdP (polymorphic VT) or a long QT because it prolongs QT interval. Will increase INR and may raise Digoxin, Diltiazem and Verapamil levels with ↓HR. Watch levels. See *BNF*.

AMITRIPTYLINE (TCA; ↑levels of NA,5HT, antimuscarinic effects). *Neuropathic pain/ migraine prevention*: AMITRIPTYLINE 10–75 mg ON, titrate dose up under specialist. For depression (specialist only): AMITRIPTYLINE 30–75 mg ON. **SE:** toxic in overdose. Always come off antidepressants gradually. Sedation, arrhythmias, ↓BP, confusion, dry mouth, urinary retention, weight gain, neuroleptic malignant syndrome, long QT. Avoid if MAOI use in past 2 weeks. Avoid with glaucoma, epilepsy, phaeochromocytoma or cardiac disease.

AMLODIPINE (dihydropyridine CCB). *Vasospasm, angina, HTN*: AMLODIPINE 5–10 mg OD PO. **SE:** low BP, reflex tachycardia, ankle oedema, leg ulcers. **Caution:** reduce Simvastatin 40 mg to 20 mg ON or use Atorvastatin.

AMOXICILLIN (broad spectrum bactericidal β-lactam). *CAP, UTI, listeria*: AMOXICILLIN 500 mg to 1 g 8 h PO/IM/IV infusion. *Severe, endocarditis*: AMOXICILLIN 500 mg 8 h to

2 g 4 h. **SE:** APX, N, V, D, cholestasis, severe rash if EBV/CMV/leukaemia. Reduce dose in renal failure.

AMPHOTERICIN B. *Systemic infection with aspergillosis, candidiasis, coccidiomycosis, cryptococcus, histoplasmosis, visceral leishmaniasis*: LIPOSOMAL AMPHOTERICIN B dose depends on formulation – see BNF. Test dose may be needed then loading dose. *Use under specialist advice only*. Highly toxic. Note liposomal form is less nephrotoxic and is dosed differently to other forms of Amphotericin which can be a source of serious errors. **SE:** fever, rigors, AKI, anaemia, phlebitis, low Mg, low K, cardiotoxic.

AMPICILLIN (broad spectrum bactericidal β-lactam antibiotic). *UTI, chest, CAP, salmonella, listeria*: AMPICILLIN 500 mg to 1 g PO/IM 6 h (oral absorption can be poor). *Severe infection, endocarditis*: AMPICILLIN 2 g slow IV 4–6 h. (Listeria meningitis treat for 21 days.) Infuse with 100 ml G5 or NS over 30 min. **SE:** APX, N, V, D, rash with infectious mononucleosis, cholestasis. Increases INR with warfarin. Avoid if diagnosis may be glandular fever type illness.

APIXABAN (Factor Xa inhibitor). *Orthopaedic VTE prophylaxis*: APIXABAN 2.5 mg BD PO duration. Hip surgery 32–38 days. Knee surgery 10–14 days. *DVT/PE*: APIXABAN 10 mg BD ×7 days, then 5 mg BD PO. *Non-valvular AF*: APIXABAN 5 mg BD PO. **SE:** bleeding, N, R. **Caution:** lower dose for AF to 2.5 mg 12 h if age >80, weight ≤60 kg or creatinine ≥133 micromol/litre or on ketoconazole, itraconazole, ritonavir, clarithromycin (see *BNF*).

ARTESUNATE. *Complicated falciparum malaria under specialist advice*: ARTESUNATE 2.4 mg/kg IV at 0, 12 and 24 h. Repeat daily until blood film clear. **SE:** QTc prolongation, bradycardia, N, V, D, H. Dilute with NS or G5. Take expert advice. If not available use IV quinine.

ASPIRIN (Cox inhibitor). *Ischaemic stroke*: ASPIRIN 300 mg for 14 days then 75 mg. *ACS/stent/IHD*: ASPIRIN 75–300 mg OD. **SE:** gastric irritation, PUD, asthma, tinnitus, toxicity. **Caution:** bleeding disorder, allergy, PUD, asthma. Check with cardiologists before stopping early post stenting.

ATENOLOL (β receptor blocker). *ACS/post MI/arrhythmias*: ATENOLOL 2.5–5 mg slow IV over 5–10 min. May be repeated after 15 min. Then ATENOLOL 25–100 mg/day. **SE:** bronchospasm, fatigue, depression, cold peripheries, ↓HR. Do not increase if CCF worsening. **Caution:** avoid in asthma, ↓HR, heart block, heart failure, pulmonary oedema.

ATORVASTATIN (HMG CoA reductase inhibitor). *IHD, ischaemic stroke, hyperlipidaemia*: ATORVASTATIN 10–80 mg OD. **Monitor:** LFTs and CK. **SE:** muscle toxicity seen with all statins – check CK (stop if >×5 increase), pancreatitis. Myopathy with macrolides or amiodarone. Liver disease, high K. Check LFT day 0, and 3 and 12 months. Check interactions.

ATROPINE. *Severe bradycardia*: ATROPINE 500 mcg (0.5 mg) every 3–5 minutes; max 3 mg. *Organophosphate toxicity*: ATROPINE 2–3 mg IV large doses needed. **SE:** mydriasis, ↑HR, N&V, dry warm skin, urinary retention, bronchodilation. Caution with MG, ileus. Do not use in asystolic arrest. **SE:** dry mouth, urine retention, and constipation. Confusion, mydriasis, dry airways, skin dryness and flushing. Angle closure glaucoma. **Cautions:** urine obstruction/ BPH. Avoid with cardiac transplant as denervated heart.

AZATHIOPRINE (purine antimetabolites). *IBD/autoimmune conditions*: AZATHIOPRINE 2–2.5 mg/kg daily PO/IV (some patients require less); adjusted according to response. **SE:** headache, myalgia, bone marrow suppression, alopecia. Commoner in those with low TPMT activity who need dose reduction. Hepatotoxicity and pancreatitis occur. Monitor LFT/FBC every 2–3 months. Myelosuppression with Allopurinol.

AZITHROMYCIN (macrolides). *RTI, CAP, syphilis, chlamydia, legionella, mycoplasma*. AZITHROMYCIN 500 mg to 1 g OD. *COPD infection prevention*: 250–500 mg three times per week long term. **SE:** N, V, R, long QT, abnormal LFTs.

BENDROFLUMETHIAZIDE (thiazide). *HTN, CCF*: BENDROFLUMETHIAZIDE 2.5–5 mg OD (standard 2.5 mg preferred). **SE:** low Na, low K/Mg, high Ca/urate/glucose, palpitations. Acute gout. Aim for K 4.0–5.0 mmol/L in cardiac patients.

BENZYLPENICILLIN (β-lactam bactericidal). *Meningococcal/pneumococcal meningitis, endocarditis, pneumococcus, cellulitis*: BENZYLPENICILLIN 1.2–2.4 g 4–6 h in 100 ml over 30 min IV with G5/NS or IM. **SE:** APX, N, V, D, R, convulsions (high dose), renal impairment. **Caution:** penicillin allergy. Not for intrathecal use.

BICARBONATE (SODIUM). *TCA overdose, severe hyperkalaemia*: 50 ml 8.4% BICARBONATE over 30–60 min or 250 ml 1.26% over 30–60 min. NB. 8.4% solution contains 1 mmol of HCO_3^- per ml and is very hypertonic and requires central venous access, so the more dilute form is preferred, which may be repeated depending on VBG, response and K. *AKI with metabolic acidosis, rhabdomyolysis, salicylate overdose with metabolic acidosis*: 500 ml 1.26% BICARBONATE or 100 ml of 8.4% over 2–4 h. Watch for overload/LVF, monitor VBG and titrate to urine pH and blood bicarbonate. *Alkaline diuresis*: 500 ml 1.26% BICARBONATE or 100 ml of 8.4% over 2–4 h until urine pH >7.5. Forced alkaline diuresis involves giving larger volumes. *DKA*: not used without senior advice.

BISOPROLOL (β receptor blocker). *Stable CCF, angina*: BISOPROLOL 1.25–10 mg PO OD. See *Atenolol* for more info.

BUMETANIDE (loop diuretic). *CCF, HTN*. BUMETANIDE 1–2 mg PO/IV OD. **SE:** diuresis, incontinence, low K, low Na, low BP, gynaecomastia, urinary retention, AKI.

CALCIUM. *K >6.5 mmol/L, severe low Ca, tetany, high Mg, CCB toxicity*: 10–20 ml 10% CALCIUM GLUCONATE/CHLORIDE with plasma-calcium/ECG monitoring. The chloride form contains more calcium but is more irritating to veins so gluconate usually preferred. Flush lines after. *Maintenance*: CALCIUM GLUCONATE 100 ml of 10% in 1 L of G5 or NS. Give 50 ml/h until symptoms resolved or [Ca] >1.9 mmol/L. $CaCl_2$ is often found as min-I-jet on arrest trolley. Use gluconate if prolonged infusion needed. **C/I:** digoxin toxicity. Do not give calcium in same line as bicarbonate or phosphate as precipitates.

CANDESARTAN (ARB). *HTN, heart failure, diabetic nephropathy, CKD with proteinuria, post MI*: CANDESARTAN 4 mg (CCF) 8–32 mg PO OD. Start low dose in heart failure. Gradually titrate dose depending on BP and symptoms. Watch U&E at 1–2 weeks. First dose ↓BP so start at night. **SE:** N, V, H, D, R, ↑K, low BP, AKI (esp. with RAS). Angioedema less common than with ACEI. **Cautions:** severe aortic stenosis (relative), renal artery stenosis (develop AKI), low Na, mitral stenosis, HOCM, ↓BP, ↑K with other potassium retaining drugs. Avoid in pregnancy as teratogen. Avoid NSAIDs.

CAPTOPRIL (ACEI). *BP, HTN, heart failure (lowest dose), diabetic nephropathy, CKD with proteinuria, post MI*: CAPTOPRIL 6.25–12.5 mg BD (max 50 mg TDS). NB. Gradually titrate dose depending on BP and symptoms. Watch U&E at 1–2 weeks. First dose ↓BP so start at night. **SE:** N, V, H, D, R, cough, angioedema, ↑K, altered taste, low BP, AKI. AKI might suggest renal artery stenosis. **Cautions:** severe aortic stenosis (relative), HOCM, low Na, ↓BP, high K with other potassium retaining drugs. Caution as teratogenic. Avoid NSAIDs.

CARBAMAZEPINE (AED) *Epilepsy*: CARBAMAZEPINE 100–200 mg 1–2 times/day, increased by 100–200 mg every 2 weeks; usual dose 1 g/d in divided doses; max dose 1.6–2 g daily in divided doses. **SE:** Sedation, Rash, SJS, oedema, low Na, N, V, vertigo, diplopia, aplastic anaemia. Can worsen myoclonic/absence seizures. Avoid with MAOIs. See *BNF* for interactions. Induces its own metabolism so levels drop at 3 weeks. Need to titrate dose. Expert advice in pregnancy.

CARBIMAZOLE (antithyroid). *Hyperthyroidism*: CARBIMAZOLE 15–40 mg/d for 4–8 weeks until euthyroid. Then reduce to 5–15 mg daily. Give for 12–18 months or CARBIMAZOLE 40–60 mg/day + THYROXINE for 18 months (block and replace). Given in divided dose. **SE:** rash, agranulocytosis. Give written warning to patient: any fever, sore throat stop drug and seek medical help. PTU preferred in pregnancy.

CARVEDILOL (β receptor blocker). *Stable CCF*: CARVEDILOL 3.125 mg od slowly up titrated to 25 mg BD PO. See *Atenolol* for C/I and SE.

CEFOTAXIME (3rd gen cephalosporin, penetrates CSF). *Bacterial meningitis, sepsis, cholangitis, epiglottitis, typhoid, UTI*: CEFOTAXIME 1–2 g slow IV/IM 6 h (meningitis 8 g/day). **SE:** R, N, V, D, *C. difficile* colitis, arrhythmias. **Caution:** reduce dose in renal failure, avoid neurotoxic drugs. See *Ceftriaxone* on penicillin allergy.

CEFTRIAXONE (3rd gen cephalosporin, penetrates CSF). *Bacterial meningitis, HACEK endocarditis, CAP/HAP, sepsis, etc.*: CEFTRIAXONE 1–2 g IM/IV BD. OD in less severe infections. **SE:** R, N, V, D, APX, pancreatitis. Avoid if history of immediate hypersensitivity or anaphylaxis to penicillin. Reduce dose in AKI/CKD.

CEFUROXIME (2nd gen cephalosporin). *Epiglottitis, pneumonia, UTI, surgical, soft tissue*: CEFUROXIME 750 mg to 1.5 g IV/IM 8 h. *UTI, chest, mild to moderate infection*: CEFUROXIME 250–500 mg BD PO. **SE:** R, N, V, D, APX, *C. difficile* colitis. See *Ceftriaxone* on penicillin allergy.

CEPHALEXIN (1st gen cephalosporin). *CAP, UTI*: CEPHALEXIN 250 mg 8 h PO (max 4 g/day) **SE:** R, N, V, APX. See *Ceftriaxone* on penicillin allergy.

CHLOROQUINE. *Non-falciparum malaria*: CHLOROQUINE 620 mg, then 310 mg after 6 h, then 310 mg on days 2 and 3; total dose 25 mg/kg of base, and PRIMAQUINE 15–30 mg OD in vivax and ovale for 14 days. Take expert guidance. Primaquine may cause haemolysis in G6PD-deficient individuals. Can worsen MG, psoriasis and epilepsy.

CHLORPHENAMINE (sedating antihistamine). *Anaphylaxis*: CHLORPHENAMINE 10 mg slow IV/IM 6 h/PRN. **SE:** sedation, blurred vision, dry mouth, retention, glaucoma. *Allergy*: CHLORPHENAMINE 4 mg 6 h PO. **SE:** antimuscarinic, sedation.

CHLORPROMAZINE (antipsychotic). *Acute psychosis/mania*: CHLORPROMAZINE 25–50 mg TDS PO/deep IM. Titrate to response (max 300 mg/d) **SE:** see *Haloperidol*.

CIPROFLOXACIN (Quinolone). *Gram-negative infections. pseudomonas, typhoid, traveller's diarrhoea, gonorrhoea, UTI, anthrax*: CIPROFLOXACIN 500–750 mg 12 h PO 400 mg 12 h IV over 30–60 min. **SE:** N, V, D, flatulence, syncope, oedema, erythema nodosum, tendonitis, long QT, insomnia, epilepsy. Avoid in pregnancy, G6PD, seizures, MG. NSAIDs, Ciclosporin. Reduce dose in AKI/CKD. Risk of theophylline toxicity, Increases INR with warfarin. ↑LFTs.

CITALOPRAM (SSRI). *Depression*: CITALOPRAM 10–60 mg OD. **SE:** N, V, H, sedation, insomnia, impotence. Low Na, hepatitis, avoid MAOIs. Slowly increase dose. Avoid abrupt withdrawal. See *Fluoxetine*.

CLARITHROMYCIN (macrolide). *UTI, CAP, pertussis, legionella, campylobacter, penicillin allergy, Lyme disease*: CLARITHROMYCIN 250–500 mg BD PO or CLARITHROMYCIN 500 mg 12 h IV. **SE:** dyspepsia, N, V, H, insomnia, porphyria, liver failure. Long QT. Inhibits p450 so ↑levels of theophylline, ciclosporin, digoxin, carbamazepine. Caution with other drugs causing long QT, porphyria, liver failure. Caution with atorvastatin and avoid with simvastatin. Review dose in AKI/CKD.

CLINDAMYCIN (lincosamide antibiotic). *TSS, Gram+ve cocci, streptococci, staphylococci, anaerobes*: CLINDAMYCIN 150–450 mg 6 h PO OR CLINDAMYCIN 0.6–2.7 g/d in 2–4 doses deep IM or IV infusions. **SE:** antibiotic-associated colitis, N, R, D, oesophagitis, jaundice, APX, SJS/TEN. **Cautions:** diarrhoea. Watch U&E and LFTs if treatment >10 days.

CLOPIDOGREL (P2Y12 receptor blocker). Prodrug: *STEMI/ACS*: CLOPIDOGREL 300–600 mg loading dose. Usual dose 300 mg PO and then 75 mg OD. *Post-TIA / ischaemic stroke*: CLOPIDOGREL 300 mg PO and then 75 mg OD. **SE:** bleeding – takes 7 days for effect to reduce. Effects reduced by omeprazole. **Caution:** active bleeding, trauma, imminent surgery. Ask cardiologist before stopping dual antiplatelet early post stenting.

CO-AMOXICLAV (AUGMENTIN). Amoxicillin and clavulinic acid. *Mild/moderate CAP, UTI, listeria*: CO-AMOXICLAV (250/125) 375–625 mg 8 h PO or CO-AMOXICLAV 1.2 g IV 8 h. **SE:** anaphylaxis, N, V, D, cholestasis, hepatitis, rash with infectious mononucleosis. **Caution:** avoid if glandular fever type illness. Increases INR with warfarin.

CODEINE (opioid). *Analgesia, diarrhoea, cough suppressant*: CODEINE 8–60 mg 4–6 h. **SE:** delirium, constipation, N, V. Beware opiate toxicity. Consider Naloxone. Some genetically predisposed to toxicity.

COLCHICINE (inhibits mitosis). *Acute gout*: COLCHICINE 1 mg stat PO then 0.5 mg 4 h (max dose of 6 mg taken or diarrhoea). A low dose COLCHICINE 0.5 mg 12 h may be given for weeks with allopurinol. *Acute and recurrent pericarditis*: COLCHICINE 0.5–2 g daily. **SE:** D, N, V, GI bleed. Toxic with Ciclosporin, Erythromycin, statin, others (see *BNF*). Avoid in pregnancy, AKI/CKD. Avoid if abnormal renal or hepatic function. Avoid with macrolide antibiotics, which alter its metabolism.

COLESTYRAMINE. *Gallstones when surgery not possible*: COLESTYRAMINE 4 g sachets BD in water (max 24 g/d). Delay taking other drugs for several hours after. **SE:** constipation. Poorly tolerated.

CO-TRIMOXAZOLE. Trimethoprim:sulfamethoxazole in 1:5 ratio (80:400). *PCP*: CO-TRIMOXAZOLE 120 mg/kg daily in 2–4 divided doses for 14–21 days usually given with steroids. *PCP prophylaxis*: CO-TRIMOXAZOLE 960 mg OD PO. **SE:** allergy, SJS, N, V, agranulocytosis, aplastic anaemia. ↑INR if Warfarin. Phenytoin, Ciclosporin, Azathioprine, Mercaptopurine, Methotrexate toxicity. Check *BNF*.

CYCLIZINE. *Severe nausea*: CYCLIZINE 50 mg slow IV/IM/PO 8 h. **SE:** sedation, dry mouth, urinary retention, N, V. Avoid in CCF/ACS.

DABIGATRAN (direct thrombin inhibitor). *Non-rheumatic AF/PE/DVT*: Adult 18–74 years DABIGATRAN 150 mg BD. Adult 75–79 years 110–150 mg BD. Adult ≥80 years 110 mg BD. PE/DVT patients need first 5 days covered with parenteral anticoagulant, e.g. LMWH. **SE:** bleeding, indigestion (try taking with food or switch to other DOAC). Active bleeding, falls, renal failure. See *BNF* or datasheet. Reduce dose with Amiodarone or Verapamil, Quinine. Do not keep in dosette box.

DALTEPARIN (LMWH). *VTE prophylaxis*: DALTEPARIN 2500 units SC pre surgery, then 2500 units OD. *Medical patients*: DALTEPARIN 5000 units SC 24 h. *NSTEMI/unstable angina*: DALTEPARIN 120 units/kg BD (max. 10000 units BD) for up to 8 days. *PE/DVT*: DALTEPARIN (FRAGMIN) 200 units/kg SC OD (max. per dose 18 000 units). **CI** and **SE**, see *Enoxaparin*.

DEMECLOCYCLINE (tetracycline). *SIADH*: DEMECLOCYCLINE 300–600 mg BD. If water restriction not tolerated or ineffective. Induces nephrogenic diabetes insipidus. **SE/cautions:** see tetracyclines. Avoid in pregnancy and children. **SE:** AKI, photosensitive rashes.

DESFERRIOXAMINE (chelating agent). *Iron, aluminium toxicity*: DESFERRIOXAMINE 15 mg/kg/h (max 80 mg/kg/24 h). **SE:** IM use can be painful, ARDS, abdominal pain, APX is rare, low BP if rapid infusion. Chelated iron causes red urine, risk of yersinia and mucormycosis infections.

DIAZEPAM (benzodiazepine). *Acute sedation/severe anxiety*: DIAZEPAM 1–5 mg PO/IV/PR depending on urgency. **SE:** oversedation is always the concern especially with parenteral administration and ensure facilities to resuscitate and manage airway are available. *Status epilepticus*: DIAZEPAM 10 mg, then 10 mg after 10 mins if needed. Give slowly at rate of 5 mg/min. If no IV access can give same dose PR with a 5 ml syringe connected to a rectal tube introduced 4–5 cm into the rectum. *Acute alcohol withdrawal/delirium tremens*: DIAZEPAM 5–10 mg TDS PO in severe cases when urgent sedation needed. Avoid neuroleptics. **SE:** dependence, tolerance, amnesia. Withdrawal symptoms.

DIGOXIN. *Rate control AF, CCF*: loading dose: DIGOXIN 0.75–1.5 mg split in 3 doses PO over 24 h, e.g. 0.5 mg × 3. Lower dose in the lean and elderly. *Urgent loading*: DIGOXIN 0.75–1 mg IV infusion over 2 h and then maintenance. Note: DIGOXIN 125 mcg PO= 80 mcg IV. Maintenance dose (125 mcg = 0.125 mg): DIGOXIN 0.125–0.25 mg OD. **SE:** arrhythmias, heart block (ensure on telemetry), fatigue, confusion. Toxicity in elderly, renal failure and low muscle mass (see *BNF*). Reduce dose. Serum levels: 1–2 mcg/L at 6 h post dose. Ensure K levels >4 mmol/L.

DILTIAZEM (calcium channel blocker). *HTN, angina, AF rate control*: DILTIAZEM 60–120 mg TDS. Long-acting forms available. **SE:** ↓HR, heart block, hypotension, flushing, constipation, ankle oedema. Inhibitor of CYP3A4. **Avoid:** heart block, shock, LVF. See *BNF* for interactions.

DOPAMINE. *Cardiogenic shock*: DOPAMINE 2–5 mcg/kg/min titrate to effect. Evidence poor. Low dose inotrope + vasodilates. **SE:** N, V, angina, ↑HR, HTN, peripheral vasoconstriction, arrhythmias, low BP. Caution if recent use of MAOI within 2 weeks. Reduce dose. Doses >5 mcg/kg/min vasoconstrict which reduces renal perfusion and may worsen heart failure. **CI:** phaeo; tachyarrhythmia. Give in G5 or NS.

DOXAPRAM (stimulant). *Hypoventilatory type 2 RF* (when decision made not for NIV/ITU): DOXAPRAM 1–4 mg/min, adjusted according to response. Monitor sats and ABG. **SE:** cardiac/neurostimulant, agitation, pyrexia, headache, ↑HR, HTN. Monitor closely on HDU/ITU. Define ceiling of care. **Caution:** avoid with cerebral oedema, stroke, IHD, epilepsy, severe HTN. Not an alternative to intubation and ventilation.

DOXAZOSIN (alpha-1 blocker). *Resistant HTN*: DOXAZOSIN 1–4 mg/day (slowly increase >max 16 mg/day split doses). **SE:** first use hypotension. Syncope, headache.

DOXYCYCLINE (tetracycline). *Severe infections, anthrax, Lyme*: DOXYCYCLINE 100 mg BD. *Falciparum malaria* (+ quinine): DOXYCYCLINE 200 mg/day for 7 days. **SE:** N, V, photosensitivity, liver toxicity. Avoid UV light. Reduced in renal failure. Avoid with milk.

ENALAPRIL (ACEI). *HTN, CCF* (start lowest doses): ENALAPRIL 2.5–40 mg/OD. See *Captopril* for info on ACE inhibitors.

ENOXAPARIN (LMWH). *VTE prophylaxis*: ENOXAPARIN 20–40 mg 24 h (20 mg in renal failure, 40 mg bd if >100 kg, higher doses weight adjusted). *STEMI*: ENOXAPARIN 30 mg IV bolus then 1 mg/kg SC BD for <8 days (<75 years) OR ENOXAPARIN 0.75 mg/kg SC BD (max 75 mg/dose) (>75 years). *NSTEMI/unstable angina*: ENOXAPARIN 1 mg/kg BD for 2–8 days (minimum 2 days). *PE/DVT*: ENOXAPARIN 1.5 mg/kg SC 24 h (renal failure 1 mg/kg SC OD). *Pregnancy + VTE*: ENOXAPARIN 40–100 mg SC BD (see *BNF*). **SE:** bleeding, low platelets (HITT), high K and osteoporosis long term. **CI:** endocarditis, trauma, epidural, lumbar puncture, bleeding disorder, peptic ulcer; recent cerebral haemorrhage; recent surgery to eye; recent CNS surgery, severe HTN, low platelets, history of heparin-induced thrombocytopenia, bleeding, HITT occurs at day 5–10 with thrombosis and a drop in platelets. Consider monitoring anti-Xa 4 h post-dose in renal failure, pregnancy, etc. **Caution:** avoid with other drugs that increase risk of bleeding.

ENOXIMONE (PD-3 inhibitor inotrope/vasodilates). *CHF*: initially ENOXIMONE 0.5–1 mg/kg (<12.5 mg/min), then 500 mcg/kg every 30 min and titrate to response. Max 3 mg/kg per 3–6 h. Avoid with HOCM/valve stenosis.

EPLERENONE (aldosterone antagonist). *CCF Class III/IV*: EPLERENONE 25–50 mg OD slowly increase. **SE:** high K, N, V, R. Watch U&E. Avoid K retaining drugs.

ERYTHROMYCIN (macrolides). *Infection*: ERYTHROMYCIN 250 mg to 1 g 6–8 h PO or ERYTHROMYCIN 12.5 mg/kg 6 h IV. **SE:** N, V, D limits use. SJS. Irritant to veins. **Cautions:** porphyria, liver failure, reduce dose with renal failure. Drugs causing long QT. Inhibits p450 enzymes, Clarithromycin better tolerated. ↑theophylline, ciclosporin, digoxin, carbamazepine levels. Myopathy with simvastatin so stop statins concurrently.

ETHANOL (alcohol). *Methanol/ethylene glycol toxicity*: ETHANOL oral (150 ml 40% Ethanol), e.g. vodka or other spirits. **SE:** ataxia, drunkenness, CNS depression. **CI:** religious reasons, seizures. Monitor blood levels. Ethanol should be titrated to a level of 100 mg/dL until ethylene glycol or methanol levels are below 20 mg/dL.

FERROUS FUMARATE. *Iron deficiency anaemia:* FERROUS FUMARATE 210 mg TDS PO. **SE:** N, V, abdo pain, diarrhoea, constipation. Toxicity in overdose.

FLECAINIDE (anti-/proarrhythmic). *SVT/VT/WPW, PAF, VT, cardiovert AF*: FLECAINIDE 2 mg/kg (max 150 mg) IV over 30 mins. Then infusion at a rate of 1.5 mg/kg/h for 1 h, reduced to 250 mcg/kg/h for up to 24 h – max cumulative dose = 600 mg. Oral therapy after senior cardiology review 150 mg PO BD. Always give with a rate control agent, e.g. beta-blocker. Monitor PR interval and ORS duration. Those with PPM/AICD should be discussed with cardiology prior to the administration of flecainide as this drug may affect the devices' ability to deliver therapy adequately. Get echo before if cardiac disease suspected. **SE:** N, V, dizziness, oedema, fatigue. Avoid if LV dysfunction (get echo). Specialist use only especially for ventricular arrhythmias. **Cautions:** LV dysfunction, heart block unless paced, heart failure. Have access to defibrillator.

FLUCLOXACILLIN (β-lactam penicillin antibiotic). _Staph. aureus infections, cellulitis, impetigo, surgical wounds,_ Staph. aureus _pneumonia, endocarditis_: FLUCLOXACILLIN 250–500 mg 6 h PO OR FLUCLOXACILLIN 1–2 g 6 h IV. **SE:** N, V, D, cholestasis, elevated LFTs, haemolysis, APX. **Cautions:** reduce dose in renal failure. Not for intrathecal use.

FLUCONAZOLE. _Oral candida_: FLUCONAZOLE 50–100 mg OD PO for 2 weeks. _Oesophageal candida_: FLUCONAZOLE 50–100 mg OD for 3 weeks PO. _Vaginal candida_: FLUCONAZOLE 150 mg PO. _Tinea pedis and related_: FLUCONAZOLE 50 mg OD 2–4 weeks. _Invasive candidiasis, cryptococcal meningitis_ (specialist input needed): FLUCONAZOLE 200–400 mg/d PO/IV for 12 weeks. **SE:** N, V, D, H, R, APX, SJS, low K. Avoid terfenadine. See _BNF_ for interactions with phenytoin, warfarin, theophylline, etc.

FLUMAZENIL (benzodiazepine antagonist). _Moderate/severe respiratory depression due to benzodiazepines_: FLUMAZENIL 200 mcg dose over 15 secs, then 100 mcg/min if required; usual dose 300–600 mcg. Max 1 mg. Do not use as diagnostic test. **SE:** N, V, flushing. Seizures, arrhythmias, agitation. Do not use if recent seizure. Consider respiratory support. **CI:** seizure or known epilepsy. Severe liver disease. Cautions with any drugs that lower seizure threshold, e.g. TCAs or that are arrhythmogenic.

FLUOXETINE (SSRI). _Depression_: FLUOXETINE 20–60 mg OD. **SE:** N, V, H, sedation, insomnia, impotence. Low Na, hepatitis, avoid MAOIs. Slowly increase dose. Avoid abrupt withdrawal. **Cautions:** long QT and drugs which lengthen QT. Any cessation should be reduced over 4 weeks or longer. **Interactions:** ↑lithium, TCA, haloperidol, carbamazepine, phenytoin toxicity, see _BNF_. Serotonin syndrome seen if given with MAOI or St John's wort.

FOLATE. _Folate deficiency_: FOLATE 5 mg PO OD for 4 months then recheck. **SE:** subacute combined degeneration of cord if a low B12 not replaced at same time.

FOMEPIZOLE (alcohol dehydrogenase inhibitor). _Methanol/ethylene glycol poisoning_: FOMEPIZOLE 15 mg/kg IV (max 1500 mg) then FOMEPIZOLE 10 mg/kg IV BD until methanol or ethylene glycol <20 mg/dL (200 mg/L) or level normal, acidosis cleared, and patient symptom-free. GIVE FOMEPIZOLE 10 mg/kg 4 h while on dialysis. **SE:** H, N, D, drowsiness and bad taste. Fomepizole is dialysable and should be given during haemodialysis.

FONDAPARINUX (Factor Xa inhibitor). _VTE prophylaxis_: FONDAPARINUX 2.5 mg SC OD (give 6 h post-op). For _PE/DVT_: FONDAPARINUX <50 kg 5 mg SC OD; 50–100 kg: 7.5 mg OD SC; >100 kg: 10 mg SC OD. _ACS_: FONDAPARINUX 2.5 mg SC OD <8 days. **Cautions:** reduce in renal failure. Bleeding disorders. **SE:** anaemia, bleeding, N, V. ↓K, ↓BP.

FOSPHENYTOIN. _Status epilepticus_: FOSPHENYTOIN 20 mg(PE)/kg at a rate of 100–150 mg(PE)/min. Reduce dose by 10–25% in elderly. PE = phenytoin equivalents.

SE: ↓BP, arrhythmias, less than with phenytoin 'purple glove syndrome'. Needs cardiac monitoring.

FUROSEMIDE (loop diuretic). *CCF/LVF*: FUROSEMIDE 40–80 mg PO/IV OD – more given as divided doses. Higher doses may be given. **SE:** diuresis, incontinence, low K, low Na, low BP, gynaecomastia, urinary retention. **Cautions:** low BP, dehydration, low K, AKI.

FUSIDIC ACID. *Staphylococcal skin infections*: FUSIDIC ACID 250–750 mg TDS PO. *Bone and joint infection, staph. endocarditis*: FUSIDIC ACID 500 mg to 1 g TDS IV. **SE:** N, V, D, H, dyspepsia. Avoid with statins as risk of rhabdomyolysis (stop statin during treatment), rarely AKI.

GANCICLOVIR. *CMV infection*: GANCICLOVIR 5 mg/kg IV BD for 14–21 days or more until adequate recovery. **SE:** myelosuppression (especially with AZT), rash.

GENTAMICIN. *Septicaemia, meningitis, biliary tract infection, pyelonephritis, endocarditis, pneumonia, prostatitis*: (TDS) GENTAMICIN 3–5 mg in 3 divided doses 8 h IV OR GENTAMICIN 5–7 mg/kg IV OD. *G+ve endocarditis or HACEK endocarditis* (with other antibacterials): GENTAMICIN 1 mg/kg 12 h IV/IM. **SE:** can worsen myasthenia and raise INR. Ensure hydrated. Ototoxicity with loop diuretics. If renal dysfunction, then prolong dosing interval and reduce dose. Avoid once daily high dose if CrCl <20 ml/min. Monitor levels. Peak dose 1 h after admin and trough just before. Multiple daily dose regimen: ensure peak = 5–10 mg/L and trough <2 mg/L. If eGFR <30 then take advice and follow local guidance on dose adjustment. Any total daily dose over 480 mg needs queried. Doses are calculated using thin weight estimate.

GLICLAZIDE (sulphonylurea). *Type 2 DM*: GLICLAZIDE 40–80 mg pre meals (max 320 mg/day). Given pre breakfast and evening meal. **SE:** hypoglycaemia, weight gain. Caution in renal/hepatic failure.

GLUCAGON (pancreatic hormone). *Hypoglycaemia protocol*: GLUCAGON 1 mg (1 unit) IM/SC repeated in 5–10 min. If no response within minutes then 20–50 ml 50% GLUCOSE IV or equivalent must be given. *β-blocker or CCB toxicity or cardiogenic shock due to low HR unresponsive to atropine* GLUCAGON 2–10 mg IV over 10 min then Infusion of 2–10 mg/h (protect airway in case of vomiting). **SE:** low K, low BP, GI disturbance. hyperglycaemia. Liver disease. Does not work if no liver glycogen reserves. Avoid with phaeochromocytoma.

GLYCERYL TRINITRATE. *Angina/LVF/HTN*: GTN: 1–2 sprays (400–800 mcg/dose) or GTN 500 mcg S/L, OR GTN 50 mg in 50 ml IV at 1–10 ml/h titrate to BP and effect. Onset 1–2 min OR GTN 5–20 mg transdermal patches per 24 h. **SE:** see *Isosorbide dinitrate*.

HALOPERIDOL. *Nausea and vomiting*: HALOPERIDOL 1–2 mg IM. *Acute psychosis/mania*: HALOPERIDOL 2–20 mg/d PO divided doses (1–10 mg elderly) OR HALOPERIDOL 2–5 mg IM (1–2 mg elderly). *Agitation in elderly*: HALOPERIDOL 0.75–1.5 mg 2–3 times a day PO. **SE:** ↑HR, low BP, HTN, QT prolonged. Dystonias, dyskinesias, blood dyscrasias, NMS. Worsening Parkinson's. Seizure. Lowest dose in elderly, acute glaucoma.

HEPARIN (UFH). Unfractionated heparin action: potentiates AT3. Use where immediate anticoagulation needed that can be quickly stopped. Time consuming, labour intensive and fluctuations outside therapeutic range in effect common. Difficult to manage well outside ITU/CCU. Needs close monitoring and supervision. Prior to treatment check

FBC (platelets), clotting screen and renal function. Dose: _VTE prophylaxis medical_: HEPARIN 5000 U SC 8–12 h. _Surgical_: HEPARIN 5000 units 2 h pre-op then 5000 U SC 8–12 h. Higher doses need monitoring of APTT. _VTE treatment_: HEPARIN loading 5000 U (10 000 U if severe PE) and then 18 U/kg/h IV. For DVT can give 15 000 U SC BD. Aim for therapeutic APTT range of 2.0–3.0. If treatment >5 days then check platelet count daily. Repeat APTT ratio every 6–8 h or after each change in rate, unless APTT ratio is >5.0 when measurement should be made more frequently (1 h after restart). **SE:** bleeding, HIT (low platelets – monitor), high K with protamine. Can be used in pregnancy. **CI:** any ↑bleeding risk. Reversal, see _Protamine_. **Systemic anticoagulation** Loading dose for patients who have not received heparin within the last 6 hours. Check baseline APTT ratio < 1.5: Give IV bolus of approx 75 units/kg (10,000 units max), rounded to nearest 2,500 units. Check APTT ratio 6 hours after starting infusion and adjust rate using the table below as a guide. Aim to keep the APTT ratio between 2.0 and 3.0 – check with your laboratory standards. If treatment >5 days then check platelet count daily. Repeat APTT ratio every 6–8 h or after each change in rate, unless APTT ratio is >5.0 when measurement should be made more frequently (1 h after restart).

APTT	Heparin sodium 1000 U/ml
>5.0	stop for 2 h; reduce by 0.5 ml/h (500 U) and recheck at 4 h
4.1–5	stop for 1 h; reduce by 0.3 ml/h (300 U) and recheck at 4 h
3.6–4	reduce by 0.2 ml/h (200 U)
3.1–3.5	reduce by 0.1 ml/h (100 U)
2.0–3.0	NO CHANGE
1.5–1.9	increase by 0.1 ml/h (100 U)
1.2–1.4	increase by 0.2 ml/h (200 U)
<1.2	give 2500 U IV bolus; increase by 0.4 ml/h (400 U)

HYDROXOCOBALAMIN. _B12 deficiency_: HYDROXOCOBALAMIN 1 mg IM × 6 doses over 3 weeks then 1 mg every 3 months for life. _Cyanide toxicity_: (Cyanokit) HYDROXOCOBALAMIN 5 g IV over 15 min, then 5 g over 15–120 mins depending on severity. **SE:** low K, iron deficiency. Monitor FBC, U&E, reticulocytes.

IBUPROFEN (NSAID). _Analgesia, anti-inflammatory: migraine_: IBUPROFEN 200–600 mg 8 h PO (max 2.4 g daily in divided doses), caution long term with NSAID. **SE:** N, V, D, R, GI bleed/ulcer, asthma, AKI. Avoid in AKI, CKD or liver disease or severe illness where AKI likely. Increased thrombotic events. Use lowest dose and shortest course. If NSAID and gastric ulcers. MISOPROSTOL 200 mcg QDS (**SE** includes diarrhoea) or PPI. **Cautions:** renal/liver disease, AKI, GI bleed.

IDARUCIZAMAB (PRAXBIND). _Life/limb/vision threatening bleeding on Dabigatran_ (Pradaxa): IDARUCIZAMAB (PRAXBIND) 2 × 2.5 mg (as 2 vials). **SE:** headache, ↓K, delirium, constipation, pyrexia, pneumonia, thrombotic risk.

IMMUNOGLOBULIN IV. _Severe infections, GBS, MG, ITP, CIDP_: IVIG 2 g/kg given as 0.4 g/kg/d for 5 consecutive days. This may be repeated after 4–6 weeks depending on indication. _Toxic shock syndrome_: IV immunoglobulin 1 g/kg day 1, 0.5 g/kg day 2 and 3 under expert advice. **SE:** N, F, H, backache in 1% in first 30 min. Some guidelines recommend screening for IgA deficiency to prevent potential anaphylaxis. Take local advice. Aseptic meningitis within 48 h, anaphylaxis, thrombotic stroke, MI and AKI can be seen. Neutropenia. **CI:** selective IgA deficiency. Watch for AKI seen in older, diabetic, dehydrated. Ensure hydrated. From the serum of at least 1000 donors screened for HIV, HTLV and hep B and C before pooling.

INDAPAMIDE (thiazide diuretic). *HTN, CCF*: INDAPAMIDE 2.5 mg OD. **SE:** See *Bendroflumethiazide* for info on thiazides.

INTRALIPID. *Lipid soluble drug toxicity*: see INTRALIPID therapy ▶ Section 14.3. **SE:** ↑TGS, acute pancreatitis, cholestasis.

IODINE (Lugol's iodine – aqueous iodine solution). *Thyroid storm*: LUGOL'S IODINE: 5–10 drops or 1 ml PO/NG every 6–8 hours can be used. It is started 1 h after the carbimazole/PTU.

IPRATROPIUM (anticholinergic). *Acute asthma, COPD, bronchospasm*: IPRATROPIUM BROMIDE 250–500 mcg via neb 6 h (air in COPD, high flow O_2 in asthma). *Chronic asthma/COPD*: IPRATROPIUM BROMIDE 20–40 mcg 6 h. Onset 30–60 min, lasts 6 h up to maximum 80 mcg 6 h. **SE:** dry mouth, ↑HR, dizziness, epistaxis. **Caution:** CCF, arrhythmias, dilated pupil if drug enters eye BPH, glaucoma.

IRON. *Iron deficiency anaemia*: FERROUS SULPHATE 200 mg BD or TDS PO, or FERROUS GLUCONATE 300 mg BD PO may be better tolerated. **SE:** N, V, D, cramps, constipation. Take with food. *Parenteral iron*: IRON DEXTRAN IV or IM. **SE:** anaphylaxis so test dose given first. Dose depends on iron stores and Hb.

ISOSORBIDE DINITRATE (NO donor). *Angina, LVF*: ISOSORBIDE DINITRATE (ISOKET) initially 2–10 mg/h, increased if necessary to 20 mg/h. *Chronic angina*: ISOSORBIDE DINITRATE 20–40 mg TDS PO in divided doses (max 240 mg/d). **SE:** headache, ↑HR, ↓BP, tolerance if continued >24 h. Avoid if low BP. Close monitoring when given IV or S/L. **Caution:** low BP, severe aortic stenosis, HOCM, tamponade, combined Sildenafil and Nitrates can cause severe ↓BP.

ISOSORBIDE MONONITRATE (NO donor). *Angina, LVF*: ISOSORBIDE MONONITRATE 20–40 mg TDS. **SE** and **CI:** see *Isosorbide dinitrate*.

IVABRADINE (funny channel blocker at SA node). *Angina with sinus rhythm LVEF <35%*: IVABRADINE 2.5–5 mg BD. Specialist use only. **SE:** ↓HR, AF, phosphenes. Avoid if HR <60/min or HR <75 and heart failure, Diltiazem, Verapamil, heart block, long QT, shock, MI.

LABETALOL (mixed α/β adrenergic blocker). *Severe HTN, urgent BP reduction, post MI*: LABETALOL 20–50 mg slow IV over at least 1 min, then repeat after 5 mins if required. Less urgent reduction Infusion 20–40 mg/h (max 120 mg/h) and titrate to target BP. Total dose 200 mg. **SE:** fatigue, depression, cold peripheries, bronchospasm. Rare hepatocellular damage. **Caution:** do not reduce BP in ischaemic stroke if not for thrombolysis unless SBP >200 mmHg and if so then slowly reduce to <200 mmHg. **SE:** asthma, ↓HR. Target BP: aortic dissection: 110 mmHg. Stroke thrombolysis: <185/110 mmHg. HTN encephalopathy: slowly lower SBP to 180 mmHg.

LAMOTRIGINE. *Epilepsy, juvenile myoclonic epilepsy*: LAMOTRIGINE 25 mg PO alt. days week 1–2 and then increase by 25–50 mg/day every 2 weeks. *Maintenance*: LAMOTRIGINE 200 mg/d (max 500 mg). **SE:** cerebellar signs, diplopia, SJS, TEN, blood dyscrasias, DIC, N, V, D, sedation. Check U&E, FBC, LFT. **Caution:** stop if rash, anaemia, bruising, fever, lymphadenopathy, sore throat – seek medical help. Slow start reduces risk of severe rash. See *BNF* for interactions. Half the dose if on Valproate, increase dose with Phenytoin and Carbamazepine. Rash common if dose increased quickly or on Valproate.

LANSOPRAZOLE (PPI): *Peptic ulcer disease, GORD/oesophagitis*: LANSOPRAZOLE 30 mg OD/BD PO/SL for 4 or more weeks. *Zollinger–Ellison syndrome*: LANSOPRAZOLE 60–120 mg/d. **SE:** abdo pain, C, D, N, V, H. Oral dispersible fast-tab format useful. PPIs can reduce effectiveness of Clopidogrel, particularly Omeprazole. Also agitation, impotence, Phenytoin toxicity. See *Omeprazole*.

LEVETIRACETAM (KEPPRA). *Epilepsy*: LEVETIRACETAM 250 mg OD/BD increasing over 2–4 weeks to 1 g 12 h (max 3 g/d). **SE:** N, V, D, H, R, nasopharyngitis, drowsiness, mood changes, dizziness, ataxia, leucopenia, rash (SJS), DRESS, low WCC, platelets. Few interactions.

LIDOCAINE (Class Ib antiarrhythmic Na channel blocker). *Cardiac arrest*: LIDOCAINE 50–100 mg (1 mg/kg) IV over 5 min, then infusion 4 mg/min for 30 min then 2 mg/min for 2 h. *Ventricular arrhythmias*: LIDOCAINE 50 mg IV over 2–5 min and then infusion as for cardiac arrest. Maximum total IV dose of 200 mg or 3 mg/kg in first hour. **SE:** slurred speech, bradycardia, twitching, coma, seizures suggest toxicity. May be beneficial in out of hospital VF cardiac arrest. **Caution:** heart block.

LISINOPRIL (ACEI). *HTN, CCF* (start lowest doses): LISINOPRIL 2.5–40 mg OD. See *Captopril* for more ACE class properties.

LITHIUM. *Mania, cluster headaches*: LITHIUM 400 mg to 1.2 g daily as a single dose or in divided doses. Aim for serum levels of 0.6–0.8 mmol/L 12 h after a dose on days 4–7 of treatment. **SE:** N, V, long QT, tremor, nephrogenic diabetes insipidus, hypothyroid. Ataxia, dysarthria, monitor U&E, Ca, PTH, TFT. Avoid dehydration. Preparations vary widely in bioavailability. Toxic levels >2 mmol/L. Hydration and haemodialysis for toxicity.

LOPERAMIDE (non-absorbed opiate). *Diarrhoea*: LOPERAMIDE 1–4 mg BD (max 16 mg/d). **Cautions:** avoid: *C. difficile* infection, intestinal obstruction, HUS. Does not cross blood–brain barrier. Use lowest dose in elderly. **SE:** N, V.

LORAZEPAM (benzodiazepine). *Acute sedation/severe anxiety*: LORAZEPAM 0.5–2 mg PO/IM/IV depending on urgency. **SE:** oversedation is always the concern especially with parenteral administration and ensure facilities to resuscitate and manage airway are available. Sedation increased if used with other sedating drugs. *Status epilepticus*: LORAZEPAM 2–4 mg slow IV (or IM) over 1 min into a large vein.

LOSARTAN (ARB). *HTN, CCF*: LOSARTAN 12.5–100 mg OD. Lower dose in CCF. More info see *Candesartan*.

MADOPAR/SINEMET. *Idiopathic Parkinson's disease* (L-Dopa + decarboxylase inhibitor (DCI)): SINEMET/MADOPAR 62.5 mg (L-Dopa 50 mg + DCI 12.5 mg) 6 hourly increased to 400–800 mg of L-Dopa per day divided in 4–5 doses. Increase slowly. **SE:** sedation, confusion, low BP, dyskinesias, nausea, vomiting (manage with DOMPERIDONE).

MAGNESIUM SULPHATE: 1 g = 4 mmol. *TdP/VT*: MAGNESIUM 8 mmol (2 g) over 15 min repeat if needed. *Acute severe asthma*: MAGNESIUM 8 mmol (2 g) in 100 ml NS over

20 min. *Pre/eclampsia*: MAGNESIUM 16 mmol (4 g) over 20 min, then 1 g/h for 24 h. *Hypomagnesaemia*: MAGNESIUM 10 mmol in 50 ml G5 over 4 h. **SE:** low BP, CNS toxicity, respiratory depression. Toxicity with renal failure. If Mg toxicity, antidote is IV Ca.

MANNITOL (osmotic diuretic). *Cerebral oedema, ↑intraocular pressure*: MANNITOL 0.25–2 g/kg, given over 30–60 min. Dose may be repeated 1–2 times after 4–8 h. **SE:** diuresis, hypovolaemia, low BP, ↑osmolarity, high Na. Max effect 90 min, rarely anaphylaxis.

MEROPENEM (Carbapenem). *Abdominal/gynae infections, CAP, diabetic soft tissue infections*: MEROPENEM 0.5–1 g 8-hourly. *Meningitis/endocarditis*: 2 g 8-hourly. **SE:** N, D, V, *C. difficile* colitis, severe low K. SJS, TEN. Monitor LFTs. High/low platelets. Reduce dose in renal/liver failure. Reduces Sodium Valproate levels. CSF penetration good. Not for MRSA.

MESALAZINE (5-aminosalicylate). *Ulcerative colitis*: MESALAZINE 4 g/day slow release. *Distal recto sigmoid colitic disease*: MESALAZINE enema 1 g PR BD. **SE:** N, H, dyspepsia, low WCC, low platelets, anaemia, rash, deranged renal and liver function.

METFORMIN. *Type 2 DM*: METFORMIN 500 mg BD to 1 g BD. **SE:** N, V, abdo pain, bowel upset, lactic acidosis. Caution if eGFR <45 ml/min/1.73 m^2. Stop if AKI, sepsis, MI, liver or cardiac failure. Use insulin if needed. Omit 48 h before giving IV radiocontrast.

METHOTREXATE (MTX) (inhibits dihydrofolate reductase). *IBD, rheumatology*: METHOTREXATE 7.5–20 mg PO/IV/IM/SC **once weekly**. **SE:** N, V, stomatitis. Give folic acid 5 mg day after MTX given. Liver toxicity, bone marrow suppression, pneumonitis. Monitor FBC and LFTS. Ensure dosed weekly and not daily. Advise must seek medical help if any fever, sore throat, bruising, mouth ulcers.

METOCLOPRAMIDE. *Severe nausea, prokinetic*: METOCLOPRAMIDE 10 mg IV/IM/PO TDS. **SE:** dystonia. Avoid in bowel obstruction. Avoid age <20 as risk of dystonia. Preferred in heart failure.

METOLAZONE (thiazide-like diuretic). *CCF*: METOLAZONE 2.5 mg OD. Very Potent often short term usage. **SE:** overdiuresis, low Na, low K. Watch fluid balance, acute gout, AKI. See *Bendroflumethiazide* for **SE** and **CI**.

METRONIDAZOLE. *Anaerobic infections, abdominal sepsis, C. difficile, giardia, amoebiasis*: METRONIDAZOLE 400–500 mg PO TDS, METRONIDAZOLE 500 mg IV 8 h, METRONIDAZOLE 1 g TDS PR. **SE:** N, V, D, liver toxicity, H, sensory neuropathy if use >4 weeks. ↑INR on Warfarin. Avoid alcohol as disulfiram effect, lithium and phenytoin toxicity, porphyria.

MIDAZOLAM. *Acute/procedural sedation/amnesia/severe anxiety/palliation*: MIDAZOLAM 1–5 mg slow IV over 2–5 min (max 7.5 mg). Lower dose in elderly. **SE:** oversedation is always the concern with IM/IV use so ensure facilities to manage ABC available. Sedation increased if used with other sedating drugs. *Palliation*: MIDAZOLAM 10 mg/24 h if ongoing agitation, SC infusion. *Status epilepticus*: MIDAZOLAM 5–10 mg IM/Buccal.

NALOXONE (NARCAN) (opiate antagonist). *Opiate-related sedation or hypoventilation*: NALOXONE 400 mcg to 2 mg IV/IM/SC. *Long-acting opiate*: NALOXONE 5–10 mg in 500 ml G5 over 4–6 h titrate to response. *Opiate reversal in palliative/chronic opiate use/*

misuse smaller doses given: NALOXONE 20 mcg repeated as needed. **SE:** N, V, ↑HR, opiate withdrawal syndrome. Use cardiac telemetry for repeated doses. IV half-life may be shorter than from opiate ingested. Consider an infusion. Consider a test dose in any suspected opiate toxicity.

NEOSTIGMINE (cholinesterase inhibitor increases Ach). *Colonic pseudo-obstruction, myasthenia gravis*: NEOSTIGMINE 2 mg IV/SC/IM over 5 min with telemetry. Repeat once if needed. **SE:** salivation, ↓HR, cramps, N, V, D, ↓BP, bronchoconstriction. Caution with asthma, recent MI, epilepsy, arrhythmias. Atropine for any significant ↓HR.

NICORANDIL (K channel activator). *Stable angina*: NICORANDIL 5–10 mg BD (5 mg dose if headache). Max 20–30 mg BD. **SE:** N, V, H, R, low BP, PUD. **Caution:** low BP, LVF.

NIFEDIPINE (dihydropyridine CCB). *HTN, Raynaud's phenomenon*: NIFEDIPINE 30–60 mg (extended release) OD PO (max 120 mg/d). *Oesophageal spasm*: NIFEDIPINE 10 mg PO TDS. **SE:** see *Amlodipine,* bradycardia, heart block, ↓BP, flushing, constipation, peripheral oedema. Inhibitor of CYP3A4. Avoid in heart block, shock. See *BNF* for interactions.

NIMODIPINE (dihydropyridine CCB). *Aneurysmal SAH, RCVS*: NIMODIPINE 60 mg 4 h PO/NG within 4 days of an aneurysmal SAH for 21 days or NIMODIPINE 1 mg/h IV infusion (0.5 mg/h if body weight <70 kg) increase after 2 h to 2 mg/h if BP stable. **SE:** HR, low BP, low platelets. See *BNF* for interactions.

NITROFURANTOIN. *UTI*: NITROFURANTOIN 50–100 mg 6 h (3 days for uncomplicated UTI, 7 days for men/complicated). *UTI prophylaxis*: NITROFURANTOIN 50–100 mg ON. Avoid in late pregnancy. **SE:** N, V, H, D, R, pulmonary fibrosis, neuropathy, brown urine. Watch LFT/resp rate. Avoid in renal failure. Can cause lupus syndrome.

(SODIUM) NITROPRUSSIDE (NO donor). Needs continuing arterial BP monitor. *Severe HTN or CCF, aortic dissection* NITROPRUSSIDE start 0.5–1.5 mcg/kg/min increasing by 0.5 mcg/kg/min steps titrate to BP and effect. Max 4–8 mcg/kg/min. Keep SBP >100 mmHg. Dissection combined with β-blockade, e.g. LABETALOL. Protect infusion from the light. **CI:** severe aortic stenosis, HCM, CKD, AKI, severe B12 deficiency, Leber's optic atrophy. **SE:** Marked ↓BP – start low dose and slowly titrate up. Overuse can lead to cyanide toxicity.

NORADRENALINE (NOREPINEPHRINE). Needs arterial BP monitoring. Potent vasoconstriction. *Shock with low systemic vascular resistance*: NORADRENALINE 0.16–0.33 ml/min (40 mcg (base)/ml) via central venous line. Titrate to response. Improves renal and mesenteric flow. **Cautions:** diabetes, ACS, resp failure. **SE:** arrhythmias, ischaemia. **NB.** 1 mg of noradrenaline base = 2 mg of noradrenaline acid tartrate.

NYSTATIN (polyene antifungal). *Oral candida*: NYSTATIN 100 000 units/ml 1 ml 6 h oral after food. *Skin rash*: cream/ointment 100 000 units QDS. Not absorbed systemically if given PO. **SE:** nausea.

OCTREOTIDE (somatostatin analogue). *Variceal upper GI bleed*: OCTREOTIDE 100 mcg stat with 25–50 mcg/h IV infusion for 3–5 days. **SE:** ↓HR, N, V, D, R, H, dizziness, hyperglycaemia, abdominal cramps. Can be used in those with IHD.

OLANZAPINE (atypical antipsychotic). *Severe nausea, severe agitation* (low dose in elderly): OLANZAPINE 2.5–10 mg IM repeat after 2 h as needed. OLANZAPINE 5–10 mg

PO OD (2.5 mg in elderly). Monitor: get ECG. **Cautions:** heart disease, seizures, depression, jaundice, myasthenia, DKA, long QT, bone marrow depression. **SE:** low WCC, ileus, resp depression, ↑lipid. Monitor lipids/glucose if long term usage. Neuroleptic malignant syndrome, acute glaucoma, SIADH, oedema, low Na. Risk of cardiovascular disease with Quetiapine. Avoid Risperidone in Lewy body disease, sleep disorder.

OMEPRAZOLE (PPI). Always ensure dyspepsia not due to gastric cancer. DU heal in 4 weeks and GU in 8 weeks so course should match this. Endoscopy in older patients and red flag symptoms. Test and eradicate HP. *Upper GI bleed*: OMEPRAZOLE 80 mg IV over 1 h then 8 mg/h IV for 72 h in G5/NS reduces rebleed rate. *Peptic ulcer disease, GORD/oesophagitis*: OMEPRAZOLE 20–40 mg OD/BD IV/ PO/SL. *Zollinger–Ellison syndrome*: OMEPRAZOLE 60–120 mg/d. **SE:** abdominal pain, constipation, diarrhoea, N, V, H. As Omeprazole oral dispersible fast-tab format useful. PPIs can reduce effectiveness of Clopidogrel particularly Omeprazole and Esomeprazole. **SE:** (omeprazole) agitation, impotence, N, V, H. Phenytoin toxicity. ↑risk of *C. difficile*.

ONDANSETRON. *Severe nausea*: ONDANSETRON 4 mg IV/IM, ONDANSETRON 8 mg BD PO (8 mg/d in liver disease). **SE:** constipation, H, flushing, hiccups. Avoid if long QT.

PABRINEX (thiamine (B1), riboflavin, pyridoxine, Vit C, nicotinamide). *Malnutrition, starvation, hyperemesis, alcoholism, beriberi*: PABRINEX (vitamin B and C) one pair of vials TDS for 1–2 days (at least 3–4 sets are given) and then oral thiamine given) then THIAMINE 100 mg TDS PO in divided doses. Give before giving PO/IV GLUCOSE. *Suspected Wernicke's syndrome*: PABRINEX 2 × pairs of vials TDS for at least 3–5 days. Be prepared to manage anaphylaxis. Dilute ampoules 1+2 with 100 ml NS or G5 give over 30 min. Then flush with a further 100 ml NS/G5.

PAMIDRONATE (bisphosphonate). *Bone metastasis/breast cancer/hypercalcaemia/ Paget's disease*: PAMIDRONATE 30–90 mg IV into large vein. **SE** and **CI:** see *Alendronate*. For raised Ca ensure well hydrated beforehand. Cancer patients need a dental check before treatment, or as soon as possible after starting treatment, to avoid osteonecrosis of the jaw.

PANTOPRAZOLE (PPI). *Upper GI bleed*: PANTOPRAZOLE 80 mg IV over 1 h then 8 mg/h IV for 72 h in G5 or 0.9% NaCl reduces rebleed rate. *Peptic ulcer disease, GORD/oesophagitis*: PANTOPRAZOLE 20–40 mg OD, PANTOPRAZOLE 40 mg slow IV OD. **SE:** abdo pain, constipation, D, N, V, H. See *Omeprazole* for more info.

PHENTOLAMINE. *Phaeochromocytoma surgery*: PHENTOLAMINE 2–5 mg IV bolus repeated if necessary. **SE:** low (postural) BP, angina, arrhythmias, chest pain, ↑HR, dizziness, malaise, D, H. **Cautions:** low BP, syncope, cataract – floppy iris syndrome.

PHENYTOIN. *Status epilepticus*: Loading dose PHENYTOIN 20 mg/kg (max dose 2 g) slow IV (max 50 mg/min) over 30–60 min then maintenance PHENYTOIN 100 mg PO/IV every 6–8 hours adjusted according to plasma levels. Rapid infusion can cause hypotension. **SE:** low BP, arrhythmias, CNS depression if given quickly. Hypersensitivity, heart. Adjust dose on levels 6 h post dose. Zero order kinetics so escalating toxicity with small dose increases. These should not exceed 50 mg if daily dose is greater than 300 mg. New steady state may take 5–7 days after dose adjustment. High pH so extravasation will cause tissue damage.

PHOSPHATE (G5 = 5% glucose, NS = 0.9% saline). *Low phosphate <0.4–0.8 mmol/L:* ORAL EFFERVESCENT SODIUM PHOSPHATE. *Phosphate <0.4 mmol/L:* PHOSPHATE infusion 9 mmol every 12 h IV. Higher doses in critical care. **SE:** low Ca/Mg, high K/Mg$^+$.

PRALIDOXIME (reactivates acetylcholinesterase). *Organophosphate, sarin poisoning:* PRALIDOXIME 30 mg/kg over 20 min and then 8 mg/kg/h up to max 12 g/24 h. Usually given with atropine. **SE:** HTN, ↑HR, diplopia, laryngospasm, H, N, V.

PRASUGREL (antiplatelet). *ACS with PCI, STEMI + PPCI, NSTEMI at time of PCI reinfarction or stent thrombosis on asp/clopidogrel, ACS + DM and PCI:* loading dose PRASUGREL 60 mg and then 10 mg OD for 1 year. PRASUGREL 5 mg OD if weight <60 kg or age >75 or ↑bleed risk. Should also take ASPIRIN 75 mg OD. **SE:** bleeding, rash, low platelets, TTP. Avoid if bleeding risk. Not for stable coronary disease. Greater risk of major bleeding than Clopidogrel. Ensure duration and dose specified in discharge letter.

PROCHLORPERAZINE. *Severe nausea/vertigo:* PROCHLORPERAZINE 12.5 mg IV/IM stat or PROCHLORPERAZINE 5 mg TDS PO. **SE:** sedation, extrapyramidal symptoms, dry mouth, urinary retention, glaucoma.

PROCYCLIDINE (antimuscarinic). *Acute dystonia:* PROCYCLIDINE 5–10 mg IV stat. **Cautions:** heart disease, HTN, psychosis, prostatic hypertrophy, pyrexia, risk of angle-closure glaucoma. **SE:** constipation, dry mouth, N, V, tachycardia, dizziness, confusion, euphoria, hallucinations, impaired memory, anxiety, restlessness, urinary retention, blurred vision, and rash.

PROPRANOLOL (β blocker). *Thyrotoxicosis, thyroiditis:* PROPRANOLOL 40 mg TDS PO. **SE:** bronchospasm, fatigue, depression, cold peripheries, ↓HR. Do not increase if CCF worsening. **Caution:** avoid in asthma, ↓HR, heart block, heart failure, pulmonary oedema.

PROPYLTHIOURACIL (PTU). *Thyrotoxicosis:* PROPYLTHIOURACIL 200–400 mg/d until euthyroid and then 50–150 mg/d. **SE:** rare hepatoxicity, low WCC, low platelets, aplastic anaemia, nephritis, lupus erythematosus-like syndromes. Monitor. PTU often used in pregnancy but can cause neonatal hypothyroidism.

PROTAMINE. *Reverse effect of LMWH and UFH:* PROTAMINE 1 mg for every 100 U of LMWH or UFH of anti-factor Xa activity in past 8 h or 1 mg of Enoxaparin. Give PROTAMINE 25–50 mg IV infusion at 5 mg/min. Max 50 mg.

PROTHROMBIN COMPLEX CONCENTRATES (PCC) (Octaplex/Beriplex). *Warfarin or any VKA antagonist reversal: life threatening active bleeding:* give with VITAMIN K 5 mg IV. *INR 2–6:* give PCC 25 units/kg. *INR >6:* give PCC 50 units/kg IV. *Intracerebral bleed on warfarin, Xa inhibitors:* PCC 50 units/kg stat don't wait for INR. (Max dose of 3000 units.) PCC given by slow IV infusion with a syringe pump. Start at 1 ml/min, increasing to max 3 ml/min as tolerated. May take 30 min. Repeat INR again at 6 h. Avoid if allergy or previous heparin-induced thrombocytopenia (HIT). If PCC not available then FFP at 15 ml/kg.

PRUCALOPRIDE (high affinity 5HT agonist). *Refractory constipation:* PRUCALOPRIDE 1–2 mg PO OD. **SE:** N, V, dyspepsia, colic, fatigue. Cautions if IHD/arrhythmias. Avoid if bowel obstruction/perforation suspected.

QUININE. *Complicated falciparum malaria. loading dose:* QUININE 20 mg/kg slow IV over 4 h (max 1.4 g). *Maintenance* (8 h later): QUININE 10 mg/kg (max 700 mg) PO/slow

IV over 4 h TDS. Dilute to 500 ml with NS/G5 by controlled IV infusion. If IV not possible then consider IM to the anterior thigh. **SE:** hypoglycaemia, arrhythmias, cinchonism with reversible hearing loss, N, V, D, visual disturbances. Send blood films. Always take expert advice. Needs ITU management if complicated. Avoid delays. Treat if suspicious. **Caution:** never give by rapid IV injection, as lethal ↓BP may result. *Uncomplicated falciparum malaria*: QUININE 600 mg/8 h PO for 7 days plus DOXYCYCLINE 200 mg OD (or CLINDAMYCIN 450 mg TDS for pregnant women) for 7 days OR ATOVAQUONE PROGUANIL (Malarone): 4 'standard' tablets daily for 3 days OR CO-ARTEM (Riamet): if weight >35 kg, 4 tablets then 4 tablets at 8, 24, 36, 48 and 60 h.

RANITIDINE (H$_2$ blocker). *Peptic ulcer disease* (4–8 weeks): RANITIDINE 50 mg IV 8 h, RANITIDINE 150 mg BD PO. **SE:** D, N, V, R, confusion, hepatitis, porphyria.

RETEPLASE (plasminogen activator fibrinolytic). *STEMI* (within 12 h of symptom onset): RETEPLASE. 1st 10 unit bolus given over 2 min; 2nd 10 unit bolus 30 min later over 2 min. NS flush before and after each bolus. **SE:** anaphylaxis, haemorrhage, angioedema. **CI:** see *Streptokinase*. Specialist use only.

RIFAMPICIN (broad spectrum anti-TB antibiotic). *Brucellosis, anti-TB drug, endocarditis, legionella, CAP*: RIFAMPICIN 0.6–1.2 g/day in 2–4 divided doses. Reduce dose in renal failure. **SE:** N, V, D, H, anorexia, red urine, tears, TTP, AKI, TEN, SJS. Potent liver p450 inducer reducing t$_{1/2}$ of other drugs. Monitor LFTs.

RISPERIDONE. *Severe agitation/aggression in Alzheimer dementia*: RISPERIDONE 250–500 mcg BD (max 1 mg BD). Monitor: get ECG. **Cautions:** see *Olanzapine*.

RIVAROXABAN (direct Factor Xa inhibitor). *VTE prophylaxis*: RIVAROXABAN 10 mg OD duration depends on surgery. *DVT/PE*: RIVAROXABAN 15 mg BD × 21 d then 15–20 mg OD depending on balance of risks. *Non-valvular AF*: RIVAROXABAN 20 mg OD if eGFR 15–49 ml/min/1.73 m^2, then reduce to 15 mg OD. **SE:** active bleeding, falls. Assess bleeding risk. Abdominal pain, N, V, H, C, D.

SALBUTAMOL (β-2 agonist). *Acute asthma, COPD, high K*: SALBUTAMOL neb 2.5–5.0 mg 6 h or every 30 min in acute severe asthma. Use with high flow oxygen in asthma, room air in COPD. SALBUTAMOL 250 mcg slow IV over 10 min when inhaled route unreliable. *Infusion*: SALBUTAMOL 3–20 mcg/min. *Chronic asthma/COPD inhaler*: SALBUTAMOL 100–200 mcg inhaled 6 h or PRN. **SE:** ↑HR, low K, tremor, headache, anxiety.

SENNA (stimulant laxative). *Constipation*: SENNA 15 mg (2 tabs) BD. **SE:** cramps, diarrhoea, low K. Avoid if bowel obstruction.

SIMVASTATIN (HMG CoA reductase inhibitor). *IHD, ischaemic stroke, hyperlipidaemia*: SIMVASTATIN 10–40 mg ON (max 80 mg). (Max dose SIMVASTATIN 20 mg with either Amiodarone, Verapamil, Diltiazem, Amlodipine and max 10 mg with a Fibrate.) Monitor: LFTs and CK. **SE:** muscle toxicity seen with all statins – check CK (stop if >5× increase), pancreatitis. Myopathy with macrolides or amiodarone. Liver disease, high K. Check LFT Day 0, and 3 and 12 months.

SPIRONOLACTONE (aldosterone antagonist). *CCF Class III/IV*: SPIRONOLACTONE 25–50 mg OD. *Ascites*: SPIRONOLACTONE 100–400 mg OD. **SE:** high K, gynaecomastia with spironolactone, N, V, R. Avoid hyperkalaemia. Watch U&E. Avoid K-retaining drugs.

STEROIDS: see *Section 22.7 below*.

STREPTOKINASE (activates plasminogen to form plasmin, which degrades fibrin and so breaks up thrombi). *Compromised PE*: STREPTOKINASE 0.25 MU over 30 min then 0.1 MU/h for 12–72 h in NS/G5. *STEMI*: (within 12 h of symptoms onset) STREPTOKINASE 1.5 MU in 100 ml of G5/NS over 60 min IV. Interactions: other antithrombotics ↑bleeding risk. **SE:** low BP, bleeding, mild ↓BP may need IV fluids and leg raising, bleeding, anaphylaxis, angioneurotic oedema, tongue swelling with alteplase especially if on ACEI. **Cautions:** not for acute stroke. Anaphylaxis, bleeding, anticoagulation, varices, aortic dissection, cavitating lung disease, heavy vaginal bleeding, stroke disease (take specialist advice), active peptic ulcer disease, recent surgery, recent trauma, severe hypertension, pericarditis, any haemorrhagic stroke. Active bleeding, trauma, malignancy. Risk of haemorrhagic stroke 0.5–1%.

SULFASALAZINE (5-aminosalicylate). *Acute attack of ulcerative colitis*: SULFASALAZINE 1–2 g QDS reducing to 500 mg QDS. Alone or with oral therapy SULFASALAZINE suppository 0.5–1 g PR BD after bowel movement. **CI:** G6PDH deficiency. **SE:** blood dyscrasias, male infertility, D, N, V, R, SJS. Monitor FBC and LFTs. Advise to report rash, sore throat, purport, bleeding, etc.

TAZOCIN (Piperacillin (penicillin antibiotic) + Tazobactam (inhibits β-lactamases)). *Pseudomonas/neutropenic sepsis*: TAZOCIN 2.25–4.5 g 6–8 h IV over 30 min. **SE:** N, V, D, R, as for benzyl-penicillin, SJS and TEN, low K, low glucose. **CI:** as for benzylpenicillin. ↓dose/frequency in renal failure.

TEICOPLANIN (glycopeptides). *C. difficile infection*: TEICOPLANIN 100–200 mg 12 h PO 10–14 days. *MRSA, severe burns*: TEICOPLANIN wt <70 kg give 400 mg 12-hrly for 3 doses then 400 mg OD. Wt >70 kg 6 mg/kg for 3 doses then 6 mg/kg OD. *Severe infections, endocarditis*: TEICOPLANIN 10 mg/kg 12-hrly for 3–5 doses then 10 mg/kg OD. *Bone/joint infections*: TEICOPLANIN 12 mg/kg 12-hrly for 3–5 doses then 12 mg/kg OD. **SE:** itch, R, D, F, H, N, V. **Cautions:** nephrotoxic and ototoxic. Plasma – Teicoplanin concentration is not measured routinely. Avoid other nephrotoxic or ototoxic drugs. Monitor hearing and LFT/U&E. Dilute in NS or G5 and give over 30 min.

TENECTEPLASE (tissue plasminogen activator fibrinolytic). *STEMI (within 12 h of symptoms onset)*: TENECTEPLASE <60 kg 30 mg, 60–70 kg 35 mg, 70–80 kg 40 mg, 80–90 kg 45 mg, >90 kg 50 mg (max dose 50 mg) given over 10 sec. **Cautions:** see *Streptokinase*. **SE:** any bleeding, angioedema, haemorrhagic stroke.

TERLIPRESSIN (synthetic analogue of vasopressin). Rapid vasoconstriction. *Variceal bleed*: TERLIPRESSIN 1–2 mg 4 h IV then 1 mg 4–6 h for 72 h or bleeding ceases. **SE:** cramps, N, V, H, uterine/bowel contraction, low Na. Low BP. Avoid if IHD/MI or arrhythmias – check ECG. Give GTN. **Cautions:** drugs with long QT, arrhythmias.

TETRACYCLINE. *Acne, tropical infections*: TETRACYCLINE 250–500 mg QDS PO. Avoid with milk or antacids. **SE:** N, V, D, H, oesophagitis. Avoid pregnancy and age <12, stains teeth, acute porphyria.

THYROID HORMONES. *Hypothyroidism*: THYROXINE 50–150 mcg/day PO. *Myxoedema coma*: THYROXINE (T4) 50–150 mcg/day. LIOTHYRONINE (T3) 5–20 mcg slow IV then 25 mcg IV BD. **SE:** start low and slow in elderly or IHD. Can precipitate CCF/angina in older patients.↑HR, arrhythmias, angina.

TICAGRELOR (blocks P2Y12 receptor). *STEMI/NSTEMI undergoing PCI*: TICAGRELOR 180 mg stat then 90 mg BD for 1 year with aspirin. **SE:** bleeding, ↑creatinine (check at 1 month), hyperuricaemia, intracranial haemorrhage. No metabolic activation.

TINZAPARIN (LMWH). *VTE prophylaxis*: TINZAPARIN 3500 U SC 2 h pre-op then OD. TINZAPARIN 50 U/kg SC, *pre-op orthopaedic* then OD. *PE/DVT*: TINZAPARIN 175 U/kg OD SC and is used in pregnancy and malignancy with specialist advice. Watch for bleeding. **CI** and **SE:** see *Heparin.*

TIOTROPIUM. *COPD*: TIOTROPIUM 18 mcg OD inhaled onset 30–60 min lasts 24 h. **SE:** dry mouth, ↑HR, dizziness, epistaxis. Dilated pupil if drug enters eye. **Cautions:** BPH, glaucoma, CCF, arrhythmias. MI < 6/12 ago.

TRAMADOL (weak opioid analgesia). *Mod./severe pain*: TRAMADOL 50–100 mg every 4–6 h, slow IV, IM or PO (max 400 mg/day, 300 mg/day in elderly). Toxicity only partially reversed with Naloxone. **SE:** see *Morphine.*

TRANEXAMIC ACID. *Acute severe bleeds, trauma patients*: TRANEXAMIC ACID 1 g IV over 10 min then 1 g slow IV 8 h (CRASH-2 trial). *Fibrinolysis, menorrhagia, hereditary angioedema, epistaxis*: TRANEXAMIC ACID 1–1.5 g PO 2–3 times a day. Caution use for gross haematuria as can clot causing obstruction. Reduce dose in renal failure. **SE:** prothrombotic, seizures, urinary clot retention and obstruction with AKI. **CI:** thromboembolic disease, DIC.

TRIMETHOPRIM (inhibits bacterial dihydrofolate reductase). *UTI/prostatitis/RTI*: TRIMETHOPRIM 200 mg BD PO for 3–7 days. ↑Resistance, ↑INR in those on Warfarin. Avoid in pregnancy and blood dyscrasias. Caution with Azathioprine, Methotrexate, Mercaptopurine. **SE:** N, V, R, TEN, ↑K.

URSODEOXYCHOLIC ACID. *PBC, PSC, gallstones, pruritus in pregnancy* (higher dose for PBC): URSODEOXYCHOLIC ACID 500 mg BD (8–16 mg/kg daily). Take with/after a meal. **SE:** R, D. **CI:** acute cholecystitis, biliary colic, colitis.

VALPROATE. *Epilepsy*: SODIUM VALPROATE 300 mg BD PO and increase over weeks to 500 mg BD (max 2 g/d). *Status epilepticus*: SODIUM VALPROATE 10 mg/kg (usually 400–800 mg) loading dose slow IV over 5 min followed by continuous or repeated infusion up to a maximum of 2.5 g/day in NS/G5. **SE:** N, V, D, R, DRESS, oedema, false +ve ketones, TEN, SJS, ammonia encephalopathy, fluid retention, liver toxicity. Rarely Parkinsonism. Avoid in fertile females as teratogenic. Haemodialysis for toxicity.

VALSARTAN (ARB). *HTN, heart failure* (start with lowest dose), *diabetic nephropathy, CKD with proteinuria, post MI*: VALSARTAN 40 mg OD PO to 160 mg BD. See *Candesartan.*

VANCOMYCIN (glycopeptides). *C. difficile infection*: VANCOMYCIN 125–500 mg PO QDS for 10–14 days. *Severe infections/MRSA*: 1–1.5 g BD IV. **SE:** stop if tinnitus develops (ototoxicity), neutropenia, nephritis, low platelets and WCC, APX. **Caution:** nephrotoxic. Caution with Gentamicin, Ciclosporin. Check renal function and trough levels every 48 h. Pre-dose ('trough') concentration should be 10–15 mg/L (15–20 mg/L for severe infections). Give slowly to avoid 'Red Man Syndrome'.

VASOPRESSIN. *Variceal bleed*: VASOPRESSIN 20 U over 15 min IV. **Cautions:** asthma, APX, angina. *Cardiac arrest*: VASOPRESSIN 40 U stat IV. No difference in outcome to adrenaline in arrest. *Pituitary diabetes insipidus*: 5–20 U IM/SC 4 h.

VERAPAMIL (dihydropyridine CCB). _Acute SVT_: VERAPAMIL 5–10 mg IV over 5–10 min (avoid in suspected VT or with beta blockers or WPW with AF). **SE:** heart block, ↓HR. Chronic constipation, low BP, ankle oedema. Avoid with VT, ↓HR, poor LV function, AF or atrial flutter and WPW, acute porphyria.

VITAMIN K. _Warfarin reversal/vitamin K deficiency_: VITAMIN K 2–10 mg by slow IV in 100 ml bag of G5. Can also give VITAMIN K 5 mg PO depending on urgency. Give lower (1 mg) doses if plan to restart Warfarin. INR takes hours to normalise. Consider prothrombin concentrates if immediate effect needed. **SE:** anaphylaxis.

VOLTAROL (DICLOFENAC) (NSAID). _Analgesia, anti-inflammatory_: VOLTAROL 50 mg TDS PO or VOLTAROL slow release 75 mg (max 150 mg daily) PO/PR in 2–3 divided doses, VOLTAROL 100 mg Suppository PR. Caution long term with NSAID. See _Ibuprofen_.

ZOLEDRONATE. _Bone metastasis/breast cancer/hypercalcaemia/Paget's disease_: ZOLEDRONATE 4 mg IV infusion in 100 ml NS over 15 min. **SE** and **CI:** see _Alendronate_. Cancer patients need a dental check before treatment, or as soon as possible after starting treatment, to avoid osteonecrosis of the jaw.

22.4 Important drug interactions and metabolism

- **Enzyme inducers** – reduce effectiveness of drug B with treatment failure: Barbiturates, Carbamazepine, chronic alcohol, Phenytoin, Rifampicin, inhaled anaesthetics.
- **Enzyme inhibitors** – increase toxicity of drug B: Amiodarone, Cimetidine, Ciprofloxacin, acute alcohol, Erythromycin, Ketoconazole, Fluconazole, Metronidazole.
- **Allopurinol and Azathioprine:** Allopurinol interferes with the metabolism of Azathioprine, increasing levels of 6-mercaptopurine resulting in serious blood dyscrasias.
- **Digoxin and Quinidine:** increase in plasma concentrations of Digoxin.
- **Sildenafil and Isosorbide mononitrate:** dramatic drops in BP and has been associated with some deaths.
- **Potassium chloride, Spironolactone, Amiloride, ACEI:** these drugs can in combination lead to severe hyperkalaemia.
- **Theophylline and Ciprofloxacin:** Theophylline toxicity.
- **Warfarin/DOAC and NSAID, Aspirin, Clopidogrel:** increased bleed risk despite no change in INR; expert assessment for combination therapy.
- **Omeprazole, Lansoprazole and Clopidogrel:** decreased efficacy of Clopidogrel and the potential for worsened cardiovascular outcomes; consider Pantoprazole or H2 blocker instead of PPI.
- **Amiodarone and Levofloxacin, Azithromycin, Clarithromycin, Erythromycin, antihistamines, antidepressants:** increased QTc and cause TdP.
- **Carbamazepine or Digoxin AND Clarithromycin, Erythromycin:** increased Carbamazepine or Digoxin toxicity.
- **Amiodarone and Simvastatin:** increased statin side-effects, e.g. rhabdomyolysis and myopathy; try Fluvastatin, Rosuvastatin, or Pravastatin.
- **Simvastatin and Amlodipine, or Verapamil or Diltiazem** (inhibit Simvastatin metabolism): with these drugs the maximum dose of Simvastatin is now 20 mg; higher doses are 'off-label'. Consider Atorvastatin.
- **IV Verapamil and IV Dantrolene:** potential risk of VF.

22.5 Potentially fatal drug errors

Potentially fatal drug errors

- Excessive opiate dosing due to unfamiliar or agents with similar names.
- Getting decimal place wrong, especially weight-adjusted dose, e.g. ×10 digoxin dose in infant.
- Giving drug of which there is a clear history of allergy.
- Giving IV potassium infusion too concentrated or too fast (max is 20 mmol/h).
- Setting pumps wrong, e.g. 100 ml/h rather than 10 ml/h.

- Giving Allopurinol + Azathioprine.
- Omitting insulin after failing to recognise diabetes.
- Prescribing Methotrexate daily instead of weekly.
- Giving drugs by wrong route in ITU, e.g. intra-arterial or into CSF; check where the line goes as IV doses into CSF can be fatal or an artery can lose a limb.
- Use of abbreviations (e.g. AZT has led to confusion between zidovudine and azathioprine).
- Not monitoring INR.
- Not detecting hypoglycaemia.

22.6 Prescribing warfarin

- **About:** It inhibits synthesis of K-dependent coagulation factors II, VII, IX, and X and natural anticoagulants protein C and protein S. Involved in multiple interactions: varying genetic metabolism, drugs, alcohol, and vitamin K intake affects efficacy. Requires frequent monitoring via INR. Takes at least 72 h to be therapeutic. Give LMWH or UFH cover until therapeutic range achieved.
- **Dosing regiment and duration:** always ask your senior if unsure – what is target range and what is duration and make sure documented in notes and discharge/clinic letter.
- **Target INR:** is 2.0–3.0 for almost all indications, though mechanical heart valves can get 2.5–3.5. Bleeding is the most significant problem and significant bleeding is seen in 3–5% per annum. Risk increases markedly after INR of 3.0 and even more so after INR >4.5. Skin necrosis is a rare but significant complication. Warfarin use is avoided in pregnancy especially in first trimester.
- **Drugs that INCREASE INR:** broad spectrum antibiotics kill vitamin K-forming bacteria leading to increased bleeding effect. Others: fibrates, thyroxine, amiodarone, fluconazole, cephalosporins, cimetidine, ethanol, fluvastatin, HMG-CoA reductase inhibitors, lovastatin, isoniazid, macrolides (clarithromycin, erythromycin), metronidazole, quinolones (ciprofloxacin), tricyclic antidepressants.
- **Drugs that DECREASE INR:** barbiturates, carbamazepine, colestyramine, cigarette smoking, St John's wort, vitamin K corticosteroids, oral contraceptives, phenytoin, primidone, rifampicin, broccoli and green vegetables. **Indications:** DVT, PE, cerebral venous thrombosis, cardiac: AF, PAF, metal valves, LV thrombus, axillary vein thrombosis, antiphospholipid syndrome.
- **Duration:** calf DVT 3/12, proximal DVT 6/12, PE 6/12, tissue heart valve 3/12. Target INR: most are 2.5 except recurrent embolic events consider 2.5–3.5. Mechanical prosthetic valves is often 2.5–3.5 with target = 3.0, but dependent on the type of valve replacement used; take specialist advice.
- **Warfarin contraindicated (relative and absolute):** pregnancy, bleeding, GI blood loss, haematuria, anaemia due to possible blood loss, haemorrhagic stroke, frequent falls, imminent need for surgery, safe compliance issues, excess alcohol intake or severe liver disease, high HAS-BLED score. The HAS-BLED score marks increased bleeding risk, but also marks those at high risk of thrombosis and often this still exceeds bleeding risk. A difficult area – for specialist assessment.

- **Side-effects:** bleeding anywhere – brain, gut, renal, spine, soft tissue. Bleed risk increases dramatically with INR >3.0. Risk highest in those new on warfarin in the first 3 months of treatment. Alopecia, skin necrosis, urticaria, anorexia, GI upset, liver disease and pancreatitis.
- **Starting warfarin safely:** informed consent for patient and clearly document target range and duration. Explain drug/food interactions – need to check INR if new interacting drugs. Avoid the high dose 10 mg: 'start low, go slow' and try a starting dose of 3–6 mg and then after this 3 mg daily. Check INR day 2–3 and adjust warfarin and most will need 3–5 mg per day. Occasionally some need very high doses for same effect. High risk give LMWH (Enoxaparin 1.5 mg/kg/day) until therapeutic INR for the first 3–5 days. Ensure follow-up with anticoagulation service. For most people once the INR is stable, the rate of INR testing can be extended to every 2 weeks and then to every 4–6 weeks.
- **Follow-up:** ensure there is definite follow-up through an anticoagulation clinic to manage the warfarin. Make sure all referrals to anticoagulation clinic have been done. Nowadays if there is a rush to anticoagulate non-rheumatic AF, consider Dabigatran or Rivaroxaban or Apixaban, which can be started immediately and are active within a few hours.
- **Tablets:** Warfarin 0.5 mg White, 1 mg Brown, 3 mg Blue, 5 mg Pink.

22.7 Steroids

Indications are wide – anti-inflammatory or to replace intrinsic steroid production: *asthma, COPD, cord compression, cerebral oedema, PMR, temporal arteritis, RA, SLE, ulcerative colitis, adrenal replacement.* For prolonged or repeated courses usually daily therapy for more than 3 months, or 3 to 4 courses per year; consider adding some bone protection, e.g. **CALCIUM 1 g/d and VITAMIN D 800 units/day**.

- **SE:** short-term: agitation, insomnia (avoid in evenings if non-urgent), agitation, psychosis; long term: weight gain, hyperglycaemia, fluid retention, ↑WCC, ↑infection risk, ↑osteoporosis + fracture risk, ↑BP, diabetes, cataracts. Prolonged courses need bone protection with Vit D/Calcium. Consider need for PPI.
- Where possible the steroids are often switched to a steroid sparing agent.

Indications and doses and steroids used

- *Acute Addison's disease*: HYDROCORTISONE 100 mg IM/IV 6 h if unwell or NBM.
- *Addison's disease maintenance:* HYDROCORTISONE 10 mg PO at 8 am, and 5 mg at 1 pm and 4 pm – double if unwell. Alternative is DEXAMETHASONE 0.75 mg OD.
- *Mineralocorticoid insufficiency:* FLUDROCORTISONE 50–100 mcg OD PO.
- *Pneumocystis pneumonia:* HYDROCORTISONE 100 mg IV 6 h up to 21 d.
- *Toxic shock syndrome, septic shock refractory to vasopressors/fluids:* HYDROCORTISONE 50 mg IV 6 h.
- *Cerebral oedema:* DEXAMETHASONE 10 mg IV then 4–8 mg BD PO/IM/IV. Dose as per indications.
- *Ulcerative colitis, acute severe asthma:* HYDROCORTISONE 100 mg IV 6 h. Use PO/IM for replacement.
- *COPD/asthma:* PREDNISOLONE 40 mg for 7–10 days.
- *Moderate ulcerative colitis:* PREDNISOLONE 40 mg 4–6 weeks reduce.
- *PMR, acute rheumatoid flare:* PREDNISOLONE 15 mg OD reducing dose over 12–18 months.
- *GCA, vasculitis:* PREDNISOLONE 1 mg/kg stat then as dictated by specialists depending on response.
- *Multiple sclerosis flare:* METHYLPREDNISOLONE 500 mg to 1 g IV OD, for 3–5 days or METHYLPREDNISOLONE 500 mg to 2 g OD for 3–5 days PO.

Steroid potency

Type	Drug	Equivalent doses	Potency	Mineralocorticoid potency
Short-acting $T_{1/2}$: 0.5 days	Cortisol Hydrocortisone	20 mg 25 mg	1 0.8	2 2
Intermediate-acting $T_{1/2}$: 1 day	Prednisolone Methylprednisolone	5 mg 4 mg	4 5	1 0
Long-acting $T_{1/2}$: 1.5–2 days	Dexamethasone	0.75 mg	25–50	0
Mineralocorticoids	Aldosterone Fludrocortisone	0.3 mg 2 mg	0 15	300 150

Index

A–a gradient, 88, 94, 113
ABCD$_2$ score, 281
ABCDE assessment, 18–19
ADAMTS13, 198
Abbreviated mental test score, 266
Abciximab, 418
Abdominal aortic aneurysm, 368
Abdominal pain, acute, 158
Abnormal gaits, 361
Acalculous cholecystitis, 184, 185
Acetaminophen, *see* Paracetamol
Acetazolamide, 273, 309, 321
Acetylcysteine (N), 340, 418
Aciclovir, 260, 418
Acid–base balance, 25
Acquired immunodeficiency
        syndrome, 224
Acromegaly, 126, 131
Activated charcoal, 325, 418
Actrapid, 137, 143, 145
Acute abdomen, 158
Acute angle closure glaucoma, 262,
        265, 321
Acute breathlessness, 90
Acute chest syndrome, 196–7
Acute coronary syndrome, 47, 50, 54
Acute disseminated
        encephalomyelitis, 306
Acute fulminant myocarditis, 76–7
Acute kidney injury (AKI), 237
Acute limb ischaemia, 366–7
Acute lung injury, 40, 100–1
Acute severe asthma, 104–5, 353
Acute severe colitis, 162–4
Acute tubular necrosis, 238
Addisonian crisis, 121
Adenosine, 65–9, 418
Adrenaline (epinephrine), 4–6,
        11, 33, 419
Adrenalitis, 121
Adult respiratory distress
        syndrome, 100
Advanced life support, 4
African tick typhus, 214
Air embolism, 363, 379, 404
Airways management, 20–1
Albumin, 24, 171, 173, 418

Alcohol
    abuse, 175–7, 276, 295
    withdrawal, 175–8, 266
Alcoholic cardiomyopathy, 85
Alcoholic hepatitis, 175
Alcoholic ketoacidosis, 176
Alendronate, 419
Allergic bronchopulmonary
        aspergillosis, 105, 421
Allergy, 29, 34
Allopurinol, 314, 419, 439, 440
Alport syndrome, 236
Alteplase, 62, 118, 419
    bleeding, 202
Alzheimer's disease, 267, 308
Amber care bundle, 387
Amiloride, 124, 135, 419
Aminophylline, 34, 103, 105, 420
    toxicity, 344
Amiodarone, 12, 31, 65, 420
Amitriptyline, 420
    toxicity, 344
Amlodipine, 83, 420
    toxicity, 332
Amniotic fluid embolism, 348
Amoebic dysentery, 121, 147, 232
Amoxicillin, 85, 102, 420, 424
Amphetamines, toxicity, 331
Amphotericin, 270–1, 358, 421
Ampicillin, 218, 421
Amyloid angiopathy, 288, 290–1
Anaemia, 191, 338
Anaphylactoid reaction, 34
Anaphylaxis, 29, 34
Aneurysm
    aortic, 254, 277, 368
    atrial septal, 283
    cerebral, 259, 290, 312
    coronary artery, 48
    left ventricular, 63
    mycotic, 85
    pulmonary artery, 99
Angina
    stable, 63–4
    unstable, 31, 54, 56
Angiography, 61
Angioplasty, 61

Anion gap, 26, 330, 336–7
Ankle/brachial pressure index, 367
Anterior ischaemic optic neuropathy
    arteritic, 319, 322
    non-arteritic, 319
Anterior uveitis, 321
Anthrax, 217
Antibiotic prescribing, 417
Anticholinergic syndrome, 329
Antiepileptic hypersensitivity
    syndrome, 278
Antiretroviral drugs, 226–7
Anuria, 237–44
Aortic dissection, 47, 74, 82
Apixaban, 378, 421, 441
Aplastic anaemia, 192
Apoplexy, pituitary, 131, 251, 260
Arrhythmias, 12–14, 50, 64, 326
Arrhythmogenic RV cardiomyopathy,
    54, 66, 86
Arsenic, toxicity, 346, 298
Arterial blood gas, 25–7, 410
Artesunate, 212, 421
Arthritis, acute, 313–15
Ascites, 179, 409
Aspiration pneumonia, 91–2, 110
Aspirin, 421
    toxicity, 343
Asthma, acute severe, 104, 353
Asystole, 6, 9
Atenolol, 49, 58, 73, 421
Atorvastatin, 60, 282, 285, 421
Atrial fibrillation, 14, 65, 72–4, 282
Atrial flutter, 14, 72–4
Atropine, 11–12, 34, 65, 71, 326,
    340, 421
Automated external defibrillator, 2–3
Automated implantable cardioverter
    defibrillator, 15, 51, 53, 63, 67
Autonomic nervous system, 251
    dysfunction, 52
AVRT/AVNRT, 68
Azathioprine, 186, 206, 315, 422
Azithromycin, 103, 422

Bacillus anthracis, see Anthrax
Bacillus cereus, 231
Bacterial meningitis, 254, 260, 269
Bag–valve mask, 14, 89
Bare metal stent, 56, 61, 200

Base excess, 26, 413
Basic life support, 2–3
Basilar artery, top of the, 285
Bell's palsy, 305–6
Bendroflumethiazide, 32, 83, 422
Benign paroxysmal positional
    vertigo, 303–4
Benzodiazepines, toxicity, 331
Benzylpenicillin, 85, 218, 219, 422
Berry aneurysm, 290, 312
Beta-blockers, toxicity, 331
Bicarbonate, 136, 140, 422
Bi-level positive airway pressure, 96–8
Bisoprolol, 32, 58, 59, 422
Bisphosphonates, 127, 367, 375
Bites (animal, human), 370
Blatchford Score, 154
Bleeding, 28, 41–3, 73–4, 99,
    151–7, 200
Blindness, 280, 319, 328
Blood gas analysis, 25
Blood transfusion, 202–6
    massive transfusion protocol, 54
Body packers, 344
Boerhaave syndrome, 47
Borrelia burgdorferi, 233
Botulism, 218, 255
BOVA score, 117
Bowel ischaemia, 166
Bowel preparation, 149
Bradycardia, 11, 65, 69–71, 326, 328
Brain abscess, 272
Brain tumour, 274, 356, 359
Brainstem, 250
    death, 392
Breathlessness, acute, 90
Broad complex tachycardia, 65–7
Brucellosis, 210, 216
Brugada syndrome, 50–1, 53, 66
Budd–Chiari syndrome, 172–3, 350–2
Bumetanide, 31, 32, 422

Calcium channel blockers, toxicity, 32
Calcium chloride, 124, 422
Calcium gluconate, 124, 422
Candesartan, 32, 422
Cannabis, toxicity, 345
Cannulae
    nasal, 89
    venous, 25

Capacity (mental) issues, 382, 384
Capnography, 4, 5, 10
Captopril, 239, 423
Carbamazepine, 423
    toxicity, 346
Carbapenem-resistant organisms, 229
Carbimazole, 130, 357, 423
Carbon monoxide toxicity, 89, 265, 333
Cardiac arrest, 1–16
Cardiac output, 45
Cardiac resynchronization therapy, 33
Cardiac tamponade, 28, 29, 76, 79–81
Cardiogenic shock, 28
Cardiomyopathy, 85
Cardiopulmonary resuscitation
    (CPR), 1–16
Cardioversion (DC), 14
Carotid dissection, 262, 264
Carotid sinus hypersensitivity, 51
Carvedilol, 32, 423
Cauda equina, 254–5, 300, 359, 407
Cavernous venous sinus
    thrombosis, 273
Cefotaxime, 181, 270, 423
Ceftriaxone, 270, 370, 423
Cefuroxime, 185, 233, 423
Cellulitis, 366, 370
    orbital, 273
Central pontine demyelination, 134
Central retinal artery/vein
    occlusion, 319
Central venous cannulation, 404
Cephalexin, 423
Cerebellum
    basics, 251
    stroke, 304
Cerebral abscess, 272
    aneurysm, 290, 312
    arterial syndromes, 284
    arteriovenous malformations, 291
    hyperfusion syndrome, 295
    malaria, 212
    oedema, 311
    tumour, 356
    venous thrombosis, 286
Cerebrospinal fluid, 407
    values, 416
CHA$_2$DS$_2$VaSc score, 73
Chest compressions, 2–8
Chest drain, 106–8, 114, 119, 396, 400–4

Chest pain, 46–8, 54, 400
Cheyne–Stokes breathing, 92
Chickenpox, 112, 219, 220, 268, 271
Chikungunya, 216
Child–Pugh Score, 183
Chloroquine, 212, 423
    toxicity, 342
Chlorphenamine, 34, 205, 341, 424
Chlorpromazine, 327, 424
Choking algorithm, 16
Cholangitis, acute, 184–5
Cholecystitis
    acute, 184
    emphysematous, 184
Choledocholithiasis, 184
Cholelithiasis, 184
Cholera, 231
Cholinergic syndrome, 329
Chronic inflammatory demyelinating
    polyneuropathy (CIDP), 298
Chronic kidney disease (CKD), 242–4
Chronic liver disease, 183, 351
Chronic obstructive pulmonary
    disease (COPD), 101–3
Ciprofloxacin, 164, 176, 423
Cirrhosis, 179, 183
Citalopram, 424
Clarithromycin, 370, 424
Clindamycin, 36, 424
Clonorchis, 185
Clopidogrel, 60, 424
Clostridium botulinum, 218
Clostridium difficile colitis, 147, 164
Clostridium perfringens, 219
Clostridium tetani, 232
Cluster headaches, 263
Coagulopathy, 41–3, 200
Co-amoxiclav, 102, 113, 424
Coarctation of aorta, 54, 75, 81–2, 84
Cocaine, toxicity, 56, 75, 81, 333
Codeine, 260, 375, 424
Coffee ground vomitus, 152
Colchicine, 78, 315, 347, 424
Colestyramine, 351, 424
Colitis, acute severe, 162, 441
Colloid cyst, 52
Colloid, fluids, 23, 31, 41, 173
Colonic pseudo-obstruction, 166
Coma, 181, 213, 256–62
Coma cocktail, 260

Commotio cordis, 54
Community-acquired pneumonia, 110–13
Complete heart block, 12, 65, 70
Confusion (acute), 265
Coning of brainstem, 309
Conn's syndrome, 81
Consolidation, lung, 119, 120, 223
Constipation, 148
Continuous positive airway pressure (CPAP), 31, 96–8
COPD, acute exacerbation, 101
Cord compression, 254, 297, 359
Coronary arteries, 45
Coronary stenting, 61
Coronavirus, 91
Coroner, referral to, 393
Costochondritis, 48
Co-trimoxazole, 113–14, 424
Cranial nerves, 250
Creutzfeldt–Jakob, 267
Crohn's disease, 162–4
Cross-matching, see Blood transfusion
Cryoprecipitate, 42–3, 195, 202, 204
Cryptococcus, 268, 271
Crystalloids, 23–4
CURB-65 score, 111
Cushing's syndrome, 81
Cyanide (toxicity), 334
Cyclizine, 161, 185, 327, 425
Cystitis, acute, 160, 229, 236, 243
Cytokines, 34–8
Cytomegalovirus, 77, 78, 162, 173, 220–1, 225–7

Dabigatran, 29, 42, 43, 74, 119, 202, 338, 425
Dalteparin, 425
Death, 387–92
Deep vein thrombosis, 114, 336
Defibrillation, 1–14, 287, 364
Dehydration, 21
Delirium, 265
    tremens, 178
Demeclocycline, 134, 425
Dementia, 225, 227, 265, 308
Demyelination, 297, 306
Dengue, 211, 215
Dermatomyositis, 256
Desferrioxamine, 425

Dexamethasone, 93, 218, 260–1, 271, 277, 302, 311, 360, 441
Diabetes insipidus, 132, 134–5, 337
Diabetes mellitus
    care in emergencies, 145
    foot infections, 142
    hyperosmolar state, 141
    hypoglycaemia, 123
    ketoacidosis, 137–41
    surgery, 142
    variable rate insulin infusion, 143
Diamorphine, 31, 47, 58–9, 339, 375–6
Diarrhoea, 147, 230–2
Diazepam, 178, 276, 425
Digoxin, 31–2, 65, 73, 425
    toxicity, 334
Diltiazem, 58, 332, 425
Diphtheria, 228, 255
Diplopia, 130, 255, 273, 284, 291, 322
Direct oral anticoagulants, 60, 74, 118–19
    toxicity, 338
Discharging patients, 380
Discriminant function, 175
Dissection
    aortic, 46, 47, 74–6
    cervical, 262, 264, 283
Disseminated intravascular coagulation, 195
Diverticulitis, acute, 167
Do not attempt CPR, 1, 387
Dobutamine, 11, 29, 33, 81
Dopamine, 31, 33, 425
Doxapram, 95, 426
Doxazosin, 82, 426
Doxycycline, 102, 112, 214, 426
Drains and tubes, 396
Driving and disease, 385
Drowning, 7, 9, 365
Drug-eluting stent, 61
Drug errors, 440
Drug interactions, 439
Dual antiplatelet therapy, 61
Duodenitis, 151
Duty of candour, 380
Dying patient, 387
Dyspepsia, 150
Dystonic reactions, 302

Early warning scores, 17
Ebola, 215–16
Eclampsia, 274, 348–9
Ecstasy (MDMA), 133, 331
Ectopic pregnancy, 10, 25, 29, 41, 51, 347
Electrocardiogram (ECG) interpretation, 64
Electrocution, 10
Embolism
    air, 363, 379
    amniotic fluid, 348
    bowel, 166
    cardioembolism, 283
    fat, 196–7, 362
    paradoxical, 115, 283
    pulmonary, 114–19, 352
    VTE prevention, 377
Emphysema, 101
Empyema, 94, 102, 114
Enalapril, 60, 426
Encephalitis (viral), 267
End of life care, 387
Endocarditis, 83, 209, 217, 279
Endoscopy, GI, 151
Endotracheal intubation, 20, 93
Enoxaparin, 58, 60, 118, 426
Enoximone, 59, 426
Enteral feeding, 24–5, 164, 373
Enteric fever, 214, 231
Epidural haematoma, 296
Epiglottitis, acute, 93
Epilepsy, 274
Epipen (adrenaline), 35
Eplerenone, 32, 59, 426
Epstein–Barr virus, 220, 268
Errors, medical, 379
Erythema migrans, 233
Erythema multiforme, 372
Erythema nodosum, 372
Erythroderma, 370
Erythrodermic psoriasis, 371
Erythromycin, 67, 228, 426
Escalation (clinical), 19
Escherichia coli infections, 230
Ethanol, 426
    toxicity, 335
Ethylene glycol, toxicity, 241, 330, 335
Exfoliative dermatitis, 370
Exploding head syndrome, 263

Extended-spectrum beta-lactamases (ESBL), 229
Extracorporeal life support, 9
Extracorporeal membrane oxygenation (ECMO), 96
Extrasystoles, 48–9

Facemasks (oxygen delivery), 88–9
Falciparum malaria, 210, 212, 224, 258–60
Falls, 49–50, 171, 243, 361
Familial Mediterranean fever, 78, 160
Fat embolism, 197, 362
Fatty liver of pregnancy, 351
Femoral vein cannulation, 406
Ferrous fumarate, 426
    toxicity, 337
Fever, 209, 210
Flecainide, 72–3, 426
Flucloxacillin, 36, 85, 229, 313, 370, 427
Fluconazole, 225–6, 271, 427
Fludrocortisone, 53, 122, 441
Fluid management, 21, 176, 240
Flumazenil, 260, 332, 427
Fluoxetine, 343, 427
Folate, 427
    deficiency, 191
Fomepizole, 335–6, 427
Fondaparinux, 58, 118, 427
Foreign bodies, ingested, 168
Fosphenytoin, 427
Fractures, in elderly, 316
Fresh frozen plasma, 42–3, 203
Frontotemporal dementia, 308
Fulminant hepatic failure, 171, 174, 351
Furosemide, 32, 428
Fusidic acid, 314, 370, 428

Gabapentin, 299, 377
Gallstones, 184–6, 352
Gamma hydroxybutyrate, toxicity, 336
Ganciclovir, 162, 173, 221, 428
Gastric lavage, 325
Gastric outlet obstruction, 161
Gastritis, 151, 338
Gastroenteritis, 159, 230
General Medical Council, 378
Gentamicin, 85, 216–17, 428
Giant cell arteritis, 319, 322
Giardiasis, 226, 231

Glandular fever, 41, 224, 227
Glasgow alcoholic hepatitis score, 175
Glasgow Blatchford Score, 154
Glasgow Coma Scale, 257
Glaucoma, 262, 265, 320–1
Gliclazide, 345, 428
Glucagon, 7, 11, 35, 65, 71, 123, 327, 331, 428
Glyceryl trinitrate (GTN), 428
Good medical practice, 378
Gout, acute, 245, 314
Graves' disease, 130
Guillain–Barré syndrome, 297

Haematuria, 84, 235, 440
Haemochromatosis, 172
Haemolytic anaemia, 191
Haemolytic uraemic syndrome, 197
Haemophilia A and B, 200
Haemoptysis, massive, 99, 216–17, 228
Haemorrhagic shock, 29, 41
Haemorrhagic stroke, 288
Haloperidol, 83, 130, 178, 267, 428
Hartmann's solution, 23
HAS-BLED score, 73
Hashimoto's disease, 128–9
    encephalopathy, 267, 269
Head impulse test, 303
Headache, 262–4
Heart block, 12, 48, 50, 63–5, 70–1
Heart failure, 29–33, 59
Helicobacter pylori, 156
HELLP syndrome, 172, 193
Hemicraniectomy, 286
Heparin, 428
    bleeding, 201
Heparin-induced thrombocytopenia, 119, 194
Hepatic encephalopathy, 181, 267, 310, 341
Hepatitis, 175
    alcoholic, 175
    viral, 174
Hepatorenal syndrome, 176, 180, 219, 409
Herniation syndromes, brain, 249, 258, 310
Herpes simplex
    encephalitis, 211, 267
    infection, 220, 226, 268

Herpes (varicella) zoster, 219
HIV, acute, 108, 113, 224
Horner's syndrome, 250, 258, 262, 321
Hospital-acquired pneumonia, 110
Human albumin solution, 173, 204, 409, 419
Hydatid disease, 184
Hydration, assessment, 21, 388–9
Hydrocephalus, 232, 260, 290, 293–5, 308–10
Hydrocortisone, 29, 33, 36, 40, 163, 205, 264, 322, 341, 353, 441–2
Hydroxocobalamin (B12), 429
Hyperbaric oxygen therapy, 88
Hypercalcaemia, 126, 355
Hypercapnia, 88, 94
Hyperkalaemia, 4, 124
Hypermagnesaemia, 135
Hypernatraemia, 133, 141
Hyperosmolar hyperglycaemic state, 141
Hyperparathyroidism, 126, 186, 205
Hyperphosphataemia, 135
Hyperpyrexia, 213, 338, 343, 365
Hypertension (malignant), 81
Hypertensive encephalopathy, 81
Hyperthyroidism, 129, 365
Hypertrophic cardiomyopathy, 86
Hyperviscosity syndrome, 355
Hypoadrenalism, 121–3, 129, 131, 133, 364
Hypocalcaemia, 7, 127–8, 347
Hypoglycaemia, 123, 140, 143–5, 173, 176, 182, 213, 257
Hypokalaemia, 25, 125, 138, 161
Hypomagnesaemia, 125, 330
Hyponatraemia, 132–4, 173, 180, 268, 293
Hypoparathyroidism, 127–8, 135
Hypophosphataemia, 135, 142
Hypothermia, 2–10, 37, 128, 363–5, 392
Hypothyroidism, 128–31, 133, 364
Hypoventilation, 26–9, 87–8, 94–8
Hypovolaemic shock, 23, 29, 36, 216, 231

Ibuprofen, 429
Idarucizumab (Praxbind), 202, 289, 338, 429
Idiopathic intracranial hypertension, 273, 310, 311, 322

Idiopathic thrombocytopenic purpura, 193
Idioventricular rhythm, 63
IgA nephropathy, 236
Immune reconstitution inflammatory syndrome, 227
Immunocompromised patients, 206
Immunoglobulin IV, 36, 77, 298, 429
Implantable cardioverter defibrillator, 15
Inclusion body myositis, 256
Incubation periods, 211
Indapamide, 430
Infectious mononucleosis, 41, 220, 224, 227
Infective endocarditis, 83, 236
Inferior vena cava filters, 119
Inflammatory bowel disease, 162, 354
Infliximab, 164, 371
Influenza, 221
Inotropes, 59, 129, 240
Insulin, 143, 330–2, 355
    toxicity, 337
Insulin–glucose euglycaemic therapy, 330
Internal capsule, 249, 252
Internal jugular vein, 228, 404
Internuclear ophthalmoplegia, 322
Intestinal obstruction, 165
Intestinal pseudo-obstruction, 166
Intra-aortic balloon pump, 11, 31, 33
Intracranial pressure, 309
Intra-lipid therapy, 7, 330
Invasive ventilation, 98
Iodine, 128, 130, 430
Ipratropium bromide, 430
Iron, 430
    toxicity, 337
Iron deficiency anaemia, 191
Irradiated blood products, 206
Ischaemic colitis, 166
Isoprenaline, 65–7, 326, 332
Isosorbide dinitrate, 430
Isosorbide mononitrate, 430
Ivabradine, 32, 430

J waves, 363
Jaundice, 38, 171

Katayama fever, 215
Kawasaki disease, 48
Kernig's sign, 257, 290
Kernohan's notch, 310
Ketoacidosis
    alcoholic, 176
    diabetic, 137
Kikuchi's disease, 209
Killip score, 63
Kussmaul's breathing, 27, 80, 90, 136, 176

Labetalol, 82, 430
Laboratory values, 413
Lactate, 10–11, 28, 36, 136, 176
Lactic acidosis, 136
Lactulose, 149, 155, 173, 176, 182
Lamotrigine, 278, 353, 431
Lansoprazole, 359, 431
Laryngeal mask, 8
Laryngectomy, 21
Lassa fever, 215–16
Lead (toxicity), 346
Left bundle branch block, 54, 57
Left ventricular aneurysm, 63
Leg pain, 366
Legionella pneumophila, 110
Lemierre's syndrome, 38, 228
Leptospirosis, 209, 217
Levetiracetam (Keppra), 277–8, 431
Lewy body dementia, 267, 308
Lidocaine, 431
    toxicity, 334
Light's criteria, 109
Limb ischaemia, 367
Lipid rescue, see Intra-lipid therapy
Lisinopril, 431
Listeriosis, 218, 270
Lithium, 431
    toxicity, 337
Liver
    abscess, 183
    failure, 171
    transplant, 341
Long QT syndrome, 50, 52, 54, 66, 67
Loperamide, 431
Lorazepam, 276, 279, 431
Losartan, 431
Low pressure headache, 265
Lower gastrointestinal bleed, 156–7

Lower motor neurone, 249
Lown–Ganong–Levine syndrome, 68
Lugol's iodine solution, 130, 430
Lumbar puncture, 407
Lung abscess, 120
Lyme disease, 77, 210, 233

Madopar, 431
Magnesium, 431
Malaria, 210, 212, 224, 258–60
Malignant cord compression, 359
Malignant hypercalcaemia, 356
Malignant hyperpyrexia, 365
Malignant hypertension, 81
Malignant MCA syndrome, 286
Malignant SVC obstruction, 358
Mannitol, 173, 260, 333, 357, 366, 431
Massive transfusion protocol, 42
Mast cell tryptase, 34
MDMA, toxicity, 133, 331
Measles, 219
Mechanical thrombectomy, 285–6
Medical errors, 379
Ménière's disease, 304
Meningitis, 269–70
Mental capacity, 384
Mental Health Act, 383
Mercury, toxicity, 346
Meropenem, 188, 217, 431
Metabolic acidosis, 25–7, 39, 90, 122, 136, 137
Metabolic alkalosis, 25–7, 161, 176
Metal (prosthetic) heart valves, 39, 40–2, 83, 289, 440
Metformin, 328, 330, 431
Methadone, 385
Methaemoglobinaemia, 345
Methanol, toxicity, 325, 330, 336
Methotrexate, 432
Methylthioninium (methylene blue), 345
Meticillin resistant Staph. aureus (MRSA), 229
Meticillin sensitive Staph. aureus (MSSA), 229
Metoclopramide, 432
Metolazone, 32, 432
Metronidazole, 143, 147, 156, 162, 184–5, 232, 432
Midazolam, 276, 390, 432

Middle Eastern respiratory syndrome (MERS), 222
Migraine, 263
    aura, 280
    vestibular, 282, 304
Miller–Fisher syndrome, 297–8
Milwaukee protocol, 269
Mitral regurgitation, acute, 63
Mobitz I and II heart block, 70
Modified Duke criteria, 85
Monoamine oxidase inhibitor (toxicity), 338
Morphine, 375, 376
Motor cortex, 249
Motor neurone disease, 307
Multiple organ dysfunction syndrome, 38, 40
Multiple sclerosis, 306
Mumps, 220
Mushroom poisoning, 172
Myasthenia gravis, 299
Mycoplasma pneumoniae, 110
Myocardial infarction, 54
Myocardial rupture, 63
Myocarditis, acute, 76
Myopathy, 255–6
Myxoedema coma, 128

Naloxone, 19, 326, 329, 332, 339, 432
Narrow complex tachycardia, 13, 68
Nasogastric tube insertion, 411
Nasopharyngeal airway, 20
National early warning scores, 17
Necrotising fasciitis, 371
Needlestick injury, 217
Neostigmine, 433
Nephritic syndrome, 239
Nephrolithiasis, 245
Nephrotic syndrome, 239
Neuro-ophthalmology, 321
Neurocysticercosis, 232
Neurogenic shock, 29
Neuroleptic malignant syndrome, 279
    toxicity, 338
Neuromyelitis optica, 207, 253, 302, 306
Neurosurgical options, 311
Neutropenic sepsis, 357
Never events, 379
Nicorandil, 433

Nifedipine, 246, 332, 349, 433
Nimodipine, 294, 433
Nitroprusside, 433
Non-convulsive status epilepticus, 278
Non-epileptic attack disorder, 275
Non-invasive ventilation, 96–8
Non-rebreather mask, 89
Non-ST elevation MI, 54
Non-steroidal anti-inflammatory
    drugs, 375
    toxicity, 338
Noradrenaline (norepinephrine),
    33, 433
Normal pressure hydrocephalus, 308
Nutritional support, 363, 374
Nystatin, 433

Obstetric cholestasis, 351
Obstructive shock, 29, 115, 363
Obstructive uropathy, 244
Octreotide, 18, 132, 147, 327, 390, 433
Oculomotor (III) palsy, 321
Oesophageal rupture, 46, 109, 114
Oesophageal variceal bleed, 151
Oesophageal varices, 151
Oesophagitis, 46–7, 150–1, 154
Olanzapine, 338, 433
Oliguria, 18, 22, 28, 29, 32, 237
Omeprazole, 434
Ondansetron, 327, 434
Opiates
    addiction and withdrawal, 384
    conversion chart, 376
    syndrome, 329
    toxicity, 260, 339
    uses, 375–6
Orbital cellulitis, 273, 320, 370
Organophosphates, toxicity, 339
Oropharyngeal airway, 19, 20, 89
Osmotic demyelination syndrome, 134
Osteomyelitis, 88, 142, 196, 313
Oxygen
    delivery devices, 89
    dissociation curve, 87
    therapy, 88

Pabrinex, 276, 434
Pacemaker, 12, 59, 71
Pain management, 374, 375
Palliative formulary, 389

Palpitations, 48, 53, 55, 68, 72
Pamidronate, 127, 355, 434
Pancreatitis
    acute, 186
    chronic, 186
Pantoprazole, 434
Paracentesis, 173, 179, 180, 409
Paracetamol, 375
    toxicity, 340
Paraquat, toxicity, 342
Paratyphoid fever, 231
Parenteral feeding, 374
Parkinson's disease, 267, 279
Pemberton's sign, 358
Penicillin allergy, 417
Peptic ulcer disease, 150–6
Percheron, artery of, 285
Percutaneous coronary
    intervention, 61
Percutaneous endoscopic
    gastrostomy, 373
Pericardial effusion/tamponade, 79
Pericardiocentesis, 14, 79
Pericarditis, acute, 47, 78
Periodic paralysis, 124, 356
Peripheral inserted central catheter
    (PICC), 374
Peripheral neuropathy, 307
PESI score, 117
Phaeochromocytoma, 82
Pharyngitis, acute, 227–8
Phenobarbital, toxicity, 344
Phentolamine, 434
Phenytoin, 276, 434
Phone protocols, 19
Phosphate, 434
Pituitary adenoma, 131
    apoplexy, 131
Plague, 216
Plasmapheresis, 130, 198, 199, 207
Platelet transfusions, 203, 366
Pleural effusion, 109, 119, 217, 223,
    228, 396
Pleurodesis, 108
Pneumonia, 47, 110
    pneumococcal, 110
    Pneumocystis, 113
Pneumothorax, 47, 106
Polymorphic ventricular
    tachycardia, 67

Polymyositis, 256
Porphyria, acute, 136
Postural hypotension, 51, 53
Postural orthostatic tachycardia
    syndrome, 51
Pralidoxime, 435
Prasugrel, 60, 435
Praxbind (idarucizamab), 429
Pre-eclampsia, 82, 349
Pre-excitation syndrome, 54
Precordial thump, 6
Prednisolone, 35, 102–5, 122, 127,
    130, 163, 353, 441–2
Pregnancy
    cardiac arrest, 10
    malaria, 212
    medical issues, 348–54
    pneumothorax, 108
Pressure sores, 395
Priapism, 197, 247
Primaquine, 213, 345
Primary cerebral lymphoma, 225, 357
Prinzmetal's variant angina, 56
Procalcitonin, 39, 111
Prochlorperazine, 137, 302, 435
Procyclidine, 303, 435
Progressive multifocal
    leucoencephalopathy, 225, 306
Propranolol, 435
Propylthiouracil, 435
Prosthetic heart valves, 39, 40–2, 83,
    289, 440
Protamine, 42, 201, 289, 429, 435
Prothrombin complex concentrates,
    42, 435
Prucalopride, 166, 435
Pseudocyst, 186–9
Pseudogout, 314
Pseudomembranous colitis,
    147–8, 162
Pseudomonas, 217
Pseudo-obstruction, 165–6
Pseudoseizures, 275
Psoriasis, 371
Pulmonary embolism, 47, 114, 352
Pulmonary haemorrhage, 92
Pulse oximetry, 14, 88, 94, 333
Pulseless electrical activity, 6
Pulseless VT, 5
Pyelonephritis, acute, 243

Pyloric stenosis, 161
Pyoderma gangrenosum, 372
Pyrexia
    after foreign travel, 210
    of unknown origin, 209
Pyridostigmine, 300

Q fever, 217
Q waves, 55, 77
Quinine, 212, 435
    toxicity, 342

Rabies, 269
Raised intracranial pressure, 309
Ramipril, 32, 59, 60
Ramsay Hunt syndrome, 283, 305
Ranitidine, 436
Rapidly progressive
    glomerulonephritis, 235–6
Recovery position, 3–6
Red cell concentrates, 203
Red eye, 320
Refeeding syndrome, 167, 363
Rehabilitation, 395
Renal artery stenosis, 82
Renal colic, 245
Renal failure
    acute, 237
    chronic, 242
Renal obstruction, 244
Renal stones, 245
Respiratory acidosis, 25–7
Respiratory alkalosis, 25–7
Respiratory failure, acute, 94
Resuscitation, 1–16
Reteplase, 62, 436
Retinal detachment, 320
Retroperitoneal bleeding, 28, 41
Return of spontaneous circulation, 10
Reversible cerebral vasoconstriction
    syndrome, 264
Rhabdomyolysis, 365
Rheumatoid arthritis, 315
Ribavirin, 216
Rickettsia, 77, 210–11, 214
Rifampicin, 85, 216, 223–4, 271, 436
RIFLE classification, 238
Risk register, 380
Risperidone, 436
Rivaroxaban, 436

Rockall score, 154
Rocky Mountain spotted fever, 214
Ruptured spleen, 41, 361–2

Salbutamol, 436
Salicylates, toxicity, 343
Sarin, see Organophosphates
SBAR, 20
Schistosomiasis, 215, 237
Sclerosing cholangitis, 185, 226
Seizures, 49, 274
Selective serotonin reuptake inhibitor,
    toxicity, 343
Self-discharging patients, 382
Senna, 436
Sensory pathways, 252
Septic arthritis, 313
Septic shock, 37
Serotonin syndrome, 329
Severe acute respiratory syndrome
    (SARS), 217
Sgarbossa and Wellen criteria, 57
Shigella, 147, 162, 214, 226, 231
Shingles (herpes zoster), 48
Shock, 27–43, 237, 326, 357, 363
Short synACTHen test, 52, 53, 122, 133
Sickle cell anaemia/crisis, 195
Sideroblastic anaemia, 192
Simvastatin, 436
Sinemet, 431
Smallpox, 209
Sotalol, 67, 73, 74
Spinal cord injury, 253–4, 300–2,
    359–60
Spironolactone, 32, 83, 124, 179, 436
Spontaneous bacterial peritonitis,
    179–83
Spontaneous intracranial
    hypotension, 265
Staphylococcal food poisoning, 230
Staphylococcus aureus, 229
Status asthmaticus, 104, 353
Status epilepticus, 274
ST elevation MI, 54
Stents
    aortic, 76
    biliary, 185
    coronary, 61
    gastro-oesophageal, 150
Steroids, 441

Stevens–Johnson syndrome, 369
Streptokinase, 62, 437
Stress test, 56, 57, 72
Stridor, acute, 93
Stroke disease, 279
    haemorrhagic, 288
    ischaemic, 282
    thrombectomy, 286
    thrombolysis, 286
Subarachnoid haemorrhage, 290
Subclavian steal, 52
Subclavian vein cannulation, 406
Subdural haematoma, 253, 259, 295
Sudden cardiac death, 49, 53, 77, 105
Suicidal risk in patients, 382
Sulfasalazine, 437
Sulphonylurea, toxicity, 345
Superior vena caval obstruction, 358
Supraventricular tachycardia, 48, 68
Surgical emphysema, 371, 404
Surgical referrals, 396
Syncope/presyncope, 49
Syndrome of inappropriate ADH,
    132–3
Syphilis, 227, 308, 408
Systemic inflammatory response
    syndrome, 37

Tachy–brady syndrome, 69
Tachycardias/tachyarrhythmias,
    12, 65
Takotsubo cardiomyopathy, 47, 86
Tamponade, acute, 51, 54, 63,
    75–7, 80
Tamsulosin, 246
Tazocin, 39–40, 102, 142, 437
Teicoplanin, 229, 313, 370, 437
Temazepam, 331
Temporal arteritis, 262, 322
Tenecteplase, 62, 437
Tension headache, 263
Tension pneumothorax, 4, 7, 91,
    98, 106
Terlipressin, 155, 437
Tetanus, 232–3, 370
Tetany, 127–8
Thallium, toxicity, 346
Theophylline, toxicity, 344, 420
Thiamine, 167, 173, 178, 434
Thrombocytopenia, severe, 192

Thrombolytic agents, 62
  bleeding, 202
  cardiac, 62
  contraindications, 62
  stroke, 286
Thrombotic thrombocytopenic
    purpura, 199
Thunderclap headache, 259, 262, 264,
    286, 290
Thyroid eye disease, 130
Thyroid storm/thyrotoxicosis, 129
Thyroxine, 129–32, 260, 437
Ticagrelor, 60, 438
Tick paralysis, 256
Tick typhus, 214
TIMI risk score, 57
Tinzaparin, 118, 438
Tiotropium, 103, 438
Torsades de pointes, 65, 67
Toxic epidermal necrolysis, 369
Toxic shock syndrome, 35, 37,
    128, 369
Toxoplasmosis, 77, 220, 225, 321
Tracheal intubation, 20
Tracheostomy, 20, 21
Tramadol, 339, 375, 438
Tranexamic acid, 41–3, 438
Transfusion, 54, 202–6
Transfusion-associated circulatory
    overload (TACO), 205
Transient apical ballooning
    syndrome, 56
Transient ischaemic attack, 279–81
Transient loss of consciousness, 49–53
Transverse myelitis, 221, 225, 302
Traveller's diarrhoea, 214
Tricyclic antidepressant, toxicity, 51,
    260, 344, 440
Trigeminal autonomic
    cephalgias, 263
Trimethoprim, 244, 347, 438
Troponin, 10, 12, 14, 28, 47, 54–6
Tuberculin test, 223
Tuberculosis, 203, 209–10, 223–5,
    237, 254
Tularaemia, 216
Tullio phenomenon, 304
Tumour lysis syndrome, 124, 128,
    135, 355
Typhoid fever, 211, 231

Ulcerative colitis, 162, 354
Upper airways obstruction, 16, 34, 91;
    see also Stridor
Upper gastrointestinal bleed, 151–6
Upper motor neurone, 249
Urinary alkalinisation, 326, 343
Urinary tract infection, 39, 236, 243
Ursodeoxycholic acid, 185, 351, 438

Valproate, 438
  toxicity, 332
Valsartan, 438
Values, normal, 413–16
Vancomycin, 85, 113, 162, 165, 438
Vancomycin resistant enterococcus
    (VRE), 229
Variable rate insulin infusion,
    143, 188
Varicella zoster, 112, 219, 220,
    268, 271
Vascular dementia, 308
Vasopressin, 33, 35, 40, 351, 364, 438
Vasopressors, 33, 37–40, 122, 311, 327
Vasovagal syncope, 50–2, 69, 386
Venepuncture, 399
Venous access, 9, 25
  central, 374, 404–6
Venous thromboembolism PE/DVT,
    46–7, 114
  in pregnancy, 352
  prevention, 377
Ventilation
  invasive, 98
  non-invasive, 31, 59, 96–8
Ventricular assist devices, 32–3
Ventricular fibrillation, 5
Ventricular non-compaction, 86
Ventricular septal defect, 63
Ventricular tachycardia, 5, 66, 67
Venturi mask, 88–9, 102
Verapamil, 69, 439
Vertigo, acute, 281, 284, 303–5
Vestibular disease, 304
Viral encephalitis, 209, 220, 252, 268
Viral haemorrhagic fever, 215
Viral hepatitis, 174, 350
Visual loss, 260, 262, 319
Visual pathway, 251
Vitamin B12 deficiency, 191–3, 253
Vitamin K, 42–3, 439

Voltarol, 375, 439
von Willebrand disease, 200

Warfarin, 118, 200, 282, 440
    bleeding, 201
Weakness, 252–3
Wells clinical model, score, 115–16
Wernicke–Korsakoff syndrome, 178
West Nile virus encephalitis, 268
WHO pain ladder, 375
Wilson's disease, 172

Wolff–Parkinson–White syndrome,
    68, 72, 74

Xanthochromia, CSF, 290, 293, 408

Zieve's syndrome, 177
Zika fever/virus, 222
Zoledronate, 439
Zollinger–Ellison syndrome, 151
Zoster, herpes, 160, 219–20, 226,
    268–71, 305, 321